Sport and Exercise Nutrition

The Nutrition Society Textbook Series

Introduction to Human Nutrition

Introduction to human nutrition: a global
    perspective on food and nutrition
Body composition
Energy metabolism
Nutrition and metabolism of proteins and amino acids
Digestion and metabolism of carbohydrates
Nutrition and metabolism of lipids
Dietary reference standards
The vitamins
Minerals and trace elements
Measuring food intake
Food composition
Food and nutrition: policy and regulatory issues
Nutrition research methodology
Food safety: a public health issue of growing importance
Food and nutrition-related diseases: the global challenge

Nutrition and Metabolism

Core concepts of nutrition
Molecular aspects of nutrition
Integration of metabolism 1: Energy
Integration of metabolism 2: Macronutrients
Integration of metabolism 3: Protein and amino acids
Pregnancy and lactation
Growth and aging
Nutrition and the brain
The sensory systems and food palatability
The gastrointestinal tract
The cardiovascular system
The skeletal system
The immune and inflammatory systems
Phytochemicals
The control of food intake
Overnutrition
Undernutrition
Exercise performance

Public Health Nutrition

An overview of public health nutrition
Nutrition epidemiology
Food choice
Assessment of nutritional status at individual and
    population level
Assessment of physical activity
Overnutrition
Undernutrition
Eating disorders, dieting and food fads
PHN strategies for nutrition: intervention at the level of
    individuals
PHN strategies for nutrition: intervention at the
    ecological level
Food and nutrition guidelines
Fetal programming
Cardiovascular disease
Cancer
Osteoporosis
Diabetes
Vitamin A deficiency
Iodine deficiency
Iron deficiency
Maternal and child health
Breast feeding
Adverse outcomes in pregnancy

Clinical Nutrition

General principles of clinical nutrition
Metabolic and nutritional assessment
Overnutrition
Undernutrition
Metabolic disorders
Eating disorders
Adverse reactions to foods
Nutritional support
Ethical and legal issues
Gastrointestinal tract
The liver
The pancreas
The kidney
Blood and bone marrow
The lung
Immune and inflammatory systems
Heart and blood vessels
The skeleton
Traumatic diseases
Infectious diseases
Malignant diseases
Pediatric nutrition
Cystic fibrosis
Clinical cases
Water and electrolytes

Sport and Exercise Nutrition

Edited on behalf of The Nutrition Society by

Professor Susan A Lanham-New
University of Surrey
UK

Dr Samantha J Stear
Performance Influencers Limited
Formerly, English Institute of Sport
UK

Dr Susan M Shirreffs
Loughborough University
UK

Dr Adam L Collins
University of Surrey
UK

Foreword by Dr Richard Budgett OBE

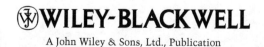
WILEY-BLACKWELL
A John Wiley & Sons, Ltd., Publication

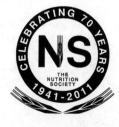

This edition first published 2011
© 2011 by The Nutrition Society

Wiley-Blackwell is an imprint of John Wiley & Sons, formed by the merger of Wiley's global Scientific, Technical and Medical business with Blackwell Publishing.

Registered Office
John Wiley & Sons, Ltd, The Atrium, Southern Gate, Chichester, West Sussex, PO19 8SQ, UK

Editorial Offices
9600 Garsington Road, Oxford, OX4 2DQ, UK
The Atrium, Southern Gate, Chichester, West Sussex, PO19 8SQ, UK
2121 State Avenue, Ames, Iowa 50014-8300, USA

For details of our global editorial offices, for customer services and for information about how to apply for permission to reuse the copyright material in this book please see our website at www.wiley.com/wiley-blackwell.

Library of Congress Cataloging-in-Publication Data

Sport and exercise nutrition / edited on behalf of the Nutrition Society by Susan Lanham-New ... [et al.].
     p.   cm. – (The Nutrition Society textbook series)
     Includes bibliographical references and index.
     ISBN-13: 978-1-4443-3468-5 (pbk. : alk. paper)
     ISBN-10: 1-4443-3468-9 (pbk. : alk. paper)
1. Exercise–Physiological aspects.   2. Sports–Physiological aspects.   3. Nutrition.   I. Lanham-New,
S. (Susan)   II. Nutrition Society (Great Britain)   III. Series: Human nutrition textbook series.
[DNLM: 1. Exercise–physiology.   2. Sports–physiology.   3. Nutritional Physiological Phenomena.
4. Nutritional Sciences.   5. Physical Fitness–physiology.   QT 260]
     RC1235.S64 2011
     613.7′1–dc23
                                            2011015206

A catalogue record for this book is available from the British Library.

This book is published in the following electronic formats: ePDF 9781444344875;
Wiley Online Library 9781444344905; ePub 9781444344882; Mobi 9781444344899

Set in 10/12pt Minion by SPi Publisher Services, Pondicherry, India

Contents

Visit the supporting companion website for this book: www.wiley.com/go/sport_and_ exercise_nutrition

Contributors

Bethanie Allanson
Sports Dietitian and Nutritionist
Australia

Dr Adrian J Allsopp
Institute of Naval Medicine
UK

Dr Keith Baar
University of California Davis
USA

Associate Professor Andrew Bosch
University of Cape Town
South Africa

Hans Braun
German Sport University Cologne
Olympic Training Centre Rhineland
Germany

Dr Elizabeth Broad
Australian Institute of Sport
Australia

Dr Nicholas A Burd
McMaster University
Canada

Professor Louise M Burke
Australian Institute of Sport
Australia

Dr Adam L Collins
University of Surrey
UK

Jeanette Crosland
Registered Dietitian and Sports Nutritionist
UK

Dr Kevin Currell
English Institute of Sport
UK

Dr Glen Davison
University of Kent
UK

Associate Professor Vicki Deakin
University of Canberra
Australia

Professor Nancy M DiMarco
Texas Woman's University
USA

Dr Joanne L Fallowfield
Institute of Naval Medicine
UK

Dr Stuart DR Galloway
University of Stirling
UK

Ina Garthe
Norwegian School of Sport Science
Norwegian Olympic Sports Centre
Norway

Professor John A Hawley
RMIT University
Australia

Neil Hopkins
Conditioning Coach and Biokineticist
South Africa

Penny J Hunking
Sports Dietitian
Energise Nutrition, UK

Professor John O Hunter
Consultant Physician Addenbrookes Hospital
and University of Cranfield
UK

Professor Asker Jeukendrup
University of Birmingham
UK

Professor Bente Kiens
University of Copenhagen
Denmark

Professor Susan A Lanham-New
University of Surrey
UK

Dr Joseph DJ Layden
Institute of Navel Medicine
UK

Dr Peter WR Lemon
The University of Western Ontario
Canada

Nathan Lewis
English Institute of Sport
UK

Bronwen Lundy
English Institute of Sport
UK

Professor Nicola Maffulli
University of London
UK

Wendy Martinson OBE
Registered Dietitian and Sports Nutritionist
UK

Shelly Meltzer
Shelly Meltzer & Associates
Sports Science Institute of South Africa
South Africa

Nanna L Meyer
University of Colorado and
United States Olympic Committee,
Colorado Springs
USA

Associate Professor David L Nichols
Texas Woman's University
USA

Dr Helen O'Connor
University of Sydney
Australia

Jeni Pearce
English Institute of Sport
UK

Dr Fiona Pelly
University of the Sunshine Coast
Australia

Professor Stuart M Phillips
McMaster University
Canada

Weileen Png
Singapore Sports Institute
Singapore

Professor Charlotte (Barney) Sanborn
Texas Woman's University
USA

Dr Susan M Shirreffs
Loughborough University
UK

Dr Richard J Simpson
University of Houston
USA

Dr Gary Slater
University of the Sunshine Coast
Australia

Karlien M Smit
Shelly Meltzer & Associates
Sports Science Institute of South Africa
South Africa

Filippo Spiezia
Campus Bio Medico
University of Rome
Italy

Dr Samantha J Stear
Performance Influencers Limited
(Formerly, English Institute of Sport, 2005–2009)
UK

Dr Trent Stellingwerff
Nestlé Research Centre
Switzerland

Professor Jorunn Sundgot-Borgen
Norwegian School of Sport Science
Norway

Professor Clyde Williams
Loughborough University
UK

Series Foreword

The early decades of the twentieth century were a period of intense research on constituents of food essential for normal growth and development, and saw the discovery of most vitamins, minerals, amino acids and essential fatty acids. In 1941, a group of leading physiologists, biochemists and medical scientists recognised that the emerging discipline of nutrition needed its own Learned Society and the Nutrition Society was established. The Nutrition Society's mission was and remains, "*to advance the scientific study of nutrition and its application to the maintenance of human and animal health*". It is the largest Learned Society for nutrition in Europe and has close to 2500 members worldwide. You can find out more about the Society and how to become a member by visiting the website at www.nutritionsociety.org.

Throughout its history, a primary objective of the Society has been to encourage nutrition research and to disseminate the results of such research. This is reflected in the several scientific meetings with the Nutrition Society, often in collaboration with sister Learned Societies in Europe, Africa, Asia and the USA, organised each year.

The Society's first journal, *The Proceedings of the Nutrition Society*, published in 1944 and recorded, as it still does, the scientific presentations made to the Society. Shortly afterwards in 1947, the *British Journal of Nutrition* was established to provide a medium for the publication of primary research on all aspects of human and animal nutrition by scientists from around the world. Recognising the needs of students and their teachers for authoritative reviews on topical issues in nutrition, the Society began publishing *Nutrition Research Reviews* in 1988. The journal

Public Health Nutrition, the first international journal dedicated to this important and growing area, was subsequently launched in 1998.

Just as in research, having the best possible tools is an enormous advantage in teaching and learning. This series of human nutrition textbooks is designed for use worldwide and this was achieved by launching the first series in multiple languages including Spanish, Greek, Portuguese and Indonesian. This fifth textbook in the series, under the Editor-in-Chief Professor Susan Lanham-New (University of Surrey), brings together the latest information on the science and practice of sport and exercise nutrition. The textbook combines the viewpoints of world-leading nutrition experts from academia and research from a practical standpoint.

Life in the world of sport revolves around training and competition. As a former athlete and having worked closely with competing athletes in my role as Chief Medical Officer for the British Olympic Team at eight Olympic Games, I know first-hand that diet is absolutely vital in supporting athletes towards their goals. To strive for performance improvements – be it skill, power, strength, speed or endurance – requires physical training, and correct nutrition is essential to this training effect. This Textbook brings together science and practice for students and those working in sports nutrition and exercise physiology and is a valuable resource to all those working in the field.

Dr Richard Budgett OBE
*Chief Medical Officer for the London 2012
Olympic and Paralympic Games*

Preface

The Nutrition Society Textbook Series was first created over a decade ago and we are indebted to Professor Michael Gibney (University College Dublin), the Founder of the Series, for his tremendous vision and hard work in those early days. The four established Textbooks: *Introduction to Human Nutrition* (IHN); *Nutrition & Metabolism* (N&M); *Clinical Nutrition* (CN); *Public Health Nutrition* (PHN) have proved to be an enormously successful venture, with sales of over 30,000 copies as of 2011 for the first editions of the four Textbooks and the second editions of IHN and N&M respectively.

It is a great honour for me to be the new Editor-in-Chief of the Series. In taking my office in 2009, I have moved quickly to establish a fifth Textbook to the Series, namely *Sport and Exercise Nutrition* (SEN). This title is unique in providing, under one single textbook, all the core aspects around the effect of nutrition on different sports and under different exercises. With the Olympic Games coming to London in 2012, our timing of this Textbook is perfect.

This NS textbook on *Sport and Exercise Nutrition* has been designed to provide the reader with the latest information on the science and practice of sport and exercise nutrition. One of the very key concepts behind SEN is the aim to combine the viewpoints of world-leading nutrition experts from both academia and research, and a practical standpoint.

Sport and Exercise Nutrition is divided into three distinct but integrated parts. At the start of each chapter there are key 'take home' messages and each chapter is concluded with a list of further reading material.

Chapters 1 to 9 cover the key components of the science that supports the practice of sport and exercise nutrition including comprehensive reviews on: nutrients both in general and as exercise fuels; exercise physiology; hydration; micronutrients; and supplements.

Chapters 10 to 14 move into focusing on specific nutrition strategies to support different types of training including: resistance; power/sprint; middle-distance/speed-endurance; endurance; technical/skill; team; and specific competition nutrition needs. The unique format of this textbook is that it breaks down nutrition support into training-specific as opposed to the traditional sport-specific support. This reflects the majority of current sport and exercise requirements of the need to undertake concurrent training and therefore facilitating targeted nutrition support to the different training components through the various macro and micro training cycles.

Chapters 15 to 25 explore some of the practical issues encountered in working in the sport and exercise nutrition field and includes key sport-related topics such as: disability sport; weight management; eating disorders; bone and gut health; immunity; injury; travel; and special populations and situations.

The NS textbook on *Sport and Exercise Nutrition* is aimed at students interested in a career in sport and exercise nutrition, along with allied sport and exercise professionals such as nutritionists, coaches, physiotherapists and doctors who need to translate or understand the science into their practice with sports, athletes and other exercise enthusiasts.

We are very honoured indeed that the Foreword for *Sport and Exercise Nutrition* has been written by Dr Richard Budgett OBE, Chief Medical Officer for London 2012 and himself an Olympic Gold Medalist as part of the British rowing coxed fours squad at the 1984 Los Angeles Olympic Games, alongside Sir Steven Redgrave, Martin Cross and the late Andy Holmes. We thank him most sincerely for his support and commitment to this Textbook venture.

The Nutrition Society Textbook Series is hugely indebted to Wiley-Blackwell, who have proved to be extremely supportive publishers and we thank Nick Morgan and Sara Crowley-Vigneau from Wiley-Blackwell, as well as Vedavalli Karunagaran from the typesetter, SPi Publisher Services, for their help with the production of this SEN book. Particular thanks are also due to the *Sport and Exercise Nutrition* specific Editors Dr Samantha Stear, Dr Susan Shirreffs and Dr Adam Collins for all their hard work. I gratefully acknowledge the encouragement of our NS President, past and present, Professor Ian Macdonald and Professor Sean J.J. Strain. I would particularly like to express my thanks to Professor Gillian Nicholls (Deputy Vice-Chancellor, University of Surrey) and Professor John Hay (Dean, Faculty of Health and Medical Sciences, University of Surrey) for their support and encouragement in the production of this book. Final thanks are due to Sharon Hui (Assistant Editor, NS Textbook Series) and Jennifer Norton (NS Business Manager) for being there every step of the

way with this Textbook and for their immense hard work in making it all possible.

I really hope that you will find the book of great use… Please enjoy!

My warm regards.

Professor Susan A. Lanham-New
Head, Department of Nutrition and Metabolism,
University of Surrey and Editor-in-Chief,
Nutrition Society Textbook Series

The Nutrition Society Textbook Series Editors

Editor-in-Chief
Susan A Lanham-New
University of Surrey, UK

Business Manager
Jennifer Norton
The Nutrition Society, UK

Assistant Editor
Sharon S Hui
The Nutrition Society, UK

1
Nutrient Basics

Adam L Collins, Penny J Hunking and Samantha J Stear

Key messages

- Eating a wide variety of commonly available foods helps ensure that all the body's needs for nutrients are met.
- Carbohydrates, both sugars and starches, are digested or converted into glucose to provide the body's primary energy fuel.
- Protein-rich foods or combinations provide all the essential amino acids.
- Alcohol is an energy-dense nutrient that should only be consumed in moderation, if at all, and should be avoided before or immediately after exercise.
- Some dietary fat is needed to provide the essential fatty acids and the fat-soluble vitamins (A, D, E and K).

- Current public health guidelines on a healthy balanced diet, alongside appropriate reference intakes for energy and individual nutrients, are useful tools in assessing dietary adequacy.
- Determination of dietary intake, both qualitatively and quantitatively, forms a key component of nutritional status assessment in athletes and non-athletes.
- An awareness of the errors and limitations of dietary assessment and its interpretation is essential if they are to be used to form the basis of change.

1.1 Introduction

A healthy balanced diet is vital for good health both from the perspective of an elite athlete and for those who enjoy working out to keep fit. Training can be optimised to help athletes and exercisers to reach their goals by making informed dietary choices. The key to making the diet healthy and balanced is to ensure it provides adequate energy from the consumption of a wide variety of commonly available foods, to meet the carbohydrate, protein and fat requirements for both health and exercise. The food we eat provides the nutrients required by the body. However, no one food or food group can provide all the essential nutrients the body requires. Athletes and exercisers should eat a variety of foods to provide all the essential nutrients to support the preparation for, the participation in, and the recovery from sports and exercise.

The body's energy supply is derived from the nutrients in the diet. Nutrients are found in differing amounts in foods and are broken down in the body to provide a certain quantity of energy, commonly expressed as kilocalories (kcal) per gram (g). The main energy-yielding nutrients in the diet are as follows.

- Carbohydrate: 3.75 kcal/g
- Protein: 4 kcal/g
- Alcohol: 7 kcal/g
- Fat: 9 kcal/g.

1.2 Carbohydrates

Dietary carbohydrate is provided by a wide variety of carbohydrate-rich food and drinks. However, all carbohydrates, both sugars and starches, are ultimately converted to and absorbed into the blood in the form of glucose, to provide the primary energy fuel. There is no universal system that can adequately describe the diverse metabolic, functional and nutritional features of the various carbohydrate foods. One of the simplest ways of classifying carbohydrates is by their structure (Figure 1.1). Basically, they can be divided into four main groups.

Sport and Exercise Nutrition, First Edition. Edited by Susan A Lanham-New, Samantha J Stear, Susan M Shirreffs and Adam L Collins.
© 2011 The Nutrition Society. Published 2011 by Blackwell Publishing Ltd.

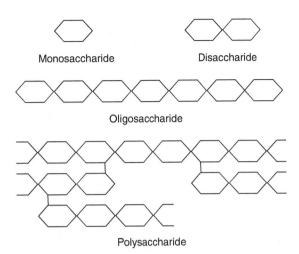

Figure 1.1 Example structure of monosaccharides, disaccharides, oligosaccharides and polysaccharides.

(1) *Monosaccharides* are single molecules of sugar: glucose, fructose and galactose. Glucose is found in most carbohydrate foods including sugars and starches. All carbohydrates are eventually digested or converted into glucose. Fructose is also known as fruit sugar and is found in fruits, vegetables and honey, and is converted into glucose by the liver. Galactose is part of lactose, the sugar found in milk and milk products.

(2) *Disaccharides* comprise two linked sugar molecules that are broken down into monosaccharides by digestion. The disaccharides include sucrose (glucose + fructose), lactose (glucose + galactose) and maltose (glucose + glucose). Sucrose (table sugar) normally comes from sugar beet and cane, but is also found naturally in all fruits and vegetables, and even most herbs and spices. Lactose is found in milk and milk products. Maltose is formed when starch is broken down.

(3) *Oligosaccharides* typically contain three to ten linked sugar molecules, which are broken down into monosaccharides by digestion. Fructo-oligosaccharides are found in many vegetables, such as Jerusalem artichoke, chicory, leeks, onions and asparagus, and consist of short chains of fructose molecules. Galacto-oligosaccharides occur naturally in beans including soybeans and consist of short chains of galactose molecules. Some oligosaccharides can only be partially digested by humans and therefore may be fer-

mented in the large intestine. The fructans, inulin and fructo-oligosaccharides, have been shown to stimulate growth of potentially beneficial bifido-bacteria.

(4) *Polysaccharides*, also known as glycans, are simply hundreds of molecules of monosaccharides joined together. Polysaccharides differ in the nature of repeating monosaccharide units, number of units in the chain, and the degree of branching. By far the most abundant polysaccharides in the diet are starches, which are simply many glucose molecules joined together. When starch is digested, it is first broken down into maltose and then into glucose.

The major difference between sugars and starches is the size of the molecule. Traditionally, foods containing significant amounts of carbohydrates have been classified according to the major type of carbohydrate they contain, which led to the simplistic division of carbohydrate-containing foods into 'simple' (mainly consisting of sugars) and 'complex' (mainly consisting of starches). This over-simplification is misleading as the majority of naturally occurring foods contain a mixture of sugars and starches. Rapidly digestible starch (RDS), as the name suggests, is rapidly digested and absorbed in the small intestine; it is found in processed food and produces a large glycaemic response. In contrast, slowly digestible starch (SDS) is found in muesli, legumes and pasta and is completely but more slowly absorbed in the small intestine, therefore generating a smaller glycaemic response.

Considering that most carbohydrates ultimately end up as glucose to provide energy fuel, there are several other factors that may be more important to athletes and exercisers. These include how rapidly the carbohydrate is converted to glucose and its appeal and practicality, all of which are specific to the individual and the exercise situation.

Dietary fibre

Dietary fibre is a generic term for a group of carbohydrates derived from the edible parts of plants that are not broken down and absorbed by the small intestine. This definition includes non-starch polysaccharides (NSP), some oligosaccharides, lignin, resistant starch (RS) and sugar alcohols. NSP comprise a complex heterogeneous range of polysaccharides contributing the largest component of fibre, mainly found in plant tissues (90% from plant cell walls). NSP can be divided into cellulose (insoluble) and non-cellulose polysaccharides (mainly soluble). The soluble components tend to increase the viscosity of the gastrointestinal contents. 'Resistant starch' is a term that describes any polysaccharide of glucose that is resistant to digestion and hence passes to the large intestine intact. There are a variety of RS classifications: RS_1 are physically inaccessible to digestion (e.g. whole grains); RS_2 are resistant granules (e.g. in unripe bananas); and RS_3 comprises retrograded amylase found in processed foods such as cooked and cooled potatoes and rice.

Dietary fibre content of food is quantified by various methods. Most UK food tables and databases have traditionally used the Englyst method, which is specifically a measure of NSP only. In 2000 the Food Standards Agency (FSA) legislated for the AOAC (Association of Analytical Communities: www.aoac.org) definition to be used, which includes NSP, RS and lignin. With this in mind, the UK estimated average requirement for fibre is derived from the Englyst method and hence would need to increase from 18 to 24 g/day if expressed as the AOAC definition.

1.3 Protein

Protein is the most abundant nitrogen-containing compound in the diet and the body. Throughout the day there is a continual process of protein turnover, with proteins being broken down and formed at the same time. The largest reservoir of protein is found in the muscles, but there is limited capacity to store new proteins. Therefore, protein intake in excess of requirements is either broken down to provide energy or stored as fat or carbohydrate.

Protein is needed for the growth and repair of tissues. During digestion, proteins are broken down into smaller units called amino acids. Amino acids are commonly described as the building blocks of protein. In chemistry, an amino acid is a molecule containing both amine and carboxyl functional groups. There are about 20 different naturally occurring amino acids, which can be combined to make a vast array of different proteins.

The terms 'essential' and 'non-essential' amino acids refer to whether the amino acid in question can be synthesised by the body at a rate sufficient to meet normal requirements for protein synthesis. There are eight essential (indispensable) amino acids for adults (isoleucine, leucine, lysine, methionine, phenylalanine, threonine, tryptophan and valine) that must be supplied in adequate amounts by the diet. Nutritionally, histidine and arginine are considered essential amino acids in human infants. After reaching several years of age, humans begin to synthesise histidine and arginine, and they thus become non-essential amino acids. The semi-essential (conditionally indispensable) amino acids can be made in the body, providing certain essential amino acids are present in the diet in sufficient amounts, for example cysteine requires methionine and tyrosine requires phenylalanine. Other amino acids, notably arginine and glutamine, are also regarded as 'conditionally essential' meaning that, during times of high utilisation, they may require repletion via the diet. For further information see Chapter 5 on protein and amino acids.

The majority of amino acids ingested by humans exist in a combined form as dietary proteins from both animal and vegetable sources. Not all proteins in the diet have the same nutritional value, since they contain different proportions of essential amino acids. The complete protein foods contain all the essential amino acids. In general, foods from animal sources contain substantial amounts of all the essential amino acids, but foods from other sources can be combined with each other to make complete protein foods. For example, the protein quality of plant products is improved when dairy products are added to a plant food and when plant-based foods, such as wheat and beans, are mixed together. Table 1.1 shows some examples of protein-rich foods or combinations that provide all the essential amino acids in sufficient amounts.

Vegetarian and vegan diets

Protein combining is not necessary in a vegetarian diet where milk, cheese and eggs are eaten, because these foods provide adequate amounts of all the essential amino acids. Strict vegetarians, and in particular vegans who eat no dairy products or eggs, need to plan their diet carefully to ensure that their combination of plant foods provides them with all the essential amino acids. However, this mixing and

Table 1.1 Complete protein foods.

Type	Examples
Dairy products	Milk, yoghurt
Eggs	Boiled, scrambled, omelette
Fish	Fresh, tinned or frozen, e.g. salmon, tuna
Meat and meat products	Beef, lamb, ham, sausages
Poultry	Chicken, turkey
Grains plus legumes	Bean curry or lentils with rice, peanut butter sandwich, bread with hummous, baked beans on toast
Grains plus nuts or seeds	Muesli mix with oats and nuts or seeds, e.g. hazelnuts or sunflower seeds, rice salad with nuts, e.g. walnuts, sesame seed spread (tahini) on bread
Legumes plus nuts or seeds	Mix of peanuts and nuts, e.g. cashews
Grains plus dairy products	Breakfast cereal and milk, rice pudding, pizza or pasta with cheese, cheese sandwich
Legumes[a] plus dairy products	Bean curry in a yoghurt-based sauce, bean chilli with cheese

[a] Legumes include pulses (e.g. peas and beans) and peanuts.
Reproduced with kind permission from Stear S. Fuelling Fitness for Sports Performance, copyright © 2004 Samantha Stear.

matching of plant foods to provide all the essential amino acids does not need to occur at the same meal but can take place over the course of the day.

1.4 Alcohol

Alcohol is an energy-dense nutrient that should only be consumed in moderation, if at all, and should be avoided before or immediately after exercise. The advice on sensible drinking exists to limit the health risks associated with excessive intakes of alcohol. In the long term, continued heavy drinking causes liver damage and other health problems. In the short term, excessive amounts of alcohol can be toxic to the individual as well as potentially dangerous to others, due to the resulting loss of coordination or self-control and behavioural changes.

Alcohol consumption may impede post-exercise recovery. Furthermore, many sports are associated with muscle damage and soft tissue injuries, either directly due to the exercise or from the tackling and collisions involved in contact sports. Although the evidence is limited, it would be advisable for athletes who suffer considerable muscle damage and soft tissue injuries to avoid alcohol in the immediate recovery phase, probably for 24 hours following the event.

Alcohol is not generally a banned substance in sport, with the exception of some sports such as fencing and shooting. It is likely that its consumption will interfere with judgement and skilled performance in sport, and in particular may increase the risk of injury. Therefore guidelines for sensible drinking should be followed at all times and especially in the period after training or competition.

In the UK, one unit of alcohol is measured as 10 ml or 8 g of pure alcohol. This equals one 25-ml single measure of whisky (ABV 40%), or one-third of a pint of beer (ABV 5–6%) or half a standard (175 ml) glass of red wine (ABV 12%). As the absolute volume (ABV) of alcohol varies between drinks, it is more accurate to calculate alcohol units using the following equation:

$$\text{Strength (ABV)} \times \text{Volume (mL)} \div 1000 = \text{No. of units}$$

For example, 1 pint (568 ml) of 5.2% strength beer = $5.2 \times 568 \div 1000 = 2.95$ units.

Based on the evidence of associated health risks the recommended maximum levels of alcohol consumption were originally set at no more than 21 units per week for men and 14 units per week for women. However, following the growing evidence of the detrimental effects on health of heavy or 'binge' drinking, the sensible drinking guidelines were switched to daily maximum intakes. For example in the UK, these guidelines state that maximum daily intakes should not exceed 3–4 units for men and 2–3 units for women.

Alcohol is a high-energy nutrient, providing 7 kcal/g, and consequently its intake should be limited so that it does not displace other nutrients or result in unnecessary additional calories.

1.5 Fat

There are many different kinds of fats, but each is a variation on the same chemical structure. All fats consist of fatty acids (chains of carbon and hydrogen atoms, with a carboxylic acid group at one end) bonded to a backbone structure, often glycerol (a backbone of carbon, hydrogen and oxygen). The main components of dietary fats and lipids are fatty acids, which vary in length from one to more than 30 carbons. A fat's constituent fatty acids may also differ in the number of hydrogen atoms that are bonded to the chain of carbon atoms. Each carbon atom is typically bonded to two hydrogen atoms. When a fatty acid has this typical arrangement, it is called a 'saturated' fatty acid because the carbon atoms are saturated with hydrogen, meaning they are bonded to as many hydrogen atoms as possible. In other fats, a carbon atom may have a double bond to a neighbouring carbon atom, which results in an 'unsaturated' fatty acid; more specifically, a fatty acid with one double bond is called a monounsaturated fatty acid (MUFA) whereas a fatty acid with more than one double bond is called a polyunsaturated fatty acid (PUFA). Figure 1.2 shows examples of the structures of a saturated, monounsaturated, and polyunsaturated fatty acid.

Fatty acids are the densest source of dietary energy, providing 9 kcal/g, but lipids also have important structural roles in membranes. A typical dietary fat contains a mixture of both saturated and unsaturated (MUFA and PUFA) fatty acids. Different foods have varying proportions of fatty acids such that the fat in meat, dairy products and coconuts is predominantly saturated fatty acid; olive and rapeseed oils have a high proportion of MUFA; and sunflower and soya oils are mostly PUFA. Essential fatty acids are a subgroup of PUFA that the body cannot make and therefore need to be supplied in adequate amounts by the diet. Essential fatty acids can be divided into two classes: the omega-3 (ω-3) and omega-6 (ω-6) fatty acids (Table 1.2).

The type of fat that dominates the diet depends on the proportion of different fatty acids present in the choice of foods consumed. The amount of dietary fat required depends on several factors including age, body size and training levels.

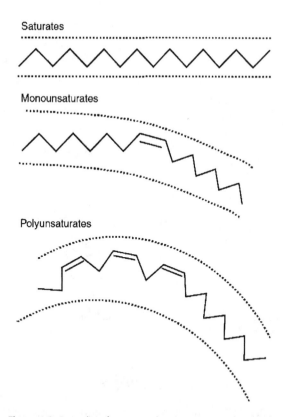

Figure 1.2 Examples of a saturated, monounsaturated and polyunsaturated fatty acid structure. (Reprinted with permission from Griffin B, Cunnane S. Nutrition and metabolism of lipids. In: Introduction to Human Nutrition, 2nd edn, Gibney M, Lanham-New S, Cassidy A, Vorster H, eds. Hoboken, NJ: Wiley-Blackwell, 2009.)

Table 1.2 Sources of essential fatty acids.

Omega-3

Oily fish, e.g. salmon, mackerel, sardines, herring, pilchards, and tuna in oil
Linseeds and pumpkin seeds
Oils, e.g. soyabean and rapeseed
Walnuts

Omega-6

Seeds, e.g. sunflower and sesame
Nuts
Oils, e.g. sunflower, safflower, corn, groundnut, sesame, rapeseed and soya oils
Polyunsaturated margarine

Reproduced with kind permission from Stear S. Fuelling Fitness for Sports Performance, copyright © 2004 Samantha Stear.

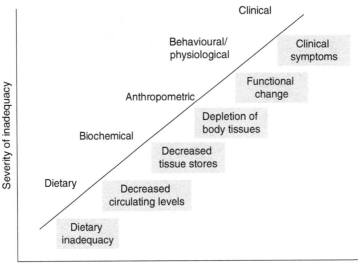

Figure 1.3 The progression of nutrient inadequacy corresponding to a change in nutritional status. (Adapted from Gibson RS. Principles of Nutritional Assessment. Oxford: Oxford University Press, 2005.)

1.6 Assessing dietary intake

When improving or maintaining nutritional health it is vital to diagnose current nutritional status as this highlights individual needs and will help determine dietary and lifestyle modifications. Accurately and reliably determining the current dietary intake identifies inadequacies (or excesses) that can give rise to biochemical, physiological, clinical and performance-related changes. The progression of any deficiency (or excess) can be detected by various means of nutritional assessment as summarised in Figure 1.3.

As depicted in Figure 1.3, the earliest detection of any inadequacy can be made through the measurement of dietary intake. However, measurement of habitual dietary intake, by its very nature, is hard to undertake as diet patterns are rarely systematic and dietary information can be highly personal. As such, all methods of its measurement are a practical compromise to one degree or another. The two basic problems to overcome are (i) accurately determining current customary food intake and (ii) converting this information into absolute amounts of energy and nutrients. Table 1.3 summarises the features of some of the commonly used dietary assessment methods. However, for clarity these will now be

discussed in more detail in the following sections by separating methods into quantitative and qualitative.

Quantitative methods
Food records and food diaries
These aim to provide a quantitative assessment of actual food intake prospectively over a period of commonly 3–10 consecutive days. The actual number of days should be realistic in terms of compliance and should usually include at least one non-working/non-training day to take into account differences in food consumption. On the simplest level, subjects record the description and timing of meals and this information is translated into nutrient composition assuming standard weights, portion sizes and composition. The validity of this method can be improved following clear instruction (verbal and written), and providing the individual with a clear form/diary on which to record the information. Developments in multimedia and communication technology (internet websites, hand-held computers, and mobile phone applications) have seen increasing use of user-friendly, menu-driven applications to help aid recording and sending of dietary intake data.

Providing the individual receives comprehensive instructions on its use, weighed food records can

Table 1.3 Summary of the uses and limitations of dietary assessment methods.

	Method	Uses and limitations
Food records	Record of all food and drink consumed over a period of time (3–10 days), usually recorded by the respondent. Food portion sizes can be estimated or quantified with use of weighing scales. Information converted to nutrient intakes using food composition database.	Can assess actual intake of individuals. More days recorded takes into account between-day variation. Can provide data on nutrient intake for comparison with reference values. Relies on high respondent compliance. May not reflect habitual intake. Susceptible to misreporting and change in eating behaviour.
Diet history/interview	Interview method. Gauge if habitual dietary habits. Portion sizes estimated possibly with use of photographs/food models. May also be incorporated with food record and/or FFQ.	Gives information on usual intake. Highlights dietary inadequacies. Can form basis of diet modification. Limited quantitative data. Reliant on skilled interviewer, can be labour intensive. Affected by honesty/psychology of respondent.
Food frequency questionnaire (FFQ)	Questionnaire comprising comprehensive list of food items coupled with frequency of intake. Can be self-administered. Can include information on usual food portion sizes.	Provides descriptive data on usual intake. Good for large groups/populations. Can allocate individuals into bands of intake. Limited individual use. Limited by suitability of food list contained. Often difficult to validate satisfactorily.

overcome errors in estimation of portion sizes and weights. Use of food photography may also be useful, either by comparing foods eaten to photographs of standard food portions, or for the individual to photograph the food eaten (aided by the advent of digital camera technology). Nevertheless, on all levels, when using food records it is important that assessors be supportive, non-judgemental and emphasise the importance of accuracy, particularly if they are to receive valid feedback and advice. Whatever the sophistication of approach, rubbish in will inevitably lead to rubbish out, so it is vital that clear instruction and clarification of entries post recording is undertaken.

The labour-intensive nature of recording food intake can give rise to errors, either in accuracy of recording or in eating behaviour. Highly composite meals are likely either to be avoided or misreported. Likewise, foods eaten outside the home, or takeaways may be vaguely reported and snacks and beverages may be omitted due to memory failure or conscious omission. Overall, misreporting of intake is a common trait as psychology has a major influence on validity, for example under (or over)-reporting may be used to prevent scrutiny or judgement by the assessor or simply to lessen the labour of recording.

Under-reporting of intake is commonly seen in obese individuals, whereas over-reporting, although less common, tends to be seen in the non-obese, particularly those who want to gain weight. Dietary surveys in athletes using food records demonstrate a typically higher energy intake compared with the estimated average requirement (Figure 1.4). Nevertheless, under-reporting can still be prevalent in athletes for the same aforementioned reasons. Determining misreporting of intake can be achieved using an independent measure of status (e.g. urinary nitrogen), although this is rarely used in practice. Comparing reported energy intake with estimated energy expenditure may be used to assess validity (i.e. under- or over-reporting), assuming the individual is in energy balance during the measurement period (i.e. 3–10 days). However, quantifying energy expenditure accurately in active individuals poses its own difficulties.

Translating food intake into nutrient intake
Even following minimal behavioural change and maximising the accuracy of portion size estimation, a further source of error when quantifying intake is made when translating food intake into nutrient composition. Nutrient intake is typically 'quantified'

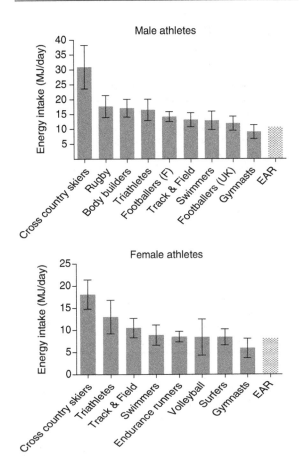

Figure 1.4 Self-reported energy intakes for male and female athletes from dietary surveys (1991–2004). EAR represents estimated energy requirement based on UK dietary reference values (Department of Health 1991). Sources of information: Farajian P *et al.* (2004) Int J Sport Nutr Exerc Metab 14: 574–585; Burke EM *et al.* (2003) Int J Sport Nutr Exerc Metab 13: 521–538; LeBlanc JCh *et al.* (2002) Int J Sport Nutr Exerc Metab 12: 268–280; Suqiura K *et al.* (1999) Int J Sport Nutr 9: 202–212; Edwards JE (1993) Med Sci Sports Exerc 25: 1398–1404; Sjödin AM *et al.* (1994) Med Sci Sports Exerc 26: 720–724; Kimber (2002) Int J Sport Nutr Exerc Metab 12: 47–62; Burke LM (2001) Sports Med 31: 521–532; Hawley JA, Williams MM (1991) Br J Sports Med 25: 154–158; Akermark C *et al.* (1996) Int J Sport Nutr 6: 272–282; Maughan RJ (1997) Br J Sports Med 31: 45–47; Lambert CP *et al.* (2004) Sports Med 34: 317–327; Filaire E, Lac G (2002) J Sports Med Phys Fitness 42: 65–70; Felder JM *et al.* (1998) Int J Sport Nutr 8: 36–48; Papadopoulou SK *et al.* (2002) Int J Sport Nutr Exerc Metab 12: 73–80; Nutter J (1991) Int J Sport Nutr 1: 395–407.

from information on the described food and amount eaten, utilising a food composition database of analysed foods. It is important that the limitations of food composition data are understood and taken into consideration when assessing the nutrient composition of the diet. Specifically, the sources of variation in the use of a food composition database can be divided into two main areas: (i) investigator error as a result of the incorrect coding of foods (i.e. matching of foods consumed with foods listed in the foods composition tables); and (ii) error due to the limitations in the food composition data itself.

Incorrect coding of foods is likely if the description of the reported food is unclear in terms of food variety, preparation and cooking method. Further complications arise from the absence of a reported food in the composition database, hence the reliance on a best match alternative which may differ in nutrient composition. Both of these sources of error can be reduced by clear instruction of the subject as well as suitable training of the assessor.

As well as limitations in the number of foods in the database, errors can arise due to the samples of food used in its construction, which may vary according to season, soil, harvesting, brand, processing additives, fortification, preservatives and cooking methods. In addition, the development of computer composition software may also be a source of error as there may be discrepancies between dietary analysis software packages.

Qualitative methods
Diet history/interview
The purpose of this retrospective technique is to gain insight into current habitual/usual dietary intake and meal patterns, typically representing intake over the previous month. The diet history technique has the advantage of obtaining information on habitual intake, with a relatively low burden on the participant, and typically high compliance. The validity of the information obtained is dependent on the memory and honesty of the participant. Psychology also comes into play as to many people disclosing their diet is highly personal and may lead to omissions (consciously or subconsciously). The validity and reliability of this technique is questionable in some populations (e.g. children, the elderly, the obese, and those with eating disorders) and is also less reliable in those individuals with erratic eating patterns (e.g. some athletes). In any situation, the quality and validity of information gained is dependent on the interviewer's skill and training.

Information on typical portion sizes can also be gained through the use of food portion photographic atlases or plastic food models. Although the main use of the information gained through the diet history is an overall picture of diet quality, if undertaken correctly it can be used to suggest dietary sources of nutrients and highlight potential inadequacies or excesses that can be addressed. The information obtained cannot be compared directly against reference intakes for specific nutrients (e.g. Dietary Reference Values or Dietary Reference Intakes), but habitual eating patterns can be compared with qualitative healthy eating guidelines. More importantly, the diet history also provides insight into the individual's lifestyle alongside eating patterns, which will help suggest changes that are both practicable and attainable.

Food frequency questionnaires

This method attempts to retrospectively assess intake of specific or all common foods over a period of 1–6 months through a self-completed questionnaire. A typical food frequency questionnaire (FFQ) will comprise two components: a list of food items and a set of frequency response categories. In order to asses total intake of all nutrients the FFQ must contain a list of all the commonly eaten foods and hence would typically be many pages in length and time-consuming to complete. Some FFQs focus only on specific foods, groups of foods, or food sources of a specific nutrient, and may therefore be shorter in length. The basic FFQ can be modified to incorporate an estimate of portion size; for simplicity this is often simplified into small, medium or large, provided there is some description of these portions (e.g. photograph or household measure). Almost all commonly used FFQs have been previously validated against either food records or with biological markers; however, the method used to validate may itself have some inherent errors.

The FFQ has the advantages that it can be self-administered, is quick and non-invasive, requires little respondent effort and has a relatively high response rate. It can also be administered by non-professional personnel, either in person or remotely. As a result, the FFQ is often the tool of choice when assessing large groups or populations. The FFQ has been used to place individuals into percentiles of intake but cannot be used to quantitatively assess individual intake, only a representation of dietary composition. Seasonal variation in habitual intake

also governs representation of the dietary data obtained from FFQ, particularly in temperate climate countries.

1.7 Dietary and healthy eating guidelines

Ascertaining adequacy of dietary intake requires an appreciation of individual requirements, some of which will be elevated in those participating in significant amounts of sport or exercise. The specific requirements for energy and nutrients in athletes will be covered in more detail in other chapters of this book. In broad terms, an appreciation of individual dietary adequacy may be gained through comparison with dietary guidelines and reference intake values based on a comparable general population. These comparators may be in the form of qualitative guidelines on overall diet composition in terms of foods and food groups, or more quantitative reference intakes associated with health for specific nutrients.

Qualitative dietary guidelines

These are developed mainly as a public health tool whereby foods are categorised into food groups and the guideline diet is then presented as suggested relative proportions of these food groups. The number and definition of food groups can vary depending on the country of origin, and typically reflects the common cultural diet in that country. In addition, the means of presenting the suggested proportions of these food groups may also vary between countries, again to better represent the eating culture. In the UK, the FSA depicts a healthy diet based on five food groups whose relative proportions are shown as segments on a plate, promoted as the 'eatwell plate' (Figure 1.5a). This plate model, manifested previously in the UK as the 'balance of good health', was chosen as a reflection of the traditional British diet (colloquially, 'meat and two veg'). In the US, the United States Department of Agriculture (USDA) Center for Nutrition Policy and Promotion endorses the My Pyramid Food Guidance System (Figure 1.5b), an update on the widely recognised food pyramid model used previously, presenting the diet as comprising six food groups. In addition to these two widely used examples of healthy eating guidelines, the FAO/WHO have devised food-based dietary

(a)

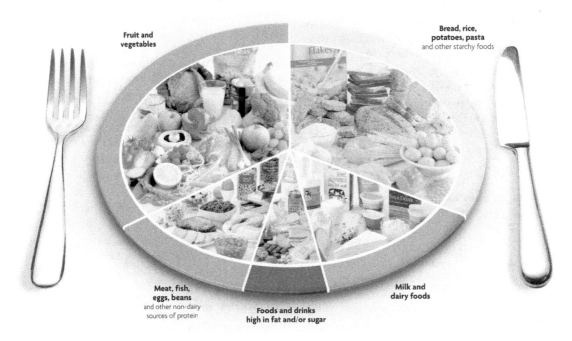

The eatwell plate

Use the eatwell plate to help you get the balance right. It shows how much of what you eat should come from each food group.

Fruit and vegetables

Bread, rice, potatoes, pasta and other starchy foods

Meat, fish, eggs, beans and other non-dairy sources of protein

Foods and drinks high in fat and/or sugar

Milk and dairy foods

Figure 1.5 (a) Current UK healthy eating guidelines manifested as the eatwell plate. (Food Standards Agency 2010, Crown Copyright 1991, Crown copyright material is reproduced with the permission of the Controller of HMSO and the Queen's Printer for Scotland.)

(b)

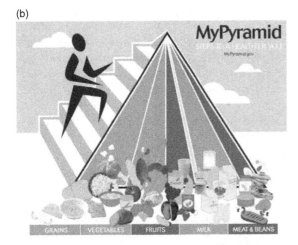

Figure 1.5 (b) Current US healthy eating guidelines comprising six food group presented as My Pyramid. (USDA Center for Nutrition Policy and Promotion.)

guidelines to accommodate cultural differences in diet for other geographical regions, including recommendations for Latin America and the western Pacific and Asian populations.

The appropriate food-based dietary guidelines from a comparable population may be used for individuals, subsequent to dietary assessment, as they can help identify food groups in excess or inadequacy and hence suggest changes for improving overall diet quality. In addition, provided overall energy intake is appropriate, adherence to these guidelines will more likely lead to adequate relative intakes of macronutrients and micronutrients.

Quantitative reference intakes

There are a set of reference values of daily intake for specific nutrients for a healthy population and these

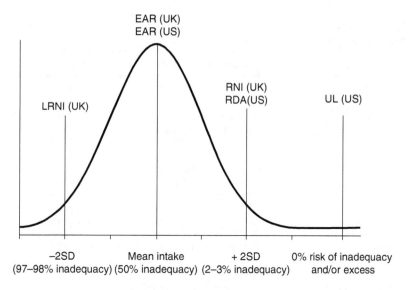

Figure 1.6 Dietary reference intakes and dietary reference values presented relative to a healthy population, where SD represents standard deviation. (Data sourced from Department of Health 1991. Dietary Reference Values for Food, Energy and Nutrients for the United Kingdom. London: HMSO. Crown Copyright 1991. Crown copyright material is reproduced with the permission of the Controller of HMSO and the Queen's Printer for Scotland.)

can be used as a benchmark to assess nutritional adequacy of an individual's assessed intake. The requirement for any nutrient can be defined as the lowest continuing intake that will maintain a defined level of nutrition for an individual within a given group or population. This criterion may differ for individuals at different life stages, for example during pregnancy, lactation, childhood/adolescence and older age.

In order to prevent confusion, it is important to be clear on the terminology with regard to recommended values of nutrient intakes. Historically, recommended intakes have been expressed as Recommended Daily Amounts in the UK and as Recommended Daily Allowances in the US, confusingly both expressed as RDAs despite slight differences in definition and actual published reference values. In the UK, since 1991 the RDAs have been superseded by Dietary Reference Values (DRVs). In the US, development of the Dietary Reference Intakes (DRIs) has expanded on the previously defined RDAs as well as the Canadian Recommended Nutrient Intakes. For the majority of nutrients, both the UK DRVs and the US DRIs are based on a healthy reference population (free from consequences of deficiency or excess), whose reported intake follows a normal distribution. The reference values for a

particular nutrient relate to the level of intake that is equal to or greater than that achieved by a set proportion of the healthy reference population. Figure 1.6 shows these intakes relative to a normally distributed intake for healthy individuals in a life stage or gender group.

For both DRVs (UK) and DRIs (US) the Estimated Average Requirement (EAR) refers to the mean intake of a nutrient within the healthy population, which relates to a 50% risk of inadequacy (i.e. only 50% of a healthy population will have a higher intake). Assuming the healthy population is normally distributed, an intake two standard deviations (2SD) higher than the EAR relates to a risk of inadequacy of only 2–3%. In the UK, this level of intake is defined as the Reference Nutrient Intake (RNI), whereas in the US this is defined as the Recommended Dietary Allowance (RDA). In the US, where an RDA cannot be determined for a nutrient, then an Adequate Intake (AI) is used as an alternative, based on the available evidence. In the UK, DRVs additionally quantify a Lower Reference Nutrient Intake (LRNI) as an intake that is two standard deviations (2SD) lower than the EAR, corresponding to a risk of inadequacy of 97–98%. Unlike DRVs, the DRIs used in the US also express values for a tolerable

Table 1.4 Comparable published reference intake values for energy and macronutrients from the UK DRVs and US DRIs. Values are presented for men and women in the age group 19–50 years unless otherwise specified.

	UK Dietary Reference Values (DRVs)		US Dietary Reference Intakes (DRIs)	
Energy (kcal/d)	EAR men	2550	EER[a] men	3067
	EAR women	1940	EER[a] women	2403
Carbohydrate (% energy intake)[b]	EAR men and women	47	Acceptable range, men and women	45–65
Fibre (g/day)[d]	EAR men and women	24	All men	38
			All women	25
Total fat (% energy intake)[b]	EAR men and women	33	Acceptable range, men and women	20–35
n-6 Fatty acids (% energy intake)[b]	Individual minimum requirement	1.0	Acceptable range, men and women	5–10
n-3 Fatty acids (% energy intake)[b]	Individual minimum requirement	0.2	Acceptable range, men and women	0.6–1.2
Saturated fat (% energy intake)[b]	EAR men and women	10	Not specified[c]	
Protein (g/day)	RNI men	55.5	RDA men	56.0
	RNI women	45.0	RDA women	46.0

[a] EER, estimated energy requirement based on an active adult, 19 years of age. For each year above 19 years subtract 10 kcal/day for men and 7 kcal/day for women.

[b] Percentage of energy intake includes energy contribution of alcohol.

[c] Recommended to be as low as possible while consuming a nutritionally adequate diet.

[d] Expressed as AOAC fibre.

Data sourced from Department of Health 1991. Dietary Reference Values for Food, Energy and Nutrients for the United Kingdom. London: HMSO. Crown Copyright 1991, Crown copyright material is reproduced with the permission of the Controller of HMSO and the Queen's Printer for Scotland. Dietary Reference Intakes for Energy, Carbohydrate, Fibre, Fat, Fatty Acids, Cholesterol, Protein, and Amino Acids (Macronutrients) (2005). National Academy of Sciences, Institute of Medicine, Food and Nutrition Board.

Upper Limit (UL) for some nutrients where excess intake may exhibit adverse effects. More recently in the UK the Scientific Advisory Committee on Nutrition have produced a draft report suggesting that the EAR for energy should be increased from the current DRV in both men and women to a level of 2104–2176 kcal/day for women and 2630–2726 kcal/day for men over 19 years of age (assessed on a median physical activity level of 1.63), an increase of 100–200 kcal/day.

For easy reference, Table 1.4 presents the current published reference intakes for energy and macronutrients from both the UK and US. Nevertheless, use of reference intakes to determine nutritional adequacy needs to be undertaken with caution. Firstly, the reference intakes will only provide a relative likelihood of adequacy based on a comparable healthy population and hence may not reflect individual requirements. For example, increased requirements for energy and some nutrients are likely in individuals who have a greater than average level of activity or participate significantly in sports and exercise. In all cases use of reference intakes to determine adequacy is wholly dependent on a robust, representative and quantitative measure of current dietary intake. This,

in itself, may be difficult to obtain to a high degree of accuracy due to inherent sources of error in methods to assess dietary intake.

1.8 Food labelling

Food labels provide valuable information about food products and, where required, provide nutritional information that can be used to make informed decisions with respect to meeting the requirements of exercise and ensuring general health. In the UK the Food Labelling Regulations (1996) make it a requirement that all manufactured foods contain certain information, but at present there is no legal requirement to provide nutrition information unless a nutrition claim is made about the product. Some common claims made on food labels are described in Table 1.5.

A nutrition claim is defined as a statement, suggestion or implication, made in any labelling, presentation or advertising of a food, that the food has particular nutritional properties. The FSA has developed guidelines for the use of certain nutrition claims in food labelling and advertising and some claims are

Table 1.5 Common claims used on food labels and their definitions and/or legal requirements.

Bio	Generally found on yoghurts. Not defined by law so open to misinterpretation and use on any food.
Free from	Ingredient is only present in trace amounts.
Fresh, pure, natural	Not defined by law so open to misinterpretation and use on any food.
Gluten-free	Those made from ingredients that are naturally free of gluten or from wheat, which has gluten extracted. Note that it is not possible to remove all gluten from wheat so these products may still contain trace amounts of gluten. The law specifies that all foods for babies less than 6 months old must indicate if they contain gluten. New laws are to be enforced from 2012 to control the phrases used on packaging stating suitable for people with gluten intolerance.
Light, lite	Not defined by law. Is often used to imply different qualities, e.g. texture, colour, or less salt, fat, or calories than similar foods.
Low fat, fat-free	The law requires these claims must not be misleading but it does not state when they can be used or specify a level of fat (except for spreadable fats).
May contain nut or seed traces	Useful for allergy sufferers.
No added sugar, unsweetened	Simply means sugar or sweetener has not been added, not necessarily low in sugar.
Organic	Originates from growers, processors and importers registered and approved by organic certification bodies.
Reduced/low salt or sodium	The law does not state how much less salt or sodium these products should contain although the FSA recommend this be 25% less than a standard product.

specifically legislated under the Food Labelling Regulations (schedule 6). These are for foods with specific nutritional uses, for reduced and low energy foods, for protein formulations (e.g. for reduced and low energy foods, protein, vitamins and minerals, and those with specific nutritional uses).

If present, nutrition information panels give valuable information on energy and nutrient values. Nutrition information is usually given in calories or grams for nutrient per recommended serving and per 100 g. The value per 100 g is the most useful for comparing foods of similar type, or when analysing total nutrient intake. Food labels in the UK are based on provisions set out by the European Commission on nutritional labelling whereby when a nutrition claim is made the nutrient label must conform to the following conditions:

- Group 1 nutrients which must be listed include energy value, protein, carbohydrate and fat.
- Where a nutrition claim is made for sugars, saturates, fibre or sodium, these Group 2 nutrients are to be listed, i.e. sugars, saturated fat, fibre and sodium.
- Where a relevant claim is made, labels must also list starch, polyols, monounsaturates, polyunsaturates, cholesterol, minerals or vitamins (present in significant amounts as defined in the regulations).

In addition to these regulations, voluntary guidelines introduced by the Institute of Grocery Distributors, a trade organisation representing UK and international food and grocery-related businesses, suggest use of the following.

- Guideline daily amounts for energy, fat and saturates.
- Per serving information for energy and fat outside the main nutritional label (e.g. on front of package).

Guideline Daily Amounts (GDAs) are based on UK DRVs and current public health targets (e.g. for sodium) and are often expressed as a single value based on a woman (or man) with an energy requirement of 2000 kcal/day. Separate GDAs may also be presented for adult men and for children. It is important to note that GDAs do not replace DRVs, particularly for micronutrients, and are designed merely to be a guide to the consumer.

In the UK, the FSA has recommended a system of 'traffic light' food labelling which provides at a glance information about the fat, saturated fat, sugars and salt content of food. Red indicates a high content, amber a medium, and green a low content. The criteria for each level are shown in Table 1.6. Some companies and supermarkets have decided to use this system, and labelling usually includes the amount of each nutrient per portion with the label. Nevertheless, some companies and retailers have not accepted this system and instead opt for a system proposed by the Food and Drink Federation based

Table 1.6 UK Food Standards Agency 'traffic light' food labelling system (values expressed as per 100 g of food unless specified).

	Green (low)	Amber (medium)	Red (high)
Fat	≤3.0 g	>3.0 g but ≤20.0 g	>20.0 g or >21 g per portion
Saturated fat	≤1.5 g	>1.5 g but ≤5.0 g	>5.0 g or >6.0 g per portion
Sugars	≤5.0 g	>5.0 g but ≤15.0 g	>15.0 g or >8.0 g per portion
Salt	≤0.3 g	>0.3 g but ≤1.5 g	>1.5 g or >2.4 g per portion

on GDAs. This system avoids the use of colour coding but provides the energy, sugars, fats, saturated fat and salt content per serving both as an amount and as a percentage of the GDA.

However, adding to the confusion is that no single labelling system has been accepted by all companies and retailers, and some companies and retailers even use a combination of two systems on the same packaging.

1.9 Perspectives on the future

The nutrient basics presented in this chapter represent understanding that has been established for some considerable time. Nevertheless, it is important to have an appreciation of the basic concepts of nutrition in order to understand how they are altered when applied to an exercise situation. Research continues to explore the interplay between nutrition and exercise, and many focus on particular nutrients or specific nutritional interventions in a very controlled experimental way, which may not translate to free living situations. In addition, the literature often assumes a level of nutrition knowledge which, if absent in the reader, can lead to misunderstanding of particular findings.

It is very important to be aware of overall nutritional adequacy and dietary requirements when extrapolating any specific knowledge into dietary advice. As described in this chapter there are a variety of ways in which dietary adequacy can be estimated, although all these methods are fundamentally flawed in some way. It is unlikely that methodological limitations in dietary assessment will be fully resolved in the future, despite advances in technology, so an appreciation of these limitations will remain vital for their correct use and interpretation.

Currently in the UK and US there are government-led nation-specific healthy eating guidelines,

which as a foundation are as applicable to the athlete or exerciser as they are for the general population. The specific energy and nutrient requirements for athletes and exercisers, when training or competing, are discussed in more detail in other chapters in this book. It is possible that the format of these guidelines may change in the future, although it is likely the fundamental message may remain similar. When considering reference intake values for nutrients, it is important to consider that these are likely to be updated periodically. Specifically, the current UK DRVs have been in place since 1991 and hence are due a revised version. However, the current US DRIs, although published in 2005, are reviewed every 5 years. It is less clear how the quality, quantity and clarity of nutritional information on food labels will change in the future as this would require agreement between retailers, manufacturers, governments, legislators and other stakeholders.

Further reading

Department of Health. Dietary Reference Values of Food Energy and Nutrients for the United Kingdom (Report on Health and Social Subjects). London: HMSO, 1991.

Englyst KN, Englyst HN. Carbohydrate bioavailability. Br J Nutr 2005; 94: 1–11.

Gibney M, Lanham-New S, Cassidy A, Vorster H, eds. Introduction to Human Nutrition, 2nd edn. Hoboken, NJ: Wiley-Blackwell, 2009.

Gibson RS. Principles of Nutritional Assessment, 2nd edn. New York: Oxford University Press, 2005.

Jéquier E. Response to and range of acceptable fat intake in adults. Eur J Clin Nutr 1999; 53 (Suppl 1): S84–S93.

Lobstein T, Davies S. Defining and labelling 'healthy' and 'unhealthy' food. Public Health Nutr 2009; 12: 331–340.

Ngo J, Engelen A, Molag M, Roesle J, García-Segovia P, Serra-Majem L. A review of the use of information and communication technologies for dietary assessment. Br J Nutr 2009; 101 (Suppl 2): S102–S112.

Otten J, Hellwig JP, Meyers LD, eds. Dietary Reference Intakes: The Essential Guide to Nutritional Requirements. Washington, DC: National Academies Press, 2006.

Poslusna K, Ruprich J, de Vries JH, Jakubikova M, van't Veer P. Misreporting of energy and micronutrient intake estimated by food records and 24 hour recalls, control and adjustment methods in practice. Br J Nutr 2009; 101 (Suppl 2): S73–S85.

Stear S. Fuelling Fitness for Sports Performance. London: The Sugar Bureau, 2004.

Tipton KD, Witard OC. Protein requirements and recommendations for athletes: relevance of ivory tower arguments for practical recommendations. Clin Sports Med 2007; 26: 17–36.

Wenk C. Implications of dietary fat for nutrition and energy balance. Physiol Behav 2004; 83: 565–571.

Websites

http://www.nhs.uk/Livewell/GoodFood/Documents/eatwellplate.pdf
http://www.mypyramid.gov/
http://www.aoac.org

2
Exercise Physiology

Susan M Shirreffs

Key messages

- Exercise physiology research has led to understanding in a wide range of areas of sports nutrition. In many instances, there is no clear boundary between exercise physiology and exercise nutrition research.
- Homeostasis is the central concept in physiology and exercise is one of the biggest challenges to homeostasis that a healthy individual can face.
- Multiple organs and organ systems of the body are affected by exercise and a number of acute responses to exercise are observed. Of particular note are those of the muscle, cardiovascular and respiratory systems and thermoregulatory processes.
- Exercise training results in a number of significant adaptations in the body. These adaptations allow improvements in functional capacity.

2.1 Introduction

Physiology is the study of body function – how cells, tissues and organs work and how they are integrated in the whole individual. The study of physiology is of central importance in medicine and the related health sciences, including nutrition. It provides a thorough understanding of normal functioning that allows a more effective insight into health maintenance and understanding of abnormal function or disease states. The scope of physiology ranges from understanding events at the molecular level (e.g. how cells sense nutrients) to the integrative physiology of organs and systems (e.g. the cardiovascular and respiratory systems). It also investigates how such events are regulated and adjust to change (e.g. in response to heat exposure or to environmental extremes such as the microgravity of space flight). The emphasis of physiology is on integrating molecular, cellular, systems and whole body function.

Exercise physiology is the study of body function in association with exercise. Again this includes the study of how cells, tissues and organs work but specifically in preparation for exercise, during exercise itself and in the recovery period after exercise. Research in the field of exercise physiology has led to understanding in a wide range of topics related to sport and exercise nutrition.

2.2 Homeostasis

Homeostasis, or the maintenance of a constant internal environment, is the central feature of the body's physiological processes. However, the human body has evolved to cope with conditions far beyond those that are normally encountered and typically we use only a small part of our functional capabilities in normal day-to-day activities. In healthy individuals, undertaking exercise can be one of the biggest threats to homeostasis. For example, there can be disruptions in blood pressure, temperature, acid–base balance, body water volume and composition.

All exercise requires increased energy supply to the muscles: if the muscles cannot meet the energy demand then the exercise cannot be performed. For both high-intensity exercise and long-duration exercise, fatigue will result if the supply of energy cannot keep pace with the demand. The limiting factors will depend on the nature of the activity and of the physiological characteristics of the individual, but exercise cannot continue past the point at which the body maintains its internal environment within the rather narrow limits of the physiological norm. The only option in this situation is to reduce the exercise intensity or to stop altogether.

2.3 Acute responses to exercise

Muscle

Muscle makes up about 40% of total body mass in a typical lean male and about 35% in a typical lean female. Each muscle contains hundreds or thousands of individual muscle cells. These specialised cells are long and thin, and are usually referred to as fibres rather than as cells. Two proteins, actin and myosin, comprise much of the muscle mass, and the interaction of these two proteins is what allows muscle cells to generate force. These proteins are arranged to form long overlapping microfilaments within the skeletal muscle fibres and these filaments can slide past each other, allowing the muscle to shorten. A number of other proteins are involved in regulating the interaction of these filaments, allowing precise control of activation and relaxation. Part of the myosin molecule functions as an ATPase, breaking down adenosine triphosphate (ATP) and so making energy available to power muscle activity. The maximum force that a muscle can generate is closely related to its physiological cross-sectional area, i.e. to the number of sarcomeres (units of contraction) in parallel. Peak velocity of shortening is proportional to muscle fibre length, i.e. to the number of sarcomeres in series. Muscles are typically arranged in opposing groups so that as one group of muscles contract, another group acting across the same joint relaxes so as not to oppose lengthening as it is stretched. The organisation of nerve impulse transmission to the muscles means that it is impossible to stimulate the contraction of two antagonistic muscles at any one time.

Exercise requires activation of several muscle groups and the extent of activation is determined by the demand placed on the muscle in terms of the force to be generated or the speed of movement. Not all the muscle fibres are used in most tasks, with only enough fibres being recruited to generate the necessary force being used: the higher the force required, the greater the number of individual muscle fibres that must be activated. Receptors in the muscle and the tendons can sense the length of the muscle and also the force being generated, allowing the brain to formulate how many fibres need to be recruited and how to coordinate the recruitment of the different muscles. Muscle fibres with the lowest activation threshold are the first to be recruited and these are fibres with a low speed of contraction and high fatigue resistance. These are the fibres used most often in daily tasks so it is sensible that they have good fatigue resistance. As the weight to be moved is increased or the power output increases (e.g. increased speed in running or cycling) progressively more motor units are recruited, and at very high forces all the fibres are likely to be active. In prolonged exercise, some of the fibres that were recruited in the early stages may become fatigued and will cease to contribute to work performance and be replaced by others. In well-trained and highly motivated individuals, it can be demonstrated that the muscle is working maximally: adding an electrical stimulus to the nerve does not generate any additional force.

Respiratory system

A key element of performance in exercise lasting more than a few minutes is the person's maximum oxygen uptake (Vo_{2max}). This represents the highest rate of aerobic energy production that can be achieved and the energy required for any power output in excess of this must come entirely from anaerobic metabolism. The importance of Vo_{2max} for endurance athletes such as marathon runners lies in the fact that endurance capacity is largely a function of the fraction of Vo_{2max} that can be sustained for prolonged periods: the higher the fraction of aerobic capacity that must be used, the shorter the time for which a given pace can be sustained. Improving performance requires either an increase in Vo_{2max}, an increase in the fraction of Vo_{2max} that can be sustained for the duration of the race, or a decrease in the energy cost of running. In practice, all these can be achieved with suitable training.

Limiting factors to Vo_{2max} have been discussed and debated over the years. The limiting factor may vary in different types of exercise, in different environments and in different individuals. Typically, the lungs are not considered to limit performance at sea level in the absence of lung disease, so attention has focused primarily on whether the limitation lies in the delivery of oxygen by the cardiovascular system or in the ability of the working muscles to utilise oxygen. However, the oxygen content of inspired air falls at altitude, leading to a fall in arterial oxygen saturation, decreased oxygen transport and a fall in Vo_{2max}. This accounts for the reduction in performance in events lasting more than a few minutes that is generally seen at altitudes above about 1500 m. Some highly trained runners show arterial desaturation in maximal exercise even at sea level and this is reversed, and Vo_{2max} increased, by breathing air with an increased oxygen content. This effect is not normally seen in trained but non-elite runners, suggesting there may be a pulmonary limitation in elite runners.

Research investigating the responses to training of the inspiratory muscles also provides some support for the idea that there may be a pulmonary limitation. For example, when the effects of 4 weeks of inspiratory muscle training for 30 min/day on cycle ergometer endurance time at 77% of Vo_{2max} were measured, untrained subjects increased their endurance time at the same power output from 26.8 min before training to 40.2 min after training. In trained subjects, who worked at a higher absolute power output, endurance time was increased from 22.8 to 31.5 min. However, it is important to note that not all research has reported the same findings so the picture is not entirely clear at present.

Cardiovascular system

The cardiovascular system's functions, amongst others, are to deliver oxygen and nutrients to all tissues of the body and to remove waste products, to control heat flux within the body, and to circulate hormones from the sites of their production to the sites of their action. There is strong experimental evidence to support the idea that limitations to oxygen delivery are imposed by the cardiovascular system and that the limitation may lie at any one or more of several stages. The key element seems to be the maximum cardiac output that can be achieved, as this is related to both Vo_{2max} and endurance performance. The size of the heart, and more specifically of the left ventricle, is also important. This determines the stroke volume – the amount of blood ejected with each beat of the heart – and the cardiac output (the product of heart rate and stroke volume) is closely correlated with both Vo_{2max} and endurance performance. In elite endurance athletes the cardiac output can exceed 40 l/min, compared with the maximum of about 20 l/min that the sedentary individual can achieve. As maximum heart rate

does not change much, this difference is accounted for almost entirely by the greater stroke volume of the endurance athlete. A high blood volume will also benefit the endurance athlete by helping to maintain central venous pressure, thus maintaining stroke volume.

The oxygen-carrying capacity of the blood is also important, and this is influenced by the haemoglobin concentration and the total blood volume. Almost all the oxygen in the blood is transported bound to haemoglobin and each gram of haemoglobin can bind 1.34 ml of oxygen. The average male has a higher haemoglobin concentration (about 140 g/l) than the average female (about 120 g/l) and so has about 15% more oxygen in the blood when it leaves the lungs. This difference accounts in part for the generally higher aerobic capacity of males and it also explains the various strategies used by athletes to increase the haemoglobin content of the blood, including altitude training, the use of agents such as erythropoietin that stimulate the formation of new red blood cells, and the use of blood transfusions prior to competition. Even though some of these strategies are prohibited by the World Anti-Doping Agency (WADA) they have been used, and almost certainly still are being used, by some athletes. The delivery of oxygen to the muscles is also influenced by the density of the capillary network within the muscles. An increase in the number of capillaries means less distance for oxygen (and substrate) to diffuse from the capillary to the mitochondria within the muscle where it is used.

Thermoregulation

The efficiency of human metabolism is only a little over 20% so almost 80% of the energy available from the catabolism of nutrients appears as heat. This is useful in a cold environment for the maintenance of body temperature but it does present a challenge in situations such as prolonged hard exercise in hot environments, where heat is generated at high rates and heat loss to the environment is more difficult. Heat stress during exercise poses a major challenge to the cardiovascular system, as in addition to continuing to supply blood to the working muscles, the brain and other tissues, there is a greatly increased demand for blood flow to the skin. This requires an increased cardiac output and also means that a significant part of the blood volume is distributed to the skin so the central blood volume is decreased. This in turn may reduce the return of blood to the heart and result in a fall in stroke volume; if the heart rate cannot increase to compensate, cardiac output will fall. If this happens there must be either reduced blood flow to the muscles, and hence a reduced supply of oxygen and substrate, or reduced blood flow to the skin, which will reduce heat loss and accelerate the development of hyperthermia. It seems likely that the temperature of the brain is the most relevant parameter, but there seems to be no set temperature at which exercise must be terminated and fatigue occurs across a wide range of core temperatures.

Sweat evaporation from the surface of the skin promotes heat loss and limits the rise in core temperature. As this occurs, there is a loss of body water and electrolytes, particularly sodium. Hypohydration and hyperthermia will both, if sufficiently severe, impair physical and cognitive function. However, low levels of hypohydration are probably of little significance in most exercise tasks. Some of the adverse effects of sweat loss can be offset by ingesting sufficient fluid during exercise to limit the development of hypohydration to less than about 2–3% of body mass. In most sporting contexts, the salt losses in sweat are small and can be replaced from food and drinks eaten after exercise. Some individuals, though, can lose large amounts of salt and there is some evidence for a link between high salt losses and muscle cramp.

2.4 Adaptations to exercise training

The aim of training is to increase functional capacity and to bring about event-specific improvements in performance. Training affects every organ and tissue of the body but the adaptation is specific to the training stimulus and to the muscles being trained. A well-designed strength training programme will have little effect on endurance and vice versa; one leg can be specifically trained for strength and the other for endurance with relatively little cross-over. Training should therefore be designed to address the event-specific limitations to performance, and this will differ between individuals as well as between events. It is important to note, however, that training is not entirely specific as the effects on the cardiovascular system will be similar whether running or cycling or any other activity is performed. The performance improvement is proportional to the training load, i.e. the intensity, duration and frequency of the training sessions. Generally the harder an athlete trains, the greater the improvements in performance that result. However, there is a limit beyond which further increases in training will result in poorer performance; this is usually referred to as an over-training syndrome, but few athletes reach this level of training.

Regular training also has important effects on the brain, though these are less well understood than many of the peripheral adaptations. One important learned response is the ability to judge pace, so that effort can be distributed evenly across the whole duration of an event. A common mistake of novice athletes is to set off too fast and then to fade badly in the later stages or to finish with too much still in reserve.

2.5 Concluding remarks

Exercise physiology, while a discipline in its own right, is intrinsically linked to many aspects of sports nutrition. An understanding of the body's physiological processes at rest, during exercise and in the recovery period after exercise is key to understanding many of the nutrition requirements of an exercising person and important in identifying nutrients that may help exercising individuals to achieve their aims, be that training adaptations, exercise performance or recovery after exercise.

Further reading

Powers SK, Howley E. Exercise Physiology: Theory and Application to Fitness and Performance, 6th edn. Sydney: McGraw Hill Higher Education, 2006.

Widmaier EP, Raff H, Strang KT. Vander's Human Physiology. The Mechanisms of Body Function, 10th edn. Sydney: McGraw Hill Higher Education, 2005.

3
Exercise Biochemistry

Stuart DR Galloway

Key messages

- Understanding some principles of exercise biochemistry is necessary to underpin knowledge of fatigue mechanisms in skeletal muscle, and informs sport and exercise nutrition strategies for combatting fatigue.
- Understanding basic control and regulation of ATP-producing pathways provides a greater insight into the potential for exercise or nutritional interventions to alter skeletal muscle metabolism.
- Knowledge of the effects of environment on metabolic responses to exercise helps to define nutritional guidelines for those exposed to harsh environmental conditions.

- Understanding the metabolic adaptations that occur in response to exercise training allows individualised nutrition strategies to be developed.
- Knowledge about the cellular/molecular drivers for adaptations in skeletal muscle metabolism with training helps to optimise current practice, and may influence future recommendations made by Sport and Exercise Nutritionists.

3.1 Introduction

Research in the field of exercise biochemistry has led to understanding in a wide range of topics related to sport and exercise nutrition. Critically, knowledge of the factors that may limit cellular metabolism and lead to local muscular fatigue (inability to sustain the intended intensity of effort) have been identified. Understanding these limiting factors has led to the development of numerous nutritional intervention strategies in an attempt to overcome limitations and ultimately improve performance or extend endurance capacity. An understanding of the impact of exercise intensity and duration on the metabolic demand for adenosine triphosphate (ATP) is key when examining substrate metabolism, when studying the impact of substrate availability/depletion on muscular fatigue, or when devising nutritional strategies for exercise.

The metabolic energy demands of jumping and throwing are very different from sprinting, middle distance running or prolonged endurance events. Therefore, different energy systems, and combina-

tions of these energy systems, are utilised to defend ATP concentration within the working skeletal muscle (Table 3.1). ATP requirement in the muscle contraction process is primarily driven by ATP hydrolysis by actomyosin ATPase, but a range of other ATPases such as calcium ATPase and sodium/potassium ATPase also have a role in the whole excitation–contraction coupling process. Therefore, maintaining and defending cellular ATP concentration is vital to delaying the onset of muscle fatigue at many sites in the whole contractile process. Indeed, maintenance of cellular homeostasis is the fundamental principle in the regulation of body functions in human physiology.

Very brief explosive contractions used in jumping and throwing require high rates of ATP utilisation and the contractions last fractions of a second (Table 3.1). The existing ATP store within the muscle may be sufficient to meet this immediate demand, but ATP re-synthesis will come from metabolism of creatine phosphate (PCr) to replenish and maintain the ATP concentration. In repeated short bouts of

Sport and Exercise Nutrition, First Edition. Edited by Susan A Lanham-New, Samantha J Stear, Susan M Shirreffs and Adam L Collins.
© 2011 The Nutrition Society. Published 2011 by Blackwell Publishing Ltd.

Table 3.1 Duration and intensity of activity (rate of ATP hydrolysis) dictates the requirement for ATP re-synthesis from a variety of metabolic substrates, which in turn determines the substrate that is metabolised.

Activity	Duration/intensity[a] of activity to be sustained	Metabolic substrate supply	Maximal rate of ATP re-synthesis possible from substrate sources[b]
Explosive events (throws/jumps)	<5 s/supramaximal	ATP/PCr	4.4
Sprinting	6–60 s/supramaximal	ATP/PCr, glycogen	3.4
Middle distance	>60 s to 5 min/maximal	PCr, glycogen, blood glucose, IMTG	1.7
Endurance	>5 min to 5 hours/ submaximal (60–85% max.)	Glycogen, blood glucose, IMTG, plasma fatty acids, amino acids	1.0
Ultra-endurance	>5 hours/submaximal (40–60% max.)	Glycogen, blood glucose, IMTG, plasma fatty acids, amino acids	0.6

[a] Intensity is relative to maximal oxygen uptake achievable in an aerobic capacity test.
[b] Indicates an approximate rate of maximal ATP re-synthesis based on mixed substrate sources. Values are (mol)(mol/min). Based on Greenhaff & Hultman (1999), © Elsevier 1999.

activity the size of the PCr store within the muscle may limit the rate of replenishment of ATP. Subsequently, creatine supplementation studies have confirmed the importance of this metabolic store in sustaining repeated short bouts of intense activity. In sprinting, the metabolic demand for ATP is met through metabolism of a combination of substrates, mainly PCr and muscle glycogen. The high rate of ATP re-synthesis required during sprinting dictates that muscle glycogen metabolism (glycogenolysis) is confined to anaerobic glycolysis occurring within the cell cytosol. Limitations in anaerobic glycogen metabolism will therefore influence the ability to sustain the rate of muscle contraction and may limit performance as fatigue ensues. As the duration of an event increases, the sustainable intensity of that activity declines. The rate of ATP re-synthesis will be met from the breakdown of other substrates such as complete aerobic oxidation of glycogen, or metabolism of fatty acids from the intramuscular triglyceride (IMTG) stores. Thus, in middle distance events a combination of anaerobic and aerobic metabolism of glycogen and glucose as well as aerobic metabolism of IMTG will contribute to the re-synthesis of ATP (Table 3.1). Factors that limit metabolism of these substrates are therefore likely to also influence performance and capacity in middle distance events. Furthermore, in more prolonged endurance events the primary pathways for replenishment of ATP will be aerobic metabolism of glycogen, glucose and IMTG as well as plasma-derived fatty acids released from adipose tissue stores. There will possibly also be a larger contribution from amino acids in more prolonged activity, particularly if there is a chronic energy deficit.

It is well established that in prolonged endurance events, in the absence of carbohydrate feeding, the muscle glycogen pool may become depleted to the point where it limits the sustainable exercise intensity. However, in trained athletes who have greater reliance on fatty acid metabolism and who also have larger muscle glycogen stores, this limitation is overcome to a certain extent, or would only occur at higher absolute work intensities. So, training adaptation and nutritional intervention may substantially alter the metabolic limitations or responses to exercise, and Sport and Exercise Nutritionists should have an understanding of these elements. The study of exercise biochemistry has not only helped our understanding of the interaction between exercise intensity/duration and substrate utilisation, but also provided great insight into the metabolic responses to environmental stresses such as heat, cold and altitude. It has also aided our understanding of the nature and time course of adaptations in metabolism that occur with exercise training. All these effects may subsequently alter nutritional requirements during exercise. By utilising knowledge of exercise biochemistry one can track metabolic responses to feeding, interpret gender differences in metabolism, and devise a variety of physical activity and nutritional approaches to weight loss/gain. Furthermore, recent advances in understanding of the cellular and molecular responses to training and nutrition have provided greater insight into the particular drivers for metabolic adaptations. It is probable that new knowledge in this area will ultimately support or refute current recommended practices in training and dietary intake strategies.

In summary, the requirement for ATP re-synthesis and the substrate metabolised to meet that demand will be dictated by the intensity and duration of activity that is being sustained. However, other factors will dictate the particular substrate(s) used, including prior diet, training status, environment, gender and genetics. The aim of this chapter is therefore to provide an overview of these key areas and to stimulate interest in exercise biochemistry. It is hoped that this brief background chapter will enable a more in-depth considered view of nutritional approaches to sport and exercise that are discussed in later chapters.

3.2 Control and regulation of metabolic reactions

The rates of metabolic reactions are influenced by many factors including substrate availability, end-product accumulation, energy requirements of the reaction, enzyme activity, or quantities of co-factor present (such as nicotinamide adenine dinucleotide in oxidised or reduced form, i.e. NAD/NADH status). Furthermore, the ability to transport substrates into the muscle as well as the temperature within the working skeletal muscle, and the hormonal milieu, will also influence substrate metabolism. Thus the rate of a reaction depends upon many different influencing factors. Exercise training status, nutritional and activity status, gender, and genetic/individual variation, all play a role in determining the diversity of the metabolic responses observed at rest and during exercise in humans.

However, it is important to know that there are some reaction steps that will proceed in one direction or another based largely upon the quantity of reactants present, or the build-up of end products. An example of this would be PCr metabolism, in which an elevation of ADP concentration will activate creatine kinase to increase metabolism of PCr and thus restore the intracellular concentration of ATP (Figure 3.1). Other key reaction steps in the pathways of carbohydrate, fat and protein metabolism are regulated in a similar manner but are also

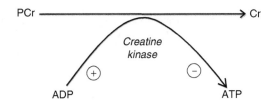

Figure 3.1 Phosphocreatine (PCr) degradation is enhanced through activation of creatine kinase by ADP. This figure only shows the reaction proceeding in one direction but the reaction is reversible.

more tightly controlled by co-factors, availability of other substrates, or hormonal influences that activate or inactivate the key enzymes involved. Usually this regulation is through phosphorylation/dephosphorylation of the inactive/active forms of the enzyme, respectively. For example, phosphorylase is activated by increased calcium (Ca^{2+}) concentration, adenosine monophosphate (AMP), inosine monophosphate (IMP), free inorganic phosphate (Pi) and adrenaline concentrations. Thus the enzyme is activated directly by muscular contraction, the intensity of exercise and the rate of ATP turnover required. This tight regulatory control is essential to effectively defend ATP concentration within contracting skeletal muscle.

By understanding how the activities of these key enzyme reaction steps are influenced, a better understanding of the impact of training and/or nutrition on flux through these metabolic pathways is gained. Furthermore, knowledge of these regulatory factors is also useful for identifying potential targets for nutritional interventions.

3.3 Carbohydrate, fat and protein metabolism

In the previous sections of this chapter it has been noted that defending ATP concentration, and thus matching supply of ATP to demand for ATP, essentially determines which substrates are metabolised. This part of the chapter covers the oxidation of carbohydrate, fat and protein fuel sources for ATP re-synthesis, and focuses briefly on the integration of metabolism of these different substrates.

Carbohydrate metabolism

Carbohydrate metabolism can be fuelled by the breakdown of glycogen stored within the contracting muscle, or from blood glucose that is transported

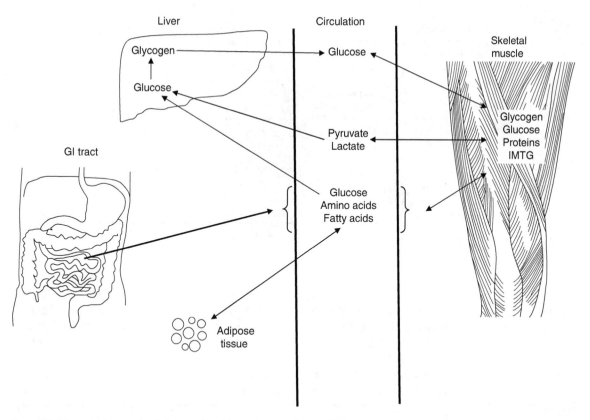

Figure 3.2 Schematic diagram of carbohydrate, fat and protein sources for metabolism.

into the muscle for oxidation, while blood glucose concentration is maintained through liver glycogen metabolism or gluconeogenesis from amino acids or lactate (Figure 3.2). These different sources of carbohydrate for metabolism and maintenance of blood glucose homeostasis are crucial since the carbohydrate stores in working muscle can typically only sustain activity at about 70% of maximal working capacity for around 90 min in a moderately active person (Table 3.2). Key steps that could limit skeletal muscle metabolism of carbohydrate include: enzymatic regulation at various stages in glycolysis/glycogenolysis, including pyruvate dehydrogenase (PDH), phosphofructokinase (PFK), hexokinase (HK), and glycogen phosphorylase (GP); low availability of muscle glycogen; limitation in glucose transport capacity into skeletal muscle (GLUT4); reduction in glucose availability in the circulation (low liver glycogen, low carbohydrate intake); and even poor transport/absorption of ingested carbohydrate

in the intestine. The integration of these factors alongside the hormonal influence of glucagon or adrenaline, which can stimulate breakdown of glycogen, all act to match substrate metabolism with demand for ATP re-synthesis. The final end product of glycolysis/glycogenolysis in the cell cytosol is pyruvate. Pyruvate either enters mitochondria and is converted to acetyl-CoA by PDH for complete oxidation in the tricarboxylic acid (TCA) cycle and respiratory chain, or is converted to lactate (if supply of pyruvate exceeds capacity for transport and oxidation in mitochondria). The lactate produced may be used as a fuel source within skeletal muscle or is released into the circulation for processing in the liver to form glucose/glycogen (Figure 3.3).

Fat metabolism

Fat may be metabolised by mobilisation of intramuscular triglyceride stores or through oxidation of plasma-derived fatty acids obtained from peripheral

Table 3.2 Estimated availability of carbohydrate and fat stores, approximate total caloric expenditure possible from these stores, and theoretical duration of exercise sustainable.

Substrate	Estimated total storage quantity[a]	Approximate total caloric expenditure possible before depletion of store	Theoretical exercise duration sustainable at moderate intensity (70–85% max.)
Muscle glycogen/liver glycogen/blood glucose	420 g	~1575 kcal	~1.5 hours
Intramuscular triglycerides/plasma FFA/adipose tissue triglycerides	14.5 kg	~130 500 kcal	~120 hours

[a] For a healthy active untrained human.

adipose tissue stores or dietary fat intake (see Figure 3.2). Clearly, the main difference between the storage of fat and carbohydrate is the size of the available store. Most adult humans have sufficient adipose tissue stores to provide an almost unlimited supply of substrate for ATP re-synthesis during exercise and could theoretically sustain over 120 hours of continuous effort (Table 3.2). In reality this is not possible as substrates are not used in isolation, and other factors would act to limit fat oxidation. It is now widely acknowledged that the key factors limiting fatty acid oxidation in skeletal muscle largely relate to three components:

(1) ability to transport fatty acids into muscle via passive diffusion as well as facilitated transport via fatty acid binding proteins (FABPpm) and carrier proteins such as fatty acid translocase (FAT/CD36), fatty acid transport proteins (FATPs) or cytosolic FABP (FABPc);

(2) transfer of activated fatty acids, derived from plasma or intramuscular triglyceride stores, across the mitochondrial membranes via carnitine palmitoyl transferase I and II (CPT I/II) with regulatory involvement from FAT/CD36 and malonyl-CoA; and

(3) enzymatic regulation of β-oxidation through mitochondrial capacity for fatty acid oxidation, typically assessed using maximal activity of L-β-hydroxyacyl CoA dehydrogenase (β-HAD).

All these components can change to improve fatty acid metabolism in trained individuals. However, there are clearly other factors involved that will influence fat oxidation in exercise such as availability of substrate (carbohydrate feeding will blunt fatty acid mobilisation and oxidation) and hormonal control (fatty acid mobilisation is increased by adrenaline due to an action on hormone-sensitive lipase), and thus intensity of exercise and duration are also critical in determining rates of whole body fatty acid oxidation. Metabolism of activated long-chain fatty acids within the mitochondrion involves the process of cleaving 2-carbon units off the chain on each pass through the β-oxidation pathway. A 16-carbon palmitate chain thus produces eight 2-carbon acetyl-CoA units for oxidation in the TCA cycle and respiratory chain (Figure 3.3).

Protein metabolism

Protein is generally overlooked as a key substrate for exercising skeletal muscle, but it is metabolised through oxidation of free amino acids derived from muscle or plasma sources. Plasma-derived amino acids include amino acids obtained from dietary intake or mobilised from other body protein stores (see Figure 3.2). Protein oxidation normally only contributes a small amount to whole body substrate oxidation (<5%) but may increase up to about 10% depending on duration of activity and energy balance. Protein oxidation will be greater as duration of exercise is increased and particularly when there is a large energy deficit, or low carbohydrate availability. Thus, similar to other substrates amino acid oxidation

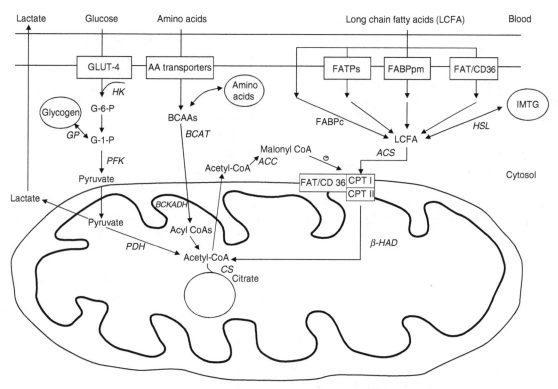

Figure 3.3 Schematic diagram of the integration of carbohydrate, fat and protein metabolism in human skeletal muscle. ACC, acetyl-CoA carboxylase; ACS, acyl-CoA synthetase; BCAA, branched chain amino acid; BCAT, branched chain aminotransferase. For explanation of other abbreviations see text.

is influenced by training status and nutritional status as well as the exercise intensity and duration being sustained. Of the 20 amino acids that contribute to normal physiological functioning, only seven of these play a role in metabolism. Glutamate, glutamine, alanine and aspartate contribute to intermediary metabolism whilst the branched-chain amino acids (isoleucine, leucine and valine) are the main amino acids catabolised as a fuel source within contracting skeletal muscle. The branched-chain amino acids are oxidised by the rate-limiting enzyme branched-chain keto acid dehydrogenase (BCKADH) to form acyl-CoAs. BCKADH is an enzyme similar to PDH and the acyl-CoA produced may be converted to acetyl-CoA for entry into the TCA cycle and respiratory chain (Figure 3.3).

Thus, the common linking product in the complete aerobic oxidation of carbohydrate, fat and protein is the formation of acetyl-CoA within the mitochondria of working skeletal muscle. This common end product from intermediary metabolism of these three

substrates enters the TCA cycle initially through conversion to citrate by the enzyme citrate synthase (CS). The key role of the TCA cycle is to produce reducing equivalents (NADH + H^+ and $FADH_2$) that subsequently enter the electron transport chain and drive oxidative phosphorylation of ADP + Pi to form ATP. In this process 'metabolic' water is produced from the combination of $2H^+$ + O_2 to form H_2O. Reducing equivalents that are formed earlier in metabolism, within the cytosol, are also able to enter the mitochondrion through the malate/aspartate shuttle (and thus help to phosphorylate ADP) unless the intensity of exercise is high.

As previously stated the requirement for ATP re-synthesis determines which substrate is utilised, and it should be acknowledged that complete aerobic oxidation of carbohydrate, fat and protein does not produce ATP at very high rates compared with anaerobic glycolysis or PCr metabolism. In particular, the rate of ATP re-synthesis from fat is slow by comparison to PCr or glycogen degradation. However, there are advantages to carrying and metabolising fat as it generates substantially more ATP per gram than carbohydrate (and is therefore an effective substrate source). This enables a substantial substrate reserve to be carried efficiently (an equivalent energy reserve of glycogen would add substantial mass and limit mobility).

3.4 Metabolic responses to environmental stress

Given that many Sport and Exercise Nutritionists will work with athletes training and competing in extreme environments, it is important to briefly describe the key metabolic considerations at environmental extremes.

Heat

In hot climates the environment may directly impact upon metabolic responses to exercise through increased stress on the cardiovascular system (loss of blood volume, and redistribution of blood volume for thermoregulation) and the resulting altered hormonal responses to exercise. Typically, heat stress (body temperature of ~40°C) leads to increased rates of muscle glycogen utilisation through an increased circulating adrenaline concentration, and has been demonstrated to result in greater type I fibre glycogen depletion. This is often associated with greater lactate efflux from working muscle into the circulation, which would suggest a mismatch in flux through glycolysis with mitochondrial functional capacity under these conditions. These observations suggest that heat stress increases anaerobic contribution to exercise, but arteriovenous oxygen balance studies refute this by demonstrating increased oxygen extraction under conditions of thermal stress.

Having highlighted that an increase in rate of glycogen degradation may occur, it is important to note that most endurance performance studies have revealed that complete depletion of muscle glycogen is not the key limiting factor during exercise in the heat. Therefore, metabolic limitations under heat stress have been put aside in favour of a focus on hydration issues for maintenance of cardiovascular function and exercise performance in the heat. Details of these aspects are covered in a later chapter.

Cold

Cold stress may not be an issue for many athletes as clothing can be worn or intensity of exercise increased to maintain core temperature and peripheral skin temperatures. Under these conditions skeletal muscle metabolism should remain unaltered. However, studies have shown variable effects on metabolism that are dependent upon the exposure temperature, whether peripheral cooling occurs, or whether core cooling occurs. If ambient temperature is cooled (to around 10°C) there can be an initial reduction in muscle glycogen usage; however, with more extreme cooling (0°C or below) an increased rate of muscle glycogen degradation has been observed with blunted fatty acid oxidation. These changes likely reflect increased sympathetic activation during exercise in more severe cold. Thus, determining optimal nutritional strategies must be specific to the conditions, clothing and effects on core and muscle temperatures. Typically, if moderate exercise intensity can be sustained, then core cooling will not occur at cool ambient temperatures, and little change in substrate metabolism will be noted. However, more extreme cold may increase reliance on muscle glycogenolysis and reduce oxidation of fat.

Altitude

At altitude the key stimulus for altered substrate utilisation is through sympathetic activation. This will lead to enhanced rates of carbohydrate oxidation compared with the same intensity of exercise conducted at sea level. The stimulus to sympathetic activation is driven by hypoxic exposure and therefore becomes greater at higher altitudes. An increase in glycogenolysis at low to moderate altitudes (<2500 m) eventually becomes an increased stimulus to utilisation of all substrates (carbohydrate, protein and fat) at high altitudes (>4000 m). This catabolic effect of high altitudes is linked to sympathetic activation and appetite suppression as well as continued high metabolic cost of activity, and thus leads to a significant negative energy balance. On prolonged exposure to high altitudes fat loss and muscle wasting has been observed. Furthermore, after prolonged exposure the muscle phenotype reflects this hypoxic challenge, with a reduced mitochondrial mass and reduced activity of the mitochondrial enzymes associated with β-oxidation, TCA cycle and the respiratory chain, and increased activity of glycolytic enzymes such as PFK.

3.5 Metabolic adaptations to training

The substrates metabolised during exercise reflect the intensity and duration of activity and the requirement for ATP re-synthesis. Typically, low-intensity exercise (<30% of maximum work capacity) relies most heavily on fat metabolism from plasma fatty acids and IMTG, moderate-intensity exercise (60–80% of maximum work capacity) relies upon the full range of available substrates including glucose, glycogen, plasma fatty acids and IMTG, whereas higher-intensity exercise (85–90% of maximum work capacity) relies more heavily on muscle glycogen stores to meet ATP re-synthesis demands (Figure 3.4).

Following an endurance training period the overall effect on substrate selection is a shift towards greater reliance on fat metabolism at the same absolute sub-maximal exercise workload compared with before training. Early studies in the 1970s revealed that these changes in metabolism were at least partly related to an upregulation of mitochondrial biogenesis that increased the size and number of mitochondria. As a result, the maximal activities of key marker enzymes such as β-HAD, CS, CPT I and cytochrome *c* were observed to increase in trained skeletal muscle. Nowadays, this greater reliance on fat oxidation during submaximal exercise is known to be driven not only by increased mitochondrial biogenesis but also by several other factors including: increased total work capacity; increased storage, mobilisation, transport and oxidation of IMTGs; reduced sympathetic activation; and changes in other hormonal responses to exercise. The hormonal changes include blunted reduction in plasma insulin and blunted rise in plasma glucagon concentration during an exercise period. After training there are also reductions in the factors influencing rates of reactions in glycolysis/glycogenolysis that lead to a reduced stimulus for activation of these metabolic pathways.

Therefore, these changes and the subsequent shift towards fat metabolism result in a reduction in glycogen utilisation as well as a reduction in plasma glucose oxidation (Figure 3.5) and consequently lactate accumulation is also decreased. Interestingly, endurance training increases the uptake and storage of muscle glycogen through increased GLUT4 expression, so a larger store of glycogen used at a lower rate means a much greater duration of activity can be sustained before depletion of glycogen stores

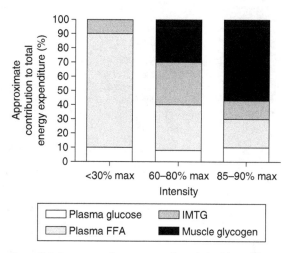

Figure 3.4 Percentage of energy expenditure derived from different substrate sources in relation to intensity of exercise. (Adapted from Romijn *et al.* 1993, © 1993 by American Physiological Society. Reproduced with permission of American Physiological Society in the format Textbook via Copyright Clearance Center.)

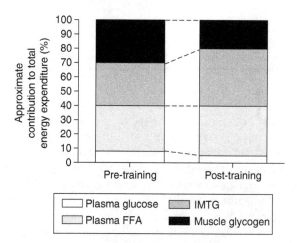

Figure 3.5 Training-induced change in percentage of energy derived from fat during moderate-intensity exercise. (Adapted from Martin 1996, with permission from Wolters Kluwer Health.)

will occur. These training-induced adaptations clearly also support effective recovery of muscle glycogen stores after exercise, if a suitable diet is consumed in a timely manner. Studies have also revealed that endurance training increases the capacity for amino acid oxidation. However, there is increased efficiency of degradation following training. This dual impact of training on amino acid metabolism has continued to cause much debate over dietary protein requirements for athletes.

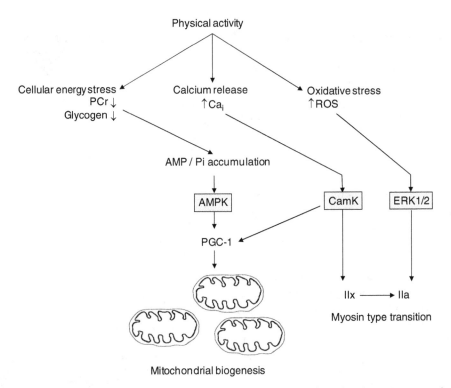

Figure 3.6 Schematic diagram of cellular/molecular drivers for metabolic adaptations in skeletal muscle with exercise. See text for explanation of abbreviations.

In addition, endurance training improves the capacity to perform high-intensity work bouts through enhanced glycogen stores and increased sympathetic activation during high-intensity efforts. Incorporation of high-intensity work bouts into a training programme has been shown to provide a further powerful stimulus to muscular metabolic adaptations. Indeed, in recent years the short time periods required to observe adaptations in skeletal muscle metabolism have been realised. This plasticity of muscle metabolism has renewed the interest in short-term training interventions that can stimulate rapid metabolic changes to occur (such as high-intensity interval training), which could be exploited to benefit athletes but also those suffering from metabolic diseases related to sedentary behaviour.

3.6 Cellular/molecular drivers for adaptations in skeletal muscle metabolism

As stated in the previous sections of this chapter the maintenance of cellular ATP homeostasis is the primary driver for substrate metabolism and fuel selection. The factors that help to regulate substrate use through effects on near-equilibrium reactions and non-equilibrium reactions in the metabolic pathways (such as ADP, Pi, Ca^{2+}, AMP, IMP, hydrogen ions (H^+), end products or substrate supply) also act as drivers for adaptation in skeletal muscle. Logically this makes sense, as a repeated stimulus that disturbs metabolic homeostasis and induces cellular stress should lead to improved capacity to cope with disturbances in homeostasis over the longer term (the basis of adaptation to exercise). Thus some insight into the cellular and molecular processes/mechanisms involved in adaptation may help to inform training and nutritional strategies for athletes.

The signal transduction pathways that lead to adaptation firstly promote transcription of genes (mRNA copies of DNA sections), and subsequently the translation of some of this mRNA into new proteins will induce a functional change (adaptation). By studying gene expression and changes in regulatory proteins, such as transport proteins or key regulatory enzymes, we can gain an insight into the effectiveness of training or nutritional interventions.

The metabolic adaptations to endurance training, and the increased capacity for fat oxidation, induced mainly through increased size and numbers of mitochondria are now more clearly understood. Cellular energy stress such as glycogen or PCr depletion impairs the ability to maintain ATP concentrations within contracting skeletal muscle leading to accumulation of AMP and IMP, which are powerful stimulators of a key enzyme called AMP-activated protein kinase (AMPK). Activation of AMPK has been shown to lead to expression of the transcriptional co-factor PPAR-γ co-activator (PGC)-1 that is responsible, along with nuclear respiratory factors, for promoting expression of mitochondrial genes. This gene expression ultimately results in formation of new or larger mitochondria. An increased size and number of mitochondria means increased capacity for oxidative substrate metabolism. Increased intracellular Ca^{2+} and factors such as reactive oxygen species (ROS) also provide stimuli to promote greater oxidative capacity of skeletal muscle fibres by promoting IIx to IIa fibre transition through increased expression of slower myosin types. Other stimuli activate expression of genes that translate proteins involved in fat metabolism and the details of these are not fully understood but may also involve AMPK (Figure 3.6).

As a result of the identification and mapping of these signal transduction pathways, nutritional and training strategies that increase or reduce cellular stress have recently been a focus of research. Training when fed or fasted, training following glycogen depletion or with carbohydrate provision, training with or without antioxidant supplementation, and many other perturbations are all being investigated. The literature in this field is still in its infancy and there is a great deal of work to be done in the future to understand the interactions between nutrition, training, and drivers for metabolic adaptations in skeletal muscle.

3.7 Concluding remarks

Exercise biochemistry and the study of metabolic pathways may seem to be a vast and complex topic to include in a sport and exercise nutrition text. However, basic knowledge of exercise metabolism alongside exercise physiology provides the Sport and Exercise Nutritionist with the ability to integrate information.

This knowledge leads to a better understanding of the science that underpins current nutritional guidelines, as well as providing the basis for development of new approaches. Detailed knowledge of local metabolic regulators that limit or promote the use of a particular substrate, and knowledge of the integration between hormonal and other factors that aid in regulation of metabolism, allows the Sport and Exercise Nutritionist to make independent informed judgements on the effectiveness of nutritional interventions.

Whilst this chapter does not touch on all relevant aspects of exercise biochemistry, it hopefully sets out the basic elements to support further reading around the topic (which should always be encouraged) and it focuses on the key aspects that are developed further within other chapters of this text.

Further reading

Brooks GA, Fahey TD, White TP. Exercise Physiology: Human Bioenergetics and Its Applications, 2nd edn. Oxford: Mayfield Press, 1996.

Burke LM, Hawley JA. Fat and carbohydrate for exercise. Curr Opin Clin Nutr Metab Care 2006; 9: 476–481.

Coffey VG, Hawley JA. The molecular bases of training adaptation. Sports Med 2007; 37: 737–763.

Flueck M. Plasticity of the muscle proteome to exercise at altitude. High Alt Med Biol 2009; 10: 183–193.

Frayn KN. Metabolic Regulation: A Human Perspective, 3rd edn. Oxford: Wiley-Blackwell, 2010.

Gibney MJ, Macdonald IA, Roche HM. Nutrition and Metabolism. Oxford: Blackwell Publishing, 2003.

Greenhaff PL, Hultman E. The biochemical basis of exercise. In: Basic and Applied Sciences for Sports Medicine (Maughan RJ, ed.). Oxford: Butterworth-Heinemann, 1999, pp 69–89.

Hargreaves M, Spriet LL. Exercise Metabolism, 2nd edn. Champaign, IL: Human Kinetics, 2006.

Hawley JA. Molecular responses to strength and endurance training: are they incompatible? Appl Physiol Nutr Metab 2009; 34: 355–361.

Hawley JA, Tipton KD, Millard-Stafford ML. Promoting training adaptation through nutritional interventions. J Sports Sci 2006; 24: 709–721.

Hawley JA, Gibala MJ, Bermon S. Innovations in athletic preparation: role of substrate availability to modify training adaptation and performance. J Sports Sci 2007; 25 (Suppl 1): S115–S124.

Holloszy JO, Kohrt WM. Regulation of carbohydrate and fat metabolism during and after exercise. Annu Rev Nutr 1996; 16: 121–138.

Holloway GP. Mitochondrial function and dysfunction in exercise and insulin resistance. Appl Physiol Nutr Metab 2009; 34: 440–446.

Holloway GP, Luiken JJFP, Glatz JFC, Spriet LL, Bonen A. Contribution of FAT/CD36 to the regulation of skeletal muscle fatty acid oxidation: an overview. Acta Physiol 2008; 194: 293–309.

Holloway GP, Bonen A, Spriet LL. Regulation of skeletal muscle mitochondrial fatty acid metabolism in lean and obese individuals. Am J Clin Nutr 2009; 89 (Suppl): 455S–462S.

Hoppeler H, Vogt M, Weibel ER, Fluck M. Response of skeletal muscle mitochondria to hypoxia. Exp Physiol 2003; 88: 109–119.

Jeukendrup AE. Regulation of fat metabolism in skeletal muscle. Ann NY Acad Sci 2002; 967: 217–235.

Jeukendrup AE. Modulation of carbohydrate and fat utilization by diet, exercise and environment. Biochem Soc Trans 2003; 31: 1270–1273.

Margaritis I, Rousseau AS. Does physical exercise modify antioxidant requirements? Nutr Res Rev 2008; 21: 3–12.

Martin WH. Effects of acute and chronic exercise on fat metabolism. Exerc Sports Sci Rev 1996; 24: 203–232.

Maughan RJ, Gleeson M. The Biochemical Basis of Sports Performance. Oxford: Oxford University Press, 2004.

Newsholme EA, Leech AR. Biochemistry for the Medical Sciences. Chichester: Wiley, 1992.

Nimmo M. Exercise in the cold. J Sports Sci 2004; 22: 898–916.

Rasmussen BB, Wolfe RR. Regulation of fatty acid oxidation in skeletal muscle. Annu Rev Nutr 1999; 19: 463–484.

Ren JM, Hultman E. Regulation of phosphorylase *a* activity in human skeletal muscle. J Appl Physiol 1990; 69: 919–923.

Romijn JA, Coyle EF, Sidossis LS *et al.* Regulation of endogenous fat and carbohydrate metabolism in relation to exercise intensity and duration. Am J Physiol 1993; 265: E380–E391.

Rusko H, Tikkanen H, Peltonen J. Altitude and endurance training. J Sports Sci 2004; 22: 928–945.

Salway JG. Metabolism at a Glance. Oxford: Blackwell Science, 1994.

Schwenk RW, Holloway GP, Luiken JJFP, Bonen A, Glatz JFC. Fatty acid transport across the cell membrane: regulation by fatty acid transporters. Prostaglandins Leukot Essent Fatty Acids 2010; 82: 149–154.

4
Carbohydrate

Asker Jeukendrup and Clyde Williams

Key messages

- Carbohydrate is stored as polymers of glucose, in plants as starch and in animal tissue as glycogen.
- Carbohydrates are classified according to their glycaemic responses, i.e. high glycaemic index (HGI) and low glycaemic index (LGI) carbohydrates.
- HGI carbohydrates are characterised by a rapid large rise in blood glucose after ingestion, whereas LGI carbohydrates are characterised by a low and even slow rise in blood glucose concentration after ingestion.
- The degradation of muscle glycogen (i.e. glycogenolysis) occurs along two major biochemical pathways: anaerobic metabolism, which occurs on the surface of the mitochondria; and aerobic metabolism, which occurs inside the mitochondria via the tricarboxylic acid (TCA) cycle.
- Carbohydrate is stored mainly in the liver and in skeletal muscles but in limited amounts when compared with the fat stores of the body.
- Fatigue during prolonged exercise is associated with the depletion of muscle glycogen stores.

- Dietary carbohydrate loading in the days before prolonged exercise increases muscle glycogen concentrations and generally results in an increase in endurance capacity.
- Muscle and liver glycogen re-synthesis can be accelerated by consuming a carbohydrate-rich diet immediately after exercise.
- Post-exercise glycogen re-synthesis begins immediately after exercise following contraction-induced activation of GLUT4 glucose transport proteins from their storage vesicles within the sarcoplasm of muscle and activation of the enzyme glycogen synthase.
- Post-exercise muscle glycogen re-synthesis is also accelerated in the presence of insulin, which indirectly results in the GLUT4 transporter proteins remaining active in glucose transport for longer than when insulin is absent.
- Muscle glycogen stores can be replenished within 24 hours when carbohydrate intake is equivalent to approximately 10 g/kg.

4.1 Introduction

Nutrition plays an essential role in the preparation for, participation in and recovery from sport and exercise. Most athletes train more than they compete and so it is important that they adopt nutritional strategies that support training and recovery and avoid dietary practices that might compromise their health. The main fuel during heavy exercise is carbohydrate, which is stored in skeletal muscles and in the liver as glycogen. It is a limited store that when depleted leads to fatigue and so it is not surprising that dietary methods to rapidly replace the glycogen stores has been the focus of much research. Increasing the glycogen stores in the days leading up to endurance

competition by consuming a high-carbohydrate diet improves endurance capacity by delaying the onset of fatigue. Even high-carbohydrate breakfasts will increase glycogen stores and improve endurance capacity during prolonged exercise. Ingesting a carbohydrate–electrolyte solution during prolonged exercise will contribute to carbohydrate metabolism and help delay severe dehydration. Athletes who avoid eating before exercise will benefit more from drinking a carbohydrate–electrolyte solution during exercise than from drinking water alone. Successful recovery from exercise, especially training, is important because it allows the athlete to sustain a consistent training programme. Of the three elements in any training programme, i.e. intensity, duration

---

Sport and Exercise Nutrition, First Edition. Edited by Susan A Lanham-New, Samantha J Stear, Susan M Shirreffs and Adam L Collins.
© 2011 The Nutrition Society. Published 2011 by Blackwell Publishing Ltd.

and frequency, it is frequency of training that results in the optimum adaptation. To be able to cope with high-intensity training each day athletes should try to replenish their glycogen stores during their recovery period. Muscle glycogen re-synthesis is most rapid during the immediate post-exercise period and so consuming carbohydrate immediately after exercise and then eating high-carbohydrate meals later in the day is the most effective recovery strategy. Many athletes train or compete twice a day and so the recovery period may be only a few hours.

4.2 Carbohydrate metabolism

Carbohydrate has been the main focus in the study of exercise nutrition and performance in the last century because carbohydrate is an essential nutrient and substrate for almost all metabolic processes. It is a relatively small store and yet it is essential for energy metabolism especially during heavy exercise because fatigue is associated with depletion of the carbohydrate stores in skeletal muscles. Carbohydrate is stored in the body in the form of glycogen in muscle and liver. Carbohydrates can provide more energy per unit of time than fats. This is why with increasing exercise intensity carbohydrate will become more and more important at the expense of fats. At low to moderate exercise intensities, most of the energy can be obtained from oxidative phosphorylation of acetyl-CoA derived from both carbohydrate and fat. As exercise intensity increases to high levels, the energy requirements cannot be met by only the oxidation of carbohydrate and fat. Carbohydrates can be used both aerobically and anaerobically. At very high intensities glycogen is rapidly broken down to pyruvate and lactate to provide energy to the working muscles.

Muscle glycogen

Glycogen is described in terms of the number of 'glucose or glucosyl units' that make up the polymer. When considering the literature values for muscle glycogen concentrations, as well as the glycolytic intermediates, it is helpful to be aware that values are reported as either wet weight (/kg w.w.) or dry weight (/kg d.w.). To obtain dry weight values, muscle samples are freeze dried before analysis. Freeze-dried muscle samples are easier to handle and analyse than

fresh samples because the process concentrates the substrate and metabolite content. In order to convert wet weight to dry weight concentrations simply multiply the wet weight value by 4.3 because the water content of human muscle is approximately 77%. The normal concentration is within the range 60–150 mmol glucosyl units/kg ww or 250–650 mmol glucosyl units/kg dw. Bearing in mind that muscle makes up about 40% of the body mass of an adult, then the total glycogen concentration is equivalent to about 550 g. Glycogen in both muscle and liver is stored with about 3 g water for every gram of glycogen. Therefore, after a period of carbohydrate loading the additional weight gain will not be entirely due to the enlarged glycogen stores but by the consequence of the presence of the additional water. As is well known, one of the advantages of glycogen as a fuel for exercise is that it can be degraded to provide energy by aerobic and anaerobic processes.

Liver glycogen

The size of the store of glycogen in the liver depends on the nutritional state of the individual. For example, in the fed state the adult liver weighs about 1.5 kg and contains approximately 80–110 g of glycogen, whereas after an overnight fast the concentration of glycogen can fall to below 20 g. Weight for weight the liver contains more glycogen than does skeletal muscle but of course there is a greater amount of skeletal muscle in the body than there is liver. Prolonged fasting may compromise the function of the brain by failing to maintain an adequate supply of blood glucose for cerebral metabolism (see below). In an attempt to maintain the supply of glucose to the blood, the liver is able to manufacture glucose from the breakdown products of carbohydrate, fat and protein metabolism. This process is called gluconeogenesis and uses metabolites such as lactate, glycerol and amino acids such as alanine to produce glucose in the liver.

Blood glucose

Liver glycogen is the reservoir from which glucose is released to maintain normal blood glucose concentrations within a fairly narrow range (4–5 mmol/l). Therefore, there is about 4–5 g of glucose within the systemic circulation. It is under the control of the hormone glucagon, which is released from the α cells of the islets of Langerhans in the pancreas when blood glucose concentrations fall. The brain, the central nervous system, blood cells and kidneys use about 75% of the available blood glucose in resting individuals. The brain and central nervous system use glucose at a rate of about 0.1 g/min, i.e. approximately 120–140 g/day; however, a fall in blood glucose concentrations to below 3 mmol/l (i.e. hypoglycaemia) may cause headaches, dizziness and feelings of weakness.

The uptake of glucose into muscle cells and adipose tissue is under hormonal control. Insulin is released from the β cells of the islets of Langerhans in response to an increase in the concentration of blood glucose. Insulin controls the uptake of glucose into adipose tissue and into muscle cells mainly during the postprandial period that follows a meal. During exercise the release of insulin is suppressed by an increase in the concentrations of the hormones noradrenaline and adrenaline, collectively called catecholamines. Even during low-intensity exercise there is an increase in noradrenaline as a result of an outflow of this neurotransmitter from the sympathetic nerve endings, whereas adrenaline release from the adrenal medulla occurs at higher exercise intensities. The inhibition of insulin secretion during exercise may be regarded as a safety mechanism that protects us from a life-threatening fall in blood glucose concentration (hypoglycaemia). For example, during prolonged submaximal exercise carbohydrate metabolism can be sustained at a rate of 2.5–3.0 g/min to the point where glycogen concentrations fall to very low values and exercise intensity cannot be maintained. If skeletal muscle had free access to blood glucose under these conditions, then there would be a rapid onset of hypoglycaemia as muscle 'soaked up' the relatively small amount of circulating glucose. One of the many metabolic adaptations to endurance training is a reduction in the contribution of blood glucose to muscle metabolism during submaximal exercise.

4.3 Dietary carbohydrate

Glycogen stores are important and depletion of these stores needs to be prevented in order to reduce fatigue. This can be done by making sure stores are optimal at the start of exercise by carbo-loading in the days before an event, by eating a carbohydrate-rich meal

(breakfast) 3–4 hours before the event and by topping up carbohydrates during a prolonged event. There are many good sources of carbohydrate, but bread, cereals, potatoes, pasta, rice, vegetables and sugars (sports drinks, gels and energy bars) are examples of popular carbohydrate-containing foods. The classification of carbohydrate foods as simple and complex was largely based on their fibre content. High-fibre carbohydrates were classified as complex whereas foods with low fibre content that contain a significant proportion of simple sugars such as glucose and fructose were described as simple carbohydrates. The common assumption was that after consuming simple, rather than complex, carbohydrates, blood glucose rises rapidly. However, this is not the case with all simple carbohydrates or, indeed, with all complex carbohydrates.

A more informative way of defining carbohydrates is one that describes the degree to which they raise blood glucose concentrations. Carbohydrates which produce a large increase in blood glucose concentration are classified as having a high glycaemic index (HGI). The glycaemic index is determined by comparing the area under a glucose–time curve following ingestion of 50 g of carbohydrate in a food. The reference value of 100 is assigned to the changes in blood glucose concentration following the ingestion of 50 g of glucose. Examples of HGI carbohydrates include white bread, rice, sweet corn and potatoes, whereas low glycaemic index (LGI) carbohydrates include apples, dates, peaches, fructose, and milk ice-cream. Fructose is a simple sugar but has a glycaemic index of less than 60. There is a clear difference between blood glucose concentrations following the consumption of the same amount of individual HGI and LGI carbohydrate foods. However, this difference is not so marked when HGI and LGI carbohydrates are part of mixed meals. Nevertheless, the glycaemic index provides additional information about a carbohydrate that may be useful when designing diets to deliver glucose rapidly to working muscles or to optimise fat metabolism.

4.4 Carbohydrate nutrition and performance

The close association between the depletion of muscle glycogen stores and fatigue during prolonged exercise (constant or intermittent) is well known. Therefore, it is not surprising that different nutritional strategies have been adopted to rapidly restore and/or increase muscle glycogen stores before exercise. These strategies are outlined along with examples of the evidence that supports their adoption.

Carbohydrate loading before exercise

It is well established that if the diet after prolonged heavy exercise is rich in carbohydrate, then supra-normal muscle glycogen stores may be achieved. Therefore, nutritional strategies have been developed to take advantage of this super-compensatory response of glycogen-depleted muscle to carbohydrate intake. The traditional method of increasing muscle and liver glycogen stores after prolonged cycling to exhaustion is to eat a diet low in carbohydrate for the first 3 days of recovery and then switch to a high-carbohydrate diet for the next 3 days. Classic Scandinavian studies in the 1960s demonstrated the link between increased muscle glycogen concentration following carbohydrate loading and improvement in exercise capacity. These pioneering studies produced the classic 7-day model of carbohydrate loading. This model consists of a 3–4 day 'depletion' phase of hard training and low carbohydrate intake, finishing with a 3–4 day 'loading' phase of high carbohydrate eating and exercise taper (i.e. decreased amounts of training). Early field studies of prolonged running events showed that carbohydrate loading enhanced sports performance, not necessarily by allowing the athlete to run faster, but by prolonging the time that race pace could be maintained.

Although this classic carbohydrate-loading pro-tocol is effective, there are also several disadvantages of this super-compensation protocol: athletes felt very fatigued after the low carbohydrate intake up to 4 days before competition, the high-fat low-carbohydrate diet that was consumed often caused gastrointestinal problems, and athletes did not like abstaining from training. A solution to these downsides came in the form of a 'modified' carbohydrate-loading strategy. The muscle of well-trained athletes has been found to be able to super-compensate its glycogen stores without a prior depletion or 'glycogen stripping' phase. For well-trained athletes at least, carbohydrate loading may be seen as an extension of 'fuelling up', involving rest/taper and high-carbohydrate intake over 3–7 days. The modified carbohydrate-loading protocol offers a more practical strategy for competition preparation, by avoiding the fatigue and complexity of the extreme diet and training protocols associated with the previous depletion phase. Typically, carbo-hydrate loading will postpone fatigue and extend the duration of steady-state exercise by about 20%, and improve performance over a set distance or workload by 2–3%.

Athletes are eager to continue training while carbohydrate loading but are concerned that this might delay restoration of their muscle glycogen stores. There does appear to be some slowing of glycogen re-synthesis during the first hour of recovery even while performing low-intensity exercise (40–50% Vo_{2max}) compared with passive recovery. However, more recent research suggests that daily 20-min sessions of light exercise (~65% Vo_{2max}) do not limit the super-compensation process; very high glycogen concentrations were found in trained individuals training for 2 hours daily at moderate intensities whilst consuming a very high carbohydrate diet.

Pre-exercise carbohydrate intake and performance

Carbohydrate consumed in the 3–4 hours before submaximal exercise of prescribed intensity usually results in an increase in endurance capacity. Early studies showed that although small amounts of carbohydrate (46 and 156 g) consumed 4 hours before intermittent cycling improved endurance capacity, a larger amount of carbohydrate (312 g) was even more effective. After consuming the larger amount of carbohydrate the exercise capacity was 15% greater (56 min) than after the water placebo (48 min). Carbohydrate intake in the 3–4 hours before prolonged exercise is especially effective if no carbohydrate can be ingested during exercise. Several competition situations may make it difficult to consume carbohydrate during exercise so a good carbohydrate meal 3–4 hours before would be important in those situations.

The ingestion of carbohydrates with different glycaemic indices will produce markedly different changes in plasma glucose and insulin concentrations. Three hours after a pre-exercise meal containing HGI carbohydrates there is suppression of fat oxidation during 60 min of submaximal treadmill running compared with a meal containing LGI carbohydrates. A greater rate of fat oxidation and lower rate of carbohydrate oxidation are conditions that would generally lead to improvement in endurance exercise capacity. Whether or not the improved endurance capacity is a consequence of sparing the limited glycogen stores in both the liver and skeletal muscle or simply in skeletal muscles has yet to be established. A pre-exercise meal of LGI carbohydrate results in a higher rate of fat oxidation because the insulin-suppressed mobilisation of fatty acids is not as great as after an HGI carbohydrate meal. Therefore the benefits of pre-exercise meals of LGI carbohydrate are probably more evident during prolonged low-intensity exercise than during high-intensity exercise.

Even when an HGI meal is consumed 3 hours before exercise not all the carbohydrate has been digested and absorbed. An HGI carbohydrate, which should deliver carbohydrate rapidly, only increases muscle glycogen by 10–15% in 3 hours (with an LGI carbohydrate meal, glycogen may not change at all). These small changes in muscle glycogen concentrations suggest that performing exercise 3 hours after a large carbohydrate meal may allow insufficient time for complete digestion and absorption of the meal. Of course, some of the carbohydrate will have been stored in the liver and so may contribute to muscle metabolism during exercise but even so 3 hours is insufficient time for the complete dispersal of ingested carbohydrate to the liver and skeletal muscles.

In summary, carbohydrate consumed in the 3–4 hours prior to an event may help to achieve the following sports nutrition goals:

- to continue to fill muscle glycogen stores if they have not fully restored or loaded since the last exercise session;
- to restore liver glycogen levels, especially for events undertaken in the morning where liver stores are depleted from an overnight fast;
- to prevent hunger (yet avoid gastrointestinal discomfort and upset during exercise);
- to improve endurance capacity during prolonged exercise.

Carbohydrate within the hour before exercise and performance

Early studies on the influence of ingesting carbohydrate within the hour before exercise suggested that this practice would reduce performance. These studies showed that there was a greater rate of glycogen degradation during exercise after ingesting a concentrated carbohydrate solution and in one study fatigue occurred sooner (19%) during cycling to exhaustion at 80% Vo_{2max}. These early studies also showed a sharp peak in blood glucose concentrations following the ingestion of the concentrated glucose solution and then a rapid fall at the onset of exercise. This phenomenon is frequently observed and is called reactive or rebound hypoglycaemia. The carbohydrate ingested before exercise causes a rise in insulin that increases glucose transport into various tissues. When exercise is started glucose uptake increases even more and the combination of insulin and contraction-mediated glucose uptake causes a rapid disappearance of glucose from the circulation. The blood glucose concentration can drop to very low levels and this hypoglycaemia was said to be responsible for the decrease in performance. However, the highly publicised recommendation of not consuming carbohydrate in the hour before exercise has not been supported by (more than 100) subsequent studies. The vast majority of studies showed that there may be metabolic effects (i.e. reduction of fat oxidation) and in some cases hypoglycaemia may occur but this did not affect performance. For most individuals the transient fall in blood glucose concentrations during the first few minutes of exercise goes unnoticed and has no influence on subsequent exercise capacity.

Whether or not individuals develop hypoglycaemia is not easy to predict but such individuals are usually aware of this and have already adopted nutrition strategies to prevent this. Such strategies could include ingesting LGI carbohydrates (such as fructose) or ingesting the carbohydrate in the last 5 min before exercise or during warm-up. Both strategies will prevent a rise in insulin and thus prevent reactive hypoglycaemia. However, as mentioned above, even when hypoglycaemia does occur this does not necessarily affect performance.

Carbohydrate intake during exercise and performance

Submaximal exercise

The ergogenic effects of consuming carbohydrate during prolonged exercise are well known. Starting in the 1920s, these effects have been extensively studied. The vast majority of studies showed the benefits of ingesting carbohydrate solutions during prolonged cycling (>2 hours) but running studies have demonstrated similar positive effects. The proposed mechanisms are maintenance of blood glucose concentration and maintenance of high rates of carbohydrate oxidation, especially late in exercise when endogenous carbohydrate sources are running low. Most studies have not seen an effect of carbohydrate intake on muscle glycogen use but there are a few studies, especially in runners, that have demonstrated a modest muscle glycogen-sparing effect.

An examination of relationship between the amount of carbohydrate ingested and the amount oxidised during prolonged submaximal exercise suggests that the maximum rate achieved is around 1 g/min (60 g/hour). The ingestion of ever greater quantities of carbohydrate did not lead to a further increase in carbohydrate oxidation during exercise. The limitation may not be gastric emptying of the ingested carbohydrate but absorption across the intestinal wall of the gut. Therefore, the optimal amount of exogenous carbohydrate that will achieve the maximum oxidation rate is around 70 g/hour. Accompanying the increased rate of oxidation of the exogenous carbohydrate is an almost complete reduction in hepatic glucose output. Thus the ingestion of carbohydrate during exercise has a glycogen-sparing effect on the liver because the exogenous carbohydrate appears to be oxidised before the endogenous stores. Late in exercise, when muscle glycogen concentrations are low, the uptake of blood glucose into muscle contributes to the high rates of carbohydrate oxidation.

More recently it was discovered that the limitation in absorption can be overcome by ingesting a blend of two carbohydrates that use different intestinal transporters for absorption. For example, glucose uses the sodium-dependent glucose transporter SGLT1. It is though that this transporter becomes saturated when large amounts of glucose are ingested. When fructose is ingested simultaneously this can increase total carbohydrate absorption because fructose uses a different transporter (GLUT5).

By using mixtures of glucose and fructose, more carbohydrate can be absorbed and utilised by the exercising muscle. This will only work when the glucose transporter is saturated and therefore high rates of carbohydrate ingestion are needed. It has been demonstrated that exogenous carbohydrate oxidation can be increased to levels of 1.75 g/min (75% more than was previously thought to be the maximum)

when large amounts of carbohydrate are ingested. Such amounts may not be practical in real life and therefore the advice is to ingest 90 g/hour of mixed carbohydrates (60 g/hour glucose plus 30 g/hour fructose). This may become important during very prolonged endurance events of 3 hours or more. It has also been demonstrated that mixtures of glucose and fructose can improve fluid delivery compared with a glucose-only solution and it can improve exercise performance over and above the effects of a single carbohydrate. In one study subjects exercised for 2 hours while ingesting glucose or glucose + fructose at a rate of 90 g/hour and then performed a time trial (approximately 1 hour). The time trial performance was improved with glucose (9% compared with placebo) and was further improved with glucose + fructose (8% better than glucose, 17% better than placebo).

Most of the studies that have shown a benefit from drinking a carbohydrate solution during prolonged exercise have used prolonged exercise to exhaustion. Even in the relatively few time trial studies the exercise duration has usually been greater than 1 hour because under these conditions muscle glycogen is severely reduced and so the benefits of drinking a carbohydrate solution are more clearly demonstrated. However, there are several time-trial studies of shorter duration (≤1 hour) that have reported improvements in performance after ingesting a carbohydrate solution when compared with a placebo solution. This is intriguing because only a small fraction of the ingested carbohydrate would have been oxidised.

In a series of studies it was demonstrated that the same performance benefits could be obtained by a carbohydrate mouth rinse where the carbohydrate is not ingested but expelled. This led to the suggestion that there must be carbohydrate receptors in the mouth that are connected to higher centres in the brain. Indeed brain imaging studies confirmed that such connections exist, as different activations patterns were seen with carbohydrate mouth rinses compared with a placebo mouth rinse. It appears that such effects are especially obvious when these studies are performed in the fasted state and the effects are less clear when a large breakfast has been ingested prior to exercise. Collectively these results suggest that there is a link between carbohydrate receptors in the oral cavity and the brain. It appears that even the promise of carbohydrate (i.e. only in the oral cavity) is enough to 'allow' athletes to select higher work rates.

Multiple-sprint exercise

Even during brief periods of maximal exercise, muscle glycogen makes a significant contribution to ATP production. Some studies have also examined the benefit of ingesting carbohydrate–electrolyte solutions during prolonged intermittent high-intensity running in an attempt to assess the applicability to sports such as football, rugby and hockey. For several of these studies the shuttle running test (LIST) was used, which requires participants to repeatedly run, walk, jog and sprint between two lines 20 m apart in 15-min blocks of activity with 3 min recovery between each block. When continued for the full 90 min the participants cover about 12 km during which they perform 66 maximum sprints and expend in total about 1300 kcal. These distances covered and energy expended are similar to those reported for mid-field players in professional football.

In one study a group of recreational football players completed five blocks of the LIST before undertaking an endurance test. This test required the subjects to continue sprinting and jogging back and forth over the 20-m course to the point of fatigue. It was demonstrated that the players could cover more distance towards the end after drinking a carbohydrate solution. In several studies it was confirmed that the distance covered was greater when the football players drank a carbohydrate solution than when they drank a flavoured placebo solution. It was also demonstrated that these effects may even be present when muscle glycogen concentrations at the start of exercise are high. Other studies have also demonstrated benefits in terms of skill and agility. Both skill and agility tend to decrease as players become fatigued and carbohydrate ingestion seems to prevent this decline compared with placebo.

The mechanisms are still incompletely understood but the majority of studies in high-intensity intermittent exercise have shown that carbohydrate feeding can reduce muscle glycogen breakdown (or stimulate glycogen synthesis between high-intensity bouts). In many sports the practical problems of ingesting carbohydrate during a game often prevent this practice from being commonly applied.

4.5 Post exercise, recovery and glycogen synthesis

It is essential that athletes who train hard and compete regularly recover quickly from training and competition. Recovery from exercise depends on the nature of the exercise, its intensity and duration, and the time between training sessions. Successful recovery involves the completion of several essential physiological and metabolic processes that act in concert to prepare the athlete for the next bout of exercise. These include rehydration, restoration of carbohydrate stores and adequate rest.

Glycogen re-synthesis

The process of glycogen re-synthesis begins immediately after exercise and is most rapid during the first hours of recovery. The uptake of glucose into the muscle takes place through specific glucose transporter proteins called GLUT4. These glucose transporters are normally stored in vesicles in the sarcoplasm of the muscle fibres. As a consequence of contractile activity and a reduction in glycogen concentration they translocate to the cell membrane where they transport glucose into the muscle cell (Figure 4.1). After exercise they slowly return to the vesicles but for the first hours after exercise there is still an increased number of GLUT4 at the cell membrane and this helps glycogen restoration. The enzyme responsible for glycogen re-synthesis is glycogen synthase, which is activated mainly as a consequence of a reduction in glycogen stores.

Thus the GLUT4 transporter proteins and glycogen synthase are probably the two most important components in the glycogen re-synthesis process. The size of the subsequent glycogen store also appears to limit further re-synthesis, i.e. there is evidence of autoregulation. In addition to the fundamental influence of muscle contraction *per se* on glucose transport and glycogen re-synthesis, the presence of insulin also makes a significant contribution to this process. Insulin contributes to glycogen re-synthesis by extending the time that GLUT4 transporters are at the cell membrane and by stimulating the translocation of more transporters from a different storage site. Thus the glycogen re-synthesis process occurs in two parts. First there is the non-insulin re-synthesis period that lasts for about an hour and is the result of muscle

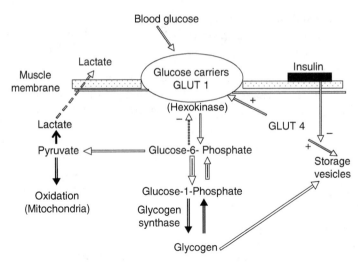

Figure 4.1 Diagram outlining the mechanisms responsible for the transport of glucose into muscle during recovery from exercise and the formation of glycogen. (Reprinted from MacLaren, 2007, p. 53, © 2007 with permission from Churchill Livingstone, Elsevier.)

contractions *per se*. The second part is a consequence of the action of insulin and this period of glycogen re-synthesis can last many hours into the recovery period. The activities of the GLUT4 transporters and glycogen synthase are increased with endurance training and decrease during a period of inactivity.

Diet and glycogen re-synthesis

The early studies on post-exercise glycogen re-synthesis recommended that the optimum amount of carbohydrate is about 1–1.5 g/kg, consumed immediately after exercise and at 2-hour intervals until the next meal. Elevated post-exercise insulin concentrations play an essential role in promoting high rates of glycogen re-synthesis. Adding protein and some amino acids to carbohydrate generally results in an increase in insulin concentrations to values that are higher than those achieved with an equal amount of carbohydrate. Some studies have suggested that consuming a carbohydrate–protein mixture immediately after exercise can increase the rate of post-exercise muscle glycogen re-synthesis beyond that which occurs with carbohydrate alone. However, in these studies the test drinks were never isocaloric and when the protein was replaced with carbohydrate, glycogen synthesis was no different or even better with carbohydrate only.

In summary, the most important factors for rapid glycogen re-synthesis after exercise seem to be the amount of carbohydrate ingested, the type of carbohydrate (HGI) and the frequency of ingestion. It is often recommended to take the carbohydrate at 30-min intervals as this seems to be more effective than larger but less regular meals. Consuming carbohydrate at a rate of 0.6 g/kg every 30 min during a 4-hour recovery period results in a maximum rate of glycogen re-synthesis of approximately 45 mmol/kg/hour. However, smaller amounts might be advisable because athletes may experience intolerable abdominal discomfort during subsequent exercise.

Muscle glycogen during training periods

Several studies have explored what is the optimum amount of carbohydrate for athletes who undertake daily training. Most studies have demonstrated that when daily exercise training is performed with a low to moderate carbohydrate diet, muscle glycogen concentrations may gradually decline. With a high-carbohydrate diet this decline may at least partly be prevented. Although very few studies have addressed this question, after several weeks of training performance appears to be better after high rather than low to moderate carbohydrate diets. Also, when training is increased dramatically (such as would be the case in training camps) and symptoms of over-reaching (over-training) are likely to develop, this may have an even greater impact. The symptoms of over-training (e.g. drop in performance, reduced mood state, sleep disturbances) can be reduced with a diet that is very high in carbohydrate (9–10 g/kg daily) compared with a normal/high carbohydrate diet (7 g/kg daily). It is always important to consider the total energy expenditure when adopting these recommendations. Carbohydrate recommendations of 9–10 g/kg daily, or even higher, are meant for athletes with very high energy expenditures of at least 5000 kcal/day. If this is applied to athletes with lower energy expenditure, it is likely that weight gain would be the result.

Recovery of performance within 24 hours

Consuming a high-carbohydrate diet during the 24 hours after prolonged heavy exercise or even without heavy exercise restores muscle glycogen concentrations to normal pre-exercise values in trained individuals. However, when athletes are allowed to eat ad libitum for 24 hours after exercise they tend to choose an intake that is insufficient to restore their muscle glycogen concentrations. Therefore, to ensure recovery within 24 hours it is essential that the amount of carbohydrate that athletes consume during the recovery period is prescribed for them and not left to their own promptings of hunger and satiety. One of the key questions is whether eating a high-carbohydrate diet that restores muscle glycogen will also restore performance? Unfortunately, there are only a few studies that have addressed this question. In one study there was successful recovery of endurance running capacity 22 hours after prolonged exercise when the runners ate a high-carbohydrate diet. The authors found that when their subjects ran for 90 min or to fatigue (whichever occurred first) on treadmill at 70% Vo_{2max} and were then fed either a diet high in carbohydrate (9 g/kg) or an isocaloric mixed diet (6 g/kg carbohydrate) during a 22-hour recovery, only those runners on the high-carbohydrate diet were able to match their previous day's run time of 90 min. Those runners who consumed the mixed diet could only manage to complete 78% of their previous day's exercise, even though their recovery diet contained their normal carbohydrate intake and the same total energy as the carbohydrate recovery diet.

The type of carbohydrate consumed during recovery may also have an influence on the rate of muscle glycogen re-synthesis and subsequent performance. Muscle glycogen re-synthesis after a 24-hour recovery from prolonged exercise was greater when subjects consumed an HGI rather than an LGI carbohydrate recovery diet. In another study this more complete

glycogen restoration resulted in a treadmill run time to exhaustion that was 12 min longer after the LGI rather than the HGI recovery. It is also interesting to note that the runners reported that they never felt hungry on the LGI diet even after the overnight fast prior to the run to exhaustion on the second day of the trial. This was not the case when they consumed the HGI recovery diet that was matched for energy and macronutrient composition with the LGI recovery diet. Therefore, it may be more effective to consume HGI carbohydrates for the first few hours after exercise and then consume LGI carbohydrate meals for the remainder of the recovery period. In this way the HGI carbohydrate will contribute quickly absorbed substrate during the most rapid period of glycogen re-synthesis and the LGI carbohydrates will provide high satiety.

These conclusions also translate to multiple-sprint or 'stop–go' sports such as football, field and ice hockey, rugby, tennis and basketball. The prolonged intermittent high-intensity exercise that is part of these sports reduces muscle glycogen stores and impairs performance as is the case in constant pace exercise. For example, the muscle glycogen concentrations of professional football players are severely reduced after 90 min of match play. It is well established that those players who begin play with modest or low glycogen concentrations cannot fully engage in the game because of the early onset of fatigue. In a study on nutrition and football-specific fitness it was demonstrated that when players consumed a high-carbohydrate diet for 48 hours before a series of football-specific tests, their endurance capacity during prolonged intermittent high-intensity treadmill running was significantly better than when a normal mixed diet was consumed.

Performance following short recovery periods

It is quite common for athletes to train twice a day with as little as 4–5 hours recovery between training sessions. In some sports athletes have to compete more than once a day and so optimal recovery is even more important than recovery between training sessions. After training or competition there will be a real need to rehydrate and to begin to replace some of the carbohydrate stores before the next session. Consuming carbohydrate beverages immediately after exercise will accelerate muscle glycogen re-synthesis during a recovery as short as 4 hours. However, even though there is solid evidence to support the benefits of drinking a carbohydrate solution immediately after exercise, there is relatively little information on the impact of this recommendation on subsequent exercise performance. In one study subjects ran on a treadmill at 70% Vo_{2max} for 90 min or to fatigue (whichever occurred first) and then were allocated to either the placebo or the carbohydrate group. The carbohydrate group ingested a carbohydrate solution that provided the equivalent of 1 g/kg of carbohydrate immediately after exercise and then again 2 hours later. The placebo group drank the same volume of flavoured coloured water at the same times as the carbohydrate group. After the 4-hour recovery, both groups ran to exhaustion at the same treadmill speeds as on the first occasion. The group that ingested the sports beverage were able to run for 20 min longer than the group who ingested the flavoured placebo solution. Even following the simple recommendation to consume about 50 g of carbohydrate immediately after exercise results in greater endurance capacity during subsequent exercise compared with consuming only water during a 4-hour recovery period.

However, ingesting a greater amount of carbohydrate immediately after exercise may not result in expected further improvements in endurance capacity during subsequent exercise. There was no difference in running time to exhaustion when runners consumed 175 g of carbohydrate or 50 g of carbohydrate during the 4-hour recovery, even though carbohydrate ingested post-exercise resulted in increased muscle glycogen concentrations after 4 hours of recovery when the runners ingested the larger amount of carbohydrate. These results are paradoxical because it would be reasonable to expect an improved exercise capacity following short-term recovery during which more carbohydrate was consumed. Possible explanations include rate-limited uptake of glucose during the recovery period and insulin-induced reduction in the availability and oxidation of fatty acids. The consumption of carbohydrate may have been sufficient to depress fat oxidation but insufficient to make up the deficit in substrate provision and so overall there was no net gain in endurance capacity.

There have been suggestions that adding protein to a carbohydrate recovery drink is of benefit as clear effects on insulin and increases in glycogen synthesis can be observed when protein is added to carbohydrate. However, studies show no difference in muscle glycogen re-synthesis rates after ingestion of carbohydrate–protein mixtures and the energy-matched carbohydrate solution or any differences in performance. Some studies report that the degree of muscle soreness experienced by their subjects is less after ingesting a carbohydrate–protein solution than after ingesting carbohydrate alone. It is difficult to offer a rational explanation for these observations in the absence of further information. At the moment it is unclear what the mechanism for the reduced soreness would be, but it will have nothing to do with protein synthesis and repair of muscle damage as this is a process that takes much longer than just a few hours.

4.6 Summary

The daily carbohydrate intake should be adjusted according to the intensity and duration of the training programme and the time available for recovery. For example, a daily carbohydrate intake of 5–7 g/kg is recommended for male athletes undertaking daily training of moderate intensity that lasts about an hour. For male endurance athletes who train for 3 hours daily or more, the recommendation is a daily carbohydrate intake of 7–10 g/kg. For rapid recovery of glycogen within a few hours it is important to ingest carbohydrate as soon as possible after exercise, the carbohydrate is best ingested at regular intervals (e.g. every 30 min), the carbohydrate should be HGI, and the amounts should equate to approximately 1.2 g/kg/hour. After the initial period LGI carbohydrates can be ingested. The amount of carbohydrate ingested has to be balanced with other macronutrients and energy balance should be maintained. Nevertheless, the consumption of an appropriate amount of carbohydrate immediately after exercise is not only essential for recovery of performance but it may also help in preventing a severe reduction in immunocompetence (see Chapter 21).

Further reading

Jeukendrup AE (ed.) Sports Nutrition: From Lab to Kitchen. Aachen: Meyer and Meyer Sport, 2010.
Jeukendrup AE, Gleeson M. Sport Nutrition. Champaign, IL: Human Kinetics, 2010.
Maclaren D (ed.) Nutrition and Sport. London: Churchill Livingstone, 2007.
Maughan R (ed.) Nutrition in Sport. Oxford: Blackwell Science, 2000.

5
Protein and Amino Acids

Peter WR Lemon

Key messages

- Amino acids are the component parts of protein and all are needed to produce body proteins. Some foods (especially vegetable sources) lack or contain insufficient quantities of at least one amino acid.
- The Protein Digestibility Corrected Amino Acid Score is a method of rating a food based on the adequacy of its amino acid content relative to human needs.
- Traditionally, dietary requirements are based on growth studies in animals or balance studies in animals or humans and more recently with metabolic tracer experiments.
- Dietary recommendations contain a safety buffer (two standard deviations above the requirement) to ensure that everyone in the population is covered.

- Amino acid needs are likely increased for many athletes (about 50–100%), but for most it is easy to obtain these quantities assuming a variety of food sources are consumed with sufficient overall energy intake. One exception is female athletes who often under-eat relative to their energy expenditure.
- Timing of amino acid ingestion relative to training and/or competition, the type of protein used and associated macronutrient intake are likely more important issues for athletes.
- Small quantities of indispensable amino acids and carbohydrate shortly before, during, immediately following, and a few hours after exercise enhances subsequent performance by speeding recovery. Some foods are likely better than others because they facilitate both muscle glycogen and protein synthesis.

5.1 Introduction

Protein is found in every cell of living organisms and is needed for all life functions, including fighting infections, transporting oxygen, catalysing metabolic reactions, building/repairing body tissues, and contracting muscles. Amino acids are the components parts of protein and as such are necessary for life. There are some 20 amino acids in proteins and all are needed for the human body to make proteins (*protein synthesis*). Generally, eight of these (*indispensable* or *essential* amino acids; Table 5.1) are most important because humans cannot produce them at a sufficient rate from precursors normally available. Further, the pool in the body is quite small so they must all be consumed regularly (at least daily) or the ability to synthesise protein is affected adversely resulting in overall impaired function. For example, an athlete consuming a diet with insufficient amino acids could experience a loss of muscle tissue (due to reductions

in growth and/or impaired recovery/repair from exercise) as well as reduced muscle function (due to reductions in hormones, substrates, enzymes and/or co-factors involved in energy-producing metabolic pathways). Obviously, this would compromise athletic performance and eventually health.

Dietary requirements for the indispensable amino acids have been determined (FAO/WHO/UNU, 2007) (Table 5.1). In contrast, minimal dietary intake is not necessary for the dispensable (non-essential) amino acids because they can be synthesised from other available precursors. However, the number of indispensable amino acids is variable because some can be produced from others (e.g. tyrosine from phenylalanine) and a number of situations (likely including exercise) can affect requirements. Functionally, all amino acids are needed for protein synthesis and under certain circumstances some dispensable amino acids become indispensable. These particular amino acids are often

Sport and Exercise Nutrition, First Edition. Edited by Susan A Lanham-New, Samantha J Stear, Susan M Shirreffs and Adam L Collins.
© 2011 The Nutrition Society. Published 2011 by Blackwell Publishing Ltd.

Table 5.1 Indispensable (essential) amino acids.

Amino acid	Requirements (mg/kg/day)[a]
Isoleucine	20
Leucine	39
Lysine	30
Methionine (10.4) + cysteine[b] (4.1)	15 (total)
Phenylalanine + tyrosine[b]	25 (total)
Threonine	15
Tryptophan	4
Valine	26
Arginine[b]	
Glycine[b]	
Glutamine[b]	
Histidine[b]	10
Proline[b]	
Serine[b]	

[a] Requirements are ~10–20% greater for children and as much as 150% greater for infants under 1 year.
[b] Conditionally indispensable.
Source: FAO/WHO/UNU (2007).

Table 5.2 Complete and incomplete protein foods.

Protein source	Limiting amino acid
Egg	None
Meat	None
Fish	None
Dairy	None
Soy	Methionine
Corn	Lysine, tryptophan
Legumes	Tryptophan, methionine or cysteine
Rice	Lysine
Wheat	Lysine

Table 5.3 Protein quality.

Food	PDCAAS[a]
Casein (milk protein)	1.0
Whey (milk protein)	1.0
Egg	1.0
Soy protein	1.0
Beef	0.92
Soybeans	0.91
Fruits	0.76
Whole wheat	0.42

[a] The Protein Digestibility Corrected Amino Acid Score is the ratio of a food's indispensable amino acid content to requirements corrected for digestibility (a value of 1 is the highest and 0 is lowest).

called *conditionally indispensable* (Reeds, 2000; Fürst & Stehle, 2004).

Although the variability of amino acid requirements among individuals is unclear, based on similar measures for protein it is generally assumed that recommendations or safe intakes are about 24% greater than requirements (FAO/WHO/UNU, 2007). In practice, dietary recommendations may vary slightly from country to country because experimental data can be interpreted somewhat differently by the respective expert committees. Importantly, the human need for dietary protein is because of the need for amino acids as well as for the nitrogen protein contains, not for protein per se.

5.2 Complete protein foods

Some foods contain all indispensable amino acids in sufficient quantities for human needs. These are called *complete protein foods*. Examples include animal sources (poultry, fish, meat, eggs and dairy products). In general, plant sources lack one or more of the indispensable amino acids (called a 'limiting' amino acid) and as a result are termed *incomplete protein foods* (Table 5.2). This means that complete vegetarians (vegans) will have more difficulty obtaining sufficient indispensable amino acids, although this

can be overcome by consuming plant sources that together contain all the indispensable amino acids (*complementary protein foods*) (Craig & Mangels, 2009; Fuhrman & Ferreri, 2010); however, the mass of food necessary to match energy expenditure for vegans could become excessive for some athletes. Some plants are nearly complete protein sources (e.g. quinoa, hempseed and buckwheat) and some are fortified into complete proteins (e.g. soy protein).

Because of the importance of dietary protein for growth and development, several methods to estimate protein quality have been utilised over the years. Examples include biological value and protein efficiency ratio, but likely the most appropriate for human use is the Protein Digestibility Corrected Amino Acid Score because it assesses whether a food contains the indispensable amino acids and in sufficient quantities for humans taking into consideration digestibility losses (Table 5.3) (Schaafsma, 2000, 2005; FAO/WHO/UNU, 2007).

5.3 Dietary requirements versus dietary recommendations

Although often misunderstood, the distinction between these two is both simple and important. As one might expect, a *dietary requirement* is the quantity of a particular nutrient needed per day. Historically, for amino acids, this has been determined in two ways:

(1) as the amount of the nutrient necessary to support maximal growth, i.e. differing doses of individual amino acids are provided separately in an animal's diet until growth is maximal; or
(2) using the nutritional balance technique in humans or animals, in which the diet is manipulated and the requirement is determined as the nutrient intake where loss from the body (by all routes) equals nutrient intake.

Both of these techniques are problematic (Kopple, 1987; Bos *et al.*, 2000): the growth approach because animals (especially laboratory rodents) may have differing nutritional needs compared with humans due to variable growth rates; the balance technique because it is laborious and expensive but also because errors tend to overestimate intake and underestimate excretion resulting in erroneously positive balances. More recently, these traditional amino acid requirement data have been supplemented with metabolic tracer results reflecting information on oxidation and synthesis (Young *et al.*, 1989; Rennie, 1999; Wagenmakers, 1999). Basically, the intake where oxidation increases and synthesis plateaus is the requirement.

In contrast, a *dietary recommendation* is the requirement plus a safety margin (typically two standard deviations above the experimental sample mean) because this ensures that essentially all the population (97.5%) will avoid deficiency symptoms (FAO/WHO/UNU, 2007). This is a statistical approach, so that even those in the population with greater requirements than the sample mean still receive sufficient intake. In fact, because the majority of individuals fall at or below the mean, many will receive adequate intake of a particular nutrient as long as they consume at least 67% of the recommendation. This concept is poorly appreciated because many assume falsely that the recommended value is the requirement!

Finally, it is necessary to express requirements and recommendations in units per kilogram body mass (g/kg/day) rather than percent energy intake (%kcal or %kJ) for several reasons. First, and most importantly, because with the latter the quantity consumed depends on energy intake which itself can be quite variable. For example, a high macronutrient percentage of a low energy intake could be insufficient, while a low macronutrient percentage of a large energy intake could be adequate. This means that macronutrient intake expressed as percent energy is essentially worthless information. Second, when expressed relative to body mass, one recommendation applies to all individuals.

5.4 Protein needs for athletes

Athletes have believed for a very long time, perhaps going back as far as Ancient Greece, that large intakes of protein are necessary for optimal athletic performance. Regardless, modern nutritionists have largely downplayed the importance of this idea. In fact, dietary protein recommendations (~0.8 g/kg/day) in many countries are not adjusted in any way for individuals who exercise regularly, not even for those involved in rigorous daily sport training (FAO/WHO/UNU, 2007; US Department of Agriculture and US Department of Health and Human Services, 2010). However, the question of dietary recommendations for athletes has remained controversial for years (Lemon & Nagle, 1981; Lemon, 1987, 1998) and a definitive conclusion on this question still remains unclear for a variety of reasons, partly due to the limitations of available experimental techniques.

Briefly, there are data indicating that some types of regular exercise (both strength and endurance) increase dietary protein needs (perhaps by 50–100%) and that some athletes benefit from protein intakes in excess of daily recommendations but there are also conflicting experimental results (Lemon *et al.*, 1992; Tarnopolsky, 2004; Rodrigues *et al.*, 2009). Further, most scientific studies have focused on protein/amino acid requirements and not athletic performance measures, which of course is the athlete's primary interest. More data examining both of these areas, especially in elite athletes, are needed to settle this issue. Unfortunately, the question is complicated further because some

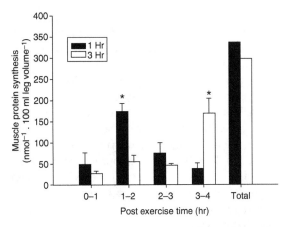

Figure 5.1 Muscle protein synthesis increases following the ingestion of an indispensable amino acid (IAA) + carbohydrate (CHO) drink (6 g IAA + 35 g CHO) ingested at either 1 hour (filled bars) or 3 hours (open bars) post exercise. Values are means ± SEM. Asterisks indicate significantly different from placebo and pre-drink values ($P<0.05$). (Adapted from Rasmussen *et al*. 2000, copyright 2000 American Physiology Society. Reproduced with permission of American Physiological Society in the format Textbook via Copyright Clearance Center.)

studies that have found greater protein/amino acid needs have been reported inadequately and/or may even have been affected by unacknowledged performance-enhancing drug use.

Although very high protein intakes (4–5 g/kg/day) in some athlete groups are common among anecdotal reports, as mentioned there is a dearth of data reporting associated performance effects in the scientific literature. Similarly, the adverse health effects of high-protein intakes (primarily kidney damage), often mentioned in the lay literature, appear to be overestimated (Poortmans & Dellalieux, 2000; Bilsborough & Mann, 2006). On the other hand, dehydration might be a real concern in athletes because high protein intakes can increase urine output substantially and, together with sweat losses, could impair performance and/or health.

Nevertheless, consuming sufficient protein to meet even the highest reported athlete recommendations (~2 g/kg/day) is not difficult assuming one eats a wide variety of foods and sufficient overall energy to match expenditure. This means it is very unlikely that obtaining adequate dietary protein is a significant concern at least for men because even a diet of only 5% protein would contain 2.5 g/kg/day protein for an 80-kg athlete consuming 16.7 MJ energy.

However, to ensure adequate protein/amino acid intake for women, more vigilance is required as many women under-eat voluntarily when involved in rigorous training (Loucks, 2004). The latter is especially critical as insufficient energy intake increases protein needs further (Lemon & Mullin, 1980; Todd *et al*., 1984) and of course minimises both training adaptations and performance.

All this means that the more important dietary issue for physically active individuals relative to protein or amino acids likely centres on other topics, such as the timing of any intake or perhaps even the type of protein consumed. Unfortunately, to date these topics have not been well studied but some information consistent with this hypothesis is available.

5.5 Dietary protein timing

Post-exercise intake

Both infusion and ingestion of amino acids (especially indispensable amino acids) after exercise increase subsequent muscle protein synthesis (MPS) compared with the same exercise alone (Tipton *et al*., 1999; Rasmussen *et al*., 2000; Tipton & Ferrando, 2008) (Figure 5.1). Further, the amino acid leucine may be a particularly effective stimulator of MPS (Devkota & Layman, 2010). Ingestion immediately after exercise seems to be best but the post-exercise window to accelerate MPS may last up to several hours (Rasmussen *et al*., 2000). This ingestion approach relative to the exercise bout should not be surprising as exercise, especially strength exercise, eating and insulin all increase MPS, likely via the upregulation of molecular cell signalling pathways involving phosphatidylinositol 3-kinase/mammalian target of rapamycin (mTor) and mRNA translation initiation and elongation (Fujita *et al*., 2007; Dreyer *et al*., 2008).

Although beyond the scope of this review, this signalling cascade is influenced by the phosphorylation of mTor and the subsequent activation of p70/p85 ribosomal protein kinase (S6K1) and eukaryotic initiation factor 4E-binding protein (4E-BP1) (Kimble *et al*., 2002). Recently, co-ingestion of protein and carbohydrate following strength exercise has been shown to increase the phosphorylation status of this protein synthetic signalling pathway, which could lead to muscle building (anabolic) effects (Koopman *et al*., 2007a; Dreyer *et al*., 2008). Further, a 12-week strength training programme (twice weekly) with immediate post-exercise co-ingestion of indispensable amino acids (15 g) and carbohydrate (15 g) resulted in greater muscle size (hypertrophy) compared with the same energy intake (isoenergetic) of carbohydrate (30 g) alone (Vieillevoye *et al.*, 2010).

There is one study indicating that if protein intake is high enough, MPS may be maximised without carbohydrate (Koopmann *et al.*, 2007b). However, co-ingesting carbohydrates and amino acids may still be the best strategy because the associated insulin release can minimise muscle protein breakdown (MPB) (Gelfand & Barrett, 1987) and of course the sum total of changes in MPS and MPB determine overall muscle development. Further, it has been known since the late 1980s that the intake of carbohydrate immediately post exercise enhances subsequent exercise performance via increased carbohydrates storage (glycogen re-synthesis) (Ivy *et al.*, 1988). A few studies have suggested that nutritional intake associated with exercise training may be even more critical in older individuals (Esmarck *et al.*, 2001; Drummond *et al.*, 2008; Koopman & van Loon, 2009), likely due to age-related insulin resistance (Fujita *et al.*, 2009a). Consequently, use of this exercise nutrient ingestion strategy could play a role in reducing the muscle wasting (sarcopenia) associated with ageing and, if so, reduce substantially a number of the health concerns experienced by today's seniors (Booth & Roberts, 2008; Johnson *et al.*, 2008).

Although determination of optimal post-exercise intakes (quantities and timing) must await further study, both ageing and protein type (see below) appear to be key factors. Regardless, the enhanced muscle protein response can occur with only small quantities of amino acids (<10 g) and carbohydrate (20–35 g). Further, the indispensable amino acids, and perhaps leucine, appear to be most important.

Intake before and during exercise

Tipton *et al.* (2001) demonstrated with strength exercise that similar small intakes of indispensable amino acids and carbohydrate shortly before exercise further enhanced the overall muscle anabolic response compared with intake after exercise and suggested this was due, at least in part, to increased amino acid delivery resulting from greater muscle blood flow during exercise. Further, Beelen *et al.* (2008) found that even in fed subjects, co-ingestion of indispensable amino acids and carbohydrate during exercise increased whole-body protein balance, primarily via an effect on MPS (Figure 5.2). On the other hand, Bird *et al.* (2006) reported reduced urinary 3-methylhistidine excretion (index of MPB) on a meat-free diet when subjects co-ingested a liquid mixture of indispensable amino acids and carbohydrate during a strength training session in comparison to intake of a placebo or either alone. Admittedly, these later data are indirect but they also suggest a reduced MPB response to strength exercise when carbohydrate and amino acids are consumed together. Moreover, there are some exercise performance results consistent with these metabolic data. For example, Berardi *et al.* (2006, 2008) found that ingestion of snacks (7 kcal/kg; 1.2 g/kg carbohydrate, 0.3 g/kg protein, 0.1 g/kg fat) before, immediately and 60 min following a 60-min cycling time trial reduced the performance decrement observed on a second 60-min cycling time trial 6 hours later compared with isoenergetic carbohydrate ingestion (Figure 5.3). Apparently, these positive protein metabolism effects of macronutrient ingestion before exercise might be limited to the immediate pre-exercise period because co-ingestion of carbohydrate and indispensable amino acids 1 hour before exercise did not increase MPS and did not reduce post-exercise MPB (Fujita *et al.*, 2009b).

Taken together these data suggest that co-ingestion of small amounts of protein or indispensable amino acids, carbohydrate and perhaps leucine shortly before, during and shortly after exercise would be a useful strategy for both muscle development and/or muscle repair not only for athletes but also for any individuals attempting to increase or maintain muscle mass, including seniors.

5.6 Dietary protein type

In addition to co-ingestion of protein or indispensable amino acids plus carbohydrate before, during and following exercise, considerable data suggest that protein type is also important for optimising the muscle response. For example, casein (a milk protein) ingestion causes a moderate and prolonged increase in blood amino acids. In contrast, whey (another

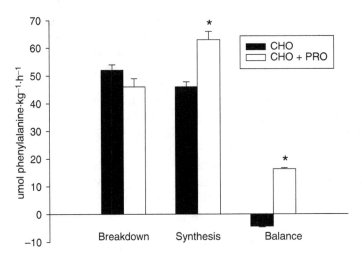

Figure 5.2 Whole-body protein breakdown and synthesis and net protein balance rates when ingesting carbohydrate (CHO) and protein (CHO + PRO, open bars) or carbohydrate alone (CHO, filled bars) both before and during strength exercise. Values are means ± SEM. Asterisks indicate significantly different from CHO ($P<0.05$). (Adapted from Beelen *et al.* 2008, copyright 2008 by American Physiological Society. Reproduced with permission of American Physiological Society in the format Textbook via Copyright Clearance Center.)

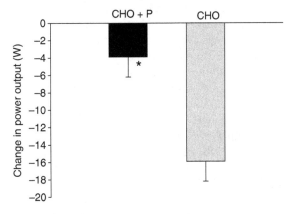

Figure 5.3 Effect of isoenergetic carbohydrate (CHO) versus CHO + protein (P) ingestion before, immediately following, and 1 hour after a 60-min time trial on a second time trial performance 6 hours later. W, watts. Asterisk indicates $P<0.05$. (Reproduced from Berardi *et al.* 2008, with permission from BioMed Central.)

milk protein) results in a more rapid but short-lived response probably due to differing absorption rates and insulin responses (Boirie *et al.*, 1997; Dangin *et al.*, 2001). Further, fish protein may be a good choice because intake of some fish produces insulin sensitivity increases, either because of their ω-3 fat content (deep ocean fish) or perhaps because of their specific amino acid profile (cod) (Lavigne *et al.*, 2000, 2001).

Milk, especially chocolate milk, is an excellent choice for peri-exercise nutrition because it has a carbohydrate, electrolyte and fluid composition that is very suitable for stimulating both muscle glycogen and protein synthesis (Elliot *et al.*, 2006; Wilkinson *et al.*, 2007). Moreover, post-exercise whey protein ingestion increases MPS following acute strength exercise (Tang *et al.*, 2007) and milk, isoenergetic whey protein, or whey and casein ingestion post exercise all lead to an enhanced hypertrophic response when combined with a strength training programme (Cribb *et al.*, 2007; Hartman *et al.*, 2007; Willoughby *et al.*, 2007). Although greater hypertrophy with milk supplementation was not observed in a study of older individuals (50–79 years) (Kukuljan *et al.*, 2009), this might be because the subjects in this investigation did not necessarily ingest the milk associated with the training bouts but rather at other times in the day. Also, a variety of investigations (Karp *et al.*, 2006; Thomas *et al.*, 2009) but not all (Pritchett *et al.*, 2009) have also demonstrated an ergogenic effect on endurance exercise performance with post-exercise chocolate milk ingestion compared with isoenergetic carbohydrate (Figure 5.4).

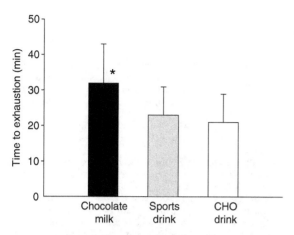

Figure 5.4 Effect of chocolate milk, sports drink or carbohydrate drink ingestion immediately following glycogen-depleting exercise on time to exhaustion at 70% maximum power 4 hours later. Asterisk indicates $P = 0.01$. (Reproduced from Thomas *et al.* 2009 with permission, © 2008 NRC Canada or its licensors.)

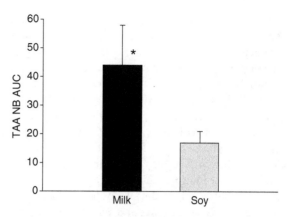

Figure 5.5 The total amino acid (TAA) net arterial–venous balance (NB) area under the curve (AUC) for 3 hours following a strength exercise session with milk or soy milk ingestion immediately post exercise. Asterisk indicates $P<0.05$. (Adapted from Wilkinson *et al.* 2007, copyright © American Society for Nutrition.)

It is likely that digestion/absorption rates are critical for the enhanced protein response with peri-exercise protein ingestion because hydrolysed protein is superior to intact protein, suggesting that amino acid availability after exercise could be the critical stimulus (Koopman *et al.*, 2009). However, some data indicate that casein stimulates muscle hypertrophy more than whey, and because whey is absorbed more quickly than casein (Cribb *et al.*, 2007; Mahe *et al.*, 1996) prolonged amino acid availability could also be important.

Limited data suggest that vegetable protein may be suboptimal relative to protein metabolism because men aged 51–69 years on a vegetarian diet during a 12-week strength study experienced reduced gains in body density, lean mass and creatinine excretion (index of total muscle mass) and a 50% reduced increase in type 2 muscle fibre area compared with a group of meat eaters (Campbell *et al.*, 1999). A number of possibilities might explain these findings, such as altered digestibility, lower amino acid score or even enhanced muscle catabolism caused by increased cortisol release associated with vegan diets (Henley & Kuster, 1994; Baglieri *et al.*, 1995; Lohrke *et al.*, 2001). Consistent with this is the observation that milk (18 g protein, 750 kJ) ingested immediately post exercise produced a greater MPS response compared with

isonitrogenous, isoenergetic and macronutrient-matched soy beverages (Wilkinson *et al.*, 2007) (Figure 5.5). This occurred despite no observed treatment differences in blood flow, insulin, glucose or indispensable amino acid concentrations. A possible explanation could involve greater amino acid availability over time with the milk treatment as soy caused a much more rapid but transient increase in circulating amino acid concentration (Bos *et al.*, 2003). In contrast, Brown *et al.* (2004) found no difference in the observed increase in lean mass with strength training in young men consuming isoenergetic bars containing soy or whey protein. These soy versus milk results are intriguing but far from definitive. Apparently, protein type does play a role in the muscle response to exercise but much more study is needed before it is possible to determine the best approach.

5.7 Summary

Protein metabolism clearly plays a central role in the response to training. Further, although dietary protein needs of athletes likely exceed those of their more inactive counterparts, obtaining sufficient overall dietary protein is rarely a concern as long as one's diet contains a wide variety of foods and adequate overall energy. This could be a concern for some female athletes because, unlike men, many women fail to adequately increase energy intake to match their training expenditures. Essentially, the major issues involving dietary protein and exercise most likely relate to the timing of intake relative to the training sessions, the type of protein/amino acids used, and the mix of nutrients co-ingested. Additional study is required to sort all this out but at present it appears that co-ingesting a mixture of proteins (or perhaps a few indispensable amino acids) and carbohydrate shortly before, during and immediately following exercise is the best approach for both muscle hypertrophy and strength gains as well as for optimal endurance performance. Regular small quantities (snacks) are sufficient and prolonged modest amino acid availability appears to be the mechanism responsible so protein types that accomplish this are most appropriate.

References

Baglieri A, Mahe S, Benamouzig R, Savoie L, Tomé D. Digestion patterns of endogenous and different exogenous proteins affect the composition of intestinal effluents in humans. J Nutr 1995; 125: 1894–1903.

Beelen M, Koopman R, Gijsen AP et al. Protein co-ingestion stimulates muscle protein synthesis during resistance type exercise. Am J Physiol 2008; 295: E70–E77.

Berardi JM, Price TB, Noreen EE, Lemon PWR. Postexercise muscle glycogen recovery enhanced with a carbohydrate–protein supplement. Med Sci Sports Exerc 2006; 38: 1106–1113.

Berardi JM, Noreen EE, Lemon PWR. Recovery from a cycling time trial is enhanced with carbohydrate–protein supplementation vs isoenergetic carbohydrate supplementation. J Int Soc Sport Nutr 2008; 5: 24. Available at www.jissn.com/content/5/1/24

Bilsborough S, Mann N. A review of issues of dietary protein intake in humans. Int J Sport Nutr Exerc Metab 2006; 16: 129–152.

Bird SP, Tarpenning KM, Marino FE. Liquid carbohydrate/essential amino acid ingestion during a short term bout of resistance exercise suppresses myofibrillar protein degradation. Metab Clin Exp 2006; 55: 570–577.

Boirie Y, Dandin M, Gachon P, Vasson M-P, Maubois J-L, Beaufrère B. Slow and fast dietary protein differently modulate postprandial protein accretion. Proc Natl Acad Sci USA 1997; 94: 14930–14935.

Booth F, Roberts CK. Linking performance and chronic disease risk: indices of physical performance are surrogates for health. Br J Sports Med 2008; 42: 950–952.

Bos C, Gaudichon C, Tomé D. Nutritional and physiological criteria in the assessment of milk protein quality for humans. J Am Coll Nutr 2000; 19: 191S–205S.

Bos C, Metges CC, Gaudichon C et al. Postprandial kinetics of dietary amino acids are the main determinant of their metabolism after soy or milk protein ingestion in humans. J Nutr 2003; 133: 1308–1315.

Brown EC, DiSilvestro, Babaknia A, Devor ST. Soy versus whey protein bars: effects on exercise training impact on lean body mass and antioxidant status. Nutr J 2004; 3: 22. Available at www.nutritionj.com/content/3/1/22

Campbell WW, Barton ML Jr, Cyr-Campbell D et al. Effects of an omnivorous diet compared with a lactoovovegetarian diet on resistance-training-induced changes in body composition and skeletal muscle in older men. Am J Clin Nutr 1999; 170: 1032–1039.

Craig WJ, Mangels AR. Position of the American Dietetic Association: vegetarian diets. J Am Diet Assoc 2009; 109: 1266–1282.

Cribb PJ, Williams AD, Stathis CG, Carey MF, Hayes A. Effects of whey isolate, creatine, and resistance training on muscle hypertrophy. Med Sci Sports Exerc 2007; 39: 298–307.

Dangin M, Boirie Y, Garcia-Rodenas C et al. The digestion rate of protein is an independent regulating factor of postprandial protein retention. Am J Physiol 2001; 280: E340–E348.

Devkota S, Layman DK. Protein metabolic roles in treatment of obesity. Curr Opin Clin Nutr Metab Care 2010; 13: 403–407.

Dreyer HC, Drummond MJ, Pennings B et al. Leucine-enriched essential amino acid and carbohydrate ingestion following resistance exercise enhances mTOR signaling and protein synthesis in human muscle. Am J Physiol 2008; 294: E392–E400.

Drummond MJ, Dreyer HC, Pennings B et al. Skeletal muscle protein anabolic response to resistance exercise and essential amino acids is delayed with aging. J Appl Physiol 2008; 104: 1452–1461.

Elliot TA, Cree MG, Sanford AP, Wolfe RR, Tipton KD. Milk ingestion stimulates net muscle protein synthesis following resistance exercise. Med Sci Sports Exerc 2006; 38: 667–674.

Esmarck B, Andersen JL, Olsen S, Richter EA, Mizuno M, Kjaer M. Timing of postexercise protein intake is important for muscle hypertrophy with resistance training in elderly humans. J Physiol 2001; 535: 301–311.

FAO/WHO/UNU. Protein and Amino Acid Requirements in Human Nutrition, 2007. Available at http://whqlibdoc.who.int/trs/WHO_TRS_935_eng.pdf

Fuhrman J, Ferreri DM. Fueling the vegetarian (vegan) athlete. Cur Sports Med Rep 2010; 9: 233–241.

Fujita S, Dreyer HC, Drummond MJ et al. Nutrient signalling in the regulation of human muscle protein synthesis. J Physiol 2007; 582: 813–823.

Fujita S, Glynn EL, Timmerman KL, Rasmussen BB, Volpi E. Supraphysiological hyperinsulinaemia is necessary to stimulate skeletal muscle protein anabolism in older adults: evidence of a true age-related insulin resistance of muscle protein metabolism. Diabetologia 2009a; 52: 1889–1898.

Fujita S, Dreyer HC, Drummond MJ, Glynn EL, Volpi E, Rasmussen BB. Essential amino acid and carbohydrate ingestion prior to resistance exercise does not enhance post-exercise muscle protein synthesis. J Appl Physiol 2009b; 106: 1730–1739.

Fürst P, Stehle P. What are the essential elements needed for the determination of amino acid requirements in humans? J Nutr 2004; 134: 1558S–1565S.

Gelfand RA, Barrett EJ. Effect of physiologic hyperinsulinemia on skeletal muscle protein synthesis and breakdown in man. J Clin Invest 1987; 80: 1–6.

Hartman JW, Tang JE, Wilkinson SB et al. Consumption of fat-free fluid milk after resistance exercise promotes greater lean mass accretion than does consumption of soy or carbohydrate in young, novice, male weightlifters. Am J Clin Nutr 2007; 86: 373–381.

Henley EC, Kuster JM. Protein quality evaluation by protein digestibility-corrected amino acid scoring. Food Technology 1994; 48: 74–77.

Ivy JL, Katz AL, Culter CL, Sherman WM, Coyle EF. Muscle glycogen synthesis after exercise: effect of time of carbohydrate ingestion. J Appl Physiol 1988; 64: 1480–1485.

Johnson AP, De Lisio M, Parise G. Resistance training, sarcopenia, and the mitochondrial theory of ageing. Appl Physiol Nutr Metab 2008; 33: 191–199.

Karp JR, Johnston JD, Tecklenburg S, Mickleborough TD, Fly AD, Stager JM. Chocolate milk as a post-exercise recovery aid. Int J Sport Nutr Exerc Metab 2006; 16: 78–91.

Kimble SR, Farrell PA, Jefferson LS. Invited Review: Role of insulin in translational control of protein synthesis in skeletal muscle by amino acids or exercise. J Appl Physiol 2002; 93: 1168–1180.

Koopman R, van Loon L. Aging, exercise, and muscle protein metabolism. J Appl Physiol 2009; 106: 2040–2048.

Koopman R, Pennings B, Zorenc AH, van Loon LJ. Protein ingestion further augments S6K1 phosphorylation in skeletal muscle following resistance type exercise in males. J Nutr 2007a; 137: 1880–1886.

Koopmann R, Beelen M, Stellingwerff T et al. Coingestion of carbohydrate with protein does not further augment postexercise muscle protein synthesis. Am J Physiol 2007b; 293: E833–E842.

Koopman R, Crombach N, Gijsen AP et al. Ingestion of a protein hydrolysate is accompanied by an accelerated in vivo digestion and absorption rate when compared with its intact protein. Am J Clin Nutr 2009; 90: 106–115.

Kopple JD. Uses and limitations of the balance technique. J Parenter Enteral Nutr 1987; 11 (5 Suppl): 79S–85S.

Kukuljan S, Nowson CA, Sanders K, Daly RM. Effects of resistance exercise and fortified milk on skeletal muscle mass, muscle size, and functional performance in middle-aged and older men: an 18-mo randomised controlled trial. J Appl Physiol 2009; 107: 1864–1873.

Lavigne C, Marette A, Jacques H. Cod and soy proteins compared with casein improve glucose tolerance and insulin sensitivity in rats. Am J Physiol 2000; 278: E491–E500.

Lavigne C, Tremblay F, Asselin G, Jacques H, Marette A. Prevention of skeletal muscle insulin resistance by dietary cod protein in high fat-fed rats. Am J Physiol 2001; 281: E62–E71.

Lemon PWR. Protein and exercise: update. Med Sci Sports Exerc 1987; 19 (5 Suppl): S179–S190.

Lemon PWR. Effects of exercise on dietary protein requirements. Int J Sport Nutr 1998; 8: 426–447.

Lemon PWR, Mullin JP. Effect of initial muscle glycogen levels on protein catabolism during exercise. J Appl Physiol 1980; 48: 624–629.

Lemon PWR, Nagle FJ. Effects of exercise on protein and amino acid metabolism. Med Sci Sports Exerc 1981; 13: 141–149.

Lemon PWR, Tarnopolsky MA, MacDougall JD, Atkinson SA. Protein requirements and muscle mass changes during intensive training in novice body builders. J Appl Physiol 1992; 73: 767–775.

Lohrke B, Saggau E, Schadereit R et al. Activation of skeletal muscle protein breakdown following consumption of soyabean rotein in pigs. Br J Nutr 2001; 85: 447–457.

Loucks AB. Energy balance and body composition in sports and exercise. J Sports Sci 2004; 22: 1–14.

Mahe S, Roos N, Benamouzig R et al. Gastrojejunal kinetics and the digestion of [¹⁵N] beta-lactoglobulin and casein in humans: the influence of the nature and quantity of the protein. Am J Clin Nutr 1996; 63: 546–552.

Poortmans JR, Dellalieux O. Do regular high protein diets have potential health risks on kidney function in athletes? Int J Sports Nutr Exerc Metab 2000; 10: 28–38.

Pritchett K, Bishop P, Pritchett R, Green M, Katica C. Acute effects of chocolate milk and a commercial recovery beverage on postexercise recovery indices and endurance cycling performance. Appl Physiol Nutr Metab 2009; 34: 1017–1022.

Rasmussen BB, Tipton KD, Miller SL, Wolf SE, Wolfe RR. An oral essential amino acid–carbohydrate supplement enhances muscle protein anabolism after resistance exercise. J Appl Physiol 2000; 88: 386–392.

Reeds PJ. Dispensable and indispensable amino acids for humans. J Nutr 2000; 130: 1835S–1840S.

Rennie MJ. An introduction to the use of tracers in nutrition and metabolism. Proc Nutr Soc 1999; 58: 935–944.

Rodrigues NR, Di Marco NM, Langley S. American College of Sports Medicine position stand. Nutrition and athletic performance. Med Sci Sports Exerc 2009; 41: 709–731.

Schaafsma G. The protein digestibility-corrected amino acid score. J Nutr 2000; 130: 1865S–1867S.

Schaafsma G. The Protein Digestibility-Corrected Amino Acid Score (PDCAAS): a concept for describing protein quality in foods and food ingredients. A critical review. J AOCA Int 2005; 88: 988–994.

Tang JE, Manolakos JJ, Kujbida GW, Lysecki PJ, Moore DR, Phillips SM. Minimal whey protein with carbohydrate stimulates muscle protein synthesis following resistance exercise in trained young men. Appl Physiol Nutr Metab 2007; 32: 1132–1138.

Tarnopolsky M. Protein requirements for endurance athletes. Nutrition 2004; 20: 662–668.

Thomas K, Morris P, Stevenson E. Improved endurance capacity following chocolate milk consumption compared with 2 commercially available sport drinks. Appl Physiol Nutr Metab 2009; 34: 78–82.

Tipton KD, Ferrando AA. Improving muscle mass: response of muscle metabolism to exercise, nutrition and anabolic agents. Essays Biochem 2008; 44: 85–98.

Tipton KD, Gurkin BE, Matin S, Wolfe RR. Nonessential amino acids are not necessary to stimulate net muscle protein synthesis in healthy volunteers. J Nutr Biochem 1999; 10: 89–95.

Tipton KD, Rasmussen BB, Miller SL et al. Timing of amino acid–carbohydrate ingestion alters anabolic response of muscle to resistance exercise. Am J Physiol 2001; 281: E197–E206.

Todd KS, Butterfield GE, Calloway DH. Nitrogen balance in men with adequate and deficient energy intake at three levels of work. J Nutr 1984; 114: 2107–2118.

US Department of Agriculture and US Department of Health and Human Services. Report of the Dietary Guidelines Advisory Committee on the Dietary Guidelines for Americans, 2010. Available at www.cnpp.usda.gov/DGAs2010-DGACReport.htm

Vieillevoye S, Poortmans JR, Duchateau J, Carpentier A. Effects of a combined essential amino acids/carbohydrate supplementation on muscle mass, architecture and maximal strength following heavy-load training. Eur J Appl Physiol 2010; 110: 479–488.

Wagenmakers AJ. Tracers to investigate protein and amino acid metabolism in human subjects. Proc Nutr Soc 1999; 58: 987–1000.

Wilkinson SB, Tarnopolsky MA, Macdonald MJ, Macdonald JR, Armstrong D, Phillips SM. Consumption of fluid skim milk promotes greater muscle protein accretion after resistance exercise than does consumption of an isonitrogenous and isoenergetic soy-protein beverage. Am J Clin Nutr 2007; 85: 1031–1040.

Willoughby DS, Stout JR, Wilborn CD. Effects of resistance training and protein plus amino acid supplementation on muscle anabolism, mass, and strength. Amino Acids 2007; 32: 467–477.

Young VR, Bier DM, Pellet PL. A theoretical basis for increasing current estimates of the amino acid requirements in adult man with experimental support. Am J Clin Nutr 1989; 50: 80–92.

Further reading

Koopman R, van Loon L. Aging, exercise, and muscle protein metabolism. J Appl Physiol 2009; 106: 2040–2048.

Rennie MJ. Exercise- and nutrient-controlled mechanisms involved in maintenance of the musculoskeletal mass. Biochem Soc Trans 2007; 35: 1302–1305.

Rodrigues NR, Di Marco NM, Langley S. American College of Sports Medicine position stand. Nutrition and athletic performance. Med Sci Sports Exerc 2009; 41: 709–731.

Tipton KD, Ferrando AA. Improving muscle mass: response of muscle metabolism to exercise, nutrition, and anabolic agents. Essays Biochem 2008; 44: 85–98.

6
Fat Metabolism

Bente Kiens and John A Hawley

Key messages

- Lipid-based fuels (i.e. adipose and muscle triacylglycerol as well as blood-borne fatty acids and triacylglycerol) provide the largest nutrient store of readily available chemical energy for muscle contraction.
- Lipid has several advantages over carbohydrate-based fuels: the energy density of lipid is higher and the relative weight as stored energy is lower. Lipid also provides more adenosine triphosphate (ATP) per molecule than glucose, although the complete oxidation of fatty acid requires more oxygen than the oxidation of carbohydrate.
- During submaximal prolonged (>90 min) exercise, both lipid and carbohydrates are oxidised by the working muscles.
- The consumption of a fat-rich diet for 5–28 days increases fatty acid availability (in blood and muscle) and results in increased rates of whole-body fat oxidation in humans.

- The decreases in whole-body carbohydrate oxidation ('glycogen sparing') and increase in fat oxidation following fat-rich diets are a function of metabolic changes within skeletal muscle. The glycogen-sparing effect may actually be an impairment of the rate of muscle glycogenolysis, an adaptation that may not be beneficial for performance of high-intensity exercise.
- Exposure to fat-rich diets are associated with insulin resistance in the liver, resulting in a failure to suppress hepatic glucose output, and an attenuation of liver glycogen synthesis. For these reasons, caution should always be exercised when sports practitioners recommend high-fat diets to athletes.

6.1 Introduction and historical perspective

At the end of the nineteenth century it was widely thought that carbohydrates (CHO) were the exclusive energy substrate for contracting skeletal muscle and that lipids were not directly oxidised by muscle during exercise but instead converted into glucose and glycogen in the liver. However, at the turn of the twentieth century, the first evidence was provided to show that both CHO and fat fuels contributed as energy sources for the muscle during submaximal aerobic exercise. Subsequently, a series of experiments published in the 1920s provided unique information on the interaction of diet and exercise. The results from these studies can be summarised as follows:

(1) both lipids and CHO are oxidised by the muscle during submaximal exercise;
(2) the preceding diet influences muscle metabolism both at rest in the post-absorptive state and during subsequent exercise;
(3) respiratory exchange ratio (RER) values increase as a function of an increase in exercise intensity, shifting towards a greater reliance on CHO as an energy source; and
(4) subjects have a low tolerance for exercise when lipids are the major energy fuel.

In the 1930s, work from researchers in Scandinavia further described how diet, training and exercise intensity and duration affected CHO and lipid utilisation. The findings from these early pioneering

Sport and Exercise Nutrition, First Edition. Edited by Susan A Lanham-New, Samantha J Stear, Susan M Shirreffs and Adam L Collins.
© 2011 The Nutrition Society. Published 2011 by Blackwell Publishing Ltd.

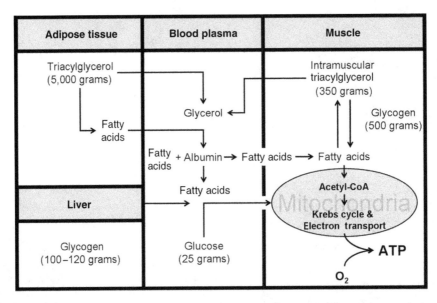

Figure 6.1 A schematic of the endogenous carbohydrate and lipid stores in an endurance trained athlete. (Redrawn and adapted from Coyle EF. Fuels for sport performance. In: Perspectives in Exercise Science and Sport Performance, Vol 10. Optimizing Sport Performance (Lamb DR, Murray R, eds). Traverse City, MI: Cooper Publishing Group, 1997, pp 96–137.)

studies were instrumental in underpinning our current understanding of muscle fuel metabolism.

The introduction of the percutaneous needle biopsy technique in the 1960s saw the beginning of the classic period of exercise biochemistry that commenced in the late 1960s and progressed through the mid-1980s. As direct measures of muscle CHO stores (i.e. muscle glycogen) were now possible, the emphasis shifted from measures of whole-body substrate oxidation (through RER values) and blood glucose concentrations towards endogenous CHO as a fuel source during exercise. During this time it was demonstrated that (i) there was an increased capacity of endurance-trained muscle to oxidise blood-borne fatty acids (FAs) and intramuscular triacylglycerol (IMTG) during submaximal exercise; (ii) there was a training-induced increased capacity for fat oxidation during submaximal exercise and a concomitant 'sparing' of endogenous glycogen stores (muscle and liver); and (iii) there was an increased exercise endurance capacity when subjects were fed CHO during prolonged submaximal exercise. In this chapter we present an overview of the sources of endogenous fat as an energy substrate for skeletal muscle during exercise, examine the effect of training on fat metabolism during exercise, and detail nutritional procedures that enhance fat utilisation and impact on aerobic exercise performance in humans.

6.2 Fat as an energy source for contracting skeletal muscle: effects of endurance training (Figure 6.1)

Lipid-based fuels, i.e. adipose and muscle triacylglycerols (TGs) as well as blood-borne FAs and TGs, provide the largest nutrient store of readily available chemical energy for muscle contraction. As an energy source, lipid has several advantages over CHO-based fuels (i.e. glycogen, blood glucose, and blood, muscle and liver lactate). The energy density of lipid is higher (37.5 kJ/g for stearic acid vs. 16.9 kJ/g for glucose) and the relative weight as stored energy is lower. Lipid also provides more ATP per molecule than glucose (147 vs. 38 ATP), although the complete oxidation of FA requires more oxygen than the oxidation of CHO (6 vs. 26 mol of oxygen per mole of substrate for glucose and stearic acid oxidation, respectively). Adipose tissue TG is the largest energy store in the body, and it has been estimated that this depot is sufficient to sustain skeletal muscle contraction for about 120 hours at marathon running pace. The size of the adipose tissue lipid pool largely depends on the fat mass of an individual. However, with extremes of body adiposity (ranging from 10 to 30% of body mass), the pool could comprise 50 000–100 000 kcal, clearly an abundance of energy! In order for this lipid to be used as a substrate for oxidative metabolism, it has to be exported from adipose tissue and transported in the blood to the active tissues where it will be utilised.

Another physiologically important store of lipid is found within the skeletal muscle (IMTG), mostly adjacent to the mitochondria: the total active muscle mass may contain up to 300 g of TG within the myocyte as lipid droplets, although this amount can vary substantially due to individual differences in fibre type (type I fibres contain a greater concentration of IMTG than type II fibres), diet and possibly training status. Finally, FA can also be derived from circulating TG (chylomicrons) and very low-density lipoproteins (VLDL) formed from dietary fat in the absorptive and post-absorptive state. In theory, if all the circulating VLDL-TG were taken up and oxidised, VLDL-TG degradation could contribute up to 50% of the lipid oxidised during submaximal exercise. The contribution from either of these different sources to energy supply, especially during exercise, depends on several factors including exercise duration, intensity, training status and gender. It is well established that the endurance-trained athlete has an increased capacity to oxidise fat for energy during exercise compared with an untrained individual. In this regard our knowledge of the regulation of cellular fatty acid uptake has dramatically increased in the past decade. Notably, FA uptake has been shown to occur as passive diffusion and facilitated diffusion by a mechanism that resembles that of cellular glucose uptake. Thus, the increased potential for FA uptake and utilisation during exercise is partly due to a training-induced upregulation of several proteins involved in skeletal muscle lipid metabolism. Despite the vast stores of endogenous lipid, FA oxidation during exercise is limited. Unlike the rate of CHO oxidation, which is closely matched to the energy requirements of the working muscle, there are no mechanisms for matching the availability and utilisation of FA to the prevailing rate of energy expenditure. There are many potential sites at which the ultimate control of FA oxidation may reside, with the relative importance of each site depending on a myriad of external factors such as the aerobic training status of the individual, habitual dietary intake, ingestion of substrates (CHO and fat) before and during exercise, gender, and both the relative and absolute exercise intensity.

6.3 Interaction of diet and exercise on fatty acid metabolism

Endogenous CHO reserves are limited, and muscle and liver glycogen depletion often coincide with fatigue during both endurance events and many team sports. Consequently, it has been speculated that an increased availability of FA in the circulation (via the consumption of a high-fat diet or a fat-rich meal) should, in theory, 'spare' endogenous CHO stores, promote lipid utilisation and improve endurance performance in trained individuals. Several exercise–nutrition interventions have received scientific investigation and these are now discussed.

Fat feeding before exercise

Many studies have investigated the effects of acute fat feeding before aerobic exercise on the subsequent rates of substrate oxidation and exercise performance. The results from these investigations are equivocal with regard to the effect of fat feeding on muscle metabolism and also performance outcomes. In early studies, fat feeding in combination with intravenous administration of heparin was shown to stimulate lipolysis, elevate plasma FA concentrations and decrease rates of muscle glycogen utilisation by as much as 40% compared with a control condition during 30 min of submaximal running. On the other hand, other investigations have reported only small differences in the rates of fat oxidation in response to high-fat meals ingested in the hours before prolonged submaximal cycling. An interesting observation from some of these reports is that most of the differences in substrate metabolism favouring fat oxidation (i.e. a lower RER) after fat feeding were only evident in the early stages of exercise, and did not result in an improved performance time.

Long- and medium-chain triglyceride ingestion during exercise

Thirty years ago the effects of ingestion of medium-chain fatty acids (MCFA) versus long-chain fatty acids (LCFA) on FA oxidation during exercise were compared. The theoretical potential of MCFA as an energy source during exercise is based on the more efficient uptake and oxidation in skeletal muscle. Lipids (~30 g) were ingested by 10 well-trained subjects 1 hour before a bout of moderate-intensity exercise lasting 60 min. LCFA ingestion increased serum TG concentrations but neither MCFA nor LCFA had any effects on the rates of whole-body FA oxidation. When more than 50 g of MCFA or LCFA were ingested, severe gastrointestinal problems were experienced by the majority of subjects, and at the time it was recommended that a maximum amount of only 30 g of ingested FA could be tolerated by most individuals. Other studies have utilised stable isotope tracers ([1-^{13}C] octanoate, [1-^{13}C] palmitate) to track the fate of ingested MCFA and LCFA on rates of fat and CHO oxidation and exercise time to exhaustion during submaximal exercise. These experiments revealed that MCFA ingestion was associated with a rise in blood ketone bodies, which are potential energy sources. On the other hand, blood ketone concentrations were unchanged with LCFA ingestion.

In contrast to LCFA, which slow the rate of gastric emptying and enter the systemic circulation as chylomicrons, MCFA are emptied very rapidly from the intestine to the liver and are quickly metabolised. In the 1990s researchers compared the oxidation of ingested MCFA with glucose during 2 hours of cycling at 65% Vo_{2max}. It was found that the contribution of MCFA and glucose to total energy requirements during exercise was similar between the two interventions. The effects of a combination of CHO and MCFA ingested during 3 hours of moderate-intensity exercise (57% Vo_{2max}) in well-trained cyclists have also been investigated. When 10 g of MCFA was co-ingested with CHO each hour, about 70% of the MCFA consumed was oxidised compared with only 33% when MCFA was ingested alone. Towards the end of exercise, the rate of ingested MCFA oxidation closely matched the rate of ingestion. Even so, the contribution of ingested MCFA to total energy expenditure was only 7%. Subsequent work revealed that MCFA ingestion had little effect on rates of muscle glycogen utilisation during 180 min of moderate-intensity cycling. Indeed, even when subjects commenced exercise with low muscle glycogen content, MCFA ingestion had no effect on CHO utilisation and even though low glycogen resulted in increased fat oxidation, MCFA oxidation was not increased. Finally, a recent study compared the ingestion of CHO (60 g/hour) with a CHO (60 g/hour) plus MCFA (~24 g/hour) solution on cycling time trial performance. Subjects completed a set amount of work equal to about 100 km as fast as possible. Compared with a placebo (178 ± 11 min), the time to complete the ride was reduced after the ingestion of both CHO (166 ± 7 min)

and CHO plus MCFA (169 ± 7 min). Thus, the addition of the MCFA did not provide any further performance enhancement over CHO alone.

To date, only one study has reported a beneficial effect of MCFA ingestion on FA metabolism and performance. In that investigation it was shown that when large doses (~30 g/hour) of MCFA were co-ingested with a 10% glucose beverage, serum FA concentrations were elevated, FA oxidation was increased, estimated muscle glycogen utilisation reduced, and 40-km cycle performance (which followed 2 hours of submaximal exercise at 60% Vo_{2max}) improved by 2.5% compared with when glucose was ingested alone. However, it should be noted that the results from this investigation are the exception. Indeed, as noted earlier, the ingestion of large amounts of MCFA (>15 g/hour) are likely to produce gastrointestinal problems in most athletes, which would be expected to be detrimental to performance. In a recent study the effect of specific structured TGs on performance was evaluated. In contrast to MCFA, which consists of three medium-chain fatty acids, the specific structured TGs combined medium-chain and long-chain FAs (MLM). This combination of fatty acid chain length has been shown to avoid gastrointestinal distress and might improve performance. Specific structured TG (MLM) together with CHO or CHO alone was administered to well-trained subjects during 3 hours' cycling at 55% Vo_{2max} followed by a time trial (~50 min duration). Exercise performance was similar in both trials. Taken collectively, the results of the studies reviewed here clearly demonstrate that there is no beneficial effect of ingestion of MCFA or specific structured TG (MLM) on endurance performance and/or exercise capacity. The lack of an effect on performance may seem surprising, but only one study actually measured the concentration of MCFA (8:0 FAs) in plasma and in that experiment it was not possible to detect 8:0 FA. The lack of an increase in plasma FA concentrations, specifically 8:0 FA, may partly explain why muscle metabolism and performance outcomes are not different.

Consumption of high-fat low-carbohydrate diets

It has long been known that modifying an individual's habitual diet can significantly alter the subsequent patterns of substrate utilisation during aerobic exercise and impact on subsequent exercise capacity and/or performance. The consumption of a high-fat (>60% of energy intake) low-CHO (<15% of energy) diet for 1–3 days markedly reduces resting muscle glycogen content and increases FA oxidation during submaximal exercise. Such a shift in substrate utilisation is commonly associated with impairment in exercise capacity In contrast to the negative effects on exercise capacity that seem to result from short-term (1–3 days) exposure to high-fat diets, there is some evidence to suggest that longer periods (5–7 days) of adaptation to high-fat diets may induce adaptive responses that are fundamentally different to the acute lowering of body CHO reserves. It has been proposed that such adaptations eventually induce a reversal of some of the mitochondrial adaptations that favour CHO oxidation and 'retool' the working muscle to increase its capacity for FA oxidation.

A frequently cited study to support the use of high-fat diets to improve athletic performance was conducted in the mid-1980s. In this investigation the effects of 28 days of a high-fat diet (85% of energy) versus a eucaloric diet containing 66% of energy from CHO on submaximal cycle time to exhaustion was tested. The high-fat diet reduced the average resting muscle glycogen content of the five trained study subjects by 47%; consequently, when cycling at approximately 63% Vo_{2max}, RER values were 0.72 (95% of energy from fat, 5% from CHO) and 0.83 (56% of energy from fat, 44% from CHO) for the high-fat and normal diets, respectively. Remarkably, the mean exercise time at this moderate work intensity was not statistically significantly different after the two dietary interventions (147 vs. 151 min for the eucaloric vs high-fat diets, respectively).

In the mid-1990s a South African laboratory used a random cross-over design to investigate the effects of 14 days of either a high-fat (67% energy) or a high-CHO (74% energy) diet in five trained cyclists. After dietary adaptation, subjects undertook a comprehensive battery of physical tests including a 30-s Wingate anaerobic test, a ride to exhaustion at about 90% Vo_{2max} and, following a 30-min rest, a further ride to volitional fatigue at 60% Vo_{2max}. Although the high-fat diet significantly reduced pre-exercise muscle glycogen content by almost 40% (from 121 mmol/kg w.w. after the normal diet to 68 mmol/kg w.w. after the high-CHO diet), mean 30-s anaerobic power was similar between the two conditions (862 vs. 804 W

for the high-fat and high-CHO diet, respectively). Neither was there an effect of dietary manipulation on the time subjects could ride at a work rate eliciting about 90% Vo_{2max} (8.3 vs. 12.5 min for the high-fat and high-CHO trials). Indeed, the only effect of the high-fat diet was to prolong submaximal endurance time during the third and final laboratory test (ride to exhaustion at 60% Vo_{2max}) from 42 to 80 min, despite significantly lower starting muscle glycogen content (32 vs. 73 mmol/kg w.w.). Such increases in endurance were associated with a marked decrease in the average rate of CHO oxidation (2.2 vs. 1.4 g/min) and a significant increase in the rate of fat oxidation (from 0.3 to 0.6 g/min). The results of this investigation are difficult to interpret because of the unorthodox study design, but they strongly suggest that submaximal exercise capacity can be preserved despite low pre-exercise muscle glycogen content when trained individuals are adapted to a high-fat diet.

Probably the longest exposure to a CHO-restricted diet was performed by a Danish group who examined diet–training interactions in two groups of 10 untrained subjects participating in a 7-week endurance training programme while consuming either a high-fat (62% energy) or high-CHO (65% energy) diet. Cycle time to exhaustion at 70% Vo_{2max} increased by 191% after the high-CHO diet, but only by 68% in those subjects who consumed the high-fat diet. These findings clearly demonstrate that a combination of training and a fat-rich diet do not reveal an additive effect on physical performance. In summary, compared with a high-CHO diet, a period of adaptation to a high-fat diet increases the relative contribution of FA oxidation to the total energy requirements of exercise by up to 40%. However, adaptation to a high-fat diet does not appear to alter the rate of muscle glycogen utilisation or improve prolonged moderate-intensity exercise. Adaptation to a high-fat diet is only likely to impact on endurance performance in sporting situations where CHO availability is limiting. More to the point, such nutritional strategies are only likely to be of benefit to a small group of highly trained endurance or ultra-endurance athletes. Although it has been suggested that as long as 20 weeks of exposure should be allowed if humans wish to adapt to high-fat diets, such a time-frame is both impractical and could pose health problems for athletes. Exposure to high-fat diets is also associated with insulin resistance in the liver, resulting in failure to suppress hepatic glucose output, and an attenuation of liver glycogen synthesis. For these reasons, caution should always be exercised when sports practitioners recommend high-fat diets to athletes.

Short-term 'adaptation' to high-fat diets followed by acute high-carbohydrate diets

Over 20 years ago it was proposed that nutritional preparation for endurance and ultra-endurance events should encompass periods of 'nutritional periodisation'. In such a scenario athletes might train for most of the year on a high-CHO diet, adapting to a high-fat diet for several days early in the week prior to a major event, then CHO loading in the final 48 hours immediately prior to competition. Such nutritional periodisation would still permit endurance athletes to train hard throughout the year and maximise their endogenous CHO stores before competition, while theoretically allowing the working muscles to optimise their capacity for FA oxidation during a major endurance race. More to the point, a short (3–5 days) period of exposure to a high-fat diet represents a practical period for extreme dietary change while minimising any potential health risks. Indeed, it appears that most of the adaptive responses that facilitate an increased rate of FA oxidation are complete after as little as 5 days on a high-fat diet, and therefore nutritional periodisation would seem a prudent and perhaps optimal strategy for endurance and ultra-endurance athletes to follow.

A series of investigations designed to determine the effects of either 5 days' adaptation to a high-fat diet (fat 4.0 g/kg/day, CHO 2.4 g/kg/day) followed by 1 day of CHO restoration, or an isoenergetic CHO (9.6 g/kg/day) diet on metabolism and/or endurance and ultra-endurance cycling performance have been undertaken by a group of Australian researchers. Competitive cyclists or triathletes with a history of regular endurance training were recruited for these studies: such individuals have the muscle adaptations which favour FA oxidation. During the initial investigation, muscle biopsies and tracer-derived estimates of blood glucose oxidation were determined. During a second study, subjects were given a pre-trial breakfast similar in size and composition to that which they might consume before a race. In addition, they

were allowed to consume CHO throughout the ride. Such nutritional practices are currently recommended by sports nutritionists. Both investigations employed the same dietary intervention protocol *before* the laboratory exercise regimen (i.e. 5-day adaptation to a high-fat or high-CHO diet followed by 1 day of CHO restoration).

In agreement with the results from earlier studies, 5 days of a high-fat diet drastically reduced resting muscle glycogen concentration. However, 1 day of a high-CHO diet was sufficient to restore muscle glycogen concentration to normal resting levels. During 2 hours of cycling at 70% Vo_{2max}, muscle glycogen utilisation was less after fat adaptation (554 to 294 mmol/kg d.m.) than after the high-CHO diet (608 to 248 mmol/kg d.m.). This glycogen 'sparing' (100 mmol/kg d.m.) occurred because the rates of FA oxidation were elevated by about 50% above the CHO trial. Yet despite such substantial glycogen sparing, the performance of a time trial undertaken after 2 hours of submaximal cycling was similar between dietary treatments.

Unfortunately, the techniques utilised in these studies did not enable the determination of whether the elevated rates of FA oxidation were due to an increase in FA release, uptake and oxidation, or an increased reliance on TG. However, despite the brevity of the adaptation period, the high-fat diet elicited large shifts in favour of FA oxidation during submaximal exercise. Such an adaptation is impressive in light of the already enhanced capacity for FA oxidation in such highly trained subjects. Because the conditions of the first trial (i.e. an overnight fast, water ingestion throughout exercise) are not commensurate with the nutritional practices of athletes, in a follow-up investigation subjects consumed a pre-trial breakfast and ingested CHO throughout the ride. As CHO ingestion effectively eliminates any rise in plasma FA concentration, an effect that can persist for several hours after ingestion, it would be expected that FA oxidation would also be suppressed during exercise. Compared with the first experiment, the overall rate of FA oxidation was lower. However, total FA oxidation was still higher after the high-fat diet compared with the high-CHO diet, indicating that there are persistent metabolic adaptations to a high-fat diet even when CHO availability during exercise is high. Although time trial performance was similar after the two dietary regimens, the results of this study provide strong evidence that the muscle can be 'retooled' to enhance FA oxidation in as little as 5 days, even when CHO is ingested before and throughout exercise. As such, this nutritional periodisation may still confer a positive benefit to those athletes involved in ultra-endurance sports lasting longer than 5 hours, when the need to conserve glycogen as long as possible is of utmost importance for performance.

In an effort to identify some of the mechanisms in skeletal muscle that might be responsible for these shifts in fuel oxidation, muscle pyruvate dehydrogenase (PDH) and hormone-sensitive lipase (HSL) activities were measured in biopsy samples taken before and after 20 min of cycling at 70% Vo_{2max} in subjects who followed the same fat-adaptation, CHO-restoration protocol. Confirming the previous results, resting muscle glycogen levels were similar after both dietary regimens, but RER values were lower during submaximal cycling after fat adaptation, which resulted in roughly a 45% increase and a 30% decrease in fat and CHO oxidation, respectively. PDH activity was lower at rest and throughout exercise at 70% Vo_{2max} (1.69 ± 0.25 vs. 2.39 ± 0.19 mmol/kg w.w./min). Estimates of muscle glycogenolysis during the first minute of exercise at 70% Vo_{2max} were also lower following fat adaptation. HSL activity tended to be higher during exercise at 70% Vo_{2max} following fat adaptation. These results indicate that the previously reported decreases in whole-body CHO oxidation and increases in fat oxidation following the fat-adaptation protocol are a function of metabolic changes within skeletal muscle. Moreover, the glycogen sparing observed in previous studies may actually be an impairment of the rate of muscle glycogenolysis, an adaptation that would not be beneficial for performance of high-intensity exercise. In support of this hypothesis, a recent study has reported that fat adaptation increased rates of fat oxidation during a 100-km time trial. However, repeated 1-km sprints (to mimic race conditions) performed at regular intervals during the 100-km ride were compromised by fat adaptation compared with an isoenergetic high-CHO diet.

The possibility exists that 1 day of CHO intake after fat adaptation might not be sufficient duration to impact on endurance performance. In another investigation, the effects of 7 days of a high-CHO diet following 7 weeks of adaptation to a fat-rich diet (62% energy) versus an isoenergetic CHO diet (65%

energy) for 8 weeks (control trail) on endurance cycling performance were determined. Pre-exercise muscle glycogen stores were significantly higher (872 ± 59 mmol/kg d.w.) after 7 days of CHO restoration compared with the control trial (688 ± 43 mmol/kg d.w.). Yet despite the higher muscle glycogen content, the impairment in endurance performance observed after the high-fat diet could not be reversed when subjects switched to the high-CHO diet during the eighth week. Even after a week of ingestion of CHO, the mean performance time was still approximately threefold lower than when the CHO-rich diet was consumed during the 8-week period. The authors concluded that 'fat adaptation impaired the utilisation of carbohydrates rather than spared carbohydrate as an energy source during exercise.'

6.4 Summary

Many nutritional–exercise manipulations have been studied in an effort to promote rates of FA oxidation, attenuate the rate of utilisation of endogenous CHO reserves and thereby potentially enhance exercise capacity and/or endurance performance. While some of the strategies (acute fat feeding before exercise, fat feeding during exercise, fat adaptation and high-fat diets) have received rigorous scientific enquiry, some so-called sports diets (i.e. the Zone diet) have not been investigated and the so-called 'benefits' of such diets are promoted purely by anecdotal testimonies of famous sports personalities. As such, these diets are not recommended to athletes.

It is evident from the literature that increased fat availability translates into higher rates of both whole-body and muscle lipid utilisation, and a concomitant 'sparing' of muscle glycogen stores during standardised submaximal aerobic exercise. However, even in the face of substantially greater rates of fat oxidation, these dietary protocols consistently fail to improve endurance exercise capacity and/or performance outcomes. Even dietary periodisation strategies, in which endurance athletes adapt their muscles to a high-fat diet over 5–6 days and then switch to a high-CHO diet and rest for 24 hours to restore muscle glycogen content (thus giving the athlete the best of both worlds in terms of potential substrate oxidation), fail to enhance endurance performance, even though fat adaptation produces a dramatic and robust retooling of the muscle to enhance the capacity for fat oxidation and 'spare' muscle glycogen. Of interest to the basic scientist is that the enhanced capacity for fat oxidation in fat-adapted trained individuals persists even in the face of super-compensation of glycogen stores and even with a high-CHO pre-event meal and the intake of substantial amounts of CHO during exercise (conditions that would normally suppress lipolysis and fat metabolism). However, a growing body of evidence now reveals that muscle glycogenolysis is impaired by dietary fat adaptation strategies. This finding, coupled with a failure to find clear evidence of benefits to prolonged exercise involving self-pacing, suggests that we are near to closing the door on this (and other dietary fat protocols) as tools to enhance exercise capacity. Indeed, we can safely conclude that those at the coalface of sports nutrition can delete fat loading and high-fat diets from their list of genuine ergogenic aids for the enhancement of endurance and ultra-endurance performance.

Further reading

Burke LM, Hawley JA. Effects of short-term fat adaptation on metabolism and performance of prolonged exercise. Med Sci Sports Exerc 2002; 34: 1492–1498.

Burke LM, Kiens B. Fat adaptation for athletic performance: the nail in the coffin? J Appl Physiol 2006; 100: 7–8.

Hawley JA, Brouns F, Jeukendrup AE. Strategies to enhance fat utilisation during exercise. Sports Med 1998; 25: 241–257.

Helge JW, Watt PW, Richter EA, Rennie MJ, Kiens B. Partial restoration of dietary fat induced metabolic adaptations to training by 7 days of carbohydrate diet. J Appl Physiol 2002; 93: 1797–1805.

Jeukendrup AE, Thielen JJ, Wagenmakers AJ, Brouns F, Saris WH. Effect of medium-chain triacylglycerol and carbohydrate ingestion during exercise on substrate utilization and subsequent cycling performance. Am J Clin Nutr 1998; 67: 397–404.

Kiens B. Skeletal muscle lipid metabolism in exercise and insulin resistance. Physiol Rev 2006; 86: 205–243.

Roepstorff C, Vistisen B, Kiens B. Intramuscular triacylglycerol in energy metabolism during exercise in humans. Exerc Sport Sci Rev 2005; 33: 182–188.

Stellingwerff T, Spriet LL, Watt MJ et al. Decreased PDH activation and glycogenolysis during exercise following fat adaptation with carbohydrate restoration. Am J Physiol 2006; 290: E380–E388.

7
Fluids and Electrolytes

Susan M Shirreffs

Key messages

- Water makes up a significant proportion (45–70%) of a person's body mass, and this water contains significant amounts of electrolytes (e.g. sodium, potassium and chloride).
- The body's homeostatic mechanisms strive to keep us in a state of euhydration (normal body water content) by balancing losses with intake. However, sweat production during exercise can present a significant challenge to this homeostatic process.

- Exercise performance appears to be unaffected by minor levels of hypohydration, but when body mass losses reach 2% or higher, then exercise performance is frequently impaired.
- Physiological disturbances such as increased body temperature and heart rate and exercise performance decrements can be minimised by utilising a hydration strategy before, during and after exercise as determined by the sweat and electrolyte losses and exercise situation.

7.1 Introduction

Body water and electrolytes

Water is the largest component of the human body and the total body water content varies from approximately 45 to 70% of the total body mass, corresponding to about 33–53l for a 75-kg man. Although body water content varies greatly between individuals, the water content of the various tissues is maintained relatively constant. For example, adipose tissue has a low water content (10%) and lean tissue such as muscle a high water content (76%), so the total fraction of water in the body is determined largely by the total fat content. Therefore, a high body fat content is related to a lower total body water content as a percentage of body mass.

Body water can be divided into two components: the intracellular fluid (ICF) and the extracellular fluid (ECF). The ICF is the major component and comprises approximately two-thirds of total body water. The ECF can be further divided into the interstitial fluid (that between the cells) and the plasma, with the plasma volume representing approximately one-quarter of ECF volume. This is outlined in Table 7.1.

However, the water in our body is not present as plain water. A wide range of electrolytes (compounds which dissociate into ions when in solution) and solutes are dissolved in varying concentrations in the body fluids. The major cations (positively charged electrolytes) in the body water are sodium, potassium, calcium and magnesium; the major anions (negatively charged electrolytes) are chloride and bicarbonate. The location of these electrolytes in the body water is not consistent throughout the body water compartments. Sodium is the major electrolyte in the ECF, while potassium is present at much lower concentrations (Table 7.2). In the ICF, the situation is reversed: the major electrolyte is potassium, with sodium found in much lower concentrations. It is critical for the body to maintain this distribution of electrolytes because maintenance of the transmembrane electrical and chemical gradients is of

Sport and Exercise Nutrition, First Edition. Edited by Susan A Lanham-New, Samantha J Stear, Susan M Shirreffs and Adam L Collins.
© 2011 The Nutrition Society. Published 2011 by Blackwell Publishing Ltd.

Table 7.1 Body water distribution between the different body fluid compartments in an adult 75-kg male.

	Percent of body mass	Percent of lean body mass	Percent of body water
Total body water	60	72	100
Extracellular water	20	24	33
Plasma	5	6	8
Interstitium	15	18	25
Intracellular water	40	48	67

Table 7.2 Concentration (mmol/l) of ions in the extracellular and intracellular body water compartments. Plasma values are given to represent the extracellular compartment. The normal ranges of the plasma electrolyte concentrations are also shown.

Ion	Extracellular fluid (plasma)	Intracellular fluid
Sodium	140 (135–145)	12
Potassium	4.0 (3.5–4.6)	150
Calcium	2.4 (2.1–2.7)	4
Magnesium	0.8 (0.6–1.0)	34
Chloride	104 (98–107)	4
Bicarbonate	29 (21–38)	12
Inorganic phosphate	1.0 (0.7–1.6)	40

paramount importance for ensuring the integrity of cell function and allowing electrical communication throughout the body.

Terminology

Euhydration is the state of being in water balance. However, although the dictionary definition is an easy one, establishing the physiological definition is not so simple. Hyperhydration is a state of being in positive water balance (water excess) and hypohydration the state of being in negative water balance (water deficit). Dehydration is the process of losing water from the body and rehydration the process of gaining body water. However, euhydration is not a steady state but rather is a dynamic state in that we continually lose water from the body and there may be a time delay before replacing it or we may take in a slight excess and then lose this.

7.2 Disturbances in body water

The balance between the loss and gain of fluid maintains body water within relatively narrow limits of around 0.5%. The main routes of water loss from

the body are the urinary system, the skin, the gastrointestinal tract and the respiratory surfaces. The primary avenues for restoration of water balance are fluid and food ingestion, with water of oxidation also making a contribution. The volumes of water that individuals obtain from food and drinks are highly variable, although it is generally reported that the majority normally comes from liquids, with a smaller though still significant proportion from solid foods.

Body water loss in humans results in fluid losses from both the ICF and ECF compartments. However, fluid losses can cause very different effects on the remaining body water pools depending on the type of water loss that occurs. Hypotonic water loss, as can occur with sweating, results in an increase in body fluid tonicity, while isotonic loss causes a net fluid loss but no increase or decrease in body fluid tonicity. Hypertonic fluid losses, as can occur with production of concentrated urine, cause a reduction in body fluid tonicity.

Sweat loss in exercise

During exercise, the production of sweat dissipates the increased heat that is produced. The sweating response is influenced by the environmental conditions, the clothing worn, the duration and intensity of exercise and by the exerciser's individual physiology. Typically, maximum sweat rates are in the order of 2–3 l/hour. Therefore, body mass reductions of up to 2–3% and more could feasibly occur in many exercise situations and reductions of this magnitude, and more, are reported in the scientific literature. However, it is important to remember that there is large inter-individual variation in sweating even when the same or similar exercise is carried out in the same conditions or when individuals are exposed to the same heat stress.

7.3 Effects of changes in hydration on exercise performance

Endurance exercise

The effects of dehydration on physiological function and exercise performance during endurance exercise have been studied generally either by inducing a certain degree of body water loss before the exercise task or by allowing dehydration to develop during the exercise. Clearly, each of these approaches may have different effects on the type of body water loss that develops (e.g. hypotonic, isotonic or hypertonic as described above). This may in turn influence the experimental findings. However, it is clear from the published literature that regardless of the approach used to induce body water loss, many of the physiological responses and exercise performance outcomes observed are remarkably similar regardless of the means by which the body water deficit is induced. Extensive reviews of the published literature examining the effects of dehydration on exercise performance have led reviewers to conclude that during exercise in a warm environment (defined as an ambient temperature >30°C), dehydration to the extent of 2–7% of body mass consistently decreased endurance exercise performance. However, the extent of the decrements in performance was highly variable, ranging from a 7 to 60% decline in performance. However, a less consistent picture was gleaned when the endurance exercise was undertaken in temperate conditions. It was concluded that, in these situations, dehydration of 1–2% of body mass had no effect on endurance exercise performance when exercise duration was less than 90 min; however, when the level of dehydration was greater than 2% of body mass and exercise duration was greater than 90 min, endurance exercise performance was impaired. Therefore, one key conclusion when endurance exercise performance is being considered is that an important level of dehydration occurs when there is water loss equivalent to 2% of body mass or higher. Dehydration to this extent generally appears to reduce endurance exercise performance in both temperate and hot environments, especially when the duration of exercise is in the order of 90 min or more. Taken together, these findings suggest that athletes may be advised to try to minimise dehydration when exercising in a hot environment (e.g. 31–32°C) for durations approaching 60 min and longer. However, when the environment is temperate (20–21°C), athletes may be better able to tolerate 2% dehydration without significant performance decrement or risk of significantly added hyperthermia compared with exercise with full fluid replacement. In cold environments, dehydration by more than 2% may be tolerable. It is very important to note that these values are average values from scientific research and there may be individual athletes who can cope with greater levels of hypohydration without impact and some athletes who

experience performance deficits with lesser levels of hypohydration.

Strength, power and sprint exercise

When body water loss has occurred, various effects on neuromuscular function and short-term power have been reported. Muscle strength during a muscle contraction is determined by the ability of the nervous system to recruit motor units in concert with the number of muscle contractile units in cross-section. Therefore, it is of interest in this section to consider whether a reduction in muscle water has the potential to alter force generation capability or energy production when maximally stimulated.

The majority of published studies indicate that dehydration, up to a loss of 7% of body mass, can largely be tolerated without a reduction in measured maximal isometric or isotonic muscle contractions. When muscle strength reductions have been noted with dehydration, the upper body muscles appear to be affected to a greater extent than the lower body muscles. Also, the published evidence suggests that there appears to be a greater likelihood of strength reduction if dehydration is induced as a result of prolonged food and fluid restriction and questions have been raised as to the role that factors other than dehydration *per se* may have on the findings reported.

When maximal aerobic power has been investigated with regard to hydration status, the findings suggest that when hypohydration of less than 3% of body mass is present there is no subsequent effect on maximal aerobic power, but when the dehydration increases to 3–5% of body mass power reductions have been recorded. Therefore, the available evidence suggests that body water loss equivalent to 3% of body mass may be the critical level when aerobic power is being considered. Also, as seems to be the case with endurance exercise performance, decrements in maximal aerobic power appear to exist with slightly lower levels of dehydration when the environmental conditions are hot.

The influence of hydration status on sprint performance has been investigated in many studies using a number of different exercise modes. It is possible that hypohydration may influence exercise performance differently depending on whether the sprinting being investigated is running (where body mass must be supported and moved) or is cycle sprinting (when this is not the case); if body mass is reduced it changes the work required for the running. That is, the decreased body mass which is typically used to define the magnitude of hypohydration may compensate for any reduced muscular strength and/or power that it causes. However, whilst this will complicate the pure science interpretation of the findings of studies investigating sprint performance, it is the situation that occurs in real athletic situations. Studies investigating sprint running performance have concluded that body mass reductions of 2–3% have no significant effect on sprint running performance. It is possible that sprinting would have been 'easier' with lower body mass, due to less mass for the runner to move. Thus, it is feasible that a reduction in physiological demand may promote improved performance, which may counteract any effects hypohydration may have on sprinting.

Sports with skill components

Many team sports such as football, rugby, basketball and hockey are stop–start in nature and consist of prolonged periods of exercise with repeated intermittent high-intensity bursts interspersed with lower intensity exercise. Successful performance in these sports involves fatigue resistance, but also relies on cognitive function for decision-making as well as proper execution of complex skills. This makes assessment of sport performance challenging to study. However, a number of protocols have been developed which have attempted, amongst other things, to investigate the effect hydration status may have on aspects of sports performance. In many of the studies undertaken in this area, the protocol involved allowing dehydration to develop in one trial and preventing it in another by provision of drinks. However, the drink provided has frequently been a specific sports energy drink and thus the influence of carbohydrate or other components in the drink on the outcomes measured cannot always be distinguished from any effects due to prevention of dehydration.

Studies investigating aspects of football performance have reported that fluid replacement with flavoured water, sufficient to limit body mass loss to 1.4%, prevented a reduction in skill performance compared with performance when body mass was reduced by 2.5%, and that body mass reductions of 2.4% and 2.1% resulted in 13% and 15% reductions in test performance in comparison with a trial when drinking resulted in a body mass reduction of only 0.7%. In a study investigating basketball performance, when body mass losses of up to 4% were created by allowing or withholding drinks during exercise in the heat prior to performing a sequence of basketball drills, it was reported that performance during all timed and shooting drills declined progressively as dehydration increased from 0 to 4% body mass loss and the performance decrement reached statistical significance at 2% body mass loss for combined timed and shooting drills.

This information on the effects of alterations in hydration status on performance in team sports or on aspects of team sports performance, together with knowledge of the effects of sweat loss in endurance and sprint, power and high-intensity endurance activities, suggests that the effects of sweating will be similar to effects in these other activities. Therefore, it is frequently generalised that a body mass reduction equivalent to 2% should be the acceptable limit of sweat losses. However, again, it must be remembered that this is an average and some people may be negatively affected with much smaller body mass losses while others may be able to cope with this body mass loss without an impact on performance.

7.4 Effects of drinking on exercise

Pre-exercise hydration

For an individual undertaking regular exercise, any fluid deficit that is incurred during one exercise session can potentially compromise the next exercise session if adequate fluid replacement does not occur. As such, fluid replacement after exercise can frequently be thought of as hydration prior to the next exercise bout. However, in addition to this, the issue of pre-exercise hyperhydration has been investigated. In a healthy individual the kidneys excrete any excess body water, and therefore ingesting excess fluid before exercise is generally ineffective at inducing pre-exercise hyperhydration.

The practice of drinking in the hours before exercise is effective at ensuring a situation of euhydration prior to exercise if there is any possibility that slight hypohydration is present. The current American College of Sports Medicine (ACSM) position stand on exercise and fluid replacement suggests that when optimising hydration before exercise the individual should slowly drink a moderate amount (e.g. 5–7 ml/kg) at least 4 hours before exercise. If this does not result in urine production or the urine is dark or highly concentrated, then more drink should be slowly ingested (e.g. 3–5 ml/kg) about 2 hours before exercise. This practice of drinking several hours before exercise gives sufficient time for urine output to return to normal. The guidelines also suggest that consuming beverages that contain some sodium and/or small amounts of salted snacks or sodium-containing foods at meals will help to stimulate thirst and retain the consumed fluids.

Hydration during exercise

The diversity of sport and exercise training and competition, including intensity, duration, frequency and environmental conditions, mean that providing specific recommendations in terms of drink volumes and compositions and patterns of ingestions is not sensible. The current ACSM position stand on exercise and fluid replacement highlights this and concludes that the goal of drinking during exercise should be to prevent *excessive* (>2%) body mass loss due to a water deficit and to prevent excessive changes in electrolyte balance. In doing this, any compromise in performance should be minimised. The ACSM also conclude that because there is considerable variability in sweating rates and sweat electrolyte content between individuals, as highlighted above, customised fluid replacement regimens are recommended to all. This is possible because individual sweat rates can be estimated by measuring body mass before and after exercise.

Post-exercise rehydration

The primary factors influencing the post-exercise rehydration process are the volume and composition of the fluid consumed and the rate with which it is absorbed into the body. The volume consumed will be influenced by many factors, including the palatability of the drink and its effects on the thirst mechanism, although with conscious effort some people can still drink large quantities of an unpalatable drink when they are not thirsty. The ingestion of solid food, and the composition of that food, are also important factors, but there are many situations

where solid food is avoided by some people between exercise sessions or immediately after exercise.

Beverage composition
Sodium

Plain water is not the ideal post-exercise rehydration beverage when rapid and complete restoration of fluid balance is necessary and where all intake is in liquid form. This was established some time ago when a high urine flow following ingestion of large volumes of electrolyte-free drinks did not allow subjects to remain in positive fluid balance for more than a very short time. These studies also established that the plasma volume was better maintained when electrolytes were present in the fluid ingested, and this effect was attributed to the presence of sodium in the drinks.

The first studies to investigate the mechanisms of post-exercise rehydration showed that the ingestion of large volumes of plain water after exercise-induced dehydration resulted in a rapid fall in plasma osmolality and sodium concentration, leading to a prompt and marked diuresis caused by a rapid return to control levels of plasma renin activity and aldosterone levels. Therefore, the replacement of sweat losses with plain water will, if the volume ingested is sufficiently large, lead to haemodilution. The fall in plasma osmolality and sodium concentration that occurs in this situation reduces the drive to drink and stimulates urine output and has potentially more serious consequences such as hyponatraemia.

As sodium is the major ion lost in sweat, it is intuitive that sweat sodium losses should be replaced. It is not logical to think that the salty water we lose as sweat would be best replaced in the body by plain water. This area has been systematically investigated and studies show that, provided an adequate volume is consumed, euhydration is achieved when the sodium intake is greater than the sweat sodium loss. The addition of sodium to a rehydration beverage is therefore justified on the basis that sodium is lost in sweat and must be replaced to achieve full restoration of fluid balance. It has been demonstrated that a drink's sodium concentration is more important than its osmotic content for increasing plasma volume after dehydration. Sodium also stimulates glucose absorption in the small intestine via the active co-transport of glucose and sodium, which creates an osmotic gradient that acts to promote net water absorption. However, this sodium, to assist intestinal absorption, can either be consumed with the drink or be secreted by the intestine. Sodium has been recognised as an important ingredient in rehydration beverages by an inter-association task force on exertional heat illnesses because sodium plays a role in the aetiology of exertional heat cramps, exertional heat exhaustion and exertional hyponatraemia.

Potassium and magnesium

Potassium, as the major ion in the ICF, has been postulated to have a role in optimising post-exercise rehydration by aiding the retention of water in the intracellular space. Potassium is lost in sweat in concentrations of about 5–10 mmol/l. Initial work using dehydrated rats supported this idea, indicating that the role of potassium in restoring intracellular volume is more modest than sodium's role in restoring extracellular volume. However, subsequent work in humans has proved to be less conclusive. Potassium may therefore be important in enhancing rehydration by aiding intracellular rehydration, but further investigation is required to provide conclusive evidence. Importantly, however, no negative effect of including modest amounts of potassium in rehydration drinks has been demonstrated and indeed potassium, in small quantities, is an ingredient in most commercially available sports drinks that suggest they have a role in post-exercise rehydration.

The importance of including magnesium in sports drinks has been the subject of much discussion. Magnesium is lost in sweat in small amounts (<0.2 mmol/l) and many believe that this causes a reduction in plasma magnesium levels that are implicated in muscle cramp. Even though there can be a decline in plasma magnesium concentrations during exercise, it is most likely due to compartmental fluid redistribution rather than to sweat loss. There does not therefore seem to be any good reason for including magnesium in post-exercise rehydration and recovery sports drinks.

Drink volume

Obligatory urine losses persist even in the dehydrated state, because of the need for elimination of metabolic waste products. The volume of fluid consumed after exercise-induced or thermal sweating must therefore be greater than the volume of sweat lost if effective rehydration is to be achieved. This contradicts earlier recommendations that after exercise athletes should match fluid intake exactly to the measured body mass loss. Studies have investigated the effect of drink volumes equivalent to 50%, 100%, 150% and 200% of the sweat loss consumed after exercise-induced dehydration equivalent to approximately 2% of body mass. To investigate the possible interaction between beverage volume and its sodium content, a relatively low-sodium drink (23 mmol/l) and a moderately high-sodium drink (61 mmol/l) were compared. Subjects could not return to euhydration when they consumed a volume equivalent to, or less than, their sweat loss, irrespective of the drink composition. When a drink volume equal to 150% of the sweat loss was consumed, subjects were slightly hypohydrated 6 hours after drinking when the test drink had a low sodium concentration, and they were in a similar condition when they drank the same beverage in a volume of twice their sweat loss. With the high-sodium drink, enough fluid was retained to keep the subjects in a state of hyperhydration 6 hours after drink ingestion when they consumed either 150 or 200% of their sweat loss. The excess would eventually be lost by urine production or by further sweat loss if the individual resumed exercise or moved to a warm environment. Whilst other studies have also shown the importance of drinking a larger volume of drink than the sweat volume lost, an interaction between sodium intake, volume intake and whole-body rehydration has not always been reported. However, it seems likely that in these studies the length of subject observation after rehydration may not have been sufficient to observe the urine production response to the treatments. Additionally, evidence has recently emerged suggesting that the rate of drinking or the rate of delivery to the intestine for absorption of a large rehydration bolus can have important implications on the physiological handling of the drink. Drinking a large volume of fluid has the potential to induce a greater decline in plasma sodium concentration and osmolality, which in turn have the potential to induce a greater diuresis by the mechanism described above.

Food and fluid consumption

There may be opportunities to consume solid food between exercise bouts, and in many situations doing so should be encouraged to meet other nutritional goals unless it is likely to result in gastrointestinal disturbances. The role of solid food intake in promoting rehydration from a 2.1% body mass sweat loss with consumption of either a solid meal plus flavoured water or a commercially available sports drink has been investigated. The urine volume produced following food and water ingestion was almost 300 ml less than that when the sports drink was consumed, resulting in a more favourable recovery and maintenance of hydration status. Subsequent studies have also highlighted a role for food products in post-exercise fluid balance restoration.

Beverage palatability and voluntary fluid intake

In the majority of scientific studies in the area, including those described above, a fixed volume of fluid was prescribed and consumed. However, in everyday situations that athletes find themselves in, intake is determined by the interaction of physiological and psychological factors. When the effect of palatability together with the solute content of beverages in promoting rehydration after sweat loss was studied, subjects drank 123% of their sweat volume losses with flavoured water and 163% and 133% when the solution had 25 and 50 mmol/l sodium respectively. Three hours after starting the rehydration process the subjects were in a better whole-body hydration status after drinking the sodium-containing beverages than the flavoured water. Similar results have been reported in other research and together these studies demonstrate the importance of palatability for promoting consumption, but also confirm earlier results showing that a moderately high electrolyte content is essential if the ingested fluid is to be retained in the body. The benefits of the higher intake with the more palatable drinks were lost because of the higher urine output. Other drink characteristics, including carbonation, influence drink palatability and therefore need to be considered when a beverage is being considered for effective post-exercise rehydration.

Further reading

Cheuvront SN, Carter R III, Sawka N. Fluid balance and endurance performance. Curr Sports Med Rep 2003; 2: 202–208.

Coyle EF. Fluid and fuel intake during exercise. J Sports Sci 2004; 22: 39–55.

Judelson DA, Maresh CM, Anderson JM et al. Hydration and muscular performance. Does fluid balance affect strength, power and high-intensity endurance? Sports Med 2007; 37: 907–921.

Sawka MN, Burke LM, Eichner ER, Maughan RJ, Montain SJ, Stachenfeld NS. American College of Sports Medicine Position Stand. Exercise and fluid replacement. Med Sci Sport Exerc 2007; 39: 377–390.

Shirreffs SM, Armstrong LE, Cheuvront SN. Fluid and electrolyte needs for preparation and recovery from training and competition. J Sports Sci 2004; 22: 57–63.

Shirreffs SM, Sawka MN, Stone M. Water and electrolyte needs for football training and match-play. J Sports Sci 2006; 24: 699–707.

8
Micronutrients

Vicki Deakin

Key messages

- Athletes may have slightly higher requirements for micronutrients involved in energy metabolism and muscle function, blood health, antioxidant and immune function than non-athletes.
- Current US/Canada Dietary Reference Intakes (DRIs) can be used for planning diets or assessing the adequacy (or inadequacy) of micronutrient intakes in athletes. DRI cut-offs are increased for iron for athletes to accommodate elevated iron requirements.
- Athletes at risk of suboptimal intakes of micronutrients are those on low-energy intakes or missing one or more food groups. Females are at highest risk because they usually eat less food than males.
- Micronutrients of known concern in 'at-risk' athletes include calcium, iron, zinc, magnesium, vitamin D and the antioxidant nutrients (vitamins C and E, zinc and possibly beta-carotene and selenium).
- Plant-based diets are unlikely to supply enough calcium, vitamin B₁₂, iron or zinc without dietary planning to improve bioavailability or without using fortified foods.

- Micronutrient deficiency can impair performance but the effects of marginal deficiency are less clear, except for iron.
- Amenorrhoea, in combination with low energy and low calcium intakes, increases the risk of stress fractures.
- Taking micronutrient supplements, either as single supplements or combined, in the absence of a diagnosed deficiency is unlikely to have any performance benefits.
- Acute strenuous exercise increases oxidative stress and the production of free radicals, which can damage cells and tissues. Taking antioxidants as supplements is unlikely to attenuate this effect, and may further increase oxidative damage and imbalance micronutrient interactions.
- Multivitamin and multimineral supplements, rather than single micronutrient supplements, may be needed in those athletes with suboptimal intakes.
- Dietary intervention to correct suboptimal micronutrient intake is the preferred approach. Using foods rather than supplements enhances nutrient bioavailability.

8.1 Introduction

The micronutrients (vitamins, minerals, electrolytes and trace elements) are required in small amounts (micrograms to milligrams) and do not provide any measurable energy or kilojoule content in foods. Micronutrients work interactively to (i) regulate energy metabolism, nervous function and muscle contraction, (ii) regulate oxidative function, (iii) maintain bone and blood health, (iv) control fluid and electrolyte balance, and (v) assist with immune function.

Micronutrients do not work in isolation. Vitamins interact with each other or with other minerals to regulate biological and metabolic processes and are grouped into fat-soluble (A, D, E and K) and

water-soluble (B complex and C) categories based on their different solubility. Minerals are grouped into macrominerals (e.g. sodium, potassium, calcium, phosphorus and magnesium) and trace elements (e.g. iron, zinc, copper, chromium and selenium). Dietary Reference Intakes (DRIs) for macrominerals are more than 100 mg/day, whereas trace elements are required in smaller quantities (<20 mg/day). Minerals, whether they exist in large amounts (such as calcium and phosphorus in bones) or in trace amounts, also regulate metabolic functions.

Micronutrients are often considered separately, which can often encourage the concept that they work in isolation. This concept is fostered by the vast array of single vitamin and mineral supplements available in the market and the often exaggerated

Sport and Exercise Nutrition, First Edition. Edited by Susan A Lanham-New, Samantha J Stear, Susan M Shirreffs and Adam L Collins.
© 2011 The Nutrition Society. Published 2011 by Blackwell Publishing Ltd.

Table 8.1 Vitamins involved in body functions that have potential implications for athletic training and performance.

	Co-factors for energy metabolism	Nervous function, muscle contraction	Blood health (red blood cell formation and function)	Immune function	Antioxidant function	Bone health	Fluid and electrolyte balance
Water-soluble vitamins							
B group							
Thiamin	✓	✓					
Riboflavin	✓	✓			✓ᵃ		
Vitamin B6	✓	✓	✓	✓			
Folic acid		✓	✓	✓			
Vitamin B12		✓	✓			✓	
Niacin	✓	✓					
Pantothenic acid	✓						
Biotin	✓						
Vitamin C			✓	✓	✓		
Beta-carotene (vitamin A)				✓	✓		
Fat-soluble vitamins							
Vitamin A				✓	✓		
Vitamin D				✓		✓	
Vitamin E				✓	✓		
Vitamin K						✓	

ᵃ Act as coenzymes for endogenous antioxidants.
Adapted with permission from Fogelholm M. Vitamin, mineral and anti-oxidant needs of athletes. In: Clinical Sports Nutrition, 4th edn (Burke L, Deakin V, eds). Sydney: McGraw-Hill, 2010.

claims of their efficacy by manufacturers. Consumers still take single vitamin or mineral supplements, particularly B vitamins, antioxidant nutrients (particularly vitamin C and vitamin E), iron and zinc, in the hope of preventing illness or deficiency, improving health or to address poor food choices. Athletes take supplements for similar reasons or to enhance sports performance or recovery.

The functional and interactive role of micronutrients in human systems is complex and not fully understood and is beyond the scope of this chapter. Comprehensive information on functions and food sources can be found in any key undergraduate nutrition textbook. In athletes, there is limited research on the micronutrient status of athletes and the effects of physical activity on micronutrient requirements. Although gross micronutrient deficiencies are rare in athletes and no different to untrained controls, there is some evidence that marginal deficiency of magnesium, iron, zinc and vitamin D can affect performance capacity.

This chapter addresses the functional and interactive role of the important micronutrients involved in energy metabolism, antioxidant function, and bone and blood health (in relation to formation and function of red blood cells) that have known or at least expected implications for athletes. Research on micronutrients and performance in athletes is not extensive and is confounded by small sample sizes, poor experimental design (often no control group), difficulties controlling for diet, and the multifactorial and interactive effects and function of these nutrients. Most research has been conducted on the potential effects of micronutrient supplementation on performance enhancement in replete or marginally depleted athletes.

The micronutrients involved in fluid and electrolyte balance (i.e. sodium, potassium and chlorine) are under homeostatic control and are addressed in Chapter 7. The micronutrients involved in immune function are considered in Chapter 21. The main functional roles of micronutrients of known relevance to athletes are summarised in Tables 8.1 and 8.2, showing the multiple roles of these micronutrients in several body systems.

Table 8.2 Minerals involved in body functions that have reported and potential implications for athletic training and performance.

	Co-factors for energy metabolism	Nervous and muscle function	Blood health (red cell function)	Immune function	Antioxidant function	Bone health	Fluid and electrolyte balance
Macrominerals							
Sodium		✓					✓
Potassium		✓					✓
Calcium		✓	✓			✓	
Magnesium	✓	✓		✓			
Trace minerals							
Iron	✓		✓	✓	✓[a]		
Zinc	✓			✓	✓[a]	✓	
Copper	✓				✓[a]		
Chromium	✓						
Selenium				✓	✓[a]		

[a] Act as coenzymes for endogenous antioxidants.

Adapted with permission from Fogelholm M. Vitamin, mineral and anti-oxidant needs of athletes. In: Clinical Sports Nutrition, 4th edn (Burke L, Deakin V, eds). Sydney: McGraw-Hill, 2010.

8.2 Micronutrients that regulate energy metabolism and muscle function

There are eight B vitamins (thiamin, riboflavin, niacin, vitamin B_6, folate, biotin, pantothenic acid, vitamin B_{12}). All are involved in the metabolic pathways for energy metabolism of the macronutrients: carbohydrate, protein and fat (and alcohol). Their primary role is to act as coenzymes, which are molecules that bind with an enzyme to activate it. Other micronutrients involved in energy metabolism include choline and the minerals iodine, chromium, manganese and sulphur. Several other minerals and trace elements, including magnesium, iron, zinc and copper, also act as enzyme activators, primarily in glycolytic and oxidative phosphorylation reactions.

Physical activity increases energy expenditure and theoretically increases the requirements and turnover of these micronutrients involved in energy metabolism. The B vitamins and zinc assist in the release of energy from carbohydrate, fat and protein. Minerals also act as coenzymes in energy metabolism, for example iodine for regulating metabolic rate in the thyroid gland, chromium for glucose metabolism and iron for cellular energy metabolism. The current data suggest that athletes have only slightly higher requirements for 'energy' nutrients than untrained controls, except for iron, levels of which are high in athletes involved in endurance training programmes.

This section considers only those micronutrients that have received the most research attention in relation to energy metabolism in athletes, namely the B vitamins, magnesium, chromium and iron.

B vitamins

Of the nutrients involved in energy metabolism, the B vitamins have received the most attention in athletes, particularly in relation to their primary and interactive role as coenzymes in carbohydrate and amino acid metabolism, the main substrates for providing energy or ATP to the muscle. Table 8.1 indicates other systems where B vitamins and folic acid have a role. For example, vitamin B_{12}, folate and vitamin B_6 are closely involved in the synthesis of red blood cells.

Suboptimal intakes and deficiencies of B vitamins are uncommon in athletes and levels are usually no different to those in untrained subjects. B vitamin deficiencies, usually reported in people with malnutrition, do not usually occur in isolation or in athletes. Subclinical B vitamin deficiencies based on low biochemical indices are more likely to occur in athletes, although there are limited studies available.

Interestingly, marginal thiamin deficiency was reported in cyclists after a simulated trial of the Tour de France. Given the high energy expenditure and high carbohydrate intakes of these athletes, rapid turnover and depletion of thiamin was not unexpected. Other B vitamins were not significantly depleted. Thiamin has a lower storage pool than other B vitamins, which explains its fast rate of depletion. For athletes participating in any long-distance event of high energy intensity, thiamin supplements or perhaps a B multivitamin supplement may be needed, if dietary intake is compromised. Subclinical thiamin deficiency is also associated with increased lactic acid levels during exercise, but marginal deficiency, induced by a thiamin-depleted diet, had no measurable effect on working capacity of exercising muscles.

Data on the effects of marginal riboflavin depletion on performance are scarce in athletes. Under situations of depletion or deficiency, urinary excretion of riboflavin decreases which conserves further loss. Although riboflavin is involved in muscle metabolism and neuromuscular function and is a co-factor in the production of the antioxidant enzyme glutathione peroxidase, no changes to muscle efficiency were reported in athletes undertaking moderate-intensity exercise after 7 weeks of a riboflavin-restricted diet. Similarly, for athletes involved in wrestling and judo with depleted vitamin B_6 status after a weight-cutting period, no effects on performance capacity in terms of anaerobic capacity, speed or strength were reported. In summary, acute or short-term marginal deficiencies of single B vitamins, identified by blood biochemical measures of their status, have no impact on performance measures. However, despite the apparent absence of a performance effect with depleted status of a single B vitamin, aerobic performance capacity may be impaired when there is combined depletion of thiamin, riboflavin and vitamin B_6. This highlights the synergistic role of the B vitamins and explains why is difficult to detect any performance effects from single vitamin depletion studies.

Do B vitamin supplements improve performance capacity?

Supplementation with either single B vitamins or multiple B vitamins can elevate biochemical or blood markers and improve a marginal to low micronutrient status, but has no significant effects on other metabolic systems or performance measures in athletes with adequate status, with few exceptions. In one study of male athletes, a combination of vitamin B_6 supplements together with other B-complex vitamins improved shooting target performance and improved muscle

irritability. These athletes had adequate vitamin B status. However, similar intervention studies in other trained athletes have reported no significant effects of vitamin B_6 or B multivitamin supplements on performance measures compared to controls.

There are only a few well-designed studies published that have investigated folic acid supplements in relation to sports-related functional capacity in athletes with adequate vitamin folate status. In these studies, folate supplementation slightly increased serum folate levels but did not affect maximal oxygen uptake, anaerobic threshold or other measures of physical performance.

In summary, based on the limited research published, vitamin B supplements taken as either single vitamin supplements or as a multivitamin B complex are unlikely to significantly affect or improve energy efficiency, oxygen uptake or performance capacity in athletes who are not deficient.

Magnesium and energy metabolism

Magnesium is a major mineral in bone and is involved in protein synthesis, enzyme action, muscle function including oxygen uptake, nerve impulse transmission, electrolyte balance and the immune system. Its role in substrate and energy metabolism in athletes has been the focus of most research in trained subjects. Strenuous exercise initiates a redistribution of magnesium in the body with a corresponding increase in magnesium loss via sweat, faeces and urine. These losses are significantly higher in athletes than untrained controls, which may increase requirements in athletes by up to 10–20% higher than usual. Magnesium deficiency, and even marginal depletion, can impair oxygen delivery and thus the ability to undertake and complete submaximal exercise, which can reduce endurance performance. Recent evidence suggests that habitual magnesium intakes of below 260 mg/day for male athletes and less than 220 mg/day for female athletes may result in magnesium deficiency. These cut-offs are slightly below the EAR (Estimated Average Requirement) for men of 330 mg/day (19–30 years) and women of the same age of 255 mg/day. The EAR is the 'amount of a nutrient consumed on an average daily basis that is estimated to meet the requirements of half the healthy individuals in a particular life stage and gender group'. This cut-off is used by health professionals to examine the probability that usual intake of a nutrient is adequate (or inadequate) in an individual subject. Clearly, the threshold of adequate intake and hence requirement in physically active individuals such as elite athletes is indicative of higher magnesium requirements than population benchmarks.

However, according to biochemical indices and dietary surveys of athletes, magnesium status appears satisfactory and is not compromised by these higher requirements, with some exceptions. Magnesium is a mineral in the chlorophyll molecule, which is used for photosynthesis in plant leaves. As expected, green leafy vegetables are good sources. As a mineral, it is absorbed from the soil and concentrates in other areas of the plant, particularly in the grain (or seed) so legumes, nuts, seeds and foods made from cereal grains (wholegrain) are rich sources. Highly processed and refined cereal grain foods are low in magnesium. Like all covalent minerals, absorption (or bioavailability) is decreased when magnesium-rich foods are consumed together with foods rich in phytates and oxalates (see Table 8.5).

Do magnesium supplements improve performance capacity?

Magnesium supplements do not consistently increase serum magnesium levels or improve physical performance in physically active individuals with low to adequate magnesium status. Magnesium supplements of 250–360 mg/day as magnesium aspartate or up to 500 mg/day as magnesium picolinate or magnesium oxide for 3–4 weeks in athletes who have low but not deficient indices of magnesium status have been shown in some studies to improve muscle function, cardiovascular function and work efficiency. Hence, there may be a beneficial effect for magnesium supplements in athletes during periods of high-intensity training involving glucose as the predominant substrate for metabolism. Nevertheless, other studies fail to show any beneficial or at least measurable enhancing effect on performance using magnesium supplements. The reason for this may be that magnesium fluxes or redistribution of magnesium associated with exercise is highly variable between individuals and seems to alter with the type of exercise performed (i.e. aerobic vs. anaerobic). Clearly, magnesium, like the B vitamins, does not work in isolation and exerts an independent effect on metabolic pathways.

In summary, magnesium supplements may be required in athletes at risk of suboptimal intakes or during periods of very high intensity workouts, when requirements are highest. The prevalence of low status is highest in the population in people consuming low energy intakes, so athletes involved in weight class sports or those who follow very low energy diets for whatever reason are likely to be at risk. Further research is needed in different groups of athletes undertaking varying levels of exercise intensities to determine the magnesium status and level of magnesium depletion at which energy systems are compromised. Adverse effects of magnesium depletion on immune function and oxidative damage also need further investigation.

Chromium and energy metabolism

Chromium is an essential trace mineral and has many roles in metabolism. In relation to sports performance, its role in enhancing the action of insulin, which is required for uptake of glucose and amino acids into the cell, has implications for enhancing glucose oxidation and recovery. Other claims in relation to its action on insulin are increases in muscle mass and strength.

It has been proposed that chromium supplementation during exercise, mainly as chromium picolinate, the most active form, enhances carbohydrate metabolism and promotes glycogen resynthesis, hence speeding up recovery of fuel reserves. Studies on these effects have not supported this hypothesis. Adding chromium picolinate to a sports drink provided no additional effect on carbohydrate metabolism above that of the carbohydrate content in the sports drink. Other claims of habitual use of chromium supplements to increase muscle mass and strength and reduce body fat have not been substantiated in well-designed studies using a control group (see Chapter 9). Athletes with restricted energy intakes are most at risk of low chromium intakes. Food sources of chromium include wholegrain cereals, eggs and poultry.

Iron and energy metabolism

Iron has many functions but is best known for its role in blood health (see following section). Iron is also a co-factor in several biochemical reactions involved in oxidative energy production, which occurs within the mitochondria, where it is a component of oxidative enzymes and respiratory chain proteins. Clearly, iron has a strong functional role in maintaining the energy release from macronutrient substrates needed to support aerobic and endurance capacity. When iron stores are exhausted, the functional iron compartment in the cells then becomes affected and the oxidative capacity of the muscle is compromised. Recent evidence suggests that even marginal iron deficiency can reduce maximum oxygen uptake and aerobic efficiency in the muscle cells (the functional site) and decrease endurance capacity (see section Does low iron status (iron depletion) affect performance and other health outcomes?, p. 74).

8.3 Nutrients involved in blood health, particularly red blood cell production and function

Physical training increases the number of red blood cells, the volume of blood plasma and can increase vascularity, which are normal physiological responses to training. Haemoglobin, the iron-containing protein in the red blood cells, transports oxygen from the lungs to the muscle cells, the site of substrate oxidation to energy. Iron is critical to the functional role of blood in oxygen transport and cellular oxidation reactions that occur in the mitochondria that generate ATP for muscle contraction. Iron is a nutrient of concern in athletes of both sexes, but particularly female athletes.

Other important micronutrients involved in blood health, in terms of the formation and function of red blood cells that may be of concern, are folate, vitamin B_{12} and the trace element copper. However, there are inadequate data on these nutrients to assess their significance in athletes. It is well established that requirements for iron are higher in athletes compared with untrained controls, although the data currently available are insufficient to allow any quantification of specific requirements for different groups of athletes. Severe deprivation of folate, vitamin B_{12} and iron results in anaemia and significantly reduces endurance performance capacity. Copper deficiency is rare. Iron deficiency, both with or without anaemia, can impair muscle function and limit work capacity, depending on the severity of the depletion and is the main focus in this section.

Iron

Iron has multiple functional roles in the body – in thyroid hormone metabolism, neural function and immune function – but its role in energy metabolism as a coenzyme (see section Iron and energy metabolism, p. 70) and blood health, particularly red blood cell production, has been the focus of research in athletes.

Role of iron in blood health and performance

In terms of performance, iron is important in maintaining energy release needed to support aerobic and endurance activity (see section Iron and energy metabolism, p. 70).

- Iron is part of haemoglobin, the protein in the blood that carries oxygen to, and carbon dioxide from, all the cells in the body. In particular, the brain has a large demand for oxygen, hence inadequate iron in the storage pool can eventually decrease haemoglobin and reduce oxygen delivery to the brain and other cells.
- Iron assists in oxygen diffusion to the cellular site of energy production.
- Iron is part of the enzymes needed to convert nutrients into energy for use by the muscles.
- Iron is needed for red blood cell production.

As iron stores deplete, the production and number of red blood cells correspondingly decreases until the point when iron deficiency anaemia occurs. Inadequate iron in the storage pool impairs red blood cell production. Anaemia is diagnosed when haemoglobin is below the reference population range and the red blood cells decrease in number and size (microcytic, i.e. small cells) and colour (hypochromic, i.e. pale in colour). Iron deficiency anaemia severely impairs aerobic and endurance capacity, work capacity and energy efficiency in trained and untrained subjects.

Is iron depletion or deficiency a common problem in athletes?

The estimated prevalence of iron deficiency anaemia in athletes is about the same as in the general population (about 3%). Although iron depletion is a continuous process, three stages of iron deficiency are now used as the current diagnostic criteria for iron deficiency in the USA. Stage 1 is diagnosed when iron stores are low (i.e. serum ferritin <12 µg/l) but there is still stainable iron in the bone marrow, the site of red

Table 8.3 Main risk factors associated with iron depletion and deficiency in athletes.

Risk factors	Reasons
Athletic/strenuous training	Increased iron (and zinc) requirements are a consequence of an increase in red cell and haemoglobin production
Growth and pregnancy	Increases iron (and zinc) requirements by stimulating an increase in red cell and haemoglobin production
Sweat loss	Iron lost from sweat can be substantial in some athletes
Blood loss	Nose bleeds, menstruation, haematoma, damage to red blood cells caused by footstrike haemolysis, losses via urine and gastrointestinal tract associated with tissue damage or ischaemia associated with strenuous exercise, ulcers
Chronic inflammatory diseases (e.g. inflammatory bowel disease and other non-infective inflammatory diseases)	Induces iron depletion and subsequent iron deficiency anaemia, if untreated
Medications	Misuse or prolonged use of anti-inflammatory medications such as non-steroidal anti-inflammatory drugs, chronic use of antacids
Inadequate total dietary iron intake and /or low nutrient bioavailability	Poor food choices, unbalanced diets, low-energy diets, vegetarian, vegan diets or high-carbohydrate diets (mainly cereal grains) which decrease iron bioavailability, low-haem iron intakes which increases bioavailability, avoidance of red meat and iron-fortified foods (e.g. breakfast cereals)

Adapted with permission from Fogelholm M. Vitamin, mineral and anti-oxidant needs of athletes. In: Clinical Sports Nutrition, 4th edn (Burke L, Deakin V, eds). Sydney: McGraw-Hill, 2010.

cell production. The point of exhausted iron stores or advanced iron depletion is termed *Stage 2 early functional iron deficiency*, which precedes *Stage 3 iron deficiency anaemia* (IDA). Stage 2 is characterised by low serum ferritin ($<12\,\mu g/l$), haemoglobin in the usual population reference range, low transferrin saturation and elevated serum transferrin receptor ($>8.5\,mg/l$) and no stainable iron in the bone marrow. The new haematological marker, serum transferrin receptor, has allowed researchers to better define the severity and stage of iron depletion.

However, the true prevalence of iron depletion (Stage 1 and Stage 2) in athletes is unknown because reported prevalence data in athletes has been based on varying serum ferritin values, an early marker for low iron stores. Most studies on athletes use ferritin levels of 20–$30\,\mu g/l$ as indicative of iron depletion or marginal iron deficiency. The lack of a definitive cut-off for ferritin for the different stages of iron depletion in early studies of athletes has therefore biased the prevalence data.

Nevertheless, three groups of athletes identified at high risk of iron depletion (based on low serum ferritin levels) are females, distance runners and vegetarians, including those who eat little red meat. The highest prevalence occurs in female and adolescent athletes,

irrespective of type of sport, age and gender. At the Australian Institute of Sport, where elite athletes live in residence with all meals provided, 19% of females and around 3% of males had ferritin levels below $30\,\mu g/l$, indicative of low, but not exhausted, iron stores. At this level, athletes are given iron supplements to help prevent further depletion.

Why are athletes at risk of low iron status?

Table 8.3 summarises the physiological and diet-related risk factors associated with the development of iron depletion in athletes. While diet is a main contributes to iron depletion, physiological and medical factors also play an important role. A combination of several risk factors explains why athletes are at high risk of iron depletion compared with non-athletes.

Hard training and growth stimulates an increase in the number of red blood cells and small blood vessels, increasing the physiological demand for iron. High iron losses associated with sweating, blood loss through injury, menstruation and foot strike haemolysis (associated with running on hard surfaces) and gastrointestinal blood loss during extreme exercise events also contribute. However, inadequate consumption of total dietary iron and low iron bioavailability are strong predictors of low iron status, especially in females.

Are iron requirements higher in athletes than non-athletes?

Athletes involved in regular high-intensity physical activity and endurance training programmes have the highest turnover of iron and hence the highest requirements. Both male and female adolescent athletes have the highest requirements because of the increased production of red blood cells and haemoglobin accompanying growth. Requirements for iron are higher in females than males to accommodate loss of iron from menstrual blood.

Average daily iron requirements and subsequent recommendations for athletes in different sports have not been established and are likely to be highly variable because of individual differences. According to nutrient reference standards, such as Dietary Reference Intakes (DRIs), recommended iron intakes for athletes are 1.3–1.7 times higher than normal population cut-offs and 1.8 times higher for vegetarians (non-athletes) to account for low iron bioavailability (see Table 8.5). Iron requirements may be even higher for female athletes who follow vegetarian-style diets. Such high requirements are unlikely to be met from dietary sources, without appropriate dietary planning.

Are iron intakes inadequate in athletes?

Suboptimal dietary iron intake is more of a determinant of low iron status in female than male athletes, because females generally eat less food and less red meat, a readily absorbable form of iron and a rich iron food source. Male athletes, especially endurance and adolescents, usually consume more than adequate iron intakes for their increased requirements but are still at high risk of low iron status. A high iron turnover, growth or low bioavailability of iron is a probable cause of low iron status in males. High-carbohydrate diets recommended for athletes undertaking high levels of physical activity are often high in naturally occurring compounds that inhibit iron absorption, particularly phytates (found in cereal grains, nuts, soya bean and its products).

Is absorption of iron from food compromised in athletes?

Two forms of iron are available from food, haem and non-haem iron. Meat, liver, seafood and poultry contain both forms whereas plant sources, mainly cereal and grains, legumes, vegetables, fruits, eggs, iron-fortified commercial foods (such as breakfast cereal)

Table 8.4 Iron-rich foods.

	Serving size	Amount of total iron (mg) per serving
Foods containing haem iron		
Liver, cooked	(75 g)	8.3
Lean, grilled beef rump steak	(100 g)	3.8
Lean, grilled trim lamb steak	(100 g)	3.5
Tuna, dark flesh	(75 g)	0.7
Lean, cooked pork, ham	2 slices (75 g)	0.6
Lean, cooked chicken (no skin)	1 small breast (75 g)	0.5
Fish, white flesh	1 average piece (75 g)	0.3
Foods containing non-haem iron		
Commercial breakfast cereal (iron-enriched)	Average serve (60 g)	5.6
Lentils, cooked	½ cup (120 g)	2.0
Baked beans in sauce	½ cup (120 g)	1.8
Nuts (cashews, almonds)	50 g	1.6–3.1
Bread (wholemeal)	2 sandwich slices (60 g)	1.4
Pasta, cooked	1 cup	1.0
Bread (white)	2 sandwich slices (60 g)	1.0
Rice, cooked	1 cup	0.7
Green vegetables (broccoli, cauliflower, cabbage, beans, peas)	½ cup (120 g)	0.5–1.5
Dried fruit (prunes, apricots)	5–6 (50 g)	0.6

Iron requirements: 8.7 mg/day for men and 14.8 mg/day for women.
Source: Data from NUTTAB, Food Standards Australia and New Zealand, 2006.

and iron supplements contain mainly the non-haem form (Table 8.4).

Haem iron is more readily absorbed than non-haem iron, which needs to be converted into a soluble form to be absorbed. Absorption of iron from non-haem food sources is highly variable and susceptible to the effects of inhibitory or enhancing factors naturally present in food (Table 8.5). In contrast, the absorption of iron from haem-iron food sources may be up to 10-fold higher than from non-haem sources, which explains why vegetarians and those on high wholegrain carbohydrate diets are at risk of low iron status.

Of the dietary enhancers listed in Table 8.5, vitamin C (ascorbic acid) is the most potent and can

Table 8.5 Components in food affecting the absorption (or bioavailability) of non-haem iron.

Promote iron absorption (by enhancing solubility)

Vitamin C-rich foods (in salad, lightly cooked green vegetables, some fruits and citrus fruit juices and vitamin C-fortified fruit juices)

Some fermented foods with a low pH (sauerkraut, miso and some types of soy sauce)

Peptides from partially digested muscle protein (i.e. 'meat enhancement factor' in beef, lamb, chicken, pork and fish)

Alcohol

Vitamin A (e.g. fats and meat) and β-carotene (e.g. green, orange vegetables and salad foods)

Citric acid (in citrus fruits)

Inhibit iron absorption (these form an insoluble salt with iron and bind it making it less soluble)

Phytate (in cereals grains, e.g. breakfast cereal, wholegrain bread; soy products, nuts and seeds)

Oxalate (in tea, spinach, rhubarb)

Polyphenolic compounds (e.g. tannates in tea, coffee, herb tea, cocoa)

Calcium (in milk and dairy foods)

Peptides from partially digested plant proteins

---

negate the inhibitory effect of phytates. When enhancers are consumed at around the same time as an iron-rich non-haem food, they reduce the iron into a more soluble form thereby favouring absorption; hence the rationale for consuming orange juice, a good source of vitamin C, with breakfast cereal, and consuming salad or tomato with bread. Even small amounts of meat, although a less potent enhancer than vitamin C, can reduce the inhibitory effect of phytates on non-haem iron absorption.

Iron absorption is also influenced by the iron status of an individual. When iron stores are saturated, iron absorption is around 5–15% from the total diet. In people with depleted iron stores or with high physiological requirements such as growth, pregnancy or lactation, iron absorption increases to around 14–16%. In athletes with high physiological requirements, the rate of absorption of iron has not been quantified. However, there is no reason why training programmes involving high physiological demands and a high iron turnover decrease iron absorption or any evidence to indicate compromised absorption in a healthy athlete.

Nevertheless low dietary iron intakes, low-energy diets and low bioavailability of iron from consuming high-carbohydrate diets are good predictors of low iron status.

Does low iron status (iron depletion) affect performance and other health outcomes?

Although it is well established that iron deficiency with anaemia impairs performance capacity, the effects on performance in the early to late stages of iron depletion without anaemia are less clear. However, recent findings in mostly untrained subjects have suggested that exhausted iron stores without anaemia had a negative impact on aerobic function and endurance capacity. These performance measures improved after repletion of iron stores. Theoretically, inadequate iron at the functional site, the tissues and cells, reduces capacity for oxidative metabolism. Even a mild shortfall in tissue iron status appears to reduce maximum oxygen uptake and aerobic efficiency. These effects have been reported in mostly untrained subjects and need to be replicated in elite athletes. The few studies undertaken on athletes to date have shown conflicting results.

Other effects of iron depletion, independent of its role in oxidative metabolism and red blood cell production, such as fatigue, altered resistance to infection, and muscle and hormone dysfunction, could also limit training capacity.

Do iron supplements improve performance in athletes without iron depletion?

The benefits of iron supplementation on performance in athletes with diagnosed iron deficiency anaemia (Stage 3) are well established. However, iron supplements do not improve performance in athletes with marginal iron depletion (Stage 1) but may have some benefit in advanced depletion or functional iron deficiency (Stage 2) where the tissue stores are low but haemoglobin levels are still in the normal range.

Are iron supplements recommended for athletes at risk of iron depletion or deficiency?

Where iron stores are exhausted, an iron-rich diet alone is insufficient to restore iron levels quickly. Iron supplements taken daily for at least 3 months in dosages of 80–100 mg elemental iron are necessary for full recovery of iron stores. Many athletes without a diagnosis of iron deficiency routinely take iron supplements at these dosages to prevent iron depletion or as a remedy for fatigue or for feeling flat and run down. Unfortunately iron supplements may do more harm than good.

The safety of long-term iron supplements at these therapeutic dosages is questionable even in apparently healthy subjects and may mimic the effects of the genetic disorder haemochromatosis. Haemochromatosis comprises a group of genetic conditions that allow iron to be indiscriminately absorbed, leading to iron overload in the tissues that results in irreversible damage. Iron supplements are contraindicated in people with haemochromatosis. The prevalence of this recessive genetic disorder is high in the white Caucasian population of northern European origin, with about 1 in 250 people who carry both genes and express the condition. The long-term consequences of this condition, if not treated, include damage to the cardiovascular system, increased risk of cancer, alterations in immune defence and high risk of infection. There is also some evidence that carriers of the gene (heterozygotes, around 10–15% of the white population) are also at increased risk of health problems, particularly cardiovascular disease.

In healthy people without the condition, iron absorption from the gastrointestinal tract is regulated by the hormone hepcidin, which maintain iron homeostasis and prevents overload. There is no physiological mechanism to excrete iron once absorbed. Hence, the consequences of taking repeated iron injections might have similar outcomes to untreated haemochromatosis and is not an uncommon practice is some sports, particularly professional cyclists. Very high serum ferritin levels have also been reported in groups of professional cyclists routinely taking high-dose iron supplements daily, which suggests some overload or possible disturbance in absorption.

Iron supplements also inhibit zinc and copper absorption, although evidence for inducing an actual zinc or copper deficiency has not been substantiated in athletes.

Other nutrients affecting red blood cells

Folate (folic acid) and vitamin B_{12} (cobalamin) are essential for the synthesis of DNA and RNA for cell division and for maturation of red blood cells. Both folate and B_{12} deficiency (and depletion) impair the production of DNA and RNA and hence red blood cell production. In the presence of deficiency, red blood cells are fewer in number and density. Vitamin B_{12} also maintains healthy nerves.

Vitamin B_{12} is only found in animal foods or products. Athletes consuming vegan diets need to eat foods either fortified with B_{12} or take vitamin B_{12} supplements or injections to maintain adequate status. It is unlikely that adolescent or adult athletes would develop B_{12} deficiency from any other cause than inadequate dietary intake, unless they have an autoimmune problem that interferes with their capacity for vitamin B_{12} absorption. Vitamin B_{12} deficiency is associated with long-standing vegan diets and with prolonged low energy intakes. Symptoms of deficiency include reduced tolerance to exercise, fatigue and several neurological symptoms including confusion.

Folate deficiency, at least at the population level, is the most prevalent of all vitamin deficiencies. Suboptimal intakes and subsequent low folate status is reported in females and in those people with a high requirement including adolescents and pregnant women. Folate may also be a nutrient of concern in young women participating in regular and intensive physical activity, but there are, to my knowledge, no recent data on biochemical status or dietary intake measures of folic acid status in female athletes. Several westernised countries are fortifying foods with folate, mainly to address the high prevalence of birth defects in pregnant women. Given the increased supply of folate in a wide range of products (particularly breakfast cereals), consumption has increased across the population (at least in Australia) and the incidence of birth defects has correspondingly declined. Whether physical activity or hard training programmes substantially increases folate requirements remains unknown.

8.4 Micronutrients involved in bone health

Although calcium is best known for its role in bone health, other factors including vitamin D, vitamin K, protein and fatty acids as well as fruit and vegetable intake, high-salt diets, caffeine and alcohol also have an influence (for more information, refer to Chapter 19). Exercise, particularly high-impact or weight-bearing exercise and to a lesser extent resistance exercise, provide some protection to bone health by improving bone mineral density (BMD). However, when exercise in combination with a low energy intake induces amenorrhoea, bone health is compromised; bone mass is lost and ultimately cannot be fully replaced. In this situation, calcium and vitamin D exert a weak effect in treatment but are essential for building bone mass and subsequently help to prevent stress fractures. Resumption of menstrual function, increasing energy availability and decreasing training load are important in protecting from further losses in BMD.

Calcium

Calcium is an important mineral for bone health. It maintains the structural or mineral content of bone and, in the presence of adequate intake, reduces bone resorption. Other functions of calcium in metabolism (in its ionised state) include regulation of muscle contraction, nerve conduction and normal blood clotting (see Table 8.2). Adequate dietary calcium during the growing years is essential for optimising peak bone mass; in adult years it helps in bone maintenance and slows the rate of bone loss. Bone loss of around 1% per year is a normal physiological process in both cortical and trabecular bone in both male and female, although women tend to lose cortical bone faster than men.

Weight-bearing or high-impact exercise, and to a lesser extent resistance exercise involving muscle pull on the loaded limb, increases bone mass at the skeletal site at which the strain is applied. Athletes who participate in impact sports like gymnastics, basketball and volleyball typically have higher BMD than sedentary controls and weight-supported sports. Weight-supported activities like swimming and cycling do not provide enough gravitational forces or mechanical loading on the skeleton to significantly improve bone mass. Reduced BMD has been reported in elite cyclists. Disrupted bone turnover that involves reduced bone formation and increased bone breakdown can occur in cyclists during stage racing. Inadequate energy intake relative to expenditure during racing (and training) may be one possible cause of low BMD among cyclists. Other causative factors implicated include low body weight, increased loss of calcium through sweat, and substantial time spent training.

Female athletes are at higher risk of low BMD, which is more strongly associated with disturbed menstrual function than low-energy diets, low calcium intakes or high calcium turnover. Female runners are a high-risk group for low BMD if they have amenorrhoea. Despite the benefits of weight-bearing exercise on bone mass, the high prevalence of amenorrhoea or oligoamenorrhoea in females involved in elite sport negates this benefit.

Consequences of inadequate calcium intake and amenorrhoea in athletes

Inadequate intakes of calcium and potentially other micronutrients involved in bone health, in combination with inactivity and low-energy diets, particularly in the bone-forming years can impair optimal skeletal development and increase the risk of stress fractures. The age of reaching peak bone mass is genetically determined and highly variable, and occurs in late adolescence or early adulthood after cessation of bone growth (between 16 and 28 years). Once peak bone mass is reached, it is mainly the mechanical forces acting on the skeleton that consolidates BMD.

The highest prevalence of stress fractures is reported in athletes with menstrual disturbances including those with delayed menarche, oligoamenorrhoea and amenorrhoea. Adolescents, irrespective of gender, are also at high risk of stress fractures during the growth spurt when BMD is lowest. In the USA, there has been a doubling of fractures in children over the last three decades, which is attributed to low levels of physical activity, suboptimal calcium intakes and subsequent low BMD. Failure to achieve peak bone mass characterised by low BMD, whether due to menstrual dysfunction or to dietary or lifestyle issues in adolescence or early adult years, may also hasten the onset of osteoporosis in later life. Although exercise offers some protection at weight-bearing sites in both adults and adolescents, it is not sufficient to negate the adverse effects of delayed menarche and the consequences of prolonged untreated amenorrhoea or oligoamenorrhoea on bone health.

In summary, a history of menstrual irregularity or delayed menarche impairs the attainment of peak bone mass and increases the risk of stress fractures, independent of calcium intake. Inadequate calcium intake, in combination with a low-energy diet during adult and adolescent years, can hasten the rate of bone loss and predispose an athlete to early osteopenia, stress factures and increase the risk of osteoporosis later in life.

Are calcium intakes inadequate in athletes?

Calcium intakes in adolescent and young adult female athletes are often far below the intakes required to optimise peak bone mass or prevent further bone loss. The prevalence of a negative calcium balance has increased in children and young females in western countries and is one reason for the increased incidence of stress fractures in children and adolescents. However, low energy availability associated with very low energy diets and amenorrhoea is a more predictive determinant of low BMD than suboptimal calcium intake.

Are calcium requirements higher in athletes than non-athletes?

Little is known about calcium requirements in physically active people, although calcium losses and bone turnover may be higher than in sedentary people. Calcium losses in sweat are substantial in men undertaking vigorous exercise (100–300 mg per session) but much less in women (around 90 mg after 1 hour of vigorous exercise). These lower values are probably associated with lower sweat rates, although few studies have been published in female athletes to confirm these differences. Calcium requirements may therefore be higher in athletes who sweat profusely. Obligatory calcium losses in urine in both men and women can be substantial (>200 mg/day) but are largely unaffected by exercise. High-protein diets, high-salt diets, smoking and alcohol increase urinary calcium excretion, although losses vary among individuals and depending on diet, lifestyle and genetic influences. There is some evidence that sports people can compensate for potentially high calcium requirements by absorbing more calcium, even with low calcium intakes. Although calcium is under homeostatic control, this mechanism does not fully compensate for very low calcium intakes or high calcium losses.

Calcium recommendations in athletes

In the absence of specific recommendation for calcium intakes for athletes, the appropriate population reference value, i.e. Adequate Intake (AI), can be used to estimate the probability of adequate (or inadequate) calcium intake in individual athletes, with caution. Population reference values for calcium have increased in western countries for all age groups over the last 10–15 years. The AI for maximal calcium retention for those aged 9–18 years is 1300 mg calcium daily, which was based on data from white females, the highest risk group. In adult females, the AI decreases to 1000 mg calcium daily. The goal for determining the AI in the USA and Canadian DRIs was to maximise calcium retention to optimise bone

health in the highest risk group. In adolescents and children, calcium retention and BMD is higher in males than females, and higher in blacks compared with whites. Hence, white females are at highest risk of negative calcium balance and poor bone health.

Where menstruation is delayed or absent, which is not uncommon in females undertaking strenuous training programmes, calcium recommendations are even higher. Although there are only a few intervention trials with calcium supplements published in athletic populations, the recommended intake of calcium for athletes with amenorrhoea is 1500 mg/day. This amount is similar to population recommendations for post-menopausal women not taking oestrogen.

Calcium recommendations may be slightly lower in blacks and males. Limited data are available on other population groups and may not truly reflect requirements. The US and Canadian DRIs for calcium are under review. Recent research suggests that the current cut-offs are an underestimate for some risk groups, particularly post-menopausal women, which could apply as well to female athletes with amenorrhoea.

Do high calcium intakes or calcium supplements improve bone health?

The best intervention strategy for improving bone health in any population group is largely unknown and influenced by many environmental, genetic, dietary and individual factors. In terms of meeting calcium recommendations, there is insufficient evidence to confirm the efficacy of using calcium-rich food sources, calcium supplements or both. Calcium supplements and/or high calcium intakes can improve calcium retention and balance. High-protein diets and high salt intakes increase calcium excretion. The current evidence favours increasing calcium intakes from food sources, which appears to increase bone accretion more than supplementation. This improvement has been attributed to the presence of coexisting nutrients in food and from better compliance with food than with taking supplements. The increased availability of calcium-fortified products, particularly products in a wide range of dairy foods and milks, should help athletes meet calcium recommendations.

For those athletes at risk of poor bone health, particularly females with menstrual disturbances or those on low-energy diets or avoiding or limiting dairy foods, calcium supplements may be needed to improve calcium retention. However, the independent benefits of calcium supplementation on increasing BMD at all stages of the life cycle are weak but may be worthwhile for some individuals but not everybody. In randomised controlled trials of pre-menopausal women without amenorrhoea, calcium supplements of around 1000 mg/day slightly increased bone mass (0–1.17% increase per year). In older post-menopausal women, calcium supplements assisted in maintenance of, but not gain in, bone mass. In a meta-analysis of randomised trials of older post-menopausal women, calcium supplements of 1000 mg/day prevented the expected 1% per year loss of both cortical and trabecular bone.

Little is known about the effects of calcium supplements or high calcium intake on improving bone mass in female athletes. In one study, supplemental calcium 800 mg/day taken for 1 year in 23 young adult female distance runners (without amenorrhoea) prevented cortical but not trabecular bone loss compared with matched controls. The average calcium intake in these women from dietary sources was close to or exceeded the AI of 1000 mg/day but energy intake in both the control and experimental group was fairly low at an average of about 1500 kcal/day. The few trials using higher doses of calcium supplements (up to 1500 mg/day) to increase BMD in amenorrhoeic athletes have shown equivocal results at different skeletal sites and may not have been conducted for long enough.

Where calcium supplementation is recommended, the amount required is dependent on the usual amounts of dietary calcium consumed and its bioavailability, which highlights the importance of using a dietitian to estimate calcium intake and food combinations to enhance bioavailability. Because of the interaction between calcium and vitamin D in bone health, a vitamin D supplement may also be needed for those athletes not exposed to adequate sunshine. Moreover, any gains in bone mass associated with calcium supplementation are not maintained after supplementation has ceased unless dietary calcium intakes are high to compensate. Clearly in the presence of amenorrhoea, other interventions including hormone replacement therapy and increasing energy availability are more important to conserving or preventing further losses in bone mass than calcium intervention alone.

Vitamin D

The prevalence of vitamin D deficiency or insufficiency has recently increased worldwide. Although the adverse effects of deficiency on bone health are well known, negative effects of deficiency on other body systems is just emerging. Low vitamin D status is expected to be highest in those athletes who train inside or have little exposure to the sun from living in high latitudes, are dark skinned, use sunscreen or wear protective clothing.

Vitamin D is both a hormone and a nutrient. It is manufactured in the liver and kidney from the action of ultraviolet (UV) rays from the sun (or other sources) reacting with the compound 7-dehydrocholesterol in the skin, where it converted to its inactive form called provitamin D_3 or cholecalciferol. Once transported to the liver, this inactive vitamin D, together with the small amount of vitamin D derived from food sources, undergoes further transformation into another form called 25-dihydroxyvitamin D_3 (also called calcidiol). This form of vitamin D_3 is finally transported to the kidney where it is converted to the primary activated form called 1,25-dihydroxyvitamin D_3 [$1,25(OH)_2D_3$] or calcitriol.

Role of vitamin D

Activated vitamin D (calcitriol) is essential in the regulation of calcium homeostasis. A deficiency results in inadequate bone mineralisation which, if prolonged, leads to rickets in children and osteomalacia in adults. Compromised vitamin D status does diminish bone health and increase fracture risk in elderly populations but whether the same effects occur in younger populations and athletes is speculative. In early studies of athletes with stress fractures, vitamin D status was overlooked as a risk factor and not measured.

However, the role of vitamin D goes beyond calcium and bone metabolism. There is now mounting evidence that vitamin D deficiency negatively influences muscle function, immune function, inflammation, cell differentiation and growth, and that deficiency increases the risk of chronic non-skeletal diseases including cardiovascular disease, hypertension and some type of cancers. Measuring vitamin D status in people with these conditions has been overlooked in clinical practice, until recently. There is also some speculation, given the multiple roles of vitamin D and the increased prevalence of vitamin D deficiency reported in several risk groups in the population (e.g. elderly in residential care, adolescents, dark-skinned and veiled women), that the recommended AI for vitamin D might be too low to maintain bone health and reduce chronic disease risk.

Vitamin D status in athletes

Only a few studies have been conducted on the vitamin D status or vitamin D intake of athletes. In these studies, 37–68% of athletes showed deficient status based on biochemical measures, which is similar to the prevalence in the general population and in the same at-risk groups. There is some evidence that those athletes who follow low energy intakes or vegan diets are also at risk of low vitamin D status but the reasons for this are unclear. Generally, dietary sources of vitamin D are a minor contributor to vitamin D status, compared with exposure to sunlight, but become a more important source during winter when the sun is not strong enough to provide enough UV rays. In Sydney, Australia during summer, exposure of the hands, face and arms for about 6–8 min daily is needed to prevent deficiency of vitamin D in light-skinned people. In winter, exposure time increases more than threefold during the hottest part of the day when the sun's rays are strongest. Individuals with darker skin need longer exposure to UV rays for vitamin D synthesis to occur than fair-skinned people. Vitamin D synthesis via the sun is not possible during most of the winter months for people living at latitudes of more than 40°N or 40°S because the sun never rises high enough to provide the direct sunlight needed. Sunscreen with an SPF of 8 or more blocks UV light needed for vitamin D synthesis.

Does low vitamin D status affect bone health and performance?

Currently, there are no known studies that have investigated the potential effects of marginal vitamin D deficiency on bone health or athletic performance. Given the multiple roles of vitamin D in human metabolism, a prolonged inadequate intake accompanied by a low biochemical status could increase the risk for stress fractures in athletes.

Are vitamin D supplements required in at-risk groups?

To potentially protect bone health and fracture risk in older people, supplementation with 1000–2000 IU vitamin D daily may be needed to prevent deficiency

Table 8.6 Recommended daily dosage of vitamin D_2 (ergocalciferol) supplements for prevention and treatment of vitamin D deficiency.

Prevent deficiency (in absence of adequate sun)	5–10 µg	200–600 IU
Reduce fracture risk (in elderly)	25 µg	1000 IU
Treat moderate to severe deficiency	75–125 µg (for 6–12 weeks)	3000–5000 IU (for 6–12 weeks)

Source: Working Group of the Australian and New Zealand Bone and Mineral Society, Endocrine Society of Australia, Osteoporosis Australia, 2005.

in those who are unable to gain adequate exposure to sunlight, particularly in the winter months (Table 8.6). The same recommendations could be applied to athletes at high risk of stress fractures or in similar environmental circumstances where exposure to sunlight is limited (e.g. female athletes with amenorrhoea). In the absence of adequate UV light or sunlight, dietary sources of vitamin D contain only small amounts of vitamin D, and are unlikely to be consumed in amounts that will maintain adequate vitamin D status. Mandatory fortification of foods with vitamin D has increased in recent times in several European countries, which is likely to improve intake from dietary sources. However, the number and range of foods fortified with vitamin D is highly variable and may not address the problem, particularly in those athletes with low energy intakes. The recommended dosage of vitamin D to prevent deficiency in the absence of adequate exposure to sunlight is 200–600 IU/day.

Once diagnosed, treatment of moderate to severe vitamin D deficiency requires vitamin D doses of 3000–5000 IU/day. Guidelines on prevention and treatment for the general population are summarised in Table 8.6. More research is needed to determine the prevalence of vitamin D depletion in athletes and the efficacy of vitamin D supplementation on infection, illness and stress fractures and BMD in trained athletes.

In summary, recommendations for improving bone health in athletes include maintenance of normal menstrual cycles (or oral contraceptive intervention), increasing dietary energy and/or calcium intake to at least meet or exceed the current recommended intakes, and adequate exposure to sunlight. Where access to sun is limiting and calcium intakes are suboptimal, a combination of vitamin D and calcium supplements may help to enhance peak bone mass in adolescents and young adults and help prevent further bone loss in adult women.

8.5 Micronutrients involved in antioxidant defence

The antioxidant properties of food containing antioxidant nutrients and the naturally occurring antioxidants present in our bodies have received considerable attention over the last few years in relation to their protective effects on several chronic diseases, for example atherosclerosis, retinopathy, muscular dystrophy, some cancers, diabetes and rheumatoid arthritis. Antioxidants provide a protective role in cells and tissues against oxidative damage from free oxygen radicals, which are formed during the reduction of oxygen in the inner mitochondrial membrane. Free radicals are generated continuously in response to the ongoing damage to cell membranes caused by metabolic processes, inflammation, and external aggravations such as exposure to cigarette smoke, sunlight and certain chemicals. These free radicals damage the membranes of susceptible cells, including muscle cells, other cells and cell components in tissues, hence their link with chronic disease.

This section considers the main dietary sources of antioxidants that have been studied in athletes (vitamins C and E) and whether taking them as supplements adds further protection to the antioxidant defence system. There is some research on the effects of vitamin E and vitamin C supplements on the antioxidant defence system although the outcomes are mixed, and suggest more harm than benefit. There is even less research on the effects of antioxidants from food sources, although the research in relation to prevention and treatment of chronic diseases has increased and looks promising. There are no or limited data on the effects of other dietary antioxidants (e.g. carotenoids, selenium and other non-nutrients such as polyphenols) on the antioxidant defence system in athletes. Zinc is one co-factor in endogenous antioxidant production and has received some recent attention, so it is considered here in relation to its role in antioxidant defence and its other functional roles relevant to athletes.

The effects of combined, rather than single, antioxidant supplements are addressed because of their interactive roles and potential additive effects on the antioxidant defence system.

Why are antioxidants important to athletes?

Acute exercise of high intensity and duration increases oxidative stress and the production of free oxygen radicals in both animals and humans. Oxidative stress is the term used to define the point at which the build-up of free oxygen radicals exceeds the capacity of the body's antioxidant defence mechanisms, allowing the free radical to react and damage cell components. Acute exercise can induce a 10–15 fold increase in the generation of free oxygen radicals. These large amounts of circulating free oxygen radicals and other reactive oxygen species react with lipid membranes, enzymes, protein receptors and DNA resulting in muscle damage and impaired muscle function. Oxidative damage is a consequence of oxidative stress and is also linked to fatigue and reduced immune function in athletes.

However, despite the potential for oxidative damage associated with acute bouts of exercise, regular physical activity has well-known beneficial and protective effects for health. This apparent conflicting situation is often termed the *exercise–oxidative stress (EXOS) paradox* yet it is not known why this paradox exists. Several researchers have hypothesised that regular physical activity induces some adaptation to the damaging effects of free radicals by recruiting more endogenous antioxidants to enhance the protective effect. Whether athletes need higher dietary antioxidants than sedentary people because of a higher turnover of oxygen radicals imposed by high-intensity training and competition is still controversial and speculative.

Sources of antioxidant micronutrients

Several dietary micronutrients support the body's endogenous antioxidant defence systems, which allow free radicals to be neutralised to help decrease oxidative damage. Antioxidants are derived from both exogenous (dietary) and endogenous (body) sources. Endogenous antioxidants include uric acid, bilirubin, plasma proteins and the enzymes superoxide dismutase, glutathione peroxidase and catalase.

Dietary antioxidants include vitamin C, vitamin E, carotenoids (mainly β-carotene), polyphenols (e.g. flavonoids), selenium, glutathione and coenzyme Q_{10}. Endogenous antioxidants are dependent on micronutrients for their activation. Zinc, copper and manganese are required for the activation of superoxide dismutase, selenium and riboflavin for glutathione peroxidase and iron for catalase, thereby exerting an indirect association with antioxidant activity. Dietary antioxidants are found mainly in plant sources including dark-coloured vegetables and citrus fruits, legumes, nuts, grains, seeds and oils. They are also added to many commercial foods to help prevent chemical deterioration (oxidation reactions from the oxygen that is either naturally present in food or from contact with the air).

Vitamin C

Vitamin C is an effective scavenger of free oxygen radicals. It acts as an electron donor to minimise damage from free radicals, maintains the activity of glutathione (an endogenous antioxidant), and recycles oxidised vitamin E for reuse by cells. High concentrations are found in white blood cells and in eye and lung tissue, where its antioxidant effects are critical for defence against free radicals produced from known environmental aggravations. Reported data on vitamin C status in athletes are scarce. The few studies published on athletes have not shown any significant differences in the urinary excretion of ascorbic acid (an indicator of depleted vitamin C status) between athletes and controls, which further suggests that training does not have any special negative effects on decreasing vitamin C status. It is unlikely that athletes will have compromised vitamin C status unless citrus fruits, fruit juices and vegetables are excluded from the diet.

Do vitamin C supplements improve performance?

The other roles of vitamin C that may have implications for performance or which influence an athlete's capacity to undertake exercise are in immune function and the synthesis of essential cell compounds (e.g. carnitine, and the catabolic hormones noradrenaline and adrenaline). Its role in wound healing and bone repair and in reducing the severity of the common cold could have implications for athletes. Theoretically, depleted vitamin C status could affect these functions.

In terms of performance capacity, a 3-week vitamin C depletion study confirmed a decrease in work efficiency, which improved after 3 weeks of vitamin C supplements 500 mg daily. However, the majority of studies on athletes using vitamin C supplements have not shown any measurable effects on performance measures including lactate threshold, oxygen uptake or heart rate, which have a link with the anabolic hormones. In these studies, none of the athletes were vitamin C depleted.

However, the use (or misuse) of a vitamin C supplement to prevent or treat the common cold cannot be ignored in athletes who may be susceptible to upper respiratory tract infections (URTIs). Three placebo-controlled trials have demonstrated a moderately favourable effect of vitamin C supplements in athletes on reducing the risk of URTIs compared with those on placebo. Subjects in all trials were trained athletes undertaking strenuous physical training. A recent Cochrane meta-analysis concluded that vitamin C supplements did not affect the incidence or duration of the common cold in the general population. There has been some support for short-term use of vitamin C supplements in decreasing the incidence of URTIs in athletes undertaking endurance training programmes, but no beneficial effects have been reported in athletes undertaking lower levels of exercise.

Prolonged use of vitamin C supplements can cause adverse effects. Recent evidence suggests that doses of 1000 mg/day can interfere with the antioxidant defence system rather than protect it (see section Zinc, p. 82) and can potentially inhibit the cellular adaptation to exercise, a normal physiological response to training. Further studies are needed on athletes to test this effect.

Vitamin E

Vitamin E is a fat-soluble vitamin that is incorporated into the lipid structures of all cell membranes, where it offers direct protection from lipid peroxidation by free radicals. It also protects vitamin A from oxidation and improves absorption of vitamin A. From an immune system perspective, vitamin E enhances cellular immunity, possibly by reducing the effects of free radicals and other reactive oxygen species (i.e. lipid peroxides) that can induce an inflammatory response. In terms of its antioxidant effects, vitamin E deficiency increases susceptibility to free radical damage in animal studies, but true vitamin E deficiency is uncommon in healthy humans. The effects of physical activity on changing the vitamin E levels in plasma and muscle are equivocal. Prolonged use of high doses of vitamin E, similar to vitamin C, can do more harm than good.

Most people have adequate vitamin E status because of the ample storage pool in the body, although dietary intakes may be low in some at-risk groups. Although vitamin E is under homeostatic control, dietary intakes determine plasma levels because there is no endogenous production. Athletes likely to be at risk of suboptimal vitamin E intake and marginal vitamin E status are those on prolonged low-fat and/or low-energy diets. The main food sources of vitamin E are unsaturated oils, margarines, nuts, seeds and wholegrain products. Vitamin E is concentrated in the germ part of the seed and is also found in small amounts in vegetables. The effect of marginal vitamin E status on the antioxidant defence system is not clear.

Do vitamin E supplements improve performance?

Vitamin E supplements alone or in combination with vitamin C do not attenuate lipid peroxidation (or cell membrane damage) during exercise. High doses of vitamin E, combined with high oxidative stress induced by acute high-intensity exercise, may create vitamin E radicals that actually initiate lipid peroxidation of cell membranes. This further damages cell membranes. Moreover, well-controlled studies have not supported the hypothesis that vitamin E supplements reduce exercise-induced muscle damage or have ergogenic effects.

Zinc

Zinc is a co-factor for the enzymes associated with the antioxidant defence system and many other systems involved in growth, energy production and immune function (see Tables 8.1 and 8.2). There are over 300 enzymes in the body that are known to be zinc-dependent. Exercise increases zinc metabolism and hence athletes have slightly higher requirements than sedentary people, because of:

- increased production in red blood cells, which take up more zinc (see section Nutrients involved in blood health, particularly red blood cell production and function, p. 72, Table 8.3);
- zinc lost from sweat, urine and faeces;
- stimulation in antioxidant activity of Zn_2Cu_2 superoxide dismutase, an endogenous antioxidant enzyme dependent on zinc;
- increased activity of other enzymes dependent on zinc (e.g. lactate dehydrogenase).

Zinc lost from sweat ranges from 0.6 to 1.4 mg/l, which translates into a 17–42% increase in the daily requirements for each additional litre of sweat lost. Mineral loss in sweat is an extrapolated measure and varies at each collection site so is not accurate, but provides a reasonable estimate of zinc loss and is used to measure relative differences between and within groups. In athletes, there appears to be a decrease in zinc (and iron) loss from sweat in the latter stages of endurance exercise which suggests some adaptation. Urinary loss of zinc appears unaffected by exercise.

Studies of zinc requirements and zinc status in athletes are limited and confounded by poor sensitivity of the biochemical markers for zinc status (i.e. serum zinc). The available research suggests that zinc status is no different from controls. Theoretically, the requirements for zinc and copper (in Zn_2Cu_2 superoxide dismutase) and selenium (in glutathione peroxidase, another endogenous antioxidant source) may be higher than normal in physically active people to support the increased activation of the antioxidant defence system.

In the general population, marginal zinc intake and low status is more prevalent in females than males because females eat less food. Adolescent girls and vegetarian women are at high risk. Inadequate protein intake, particularly red meat, and high fibre intakes are associated with suboptimal zinc intakes. Like iron, zinc is subject to similar interference from inhibitory components in food (e.g. phytate, tannate) that decrease bioavailability (see Table 8.4). According to nutrient reference standards, vegetarians may require as much as 50% more zinc than non-vegetarians because of either low intake or poor bioavailability. Because of low bioavailability and losses, requirements may be even higher in vegetarian athletes undertaking strenuous training programmes.

Does zinc deficiency or insufficiency affect performance and antioxidant function?

It is well documented that severe zinc deficiency inhibits growth and delays secondary sexual development in adolescents and can impair the immune response. The effects of mild zinc deficiency are less clear in the general population and have been rarely studied in athletes. In one study, where mild zinc deficiency was induced, total work capacity declined and lactic acid levels increased in response to exercise, but peak performance was not affected. This may have been linked to the role of zinc in energy metabolism and decreased activity of the zinc-dependent enzyme lactate dehydrogenase, involved in lactic acid metabolism.

Although some studies suggest that zinc supplements may influence the recruitment of fast twitch muscle fibres, there is no measurable ergogenic effect of zinc supplements in individuals consuming diets adequate in energy and nutrients. Any benefits of zinc supplementation on the antioxidant defence system are unknown and have not been studied. Nevertheless, the misuse of zinc supplements by athletes may be of concern (see section Potential adverse effects of vitamin and mineral supplement use in healthy people, p. 83).

Are antioxidant requirements higher in athletes than non-athletes?

Current evidence supports a slightly higher oxidant requirement in athletes than non-athletes but there are insufficient data to quantify the amounts required. Population nutrient standards (e.g. EAR/AI) are unlikely to match these higher requirements in individuals undertaking repeated strenuous exercise. Recent evidence from epidemiological studies on chronic disease intervention suggests that dietary sources of antioxidants are preferable to single or combined antioxidant supplements and do not initiate the pro-oxidative or damaging effect associated with high doses of vitamin C and vitamin E supplements (see following section). The protective effect of diets rich in antioxidants is not simply attributed to antioxidants in isolation. Fruit, vegetables and wholegrain cereals contain other compounds that have protective physiological functions.

A low-dose antioxidant supplement containing several antioxidants together may be warranted in athletes who have difficulty meeting their higher antioxidant requirements from food. Moreover, there is no clear evidence to suggest that an athlete will benefit from high dosages of antioxidant supplements, despite the theoretical basis.

Do antioxidant supplements improve oxidative defence systems?

Antioxidant supplements (particularly vitamins E and C) are touted by manufacturers as a means to reduce or eliminate oxidative damage from free radicals. Because of their antioxidant properties, taking these and other antioxidant supplements might protect against the damaging effects of free radicals and other reactive oxygen species, induced during strenuous exercise. However, free radicals are an important stimulus for skeletal muscle adaptations. A balance between the pro-oxidative and antioxidative state is required for cell signalling and adaptation to exercise. A pro-oxidant accelerates oxidative damage. The recent findings from several studies have shown that antioxidant supplements (i.e. vitamins C and E) can blunt these positive adaptations to exercise and may actually counteract the known beneficial effects of regular physical exercise.

Moderate doses of vitamin C and vitamin E supplements in the usual recommended dosages (i.e. 1000 mg/day of vitamin C and 500 IU/day of vitamin E) have the potential to cause more harm than good in attenuating the oxidative damage induced by exercise. Vitamins taken as supplements in these dosages favour a pro-oxidant rather than an antioxidant effect. The levels or dosage and combination of antioxidant supplements needed to alter the antioxidant/pro-oxidant balance into one that is favourable for reducing oxidative stress induced by exercise is still unknown. Until further research is undertaken, prolonged use of moderate- to high-dosage supplements of vitamin E and vitamin C is not recommended.

8.6 Potential adverse effects of vitamin and mineral supplement use in healthy people

For those athletes who have poor dietary habits and miss one or more food groups, a multivitamin and multimineral supplement may be worthwhile for preventing further depletion or maintaining status, particularly during periods of high training intensity or growth. Prolonged use of any single vitamin or mineral supplement without a diagnosed deficiency may do more harm than good and interfere with the balance and interaction of other micronutrients.

Table 8.7 Potential adverse effects associated with misuse of commonly used vitamin supplements.

	RNI (~19–50 years)	RDI/RDA (19–30 years)	UL*	Potential health consequences, nutrient interactions and side effects of habitual excessive supplement intake (at intakes above UL)
Water-soluble vitamins				
Thiamin (mg/day)	0.4 mg/1000 kcal	1.2 (M)	NP	None known. Considered safe at 50–100 times RDA
		1.1 (F)		Associated with strong-smelling urine
Riboflavin (mg/day)	1.3 (M)	1.3 (M)	NP	None known. Considered safe at 100 times RDA
	1.2 (F)	1.1 (F)		Yellow discoloration of urine which is harmless
Vitamin B$_6$ (mg/day)[a]	15 µg/g protein	1.3 (M and F)	50	Sensory neuropathy. The effects of doses >200 mg/day are potentially irreversible after withdrawal
Niacin (nicotinamide and nicotinic acid) (mg/day)[a]	6.6 mg/1000 kcal	1.3 (M) 1.2 (F)	35 nicotinic acid 900 nicotinamide	Once used therapeutically to lower serum cholesterol. Flushing of face, arms and chest, risk of liver damage, glucose intolerance, blurred vision, itching, burning and tingling sensations (more pronounced with nicotinic acid than nicotinamide)
Folate (folic acid) (µg/day)[a]	200 (M and F)	400 (M and F)	1000	Masks symptoms of vitamin B$_{12}$ deficiency by inhibiting formation of megaloblasts that indicate B$_{12}$ deficiency. Risk of neurological damage, potential interference with zinc metabolism and consequent risk of inducing zinc deficiency
Vitamin B$_{12}$ (cobalamin) (µg/day)	1.5 (M and F)	2.4 (M) 2.0 (F)	NP	None known
Vitamin C (mg/day)[a]	40 (M and F)	90 (M) 75 (F)	NP but 1000 mg/day accepted as a prudent limit	Can act as a pro-oxidant and accelerate oxidative damage and may blunt the adaptive effects of the antioxidant system that occurs in people undertaking regular physical activity at intakes as low as 1000 mg/day. Nausea and diarrhoea, abdominal cramp and nose bleed, increased risk of kidney stones in susceptible people at intakes >2000 mg/day. Enhances iron absorption from non-haem food: risky for people with haemochromatosis
Beta-carotene (vitamin A) (pro-vitamin A)	NA	NP	NP	Excess storage under the skin causes yellow discoloration, which is harmless and transient on withdrawal; can occur from consuming large amounts of carrot juice
Fat-soluble vitamins				
Vitamin A (retinol equivalents preformed vitamin A) (µg/day)[a]	700 (M) 600 (F)	900 (M) 700 (F)	3000 (preformed)	Risk of spontaneous abortion and birth defects, loss of appetite, blurred vision, hair loss, abdominal pain, nausea, diarrhoea, liver and nervous system damage. Known toxicity from eating excessive liver or kidney
Vitamin D (IU/day)[a]	0 (if exposed to sun)	600	4000	Interferes with calcium homeostasis and can induce hypercalcaemia and hypercalciuria and increased risk of kidney stones in susceptible people, and calcium deposits in soft tissue. Irreversible renal and cardiovascular damage if prolonged

Table 8.7 (Cont'd)

	RNI (~19–50 years)	RDI/RDA (19–30 years)	UL*	Potential health consequences, nutrient interactions and side effects of habitual excessive supplement intake (at intakes above UL)
Vitamin E (α-tocopherol equivalents = total tocopherol)[a]	>4 mg/g PUFA (M) >3 mg/g PUFA (F)	300 mg/day (M and F)	1000	Inhibits blood clotting, increased risk of haemorrhage and stroke, interferes with vitamin K and vitamin A absorption Risk of pro-oxidative effects. High doses of α-tocopherol combined with high oxidative stress may create α-tocopherol radicals that may initiate processes of lipid peroxidation by themselves

[a] Adverse effects reported with supplement use.

* UL refers to RDI/RDA values only.

NP, not possible to set; NA, not available; RNI, Reference Nutrient Intake (UK); RDA, Recommended Dietary Allowance (USA/Canada); RDI, Recommended Dietary Intake; UL, upper intake level for adults.

Adapted from Institute of Medicine of the National Academies: Dietary Reference Intakes for calcium and vitamin D: Brief report, November, 2010 http://www.iom.edu/~/media/Files/Report%20Files/2010/Dietary-Reference-Intakes-for-Calcium-and-Vitamin-D/Vitamin%20D%20and%20Calcium%202010%20Report%20Brief.pdf accessed on 12th April 2011; Nutrient Reference Values for Australia and New Zealand Including Recommended Dietary Intakes. National Health and Medical Research Council, Canberra, Australia, 2006; and Department of Health: Report on health and Social subjects 41. Dietary Reference Values for food energy and nutrients for the United Kingdom, Committee of Medical Aspects of Food Policy, 1991.

Some vitamins and mineral supplements, if misused, have adverse side effects that may not be reversible (Tables 8.7 and 8.8). The DRIs can be used as a benchmark for assessing the risk of adverse effects. The tolerable upper intake level (UL) is the highest daily intake likely to pose no risk of adverse effects for almost all healthy individuals according to life stage and gender. It takes into account all contributing sources of a nutrient derived from food, fortified foods, water and supplements. As intake increases above the UL, the risk of adverse health effects increases.

Adverse effects of excess vitamin and mineral intake from food sources are highly unlikely. Adverse effects are reported with supplements of most fat-soluble vitamins, except vitamin E (Table 8.7). Chronic supplementation of vitamin D at very high levels can interfere with calcium metabolism and induce hypercalcaemia, hypercalciuria and formation of calcium deposits in soft tissue. Adverse effects of water-soluble vitamin supplements are less frequent than those of fat-soluble vitamins because they have a minimum storage pool. Nevertheless, vitamin C, vitamin B$_6$ and niacin taken in large doses have reported toxic effects.

Because minerals are mostly under homeostatic control, severe toxicity from taking supplements is rare. High mineral supplement use may interfere with nutrient absorption at the intestinal mucosa. For example, chronic use of elemental iron supplements at doses of 80–100 mg/day, the usual dose for treating iron deficiency, can interfere with copper and zinc absorption and increase the risk of zinc deficiency. Conversely, zinc supplements as low as 50 mg/day decrease both copper and iron absorption and at higher doses (160–660 mg/day) can induce anaemia and abnormal copper status and alter the immune response (Table 8.7). Interestingly, zinc supplements are linked to bone loss in women with osteoporosis, although well-designed randomised controlled trials are needed to confirm this association in athletes. This evidence suggests that a surplus of one trace element may cause marginal deficiency of another, especially when the intake of the latter is marginal. High calcium intakes taken as supplements may enhance the adverse side effects of vitamin D. Although there is no published UL for calcium supplement use, 1000 mg/day (the usual dosage provided in calcium supplements) is accepted as a prudent limit (Table 8.7).

Given the multiple roles of vitamins and minerals in different body systems, prescribed doses of multivitamins or multiminerals taken as directed (although they may not be needed) are considered

Table 8.8 Potential adverse effects associated with misuse of mineral supplements.

	RNI (~19–50 years)	RDI/RDA (19–30 years)	UL*	Potential health consequences, nutrient interactions and side effects of habitual excessive supplement intake (at intakes above UL)
Macrominerals				
Calcium (g/day)	700 (M and F)	1000 (M and F)	2500	Interferes with iron, zinc and magnesium absorption. Calciuria and risk of kidney stones in susceptible people
Trace minerals				
Magnesium (mg/day)	300 (M and F)	400 (M) 310 (F)	350a	May impair immune function and promote oxidative damage. Nausea, diarrhoea and abdominal cramps
Iron (mg/day)	8.7 (M) 14.8 (F)	8 (M) 18 (F)	45	Contraindicated in people with haemochromatosis. High ferritin levels from supplements reported in cyclists taking prolonged large doses as a prophylactic. Chronic use of iron supplements (80–100 mg/day) can inhibit zinc and copper absorption and increase risk of zinc deficiency. Therapeutic doses of iron supplements for diagnosed deficiency often not well tolerated by some people: constipation, black stools, abdominal discomfort, some complaints of diarrhoea, nausea and vomiting. Most side effects resolve when taken with food. Can act as a pro-oxidant and cause damage to heart, central nervous system, liver and kidneys. Increased risk of cancer in people with haemochromatosis
Zinc (mg/day)	9.5 (M) 7.0 (F)	11(M) 8 (F)	35	Low toxicity: nausea, vomiting, diarrhoea and lethargy reported at therapeutic doses >1000 mg/day. Chronic use at therapeutic doses (160–660 mg/day) may induce iron deficiency anaemia, abnormal copper status and alter the immune response
Chromium (μg/day)	NA	35 (M) 25 (F)	NP	Interferes with iron absorption, no other known symptom
Selenium (μg/day)	75 (M) 60 (F)	55 (M and F)	400	Vomiting, nausea, weakness, cirrhosis of the liver. Skin rashes, brittle hair and nails

a Excludes food and water sources and represents intake from a supplement only.

* UL refers to RDI/RDA values only.

NP, not possible to set; NA, not available; RNI, Reference Nutrient Intake (UK); RDI, Recommended Dietary Intake; RDA, Recommended Dietary Allowance (USA/Canada); UL, upper intake level for adults.

Adapted from Institute of Medicine of the National Academies: Dietary Reference Intakes for calcium and vitamin D: Brief report, November, 2010 http://www.iom.edu/~/media/Files/Report%20Files/2010/Dietary-Reference-Intakes-for-Calcium-and-Vitamin-D/Vitamin%20D%20and%20 Calcium%202010%20Report%20Brief.pdf accessed on 12th April 2011; Nutrient Reference Values for Australia and New Zealand Including Recommended Dietary Intakes. National Health and Medical Research Council, Canberra, Australia, 2006; and Department of Health: Report on health and Social subjects 41. Dietary Reference Values for food energy and nutrients for the United Kingdom, Committee of Medical Aspects of Food Policy, 1991.

safe and unlikely to substantially upset the balance of other micronutrients. Many multivitamin and multi-mineral supplements may also contain other herbal or non-nutrient ingredients that often claim functional or physiological improvements to health or performance without having been subjected to appropriate scientific testing to confirm their efficacy. Of even greater concern is that traces of substances prohibited by the World Anti-Doping Agency, including ephedrine and pro-hormones (e.g. steroid-related compounds including androstenedione, dehydroepiandrosterone and 19-norandrostenedione), have been detected in several supplements targeted at sports people, including vitamins and minerals. These results were derived from a study in 2004 of over 600 supplements from 215 suppliers in 13 countries and analysed in a laboratory accredited by the International Olympic Committee. Whether the presence of these prohibited substances came from inadvertent contamination at manufacture, poor quality control or inappropriate labelling was not clear.

Most countries, including westernised countries, do not have adequate quality control testing of supplements from locally produced or imported products. Further information on contamination from supplements can be found in Maughan (2005) and Geyer *et al.* (2008). An athlete competing in sports that apply anti-doping codes is personally liable for ingesting a prohibited substance regardless of the source. For more information about risks associated with different ingredients in multivitamin and multimineral supplements, athletes should contact the anti-doping agencies in their country.

8.7 Summary

Vitamins, minerals and trace elements have multiple and synergistic functions across many body systems. When deficiencies occur for whatever reason, more than one vitamin and/or mineral is usually responsible. Physical activity increases the metabolic requirements for vitamins and minerals associated with energy metabolism (particularly B vitamins, magnesium, chromium and iron). Prolonged aerobic exercise increases red blood cell mass and the requirements for nutrients involved in red blood cell production and haemoglobin synthesis (e.g. iron, vitamin B_{12} and possibly folate). Current evidence supports a higher antioxidant requirement in athletes than non-athletes to help reduce oxidative damage induced by short-duration exercise. Population nutrient references (i.e. EAR/AI) are unlikely to match these higher requirements.

Because of the multiple functional interactions between micronutrients, it is not possible to quantify micronutrient requirements of athletes, except for iron, which has been extensively studied. Recommended iron requirements for athletes are 1.3–1.7 times higher than population nutrient references. Measures on micronutrient status and supplementation trials are needed to evaluate whether normal dietary intakes of other micronutrients in athletes are sufficient to cover their increased requirements.

Micronutrient deficiencies are rarely reported in athletes. Athletes at risk of deficiency are those who restrict energy intakes or avoid one or more food groups or in exceptional circumstances or extreme endurance events. Marginal micronutrient depletion is more common. Based on biochemical markers of nutrient status, the vitamins of concern in at-risk groups are folate, thiamin, vitamin B_6, vitamin B_{12}, and, more recently, vitamin D. Minerals known to be of concern are calcium, zinc, iron and magnesium.

Calcium and iron require special attention in athletes. Low calcium intakes result in a negative calcium balance and an increased risk of low BMD, which is associated with a corresponding increased risk of stress fractures. Amenorrhoea, delayed menarche or menstrual irregularities, a common problem in elite athletes, in combination with low-energy diets (or low energy availability) and low calcium intakes increases the risk of stress fractures and risk of osteopenia and osteoporosis in later life.

Suboptimal intakes of iron are evident in athletes who follow low-energy diets, very high carbohydrate diets, fad diets and vegetarian-style diets. Yet many athletes, irrespective of gender, have high iron intakes and still battle with iron depletion. The reasons for this are usually low bioavailability of iron or very high requirements and turnover associated with intense training programmes or growth.

Overt nutrient deficiencies can affect performance capacity. However, marginal micronutrient deficiencies do not consistently impair physical work capacity, except perhaps for iron. It is not known the point at which depletion of one or several nutrients might affect performance or health because insufficient studies of biochemical markers of micronutrient status have been conducted in athletes. Athletes identified at risk of iron, vitamin B_{12}, vitamin D and possibly zinc depletion, based on a medical or nutrition assessment, may benefit from a blood test to confirm status. The rationale for using routine biochemical screening for at-risk athletes for marginal depletion of water-soluble vitamins, magnesium or other trace elements is not justified.

Studies on athletes with adequate nutritional status do not conclusively show that micronutrient supplementation benefits physical performance. The evidence is limited and biased by poor research design, small sample size and the multiple interactions of nutrients in different systems, which are often overlooked and confound interpretation of any real effect.

Vitamin and mineral supplements are frequently used by competitive and recreational athletes and may have adverse reactions with prolonged use or upset the natural physiological balance and interaction between micronutrients. High intake of single micronutrients may lead to physiological disturbances, especially if the diet is inadequate. Supplementation with vitamin C may decrease the incidence and duration of URTIs but evidence is equivocal and often associated with misuse and excessive intake. Contrary to popular belief, adverse effects are reported with excess supplement use of vitamin C and other water-soluble vitamins, vitamin B_6 and niacin. Whether antioxidant supplements such as vitamins E and C attenuate oxidative damage induced by exercise of high intensity is still questionable. Even in moderate doses these supplements can act as pro-oxidants and exacerbate oxidative damage rather than protect against it. If, for any reason, an athlete wants to use micronutrient supplements as a precaution without a diagnosed deficiency, a multivitamin/multimineral supplement at the recommended dosage is likely to be both safe and adequate for optimal sports performance.

Because of a wide safety margin, the appropriate DRI cut-offs for vitamins and minerals may still be used for individual athletes when assessing the probability of adequacy (or inadequacy) of miconutrient intake or planning diets, although with caution. Until research suggests otherwise, dietary intervention to correct suboptimal micronutrient intakes is the preferred approach, rather than supplements. Using food rather than supplements has the added benefit of nutrient density and improved bioavailability without the potential risk of adverse side effects from misuse of supplements.

Further reading

Cumming RG. Calcium intake and bone mass: a quantitative review of the evidence. Calcif Tissue Int 1990; 47: 194–201.

Deakin V. Prevention, detection and treatment of iron depletion and deficiency in athletes. In: Clinical Sports Nutrition, 4th edn (Burke L, Deakin V, eds). Sydney: McGraw-Hill, 2010.

Dietitians of Canada, American College of Sports Medicine, American Dietetic Association. Joint position on paper: Nutrition and athletic performance. Med Sci Sports Exerc 2009; 41: 709–731.

Douglas RM, Hemilä H, Chalker E, Treacy B. Vitamin C for preventing and treating the common cold. Cochrane Database Syst Rev 2007; (18): CD000980.

Evans WJ. Vitamin E, vitamin C, and exercise. Am J Clin Nutr 2000; 72 (Suppl): 647S–652S.

Fogelholm M. Indicators of vitamin and mineral status in athletes' blood: a review. Int J Sport Nutr 1995; 5: 267–286.

Fogelholm M. Micronutrients: interaction between physical activity, intakes and requirements. Public Health Nutr 1999; 2: 349–356.

Fogelholm M. Vitamin, mineral and anti-oxidant needs of athletes. In: Clinical Sports Nutrition, 4th edn (Burke L, Deakin V, eds). Sydney: McGraw-Hill, 2010, pp 268–294.

Geyer H, Parr MK, Koehler K, Mareck U, Schanzer W, Thevis M. Nutritional supplements cross contaminated and faked with doping substances. J Mass Spectrom 2008; 43: 892–902.

Institute of Medicine. Dietary Reference Intakes for calcium, phosphorus, magnesium, vitamin D, and fluoride. Washington, DC: National Academy Press, 1997.

Institute of Medicine. Dietary reference intakes for vitamin A, vitamin K, arsenic, boron, chromium, copper, iodine, iron, manganese, molybdenum, nickel, silicon, vanadium and zinc. Washington, DC: National Academy Press, 2000.

Lukaski HC. Magnesium, zinc, and chromium nutriture and physical activity. Am J Clin Nutr 2000; 72 (Suppl): 585S–593S.

Lukaski HC. Vitamin and mineral status: effects on physical performance. Nutrition 2004; 20: 632–644.

Manore MM. Effect of physical activity on thiamine, riboflavin, and vitamin B-6 requirements. Am J Clin Nutr 2000; 72 (Suppl): 598S–606S.

Maughan RJ. Contamination of dietary supplements and positive drug tests in sport. J Sports Sci 2005; 23: 883–889.

Nielsen FH, Lukaski HC. Update on the relationship between magnesium and exercise. Magnes Res 2006; 19: 180–189.

Peake JM. Vitamin C: effects of exercise and requirements with training. Int J Sports Nutr Exerc Metab 2003; 13: 125–151.

Sanders EM, Nowson CA, Kotowicz MA et al. Calcium and bone health: position statement for the Australian and New Zealand Bone and Mineral Society, Osteoporosis Australia and the Endocrine Society of Australia. Med J Aust 2009; 190: 316–320.

Weaver CM. Calcium requirements of physically active people. Am J Clin Nutr 2000; 72 (2 Suppl): 579S–584S.

Weaver CM. Current calcium recommendations in North America. Asia Pac J Clin Nutr 2008; 17 (Suppl 1): 30–32.

Whiting SJ, Barabash WA. Dietary Reference Intakes for the micronutrients: considerations for physical activity. Appl Physiol Nutr Metab 2006; 31: 80–85.

Willis KS, Peterson NJ, Larson-Meyer DE. Should we be concerned about the vitamin D status of athletes? Int J Sport Nutr Exerc Metab 2008; 18: 204–224.

Working Group of the Australian and New Zealand Bone and Mineral Society, Endocrine Society of Australia, Osteoporosis Australia. Vitamin D and adult bone health in Australia and New Zealand: a position statement. Med J Aust 2005; 182: 281–285.

9
Supplements and Ergogenic Aids

Hans Braun, Kevin Currell and Samantha J Stear

Key messages

- Dietary supplement use in athletes is widespread. Higher supplement use can be expected with increasing performance level and age.
- Popular dietary supplements include multivitamins, vitamin C and some minerals, but the popularity of products differs between sports and/or countries.
- Coaches, parents and physicians are significant sources of information about the use of supplements.
- Supplementing the diet does not make a bad diet better and the excessive intake of some supplements can do more harm than good.
- Indiscriminate use of supplements is unwise due to potential health, contamination and inadvertent doping risks.
- There is a placebo effect surrounding the use of dietary supplements on sports performance, with the placebo response differing between individuals.

9.1 Introduction

The use of dietary supplements (DS) in sport is widespread. However, UK Sport, amongst other sporting authorities including the International Olympic Committee (IOC) and the World Anti-Doping Agency (WADA) advise athletes not to take supplements due to the associated risks and provide resources to help the sporting community make informed choices by better understanding the risks involved. Other leading sports authorities and organizations (e.g. FIFA, ACSM) also recommend that 'athletes should ensure they have a good diet before contemplating supplement use'.

In the USA, the medical division of the US Olympic Committee (USOC) provides supplementation guidelines for athletes, coaches and healthcare professionals based on the goal of providing safe intakes of individual nutrients to promote healthful training regimens and recovery periods. In conclusion the USOC states that:

'the use of supplements is appropriate only in conjunction with a good diet. Dietary evaluation should

be made by a qualified health professional and food intake patterns should be adjusted if necessary to promote optimal health. If a thorough dietary evaluation is not possible and cursory review of the athlete's dietary habits indicates possible reason for concern, prophylactic supplementation may be desirable'.

UK Sport's resource 'Sports Supplements and the Associated Risks' takes this a stage further in its conclusion, stating that 'whilst a healthy, balanced diet remains the best way to achieve sufficient levels of vitamins, minerals and other nutrients, some supplements do have a place in high performance sport for some athletes'.

However, across the globe, many athletes, even at the elite level, have a low level of nutritional knowledge, not too dissimilar to the general population. Furthermore, very few athletes have access to a qualified dietetic/nutritional professional for dietary evaluation and nutritional counselling. A recent study in German athletes showed that only 54% of German Olympic athletes and 18% of young elite athletes had received an individual nutritional

Sport and Exercise Nutrition, First Edition. Edited by Susan A Lanham-New, Samantha J Stear, Susan M Shirreffs and Adam L Collins.
© 2011 The Nutrition Society. Published 2011 by Blackwell Publishing Ltd.

consultation and therefore their knowledge about what constitutes an optimal habitual diet may be limited (H. Braun, personal communication).

A varied well-balanced diet that meets the energy demands of training should provide adequate amounts of all the essential nutrients. However, sometimes this is not possible, and in some situations obtaining sufficient amounts from the diet is often not so straightforward. Consequently, many athletes take DS in the hope that it will compensate for poor food choices and make up for vital nutrients that they feel are potentially lacking in their diet.

What are dietary supplements?

'Dietary supplements', 'functional foods', 'nutraceuticals', 'ergogenic aids' and 'sports supplements' are just some of the terms used interchangeably within both scientific publications and the sporting arena. The term 'dietary supplements' implies that it is something which supplements the diet.

The Oxford English Dictionary definition of a supplement is 'something added to supply a deficiency'. However, this definition is inconsistent with the majority of DS usage, with many supplements, or their individual ingredients, being nutrients or food chemicals for which the body does not have an estimated or theoretical requirement. Thus, there are clearly other factors that underpin their use by athletes.

According to the US Food and Drug Administration (FDA):

'a dietary supplements is a product (other than tobacco) that is intended to supplement the diet and bears or contains one or more of the following dietary ingredients: a vitamin, a mineral, a herb or other botanical, an amino acid, a dietary substance for use by humans to supplement the diet by increasing its total daily intake, or a concentrate, metabolite, constituent, extract, or combination of these ingredients'.

This differs slightly from the definition provided by the European Food Safety Authority (EFSA), which uses the term 'food supplement':

'A Food Supplement is a concentrated source of nutrients or other substances with a nutritional or physiological effect whose purpose is to supplement the normal diet. They are marketed in dose form i.e. as pills, tablets, capsules, liquids in measured doses etc'.

Furthermore, EFSA states that:

'Supplements may be used to correct nutritional deficiencies or maintain an adequate intake of certain nutrients. However, in some cases excessive intake of vitamins and minerals may be harmful or cause unwanted side effects; therefore, maximum levels are necessary to ensure their safe use in food supplements'.

The European Commission has established harmonised rules to help ensure that food supplements are safe and properly labelled. In the EU, food supplements are regulated as foods and the legislation (Directive 2002/46/EC; www.efsa.europe.eu) focuses on vitamins and minerals used as ingredients of food supplements. Nutrients other than vitamins and minerals, or other substances with a nutritional or physiological effect, are being considered for regulation at a later stage when adequate and appropriate scientific data about them becomes available. Until then national rules concerning nutrients or other substances with nutritional or physiological effect may be applicable.

The regulatory environment is under constant progressive change, but legislation differs across countries. Although the DS category is subject to strict regulations, it has historically suffered from poor policing of claims. In general, the food industry firmly adheres to local legislation, but this is not always seen to be the case for some DS manufacturers that appear to 'sit outside' the food industry. Increasingly strict monitoring by regulatory bodies in the USA, Europe, Asia and Oceania will hopefully improve the situation.

9.2 The dietary supplements market

Globally the DS market is estimated to be greater than US$60 billion. The largest DS market is the USA at US$23.7 billion with a predicted compound annual growth rate of 5% for the 5-year period 2008–2013 from the latest calculations. Figure 9.1 shows the

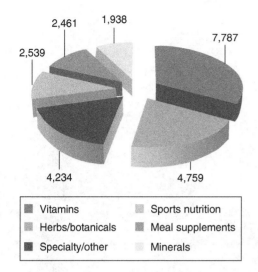

2,461   1,938
2,539   7,787

4,234   4,759

- ■ Vitamins   ■ Sports nutrition
- ■ Herbs/botanicals   ■ Meal supplements
- ■ Specialty/other   ■ Minerals

Figure 9.1 US dietary supplement market. (Data from Rea & Ooyen 2009.)

split of the main supplement subgroups for the largest DS market in the USA. In terms of this analysis the subgroups are split according to the following descriptors.

- 'Herbs/botanicals' include single or multi-herb DS made primarily from plants or plant components.
- 'Sports nutrition' subcategory includes pills, powders/formulas and sports supplement drinks (excluding carbohydrate/electrolyte 'sports drinks') that are formulated to enhance physical activity.
- 'Meal supplements' include shelf-stable liquid nutritional formulas primarily to substitute, but sometimes supplement, a meal (e.g. weight-loss formulas).
- 'Specialty' includes those DS that do not fit into other categories, e.g. glucosamine, melatonin, probiotics/prebiotics, DHEA, fish CoQ10, 5HTP, colostrum, enzymes, hormones.

In terms of growth, 'specialty' is growing the most at around 11%, followed by 'sports nutrition' at around 8%, with the rest exhibiting slow growth at around 4%.

The total size of the DS market in the EU is esti mated to be around €5 billion, with people from the UK estimated to spend around £335 million per annum (Mintel, 2009). About 50% of the products in the EU contain vitamins and minerals, while supplements containing other substances have a market share of 43% (about €2.15 billion). The growth of

the market (1997–2005) for food supplements containing other substances varies enormously between the European countries and ranges from 20% in the UK to 219% in Poland. The number of substances other than vitamins and minerals used in food supplements on the European market is estimated to be over 400.

Furthermore, products or substances do not have the same popularity across countries. For example, fish oils constitute over 40% of the market of other substances in the UK, but under 3% in Spain and Italy. Probiotics account for 44% of the market in Italy but only 1% in the UK. Herbal products (e.g. ginkgo, ginseng, St John's Wort, echinacea and garlic) make up 75% of the market in the Netherlands, 40% in France, and 16% in the UK. Figure 9.2 shows the range of popular DS bought in the UK.

9.3 Prevalence of dietary supplement use

Surveys show that nearly half of all athletes use supplements, with their popularity varying widely between different sports and between athletes of differing ages, performance levels and cultural backgrounds. In some sports, particularly strength and power sports, supplement usage is so common it is perceived as the norm.

According to a Target Group Index survey, supplement use in the general population is different between countries (www.tgisurveys.com). While supplement use in Thailand is lowest (1%), the prevalence is higher in France and Germany (25%), Northern Ireland (39%), Great Britain (42%), Ireland (44%), USA (56%) with the highest levels in Croatia (64%) and Serbia (70%). A meta-analysis of 51 studies on supplements, involving more than 10 000 athletes at all levels and participating in 15 sports, found that the mean prevalence of supplement use among all subjects was 46%, with 'study groups' ranging from 6 to 100% (Sobal & Marquardt, 1994).

Studies on UK athletes found similar supplement use. One study found that 59% of UK athletes used at least one supplement (Petroczi & Naughton, 2008), with another showing 62% DS usage in British junior national track and field athletes (Nieper et al., 2005). A study of DS usage in 286 British Olympic athletes, competing at the 2004 Athens Olympics, found that

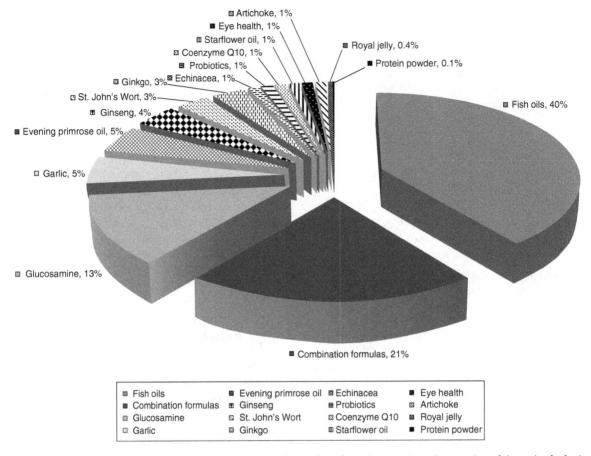

Figure 9.2 legend:

▣ Fish oils	▨ Evening primrose oil	▩ Echinacea	▪ Eye health
▪ Combination formulas	▦ Ginseng	▤ Probiotics	▨ Artichoke
▣ Glucosamine	▨ St. John's Wort	▨ Coenzyme Q10	▨ Royal jelly
▢ Garlic	▨ Ginkgo	▥ Starflower oil	▪ Protein powder

Figure 9.2 An example of popular dietary supplements bought in the UK. (Data from Characteristics and perspectives of the market for food supplements containing substances other than vitamins and minerals. © European Union 2008. http://ec.europa.eu/food/food/labellingnutrition/supplements/documents/2008.)

53% declared taking supplements on their medical preparation forms, with DS usage being more common in female (59.3%) than male (48.5%) athletes (Stear *et al.*, 2006).

It seems probable that DS usage by elite athletes exceeds that of college athletes, which in turn exceeds that of high school athletes. Furthermore, there is good evidence that DS use increases with age both in elite athletes (Maughan *et al.*, 2007) and in the general population. A difference in general DS usage between gender has only been found in a few studies. However, a gender difference in supplement use might exist for certain supplements (e.g. creatine, protein, vitamins, iron) or for specific sports. Consequently, a higher DS usage can be expected with increasing age and the performance level of the athlete.

Furthermore, not only is supplement usage common, but all too often the recommended doses are exceeded. Sometimes this is simply an attempt to outdo what the athlete believes their opponent is taking. However, more does not necessarily mean better, and in the case of some supplements, such as the fat-soluble vitamins (A, D, E and K) and iron, more can be toxic. Therefore, caution is advised surrounding excessive intakes of some DS as they may do more harm than good.

9.4 Common sports nutrition supplements

The list of supplements and ergogenic aids used within the exercise and sporting environment is exhaustive. Supplements also come in many forms

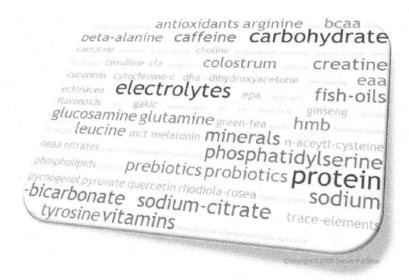

Figure 9.3 Tag cloud of popular sports nutrition supplements. (Reproduced with kind permission. Copyright © 2009 Samantha Stear.)

and guises. Figure 9.3 illustrates some of the most popular DS used in the sport and exercise arena. By using a 'tag-cloud' the most popular DS in terms of efficacy can be illustratively ranked: the largest font size (carbohydrate, electrolytes and protein) represent the most efficacious down to the smallest font size (e.g. bee pollen, glandular and yucca) representing the least efficacious.

Among 32 studies reviewed in 1994, multivitamins were the most popular DS, followed by vitamin C, iron and B vitamins (Sobal and Marquart, 1994). This seems to continue to be the trend. A study of DS usage in 286 British Olympic athletes found that vitamin C (65% of supplement users) was the most common DS declared by athletes followed by multivitamins and minerals, iron, protein supplements, vitamin E, selenium and zinc (Stear et al., 2006). A more recent, larger study that analysed questionnaires from 874 UK athletes, where 520 athletes (~60%) declared DS use (Petroczi et al., 2008), found that the most common DS were multivitamins (73%) and vitamin C (71%), followed by creatine (36%), whey protein (32%), echinacea (31%), iron (30%), caffeine (24%), magnesium (11%) and ginseng (<11%).

A study of 113 German Olympic athletes found magnesium to be the most popular (81%), followed by vitamin C (59%), multivitamins (52%), iron (50%) and zinc (42%), while ergogenic aids such as creatine (20%) and caffeine (6%) were rarely used (Braun et al., 2009a). Further, examination of the popularity of magnesium found it to be one of the most common DS in Germany, Portugal and Poland (~80% usage), but it is less popular in the UK and Norway (~10%). Despite the different evaluation questionnaires used in these studies, the popularity of magnesium does seem to vary widely between countries.

DS usage patterns vary across countries, athletic level and sports. The popularity of certain types of DS demonstrates that athletes may often be more motivated by health rather than the ergogenic benefits of some DS. However, some sports foods, such as carbohydrate/electrolyte 'sports drinks', have become so common in the sporting environment that athletes no longer perceive these as DS and hence the recording of their usage amongst studies may be inconsistent.

9.5 Reasons for dietary supplements usage

Athletes should always consider the issues of efficacy, safety and legality/ethics associated with DS products prior to deciding on their use. Unfortunately, all too frequently, specific information is limited. Studies examining the performance-enhancing effects of the vast array of supplements are relatively few, especially investigations relevant to real-life sports events and elite athletes. Studies involving specialised subpopulations such as paralympic athletes are particularly rare, and subsequent decisions regarding efficacy must often be extrapolated from the best available research rather than clear-cut evidence.

Common explanations to justify the use of DS by athletes include:

- to prevent or treat a perceived nutrient deficiency, particularly when requirements for a nutrient are increased (believed or real) by their training programme;
- to provide a more convenient form of nutrients in situations where everyday foods are not practical, particularly to address nutritional needs/goals around a training session;
- to provide a direct ergogenic (performance-enhancing) effect;
- because they believe every top athlete is consuming it and they cannot afford to miss out.

Interestingly, studies also found that large numbers of athletes report using supplements, and do so just because others (e.g. colleagues, coaches) recommend them. Even if the key rationale behind DS use cannot be identified, it seems that health and performance-related reasons are the most popular. However, this might be different according to type of product (vitamins vs. carbohydrates), moment of use (daily use vs. competition), age or gender.

It is important to note that the decision to use supplements is not always a rational one. Even when athletes are informed that their diet is sufficient or that the nutrient status of their body's stores is normal (e.g. iron stores), they still continue to take DS perhaps as a form of 'just in case' insurance.

9.6 Who recommends dietary supplements

Among the many support staff working with athletes, coaches seem to be an important source of information on DS. While adult athletes also report health professionals (physicians, physiotherapists, dietitians/nutritionists) as influential, young athletes state their parents to be an important source of information on DS. Other influential factors include marketing and advertising of supplements, which is dependent on the sport and/or media where it is published (e.g. muscle-increasing supplements in bodybuilding magazines). Based on such findings, it seems necessary to educate not only athletes but also coaches, parents and health professionals about the use of supplements alongside associated risks and benefits.

9.7 Efficacy of dietary supplements

Evaluation: levels of evidence

When deciding on the efficacy of a supplement it is important to look at the level of evidence available to support supplement efficacy. The traditional view of evidence is based on four levels.

- *Level 1: anecdotal evidence or expert opinion.* This is common in the supplement marketplace, particularly when high-profile athletes promote the use of a particular supplement.
- *Level 2: case series or observational studies.* Less common in the supplement research literature.
- *Level 3: randomised controlled trials.* The most common type of research undertaken in the supplement literature. However, it is key that the research is of suitable quality (Table 9.1).
- *Level 4: systematic reviews and meta-analysis.* The highest level of evidence to show efficacy of a supplement. However, these are rare and may not always be available, especially for newer supplements which appear on the market.

When assessing whether there is evidence to support the use of a supplement, the research should be at level 3 or 4. Caution should be taken when using the supplement if the research is only at levels 1 and 2. In addition, Table 9.1 outlines some of the other key factors that need to be taken into consideration when assessing a research paper on DS.

Recent advances in technology have resulted in an increase in the amount of *in vitro* research being conducted and subsequent claims regarding supplement use. This is important evidence to consider and should not be dismissed. However, quite often when looking at the body as a whole, the supplement may work differently from what may happen *in vitro* (Table 9.2).

Table 9.1 Factors to consider when assessing a research paper on sports supplements.

Factor	Considerations
Participants	Are they similar to the athletes you want to use the supplement with? Consider age, gender and training status
Type of performance test	Is the test valid and reliable?
Control of the study	Is the study well controlled? Does it account for factors such as diet, training and sleep?
Design of the study	Is the study placebo-controlled and double-blinded? Are there enough participants to provide statistical power? Does the design simulate real life? Is the supplement given acutely or chronically?
Supplements	Has the supplement(s) been analysed to prove ingredient composition and tested for contaminants particularly WADA banned substances?
Funding source	Is the research funded by an organisation with a vested interest in the outcome of the research?

Table 9.2 Questions to consider when deciding if a supplement will work.

Does the supplement get broken down in the mouth?
Does the supplement interact with receptors in the mouth?
How is the supplement absorbed in the gastrointestinal system?
Once absorbed does it get to the site of action?
Is the amount absorbed enough to provide a performance-enhancing effect?
Is the amount which reaches the site of action enough to provide a performance-enhancing effect?
Are there other confounding factors to consider?

Finding proof of efficacy

Measuring performance

The ideal use of supplements should be based on scientific evidence which supports a performance-enhancing effect of the supplement. However, measuring performance in a scientific controlled manner is difficult and open to debate. There are three things which need to be considered when evaluating sports performance research.

- Validity: is the protocol measuring the type of performance desired?

- Reliability: can the test be repeated with only a small variance in performance?
- Sensitivity: is the test able to detect a change in performance which has both practical and statistical significance?

In linear-based sports such as running and cycling there has been much debate about how best to measure performance.

- *Time to exhaustion trial.* The traditional method of measuring performance is a steady-state time to exhaustion (TTE) trial, originally derived from animal studies. These TTE trials provide an excellent way within which to control many external variables. However, they have limited authenticity to actual sports performance as the aim of no sporting event is to perform to exhaustion. There is an argument that in events such as a marathon the race is won by the person who can hold the greatest pace for longest, which may provide some support for the validity of a TTE trial. However, remaining at a single pace will eliminate the role of pacing in performance, which is a key aspect of sports performance. TTE trials tend to have a high coefficient of variation (CV), with values of greater than 10% generally being reported in the literature.
- *Time trials.* Time trials are more representative of sports performance and therefore are more valid measures of performance. They also tend to have a lower CV, with values between 1 and 5% regularly being reported in the literature.

For sports which are more complicated and where performance is not necessarily determined by physiological outcomes (e.g. football and tennis), it is key to ensure that actual outcomes measured affect the performance outcome. For instance in football, skill performance and perception of patterns of play are important constructs to consider when assessing the performance effects of a supplement. Table 9.3 outlines the key factors that need to be controlled when trying to measure performance.

True performance effects

In order to find a true performance effect of a supplement it is important to understand what is the smallest worthwhile effect that will lead to an improvement in performance. The difference between coming first and second in a race is often much less than 1% of the

Table 9.3 Factors to control when performance is being measured.

Factor to control	Reason
Familiarisation	Reliability increases with increased exposure to the protocol
Verbal encouragement	If this was not standardised, then this could affect the performance outcome
Music	Music affects performance and ideally should not be available during a performance trial
Feedback	Minimal feedback should be provided so as not to influence performance in subsequent trials
Measurements	Taking physiological measures during performance may disrupt performance

overall time of the race. This is such a small difference that it can frequently not be detected by traditional methods of performance testing and statistical analysis. These small differences between winning and losing are an important factor when considering a supplement. Quite often a coach and athlete will be unconcerned with statistical significance if they believe that there may be a chance of improving performance.

Disadvantages

When the evidence has been collected to show a possible benefit to performance, it is absolutely critical that any side effects are considered and the negative aspects of using the supplement are also considered. If there are any known effects that are detrimental to the athlete's health, these must be explored and controlled for.

While any negative health effects are a priority, it is also important to consider other factors.

- *Cost*: quite often supplements can be costly, particularly those which are for chronic use.
- *Doping*: will there be any inadvertent positive doping test using the supplement?
- *Interaction with other supplements*: while some supplements work in synergy, others may interact to provide negative outcomes.
- *Adaptation to training*: some supplements can interfere with the natural adaptation to training.
- *General diet*: supplements should not be used as a method to support a poor diet. Athletes may want to use supplements to avoid having to eat appropriately.

- *Performance*: some supplements which have side effects such as weight gain may not be appropriate in some sports.

9.8 Classification of dietary supplements: the APRID framework

There are numerous methods for classifying supplements, including those based on their effectiveness. Therefore, because of the vast array of supplements it is often felt useful to provide practitioners working alongside athletes with a classification framework as guidance. Many of the Olympic training centres and institutes of sports across the world have devised their own supplement frameworks. Probably the most well-known supplement programme is that of the Australian Institute of Sport (AIS), comprising a ranking system for supplements and sports foods (www.ausport.gov.au/ais/nutrition/supplements/overview). In consideration of ongoing scientific research and increasing innovation and development in the sports nutrition industry, all supplements frameworks are working documents that are accurate to the date of the most recent update.

The APRID framework, devised by Stear and Currell, initially for use by performance nutrition practitioners working at the English Institute of Sport, UK, divides supplements into five categories.

A   Acceptable: these supplements have a proven performance or health benefit with evidence available at level 4.

P   Physiological: these supplements have a clear physiological rationale as to why they would improve performance or health. However, the performance or health outcomes are not proven. Evidence is generally at level 2 and 3.

R   Research: the performance, health and physiological evidence is unclear. However, there is anecdotal evidence from practice that the supplements may be of benefit. Evidence is at level 1 and 2.

I   Ineffective: there is no rationale for using the supplement.

D   Disallowed: these supplements are either directly banned and on the WADA Prohibited Substances List, or are deemed to be a high risk for a positive doping case, and therefore should not be used by athletes.

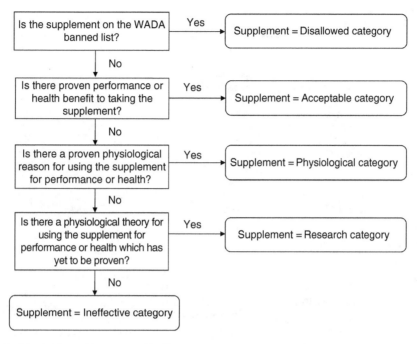

Figure 9.4 Schematic of the decision making-process utilised in APRID.

The APRID framework utilised many learnings from the excellent AIS supplement programme, localising and adapting it to meet the specific status and needs of both athletes and practitioners in the UK at the time of its inception. In addition, the APRID framework was developed from the Strength of Recommendation Taxonomy (SORT) developed by the American Board of Family Practice (Ebell *et al.*, 2004) (Figure 9.4).

Table 9.4 provides an overview of the APRID framework as an example of a current classification framework. As a working document it was designed as a resource for sports medicine and sports science practitioners that could be continually updated with the latest scientific research evidence along with any relevant WADA rulings. However, it was not made widely available, in the hope of limiting overuse and misuse by some vulnerable athletes.

The APRID framework provides a ranking system for sports foods, DS and ergogenic aids, based on a risk–benefit analysis of current evidence from both scientific research and clinical dietetic practice. The framework's five hierarchical groups provide practitioners with guidance of an evidence-based 'freedom to operate' within those groups. For the top three

groups (A, P and R), further information on each of the sports foods and supplements is provided within the full framework and includes a brief description, performance or health uses of the supplement, physiological rationale behind the supplement, key supporting evidence, suggested protocol(s) including recommended dosage, proposed methods for monitoring effectiveness, and a column for individual practitioners to add further comments. The key individual supplements or groups of supplements are reviewed in the following sections.

'Acceptable' category

In the APRID classification, the category 'Acceptable' gives practitioners freedom to operate with these sports foods and supplements, if deemed useful and appropriate for the athlete in question. However, this in no way means that all athletes should use, or indeed will see a benefit from, this group of supplements. Consideration still needs to take into account key factors, including the level of evidence supporting the supplements, the source of evidence (clinical or sports science), and the athlete's needs and requirements. For this group of 'Acceptable' sports

Table 9.4 APRID: an example of a dietary supplement classification framework.

Acceptable	Physiological	Research	Ineffective	Disallowed
Scientific research has shown a clear performance or health benefit to the supplements use.	There is a clear physiological rationale for using the supplement. However, the performance or health outcome research is unclear.	The physiological and performance/health outcome are unclear. However, there is practitioner based evidence that there may be a benefit to using the supplement in elite sport. Evidence must be gathered by the practitioner for its use.	There is no clear physiological, performance or health benefit to using the supplement.	These DS supplements are either directly banned and on the WADA Prohibited Substances List, or are deemed to be a high risk for a positive doping case, and therefore should not be used by athletes.

Acceptable	Physiological	Research	Ineffective	Disallowed
Sports Foods	**Antioxidant**	**Antioxidant**	**Examples of ineffective**	**Prohibited supplements:**
Carbohydrate drinks, powders, gels and bars	**Cardiovascular effects**	Cysteine	Bee pollen	Anabolic Agents
Carbohydrate-electrolyte 'sports' drinks ad powders	Arginine/Citrulline	Green Tea extract/EGCG	Chromium picolinate	Anti-oestrogenic Agents
Carbohydrate & Protein 'recovery' drinks, powders and bars	**Buffer capacity**	Quercitin	Coenzyme Q10	Beta-2 Agonists
Electrolyte replacements	Beta-Alanine/Carnosine	Resveratol/Grape seed extract	Cordyceps	Diuretics & other Masking Agents
Protein powders, drinks and bars	**Muscle growth and repair**	**Cardiovascular effects**	Cytochrome C	Hormones & related substances
Liquid Meal Supplements	Branched Chain Amino Acids	Carnitine/GPLC	Dihydroxyacetone	Tribulus terrestris & other herbal testosterone supplements
Performance	Essential Amino Acids (EAA)	Nitrates	Gamma-oryzanol & ferulic acid	Ephedra
Caffeine	Hydroxy methylbutyrate (HMB)	Polyphenols (Pycnogenol, Green tea)	Inosine	Strychnine
Creatine	Leucine	**Buffer capacity**	Lecithin	
Sodium Bicarbonate			Pangamic acid (B$_{15}$)	**Substances banned in competition only:**
Sodium Citrate	**CNS effects**	**Muscle growth and repair**	Phosphate Salts	
	Branched Chain Amino Acids		Polylactate	Alcohol & Beta Blockers – prohibited in certain sports
Health		**CNS effects**	Pyruvate	
Fish Oils	**Health**	Phospholipids (PC/Choline, PS)	Ribose	Cannabinoids
Iron	Colostrum	Tyrosine	Wheat germ oil	Corticosteroids
Multi-antioxidants	Glucosamine		Wobenzym & Phlogenzym	Narcotics
Multi-minerals	Glutamine	**Health**	Yohimbine	Stimulants
Multi-vitamins	Individual minerals	Echinacea	etc…	
Prebiotics	Individual vitamins	Melatonin		**Prohibited Methods:**
Probiotics		**Other**		Enhancement of Oxygen Transfer
	Other	CLA		Chemical & Physical Manipulation
		Flavones		Gene Doping
		Medium-chain triacylglycerols (MCT)		

EGCG, epigallocatechin-3-gallate; GPLC, glycine propionyl-L-carnitine; PC, phosphatidylcholine; PS, phosphatidylserine.

foods and supplements, it is felt that there is substantial supporting evidence (level 4) from scientific research and/or clinical practice to show a performance or health benefit in some athletes in some circumstances. Consequently, qualified sports dietitians/ nutritionists need to use their knowledge, judgement and discretion in light of current clinical and scientific evidence before recommending that any DS be included in the athlete's diet plan. It should also be noted that some DS are not necessarily better than food-based solutions, but may just provide an alternative solution for certain situations.

Included within the 'Acceptable' group are 'sports foods', including drinks, powders, bars and gels, that are felt to provide a useful, practical, portable and timely source of energy and nutrients and therefore have a genuine role to play in supplementing the diet during both training and competition. Also within this group are a few ergogenic aids, which are listed under the subheading of 'performance' as substances that aim to enhance performance. The three key ergogenic aids included here are caffeine, creatine and the buffers sodium bicarbonate and sodium citrate; these have all been shown to be potentially beneficial for certain athletes and were accordingly recognised in the two most recent IOC Sports Nutrition Consensus Conferences in 2003 and 2010. However, the long-term effects of all the ergogenic aids are still unclear, so caution is still advised regarding their use. Finally, within the 'Acceptable' group are some DS listed under the banner of 'health' that may provide some health benefits to athletes with limited risk. The key acceptable sports foods, supplements and ergogenic aids are reviewed below.

Sports foods

Several nutritional sports foods and supplements are effective at influencing energy supply, with the most obvious example being carbohydrate supplements. More detailed information regarding the key nutrients and ingredients in sports foods can be found in specific chapters: carbohydrates in Chapter 4, protein in Chapter 5, fluid and electrolytes in Chapter 7 and micronutrients in Chapter 8. In addition, readers are specifically referred to Part 2 of this book (Chapters 10–14) where the specific nutrition strategies including key supplements are reviewed in terms of how they support different types of training, including resistance, power/sprint, middle-distance/speed-endurance,

Table 9.5 Sports foods.

Food	Reason for use
Carbohydrate drinks, powders, gels and bars	Energy supply and glycogen re-synthesis
Carbohydrate/electrolyte 'sports' drinks and powders	Energy and electrolyte supply
Carbohydrate and protein 'recovery' drinks, powders and bars	Post-exercise recovery
Electrolyte replacements	Electrolyte replacement
Protein powders, drinks and bars	Post-exercise recovery and protein supply
Liquid meal supplements	Provision of vital nutrients and additional energy

endurance, and technical/skill. The key sports food listed within the Acceptable group of the APRID framework are shown in Table 9.5 with their principal reason for use.

The use of sports foods to achieve sports nutrition goals is well supported in both the scientific literature and practical application. Sports foods provide a convenient, practical, portable and timely source of energy and nutrients to help supplement the diet during both training and competition. Sports foods come in array of forms, primarily drinks, powders, bars and gels, to cater for both specific time of use (before, during or after exercise) and differences in individual tastes and preferences. Sports foods are particularly useful when travelling, access to food is limited, time is restricted or appetite is suppressed, or to help avoid gastrointestinal issues associated with exercise and/or nerves.

Typically, sports drinks and powders provide a source of fluid and energy with carbohydrate and/or protein in a 'fluid' form, sports bars a compact source of energy with carbohydrate and/or protein in a 'solid' bar form, while sports gels provide a more concentrated source of energy with carbohydrate and/or protein in a 'semi-solid' gel form. Typically, the fat and fibre content is low or negligible in order to provide an easily digestible source of nutrients. Some bars and gels also include additional ingredients depending on proposed reason for use, with common inclusions being vitamins and minerals, electrolytes and caffeine. As always athletes should experiment with sports foods during training to individualise use, discover preferences and assess tolerances prior to use in a competition setting.

Table 9.6 'Performance' supplements.

Supplement	Performance uses	Physiological rationale
Caffeine	Endurance performance	CNS effects, improved exogenous carbohydrate use, higher fat oxidation
	Cognitive performance	Improves alertness and vigour
Creatine	Strength and muscle mass gains	Increases muscle creatine stores. Enables the athlete to maintain a greater training load
	Hyperhydration	The increases in muscle creatine stores increased intracellular fluid
Sodium bicarbonate	Improvement in performance over times ranging from 40 s to 10 min	Increase in the hydrogen ion diffusion gradient from muscle to plasma
	Hyperhydration	High sodium load expands plasma volume
Sodium citrate	Improvement in performance over times ranging from 40 s to 10 min	Increase in the hydrogen ion diffusion gradient from muscle to plasma
	Hyperhydration	High sodium load expands plasma volume

Table 9.7 Caffeine content of common drinks.

Standard drink (250 ml cup)	Caffeine content (mg)
Instant coffee	50–70
Brewed/filter coffee	60–120
Tea	10–50
Hot chocolate	8–15
Cola	20–50

Reproduced with kind permission from Stear S. Fuelling Fitness for Sports Performance, copyright © 2004 Samantha Stear.

Liquid meal supplements

Liquid meal supplements are available in ready-to-drink or powder form and are typically carbohydrate-rich, moderate-protein and low-fat and frequently fortified with key vitamins and minerals. Therefore they provide a compact, portable, non-perishable and convenient meal replacement or supplement that provides energy, macronutrients and micronutrients. Liquid meal supplements are useful for athletes who need a convenient way to increase energy intake such as during growth spurts, heavy training loads, or while trying to increase lean body mass. Other common uses include as a pre- or post-exercise snack and as a meal replacement to help with weight management and/or help with gastrointestinal issues associated with exercise and/or nerves.

Performance supplements

Table 9.6 provides a summary of the performance supplements listed within the Acceptable category of the APRID framework.

Caffeine

Caffeine (trimethylxanthine, $C_8H_{10}N_4O_2$) is one of the most widely used aids in everyday life and sport.

Some reports suggest that 90% of the world's adult population consume caffeine in their everyday diet. Caffeine can be found in many foods and drinks, including coffee, tea, colas and chocolate. Table 9.7 shows the caffeine content of some common drinks. These traditionally available sources typically provide around 50–150 mg caffeine. However, it is also possible to find products that provide 300–500 mg of caffeine per serving.

Between 1980 and 2003, a caffeine level in the urine above 12 mg/l was not permitted during competition and would result in a positive doping test. These levels were intended to discourage the intake of large amounts of caffeine, which in general was achieved by taking about 500 mg caffeine in a short time. Although caffeine is indeed a drug that is weakly addictive, it is both socially acceptable and unrealistic to try to control it. Therefore, due to the wide availability of caffeine in drinks and foods, it is difficult but not impossible to have a caffeine level that exceeds the permissible limit just from a normal diet. Primarily as a result of this, the WADA decided to remove caffeine from the list of banned substances with effect from January 2004, although its use is still being monitored.

Over the last few decades research has shown that ingesting caffeine prior to exercise can have an ergogenic effect on many different types of sporting performance, with clear evidence of an improvement in performance in events lasting more than 1 min. Caffeine appears to exert positive effects on exercise capacity during prolonged submaximal exercise (>90 min), sustained high-intensity work (20–60 min) and short-duration supra-maximal exercise (1–5 min). Doses as low as 1.5 mg/kg taken 45–60 min prior to the start of exercise have been shown to improve performance compared with placebo. During longer duration events lasting more than 60 min, caffeine ingestion during exercise has also been shown to improve performance. More recent research has shown that caffeine is able to improve performance in team/field events such as rugby and football and others such as court and racquet sports where there is a cognitive component to performance. However, the evidence supporting an ergogenic effect of caffeine during high-intensity exercise lasting less than 1 min is less clear.

Part of caffeine's intrigue is that we still do not know with any certainty the exact mechanism by which caffeine enhances performance, with a number of possible effects on different body tissues. Potential sites of action of caffeine to explain the ergogenic effects seen include the central nervous system, metabolism, or directly effects on the muscle itself. A traditional approach for investigating the mechanisms responsible for caffeine's effect on performance is to examine fat metabolism and glycogen utilisation. While there has been some suggestion that caffeine can increase fat metabolism and therefore spare muscle glycogen, recent well-controlled studies have shown this not to be the case. However, there is some evidence suggesting that caffeine can improve the exogenous oxidation of ingested carbohydrate when the caffeine is co-ingested with carbohydrate during endurance exercise. Further evidence has suggested that large doses of caffeine ingested after exercise can enhance muscle glycogen repletion.

Potentially the most significant effect of caffeine is its action as an adenosine antagonist. Increases in adenosine in the brain can lead to decreased arousal and an increased drive to sleep. Caffeine competes with adenosine to interact with the adenosine receptors and therefore prevent the negative effects of adenosine on the brain. Evidence also suggests that caffeine can decrease the perception of effort during exercise, with many studies showing a lower rating of perceived exertion (RPE) score during exercise when caffeine is ingested. Caffeine ingestion also seems to decrease the perception of pain during exercise.

For those who are habitual users of caffeine there is still likely to be an effect of caffeine on performance. Research has shown caffeine improves performance in both habitual and non-habitual caffeine users. However, the response to caffeine does appear to be very individual, and does not appear to be related to the habitual amount of caffeine consumed. Furthermore, individuals respond differently to caffeine, as with many drugs, across a range from positive to negative outcomes, with some body tis-

sues becoming tolerant to repeated caffeine use while others do not. Caffeine can produce limiting side effects in some individuals, such as insomnia, headaches and abdominal discomfort, as well as muscle tremors and impaired coordination at high doses. Therefore, as always, it is important to experiment with caffeine during training, before contemplating using it during competition.

Furthermore, the mild diuretic effect of caffeine is often cautioned as a potential cause of dehydration. However, small to moderate doses of caffeine have only a minimal effect on urine losses or overall hydration in habitual consumers and, besides, common caffeine-containing drinks (coffee, tea and colas) actually provide a significant source of fluids in many people's diets.

Creatine

Creatine is involved in the regulation of cellular energy demand. Creatine is a naturally occurring compound and is derived from three amino acids found in large amounts in skeletal muscle. Muscle creatine content varies between individuals. Typically a carnivorous diet provides about 1–2 g of creatine daily, but vegetarians will get virtually no creatine from their diet and have reduced body creatine stores, suggesting that endogenous production cannot totally compensate for a lack of dietary intake.

Creatine monohydrate is the most common creatine supplement used. Creatine supplementation can increase muscle creatine and phosphocreatine content by approximately 20%. Research has shown that oral creatine supplementation can maximise muscle creatine levels using two regimens: (i) a loading dose of 20 g/day for 4–5 days followed by a maintenance dose of 2–3 g/day; or (ii) a maintenance dose of 2–3 g/day for approximately 30 days. Strategies to enhance creatine loading outcomes include co-ingestion with a substantial amount of carbohydrate (around 50–100 g) and exercise. Once the muscle creatine levels have been maximised, it will take around 4 weeks to return to resting levels. However, continuing with a daily maintenance dose of 2–3 g will help sustain the elevated levels. However, it is also important to note that there is considerable variability in response to creatine supplementation, with some individuals considered non-responders.

The most recognised fuel role of phosphorylated creatine is as an immediate and short-lived source of phosphate to regenerate ATP. In the first few seconds (up to 10 s) of sprint or high-intensity exercise, creatine phosphate is the most important fuel source. Consequently, supplementation regimens that maximise muscle creatine levels can lead to improved performance of repeated high-intensity exercise, increased strength and lean body mass, and enhanced fatigue resistance for exercise activities lasting 30 s or less, particularly when combined with progressive resistance training.

Therefore creatine can be used in many training programmes including resistance, interval and sprint, and also during sports involving intermittent work patterns such as team/field/court including racket sports. Conversely, there is no clear evidence for benefits of creatine supplementation for aerobic or endurance performance, bar the potential associated benefit arising from enhanced glycogen storage.

The mechanisms through which creatine supplementation improves exercise performance and body composition include metabolic enhancements, molecular adaptations and reduced muscle damage. However, creatine supplementation does not appear to result in increased skeletal muscle protein synthesis.

The long-term consequences and any associated concerns with creatine supplementation are poorly understood. However, the associated acute weight gain with creatine loading, possibly representing water gain, may actually be counter-productive for those athletes where power-to-weight ratio is a key performance influencer or a target weight is required for a specific weight classification. There are also anecdotal reports of increased risk of muscle cramps, strains and tears, but this has not been substantiated through studies on creatine use. Furthermore, despite published allegations of detrimental effects of oral creatine supplementation on liver metabolism, long-term supplementation studies in humans (up to 5 years) have failed to show any significant increase in plasma urea or liver enzyme activity throughout the duration of creatine supplementation, with values remaining within the normal range corrected for age.

However, even if there is no health risks associated with oral creatine supplementation, it is safer to remain cautious when creatine is administered chronically. Furthermore, it is recommended that creatine supplements should not be used by individuals with pre-existing renal disease or those with a potential risk for renal dysfunction (diabetes, hypertension, reduced glomerular filtration rate). Care should also be taken regarding the purity of creatine supplements and, where possible, analytical tests should be performed to prove the nutraceutical composition as safety cannot always be assured in some creatine supplement preparations.

Sodium bicarbonate

Sodium bicarbonate ($NaHCO_3$) is regularly used to enhance athletic performance, is used in some baking processes, and can also be used as an antacid. Research has shown that using an acute dose of sodium bicarbonate prior to sporting events that are high intensity lasting 40 s–10 mins can lead to an improvement in performance by helping resist fatigue caused by changes in acid–base balance. Research has shown improved performance in several sporting events, including 400–800 m running, 200 m freestyle swimming, and for repeated sprint performance in team/field/court including racket sports. Conversely, over more prolonged exercise of lower intensities sodium bicarbonate does not seem to have any effect on performance.

Typically, resting human arterial blood pH is about 7.4, slightly alkalotic, but after strenuous exercise may fall to around 7.1, while muscle pH decreases to about 6.8. Buffers such as sodium bicarbonate and citrate (see below) will increase the buffering capacity by increasing the amount of bicarbonate (for example) that can be utilised, say by increasing pH to 7.5.

In this instance, sodium bicarbonate and citrate are acting as extracellular buffers of hydrogen ions. During high-intensity exercise hydrogen ions are produced, seemingly as a by-product of high rates of glycolysis. This increase in hydrogen ion production during high-intensity exercise is one of the causes of fatigue. Ingesting sodium bicarbonate has been shown to increase blood bicarbonate concentration, thereby increasing the buffering capacity of the blood. This increase in blood bicarbonate increases the hydrogen ion gradient between the blood and within the muscle cell. This allows more hydrogen ions to be removed from the muscle, therefore delaying fatigue. This will also lead to an increase in lactate removal from the muscle and an increase in plasma lactate concentration, often seen with sodium bicarbonate supplementation. Ingestion of sodium bicarbonate can lead to quicker recovery in acid–base balance after exercise. This may be significant for events where there is multiple events or rounds in one day.

The most common dosing regimen in the research setting is to provide 300 mg/kg 90 min before the start of exercise, although in practical terms the dose is likely to vary from person to person; some athletes, through experimentation, have found it easier to spread the sodium bicarbonate dosing over a longer period of around 2–3 hours. Some research suggests that doses as low as 200 mg/kg will lead to an increase in blood buffer capacity.

A longer-term loading protocol of 500 mg/kg per day spread over the day or chronically for 2–3 days may provide a more sustained increase in blood pH, with benefits maintained for at least 1 day following the last sodium bicarbonate dose. This dosing protocol may be useful to athletes who compete in a series of events spread over a couple of days, by replacing the need to undertake multiple acute dosing protocols or having to choose which event to use sodium bicarbonate. This chronic dosing protocol may also be an alternative for athletes who suffer with gastrointestinal problems following large acute intakes, as this method means the sodium bicarbonate dosing can be stopped the day before the athlete's event. Buffering agents should generally be taken with 1–2 l of water, preferably with some carbohydrate, to reduce gastrointestinal problems attributable to osmotic diarrhoea.

Chronic or repeated use of sodium bicarbonate can also be used as a training aid. Sodium bicarbonate may increase the effectiveness of the training sessions when used around high-intensity exercise. This approach allows the athlete to obtain, and sustain subsequent, greater training intensities than without supplementation, leading to an improved training response. Supplementation of around 400 mg/kg prior to a high-intensity training session may also lead to adaptation within the muscle, allowing greater transport of hydrogen ions out of the muscle.

Some undesirable gastrointestinal side effects, such as bloating, nausea and diarrhoea, are commonplace when ingesting sodium bicarbonate at large doses. However, this reaction is very individual and athletes need to work through dosing protocols including other dietary intakes, such as optimal nutrient intake options, prior to and during dosing periods with a qualified sports dietitian/nutritionist.

Sodium citrate

Sodium citrate has also been used as a buffer in a similar manner to sodium bicarbonate. It works in a similar way to that of sodium bicarbonate by increasing the pH of the blood and therefore increasing the pH gradient between exercising muscle and the blood. A number of studies have shown that supplementation with sodium citrate can lead to an improvement in performance, particularly in shorter-duration events lasting less than 10 min. However, the evidence for the positive impact upon exercise performance is not as conclusive as sodium bicarbonate. Typical dosing protocols tend to be in the range 300–600 mg/kg, taken 1–2 hours prior to exercise. Again, buffering agents should be taken with 1–2 l of water, preferably with some carbohydrate, to reduce gastrointestinal problems attributable to osmotic diarrhoea. However, one advantage of sodium citrate over sodium bicarbonate is a reduced likelihood of gastrointestinal distress.

More recent research has investigated the effect of sodium citrate in hyperhydration prior to prolonged exercise in the heat. Ingesting large quantities of trisodium citrate, providing approximately 160 mmol/l of sodium 90 min prior to prolonged exercise in the heat, can increase time to exhaustion in both men and women. This effect appears to occur by delaying the point at which plasma osmolality begins to increase and therefore cause fatigue.

It is important to note that although sodium bicarbonate/citrate are not banned by anti-doping laws, their use may result in acute changes in urinary pH. Consequently, it may take several hours for an athlete's urine to return to what is considered an acceptable pH range.

Health supplements

In some instances, where there is an established deficiency of an essential nutrient, supplementing the diet with food or dietary supplements to correct the deficiency can be beneficial. However, exceeding the nutrient requirements is not necessarily a good thing. More detailed information regarding the key nutrients and ingredients proposed to have particular health benefits can be found elsewhere in this book (micronutrients in Chapter 8, gut health in Chapter 20, immunity in Chapter 21, and travel in Chapter 22). At present, the health supplements listed within the Acceptable group of the APRID framework are shown in Table 9.8 with their principal reason for use.

Table 9.8 'Health' supplements.

Supplement	Health use
Multivitamins	Vitamin supply for health. Support restricted diet or correct micronutrient deficiencies
Multiminerals	Mineral supply for health. Support restricted diet or correct micronutrient deficiencies
Multi-antioxidants	Antioxidant supply for health. Support immunity and health particularly during increases in training stress: training load, altitude, heat, pollution
Fish oils	Supports joint, cardiovascular and respiratory health. Rich source of essential fatty acids
Iron	Supplement for deficiencies, poor iron stores and anaemias
Prebiotics and probiotics	Gut health

Table 9.9 Diets with a higher risk of nutrient deficiencies.

Low in energy for weight loss
  -Especially if followed for a long period
Omitting foods or food groups
  -Likes/dislikes
  -Vegetarians and vegans
Lacking in a particular type of food
  -Allergy or intolerance
Erratic and unbalanced
  -Restricted food intake
  -Disordered eating

Reproduced with kind permission from Stear S. Fuelling Fitness for Sports Performance, copyright © 2004 Samantha Stear.

Multivitamins and multiminerals

Although micronutrients are reviewed in detail in Chapter 8, micronutrient supplements also warrant a brief mention here. Multivitamin and multimineral supplements comprise a broad range of low-dose formulations of vitamins and minerals. There is no sound evidence to suggest that supplementation with vitamins and minerals enhance exercise performance, unless they are needed to correct a pre-existing deficiency. Any marginal deficiency will only have a small impact on body function but may impair exercise performance, especially in individuals where more than one micronutrient is compromised. In theory, it is possible to be deficient in any of the micronutrients, but in practice deficiency is generally uncommon with the exception of calcium, iron and vitamin D.

Athletes who have restricted diets may put themselves at risk of inadequate micronutrient intakes. Table 9.9 lists common dietary situations where there is a higher risk of nutrient deficiencies. Athletes whose diet puts them at risk of nutrient deficiencies should seek advice from a Sports Nutrition professional. When food intake cannot be sufficiently improved, for example during extensive travel particularly when there is a limited supply of 'safe' food, then a low-dose multivitamin and multimineral supplement may be useful. However, single targeted nutrient supplements should only be taken under medical supervision for an established nutrient deficiency.

Other health supplements

Both heavy exercise and nutrition exhibit separate influences on immune function. Although modest exercise is good for the immune system, very strenuous and prolonged training is associated with depressed immune function. An inadequate diet or inappropriate food choices on top of hard training will further depress immune function. Although the effect of hard training on immune function is generally fairly small, any illness that interrupts training or prevents an athlete competing can be disastrous to the individual concerned.

Consequently, several supplements such as high doses of antioxidants, fish oils, glutamine, zinc and probiotics are promoted as being 'immune-enhancing', despite lack of unequivocal supporting evidence, primarily due to the difficulty of assessing efficacy. Although it is difficult to prove a causal link between certain nutritional interventions and enhanced immunity, it was felt at the time of publication that the supplements listed under Health in the Acceptable group of the APRID framework could be used in moderation by athletes to potentially provide some 'immune support' around times of competition and intense training, without any obvious detrimental effect on health. Antioxidants, fish oils and probiotics are reviewed specifically in Chapter 21. Specific antioxidants where there is some supporting research evidence in terms of their potential roles as ergogenic aids are discussed below (see p. 105). Probiotics and prebiotics are discussed further in Chapter 20 and in particular in Chapter 22 on travel. Iron is covered in detail in Chapter 8.

Fish oils

Fish oils contain the long-chain unsaturated omega-3 (ω-3) fatty acids eicosapentaenoic acid (EPA) and docosahexaenoic acid (DHA), although the amounts and concentrations of these fatty acids vary according to origin (e.g. type of fish, season and geographical location). Many commonly available fish oil supplements contain about 30% EPA plus DHA, with more concentrated sources being available, and all forms have good bioavailability. Typical daily dietary intakes of EPA and DHA are usually below 200 mg/day, which is less than the recommended levels of around 500 mg/day and therefore supplements can make a useful contribution to meeting recommended ω-3 intake levels.

Exercise or athlete-specific benefits of fish oils are inconclusive due to inconsistencies between studies. Typically both moderate (1.8 g/day) and high (4 g/day) doses of EPA plus DHA are used, over several weeks or months. There is some evidence to suggest that fish oils may improve metabolic changes that occur with exercise, and may be particularly beneficial in preventing bronchial irritation caused by particle pollutants. Furthermore, it is felt that supplementation may provide some protection against exercise-induced bronchoconstriction (EIB) and asthma-type symptoms in athletes. In one study, a high dose (3.2 g EPA plus 2.0 g DHA daily) for 3 weeks markedly improved lung function after exercise in non-atopic elite athletes with EIB and in asthmatic athletes (Mickleborough et al., 2006). In addition, recent cell culture work suggests that EPA rather than DHA may be responsible for the beneficial effects seen in individuals with EIB and asthma-type symptoms, but further research is warranted.

'Physiological' and 'Research' categories

By splitting the next most efficacious sports foods and supplements into either the 'Physiological' category, where evidence is generally at level 2 and 3, or the 'Research' category, where evidence is generally at level 1 and 2, the APRID framework recognises that not all supporting evidence is similar in nature and hence the need for practitioners to be allowed freedom to operate with these sports foods and supplements if deemed useful and appropriate for the athlete in question.

For example in some instances, the supporting evidence may be from less well trained populations and so it is possible that the performance benefits may not translate into benefits for trained individuals and elite athletes. Conversely, some research may not be able to show statistically significant performance outcomes, but any small potential performance enhancement may warrant further individualised investigation, providing it is felt that use of the product will not be detrimental to health.

For the group of 'Physiological' sports foods and supplements, it is felt that although there is a physiological rationale for using the supplement, the supporting evidence for a performance or health outcome is unclear. In contrast, for the group of 'Research' sports foods and supplements, it is felt that both the physiological and performance/health outcomes are unclear. However, for this 'Research' group of supplements, there may be some practitioner-based supporting evidence of a benefit when using the supplement in elite sport. Therefore, practitioners wishing to use supplements within this 'Research' group must do so only under the scope of a defined research protocol, where use of the supplement can be closely monitored and further supporting evidence can be gathered. The key 'Physiological' and 'Research' sports foods, supplements and ergogenic aids are briefly reviewed below.

Antioxidants

'Antioxidants' can be seen as an umbrella term for many different supplements currently available to athletes. In this section the focus is on antioxidants that are not classified as vitamins and some research has been conducted into their use as ergogenic aids. Antioxidants can be seen as supplements that help the body cope with the oxidative stress caused by exercise. Oxidative stress can lead to fatigue during exercise by influencing many sites both within and outside of the muscle itself, such as mitochondrial function, blood flow and the contractile mechanisms of the muscle. However, oxidative stress is also important in the adaptation of the body to muscle and therefore care must be taken when using antioxidants as a chronic supplement that no harm is done to the training adaptation.

A number of herbal and plant extracts have been investigated for their ability to delay fatigue during exercise. Animal-based research has shown that green tea extract, particularly the active component epigallocatechin-3-gallate, can delay fatigue during prolonged exercise after 8–10 weeks of supplementation. These performance effects found in animal models seem to be mediated by an increase in fat oxidation and a sparing of muscle glycogen during exercise. Very few data are available in human studies to confirm these findings from animal models. However, there is some evidence in humans that green tea extract does increase fat oxidation during prolonged exercise after only 1 day of supplementation. This warrants further investigation in human models.

Other polyphenol-based supplements such as capsaicin (a component of red chilli peppers) and quercetin have been shown to delay fatigue during prolonged exercise in animal models. However, once again the human studies to date have been mixed. Quercetin has received most attention, with some studies showing an improvement in performance with quercetin supplementation whilst others show no effect, possibly due to many differences in the methodologies used.

Cysteine is a non-essential amino acid and is an important precursor of the tripeptide glutathione, along with glycine and glutamic acid. Studies of cysteine infusion during prolonged exercise have shown delay in fatigue, and these effects positively related to the aerobic capacity of the athletes. However, oral intake of cysteine in the doses needed to exhibit a performance effect can cause severe diarrhoea and gastrointestinal stress.

Some polyphenols and antioxidants have been shown to both improve (resveratrol and quercetin) and inhibit (vitamin C) the adaptation to aerobic training. Resveratrol is a polyphenol found particularly in the skins of grapes. It is suggested that resveratrol ingestion increases the expression of the protein SIRT-1 within the muscle which interacts with PGC1-α to lead to an increase in mitochondrial area and activity within muscle cells, leading to an improvement in performance. Quercetin supplementation has also been shown to increase mitochondrial biogenesis in both animal and human models. This may have benefits for many athletes, although this needs to be further investigated.

Cardiovascular effects
Blood flow
There are a number of supplements that have been claimed to enhance blood flow to the working muscle, including the amino acids L-arginine (precursor of L-citrulline) and L-carnitine, nitrates

and various polyphenols. These various supplements are claimed to influence the production of nitric oxide (NO), which has an essential role in regulation of capillary blood flow. NO may also directly affect oxidative phosporylation, essentially increasing the efficiency of oxidative phosphorylation.

NO is synthesised in the endothelium from L-arginine by the enzyme nitric oxide synthase. Direct infusion of L-arginine appears to increase vasodilation of the capillaries within muscle. However, when L-arginine is given orally this effect does not appear to occur either with acute or chronic supplementation, as blood flow during aerobic exercise is sufficient under normal conditions. Arginine can also remove ammonia from the blood, which may be important in recovery from hard training. In addition, ingestion of arginine may also help muscle recovery by stimulating the secretion of growth hormone.

Furthermore, recent evidence suggests that supplementation with citrulline may be more effective at increasing plasma arginine concentration than ingestion of arginine itself. However, there is currently no conclusive evidence that citrulline ingestion enhances exercise performance.

Recent research has proposed the supplementation of nitrates to enhance NO production. Dietary nitrate can be converted to nitrite, which can in turn be reduced to NO in blood and various tissues. Nitrate supplementation can lead to a decrease in blood pressure, a decrease in oxygen use during moderate-intensity exercise and ultimately an increase in time to exhaustion during intense exercise. It appears that this effect can occur with both supplementation and a dietary increase in nitrate ingestion.

There are a number of studies which suggest that various polyphenols such as pycnogenol and green tea extract can increase endothelium-dependent blood flow by influencing the production of NO by nitric oxide synthase. This is primarily by acting as an antioxidant, since oxidative stress has been shown to promote the breakdown of nitric oxide synthase. However, very little research has been conducted in human exercise models and at present there is no evidence of a performance effect due to increased blood flow with polyphenol supplementation.

Carnitine
L-Carnitine is synthesised from the amino acids lysine and methonine. It is essential for fatty acid

transport into the mitochondria from the cytosol within muscle cells, with free carnitine possibly being a rate-limiting step in fatty acid metabolism. L-Carnitine is found naturally in the human diet, particularly in red meat and dairy products.

There has been some suggestion that supplementation with L-carnitine can increase fatty acid transport into the mitochondria leading to an increase in fatty acid oxidation. This could be of benefit to endurance athletes as increasing fatty acid oxidation can often lead to sparing of muscle glycogen stores and in turn improve performance. There have also been suggestions of benefits for weight management.

Despite the possibility that L-carnitine supplementation may increase fatty acid metabolism through increasing free carnitine in the muscle, there is very little evidence that this actually occurs. It appears that supplementation with L-carnitine does not lead to an increase in free carnitine within the muscle cell and does not have any effect on exercise metabolism. When ingested in conjunction with a large high-glycaemic-index carbohydrate beverage, carnitine is better retained within the body. In hyperinsulinaemic conditions, carnitine supplementation can increase free carnitine within the muscle cell, leading to an increase in fat oxidation at rest.

Glycine propionyl-L-carnitine (GPLC) supplementation may lead to an increase in plasma nitrate and nitrite. This may increase blood flow to the working muscles and enhance exercise performance. While there has been limited research conducted in this area, there is some evidence that 4.5 g of GPLC supplementation taken 90 min prior to repeated sprint-type exercise can improve peak power during exercise and decrease lactate accumulation in the blood. However, other studies have shown no effect of GPLC on exercise performance.

Buffer capacity
β-Alanine and carnosine

Carnosine is a dipeptide of β-alanine and histidine. β-Alanine is a naturally occuring amino acid that is an important precursor of carnosine, and is generally thought to be the rate-limiting step in the production of carnosine.

Carnosine is abundant in human muscle tissue, with very little found in other tissues. Some reports suggest that up to 99% of the body's carnosine stores can be found in skeletal muscle. However,

the concentration of carnosine in type II muscle fibres is thought to be 1.5–2 times higher than that in type I fibres. There are a number of roles which carnosine plays within skeletal muscle. The histidine-located imidazole ring in the carnosine molecule has an acid dissociation constant (pK_a) of 6.83. A buffer is most effective within the muscle cell when its pK_a is in the pH range 6.5–7.1. Therefore, as the pK_a of carnosine lies within the pH range that exists in skeletal muscle between rest and exercise, one of its important roles is as an effective intracellular pH buffer. Carnosine can also act as an antioxidant, a chelator of metals and an anti-glycation agent.

When β-alanine is ingested as a supplement it can increase muscle carnosine content. Ingestion of daily doses of around 100 mg/kg (4–7 g/day for an average athlete) leads to a 60% increase in muscle carnosine content after 4 weeks and an increase of 80% after 8 weeks. This increase in muscle carnosine content seems to be independent of muscle fibre type and initial muscle carnosine content. Research studies suggest that muscle carnosine levels remain elevated for up to 9 weeks after β-alanine supplementation is discontinued.

Supplementation with β-alanine appears to improve performance during high-intensity exercise or repeated bouts of maximal muscle contractions. Some evidence suggests that β-alanine supplementation can also increase ventilatory threshold and physical work capacity. The likely mechanism for this improvement in performance is the increased buffer capacity with the increase in muscle carnosine content.

Supplementation with β-alanine can also help to support a strength training programme. Athletes who supplement with β-alanine have been shown to be able to undertake a greater training load than those who supplement with placebo; this seems to be particularly the case when β-alanine is combined with creatine supplementation. Over time this will allow greater gains to come from the training regimen.

Some people may experience paraesthesia with ingestion of large amounts of β-alanine. When β-alanine is ingested in amounts greater than approximately 800 mg, circulating β-alanine concentrations can be greatly increased leading to sensitisation of neurones involved in neuropathic pain. Therefore, doses of β-alanine should be split throughout the day, ingested with food or taken using a sustained-release formula, to allow for slow and steady absorption of β-alanine. There do not appear to be any changes in body weight as a consequence of β-alanine supplementation.

Muscle growth and repair
Branched-chain amino acids, essential amino acids and leucine

Branched-chain amino acids (BCAAs) comprise the three essential amino acids leucine, isoleucine and valine. BCAAs, as well as the other essential amino acids, have been suggested as important supplements for influencing post-exercise protein synthesis. In particular, leucine is an important regulator of the protein kinase mTOR (mammalian target of rapamycin). It appears that leucine interacts with mTOR to activate the signalling cascade which leads to an increase in protein synthesis. Leucine alone can stimulate the activation of mTOR to a similar degree as a mixture of amino acids or protein alone. It is unclear as to whether it is the intracellular or extracellular concentration of leucine that is important in regulating the activation of mTOR. However, there is little evidence that supplementation of leucine in addition to protein can further stimulate protein synthesis. There is some evidence that supplementation with BCAAs before or after exercise can lead to a decrease in the delayed-onset muscle soreness produced as a consequence to exercise.

The amount of BCAA recommended is 0.03–0.05 g/kg per hour or 2–4 g/hour ingested repeatedly during exercise and recovery, preferably taken as a drink. Large doses (~30 g/day) are well tolerated, although they may be detrimental to performance due to increased production of ammonia by the exercising muscle.

Hydroxymethylbutyrate

β-Hydroxy-β-methylbutyrate or β-hydroxy-β-methylbutyric acid, commonly abbreviated as HMB, is a metabolite of the essential amino acid leucine, is synthesised in the body, and plays a part in protein synthesis. It has been proposed that it positively influences muscle protein metabolism, leading to claims that HMB decreases protein breakdown associated with heavy training and increases lean body mass and strength. The proposed mechanisms of action include increased sarcolemma integrity via conversion to hydroxymethylglutaryl (HMG)-CoA, enhanced protein synthesis via the mTOR pathway, and depression of protein degradation through the ubiquitin pathway. Consequently, it has been suggested that the anti-catabolic effects sometimes associated with leucine supplementation during exercise stress are mediated by HMB.

Interest in HMB supplementation stemmed from studies in rats, but studies in humans have produced equivocal results. It is hypothesised that benefits from supplementing with HMB may be greater in the early phases of a new training programme or when previously untrained individuals undertake resistance training. The human body produces about 0.2–0.4 g/day. Typical HMB supplementation doses are 1–3 g/day, usually divided into two or three doses of about 1–1.5 g per dose.

Central nervous system effects
Branched-chain amino acids

The three BCAAs are leucine, isoleucine and valine. Some research has suggested that BCAA ingestion can lead to a delay in fatigue by influencing central fatigue. BCAAs ingested during exercise may decrease RPE score and increase time to exhaustion, particularly in hot environments. However, not all research studies show an effect of BCAA supplementation during exercise, with those which do tending to come during exercise longer than 1 hour in duration and when carbohydrate is not given alongside the BCAA.

During exercise overall fatigue can occur due to central fatigue caused by an increase in the neurotransmitter 5-hydroxytryptamine (5-HT) within the brain. 5-HT is synthesised from the amino acid tryptophan, which crosses the blood–brain barrier into the brain and is converted into 5-HT by the enzyme tryptophan hydroxylase. Tryptophan is transported around the body bound to albumin and is transported across the blood–brain barrier in competition with BCAAs. During prolonged exercise in particular, BCAAs are taken up by the working muscle and tryptophan becomes unbound from albumin due to the increased demand for albumin to transport free fatty acids. This increases the ratio of free tryptophan to BCAA, leading to an increase in transport of tryptophan across the blood–brain barrier. This leads to an increase in 5-HT within the brain causing fatigue. The direct effect of BCAA ingestion on tryptophan transport into the brain is yet to be shown in humans but does seem to occur in animal models.

Phospholipids

Phospholipids are components of all biological membranes. Some research has investigated the effects of phosphatidylcholine (PC) and phosphatidylserine (PS) on exercise performance. PC can be a source of choline, which in turn is an important precursor of the neurotransmitter acetylcholine. The rate of synthesis of acetylcholine can be influenced by the concentration of free choline in plasma. During intense exercise of long duration, such as a marathon or triathlon, free choline can decrease by up to 40%. Supplementation with a source of choline can help to prevent the decrease in free choline seen during certain exercise modes, with PC seemingly more effective than choline salts in increasing free choline concentrations. However, there is very little evidence that preventing this drop in free choline will influence exercise performance.

PS is found in most biological membranes within the human body and has a role to play in modulating enzymatic reactions, membrane receptor activity and various signalling pathways within the cell membrane. PS supplements are generally derived from soy. PS supplementation may influence the cortisol response to exercise, suggesting it may have some role in athletes who are undertaking heavy training loads. However, these data are far from conclusive and further research needs to be conducted in this area.

Tyrosine

Tyrosine is an amino acid involved particularly with the synthesis of neurotransmitters such as dopamine. Dopamine competes with the neurotransmitter serotonin to cross the blood–brain barrier. Serotonin is a neurotransmitter of fatigue and fatigue can theoretically be delayed if more dopamine is available to compete with serotonin as it crosses the blood–brain barrier.

There is some evidence that supplementation with tyrosine can lead to an increase in dopamine. This in turn may lead to an improvement in mood state. It appears that tyrosine supplementation may be effective in improving cognitive function in environmental extremes such as cold exposure. Research investigating the effects of tyrosine on endurance performance currently shows no effect on performance.

Health

As discussed earlier in the section on 'Health supplements' (p. 103), in some instances where there is an established deficiency of an essential micronutrient, supplementing the diet with food or dietary supplements to correct the deficiency can be beneficial. Vitamins and minerals are covered in more detail in Chapter 8. In addition to 'health' supplements being promoted for immune-supporting benefits, there are also many that are marketed as beneficial for joint health to support the wear and tear caused by overuse during strenuous training. The main supplements promoted for joint health include antioxidants, fatty acids, vitamins B_3, B_5 and D, calcium, boron, proteolytic enzymes, glucosamine, chondroitin, methylsulphonylmethane, S-adenosyl methionine, type 2 collagen, hyaluronic acid and soy isoflavones. However, most have been shown to be ineffective. Healthy bones need an adequate supply of calcium and vitamin D, but these are normally supplied from a healthy balanced diet and so supplementation is generally not necessary. For further information see Chapter 19.

Colostrum

Bovine colostrum is milk produced in the first 2–3 days after the birth of a calf. During this period the milk produced by a cow has a higher content of certain immune, growth and antimicrobial factors than standard milk. The purpose of bovine colostrum is to provide transfer of immunity and growth factors from the cow to the calf during the early stages of development. Colostrum has been used as a DS in both clinical and athletic settings.

Sports performance research investigating the effect of chronic bovine colostrum supplementation has failed to show any conclusive evidence that colostrums can improve performance. There is inconsistent evidence for improvements in strength and power performance with colostrum supplementation. Research in this area has used a range of methodologies and subjects, making it difficult to confirm the effect of colostrum on strength and power performance. There is some evidence to suggest an improvement in buffering capacity with colostrum supplementation. Nevertheless, there does not seem to be an effect of colostrum supplementation on anaerobic exercise performance.

Colostrum supplementation up to 20 g/day has been shown to enhance high-intensity exercise performance after 2 hours of steady-state exercise. However, increasing the dose above this does not appear to confer a greater benefit on performance. In fact doses smaller than 20 g/day have been shown to improve performance in a 40-km time trial performance when taken for 5 weeks.

Colostrum's effect on endurance performance may be more relevant during periods of hard intense training which can be commonplace, particularly in elite endurance athletes. Increasing evidence suggests that supplementation with colostrum at intakes of 10 g/day or less decreases the suppression of the immune system seen with prolonged or intense exercise. There is little evidence to suggest that this support of the immune system reduces the risk of infection in athletes, although there is some evidence in healthy subjects and children that colostrum supplementation may reduce the risk of an upper respiratory tract infection. Further information on the relationship between colostrum and immunity can be found in Chapter 21.

Some reports suggest that bovine colostrum supplementation can support gastrointestinal health and integrity. While the mechanisms remain to be elucidated, colostrum's effect on gastrointestinal health and integrity may be particularly relevant during periods where there is significant inflammation within the intestine. Human research investigating the effect of colostrum on gastrointestinal health is far from conclusive when the intestine is in a healthy state. To date there is no evidence to suggest an effect of colostrum supplementation on gastrointestinal health during exercise.

Bovine colostrum does contain higher concentrations of insulin-like growth factor (IGF)-1 than standard milk. According to the WADA, IGF-1 is seen as a prohibited substance. Early research suggested an increase in serum IGF-1. However, an increasing body of evidence has shown that supplementing with colostrum for 4–8 weeks has no effect on serum IGF-1 and does not lead to a positive anti-doping test.

Glucosamine

Glucosamine ($C_6H_{13}NO_5$) is an amino sugar and a primary building block of proteoglycans. Glucosamine supplements are marketed as a treatment for osteoarthritis. Glucosamine is available as oral supplements, with commonly sold forms being glucosamine sulphate and glucosamine hydrochloride. Most supplements have approximately 90% gastrointestinal absorption, followed by absorption

by several tissues including bone and articular cartilage. Glucosamine is often sold in combination with other supplements such as chondroitin sulphate and methylsulphonylmethane. Although chondroitin sulphate has been widely used alongside glucosamine as a DS for the treatment of osteoarthritis, a comprehensive scientific review has recently deemed it ineffective.

There is some evidence that regular (once or twice daily) long-term (about 2–6 months) treatment with glucosamine and chondroitin sulphate can delay progression and/or provide subjective relief in individuals with osteoarthritis, but in athletic populations there is conflicting evidence as to its effectiveness and very limited systematic research. Glucosamine tends to work chronically, so it may take weeks to months before improvements in symptoms are noticed.

Glucosamine sulphate and chondroitin are marketed to athletes for use in the modification of acute cartilage damage after an acute injury or cartilage damage due to repetitive load from training. This is based on the hypothesis that glucosamine and chondroitin sulphate may stimulate chondrocytes to repair damaged cartilage more efficiently and completely. However, there is currently inconclusive evidence to support the use of these supplements in athletes including no data on the long-term effects of supplementation.

Glutamine

Glutamine is a non-essential (dispensable) amino acid that under certain circumstances can become indispensible and so is often classed as 'conditionally indispensable'. In human blood, glutamine is the most abundant free amino acid, with a concentration of about 500–900 μmol/l. However, during prolonged or strenuous exercise, the concentration of glutamine in the blood is decreased, often substantially (Castell, 2003).

In endurance athletes, this decrease seems to occur concomitantly with relatively transient immune depression. Glutamine is used as a fuel by some cells in the immune system. Provision of glutamine supplements has shown some beneficial effects on some aspects of immune cell function in clinical studies, and a decrease in self-reported incidence of illness in endurance athletes (Castell, 2003). However, there is no firm evidence as to precisely what aspects of the immune system are affected by glutamine feeding during the transient immune depression that occurs after prolonged and strenuous exercise. Together with the difficulty in proving a causal link between certain nutritional interventions and enhanced immunity, the evidence regarding the benefit of glutamine supplements remains inconclusive. Further information regarding glutamine and immunity can be found in Chapter 21.

Echinacea

Echinacea is a genus of plant species (coneflower). Echinacea supplements are marketed as immune-enhancing. Further information regarding echinacea and immunity can be found in Chapter 21.

Melatonin

Melatonin (*N*-acetyl-5-methoxytryptamine) is a naturally occurring compound found in animals, plants and microbes. In humans, circulating levels of the hormone melatonin vary in a daily cycle, thereby allowing entrainment of the circadian rhythm of several biological functions. Melatonin supplements are available over the counter in the USA, but the sale of the hormone remains illegal or requires a prescription in many other countries. Further information regarding melatonin can be found in Chapter 22.

Other

Conjugated linoleic acid

Conjugated linoleic acid (CLA) is the term for a series of structural and geometric isomers of linoleic acid. There are many possible forms of CLA, with *cis*-9, *trans*-11 CLA being the most abundant in nature. CLA supplements are generally an equal mixture of *cis*-9, *trans*-11, *trans*-10, *cis*-12 CLA. Consequently, some forms of CLA are better than others. In general the recommended dose of CLA is around 3.2 g/day, which has been shown to aid modest body fat loss in some instances.

CLA supplements are marketed as able to enhance fat metabolism during low- to medium-intensity exercise. The mechanisms proposed for this action include decreasing lipid uptake via increased expression/activity of SCD1 enzyme, increasing energy expenditure through increased expression of UCP2, and increasing fatty acid oxidation via increased expression of CPT enzyme.

Amongst the most controversial and highly studied physiological effects of CLA is its influence on body composition. Although CLA has been shown to be an effective supplement for reducing fat mass in various animal models (mice, rats and pigs), results in humans who exercise regularly have been inconsistent. Animal studies have also shown that the effects on body composition are isomer specific, with the *trans*-10, *cis*-12 CLA isomer identified as the form associated with a decrease in body fat.

Medium-chain triglycerides

Medium-chain triglycerides (MCT) are fats composed of medium-chain fatty acids with a chain length of 6–10 carbon molecules. MCT are digested and metabolised differently than long-chain fatty acids that are the main source of dietary fat intake in humans.

MCT supplements are marketed as an easily absorbed and oxidised fuel and fat source that are unlikely to lead to body fat deposition. Furthermore, it is felt that MCT may be able to provide a fuel source during endurance and ultra-endurance events, and assist by sparing glycogen to prolong the availability of endogenous carbohydrate stores. Co-ingestion of MCT with carbohydrate increases the rate of MCT oxidation. However, studies in humans have produced inconsistent results. Furthermore, caution is advised over high intakes ($>30\,g$) due to the increased risk of gastrointestinal distress that could be detrimental to exercise performance. Medium-chain fatty acids are covered in greater detail in Chapter 6.

'Ineffective' and 'Disallowed' categories

Supplements listed in the 'Ineffective' category, where there is no current rationale for use, have shown no or weak effects on sports performance and/or health. However, the DS listed in the 'Ineffective' category in Table 9.4 are just a few examples of the many ineffective DS promoted to athletes. Furthermore, in some cases, these DS have been shown to impair sports performance and/or health. Athletes are discouraged from using supplements in this 'Ineffective' group until further studies on both their efficacy and health consequences are available.

All supplements listed in the 'Disallowed' category should not be used by athletes. These 'Disallowed' DS supplements are either directly banned and on the WADA Prohibited Substances List, or are deemed to be a high risk for a positive doping case, and/or might cause negative health consequences.

9.9 Supplement assessment and monitoring in practice

Many of the Olympic training centres and institutes of sports across the world have devised their own supplement frameworks to classify and rank DS according to their efficacy from the latest scientific and/or clinical evidence. Therefore, it is important that practitioners across the world understand and work within the supplement policies and frameworks of the sports authorities within their own countries.

The APRID framework, devised by Stear and Currell, is simply an example of one such classification, and in this instance was devised for use by practitioners and not as a 'shopping-list' for athletes. The ranking merely gives practitioners guidance on the extent of 'freedom to operate'. Hence, just because a DS is listed in the 'Acceptable' category does not mean all athletes should be allowed free usage. Consideration still needs to take into account key factors, including the level of evidence supporting the supplements, the source of evidence (clinical or sports science), and the athlete's needs and requirements. Consequently, practitioners need to use their knowledge, judgement and discretion in light of current clinical and scientific evidence. The following list provides an example of some further guidance on approach to supplement use with athletes.

(1) Athletes can be identified as potentially requiring supplements by various support staff (e.g. technical coach, dietitian/nutritionist, physiologist, strength and conditioning coach).
(2) Athletes requiring clinical supplement support should only do so under referral and guidance by a medical practitioner, and if relevant with approval from the sport's chief medical officer (CMO).
(3) All athletes identified as potentially thought to benefit from DS or ergogenic aids should be referred to a qualified health professional, preferably an accredited sports dietitian/nutritionist for a full dietary evaluation.
(4) A qualified sports dietitian/nutritionist can help clarify and identify any supplement needs and where appropriate provide advice on the type, dosage, timing, frequency and duration of supplementation.

(5) All supplement recommendations should also be approved by the athlete's medical practitioner/CMO in accordance with the country's own sports authorities supplement policies.
(6) Ideally, any performance, clinical or physiological monitoring of the DS should be discussed with the athlete's key support staff (e.g. coach, medical practitioner and dietitian/nutritionist), prior to arranging external tests.
(7) Any physiological tests to monitor the impact of DS on performance should preferably be carried out by a physiologist, with the test protocols discussed with all key associated members of the athlete's support team.
(8) The role of a qualified sports dietitian/nutritionist is primarily to make the practical recommendations (type, dosage, timing, frequency and duration) in conjunction with the medical practitioner/CMO, the role of other interdisciplinary support team members (e.g. physiology, strength and conditioning coach) being to help monitor the impact of the DS.

9.10 Risks and benefits of dietary supplements

Despite the fact that information regarding the efficacy of DS is sometimes lacking, athletes often use DS with an expectation of performance and/or health benefits. DS cannot simply be classified into two groups of useful/not useful or risky/beneficial. In fact, it is a question of individual circumstances and response to a supplement. However, before athletes consider using a DS, they should ensure their diet is optimised as well as sport specific if appropriate.

Following earlier sections in this chapter where some of the potential benefits of some DS were reviewed, it is timely to also understand the potential risks involved with DS usage. Unfortunately, because it is not possible to offer a general risk assessment on DS use, the following sections aim to help identify and assess the potential risks, and to balance these with the potential benefits.

Health risks of dietary supplements

DS use is widespread in athletes and the general population, with vitamins and minerals being particularly popular. In addition to the popularity of DS, there has also been an increase in the fortification of food in recent years. Drinks, yoghurts, cereals and many sports foods can be found fortified with micronutrients, so it is important to consider whether all this fortification could be detrimental. Indeed, prolonged use of any single vitamin or mineral supplement, in the absence of a clinically diagnosed deficiency, may not only do more harm than good but may also interfere with the balance and interaction of other micronutrients.

Decisions regarding safety should also examine the possibility of taking a 'toxic' dose of a compound either through indiscriminate supplement use or the belief that 'if a little is good, more is better'. Furthermore, safety issues should take into account any medical concerns that may conflict with sports nutrition goals or advice. For example, recommended protein requirements are reduced in diabetes; hypertension may have implications for sodium intake; and some medical conditions may contraindicate the use of caffeine. Supplement dosages for special groups such as wheelchair athletes may also need to be altered because of decreased active muscle mass.

Recently, institutions such as the US Institute of Medicine's Food and Nutrition Board (FNB), the European Food Safety Authority (EFSA) and the UK Expert Group on Vitamins and Minerals (EVM) summarised their opinions on the safety of vitamin and mineral intakes particularly from supplementation or fortification. Consequently, tolerable Upper Intake Levels (UL) or Safe Upper Levels (SUL) for vitamins and minerals have been established.

The UL is defined by EFSA as the 'maximum level of total chronic daily intake of a nutrient (from all sources) judged to be unlikely to pose a risk of adverse health effects to humans'. Furthermore, as intakes increase above the UL, the risks of adverse health effects also increase. However, it is important to note that the ULs provided are not based on precise measurements and are more an approximation dependent on the availability and quality of data. Critics of the UL list several limitations, including lack of well-designed human studies; lack of exposure and intake data in epidemiological studies; over-interpretation and usefulness of epidemiological data with regard to safety; lack of data in children; insufficient data on the variability of the sensitivity of individuals to adverse effects; and its dependency on various factors such as age, gender, body weight, lean body mass and genet-

ics. Furthermore, specific UL and SUL for athletes or active people are not available. Further detailed information regarding potential adverse effects including UL values is provided in Chapter 8.

In addition, there are also health risks associated with poor manufacturing practice. It should also be noted that a growing number of reports have discovered products containing harmful impurities like glass, lead or animal faeces. Other reports show that products may not contain an adequate dose of the labelled ingredients. Furthermore, the FDA regularly reports on products found to contain effective amounts of prescriptive drugs, which could lead to detrimental side effects. Another potential health risk is from contamination or fake DS as discussed below.

Contamination, fake and doping

Consideration of the safety and purity of DS also needs to consider the risk of consuming contaminants that are either directly harmful or banned by the anti-doping codes under which elite sport is organised. It is important to note that elite athletes remain solely responsible for any prohibited substances found in their system (strict liability). Therefore, the ethical/ legality issues of sport can be contravened either by deliberate use of over-the-counter compounds that are prohibited by such codes (e.g. prohormones and stimulants) or by inadvertent intake of these products when they are hidden in supplements.

Consequently, one of the key factors that elite athletes need to consider in negotiating the complex world of supplements and sports foods is whether the consumption of these products could lead to an inadvertent case of doping. DS frequently contain one or more different products, some of which are banned by WADA. For example, in 1996, prohormones (anabolic androgenic steroids) became popular in the US dietary supplement market, but belong to the class of anabolic agents and so are banned by WADA.

Following the wave of nandrolone findings in the late 1990s, several studies have sought to explore the extent of contamination. These studies have shown that many DS are mislabelled or do not reflect the true ingredients, demonstrating insufficient quality control in the production process. Therefore, concern was raised regarding the potential for contamination from doping substances that were not declared on the label but which would lead to a positive doping test.

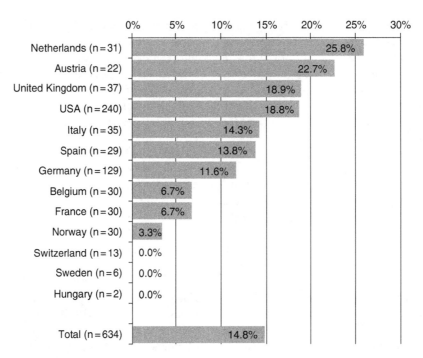

Figure 9.5 Nutritional supplements containing prohormones in relation to the total number of supplements purchased in different countries. (Data from Geyer *et al.*, 2004.)

In 2000–2001, following several positive doping cases, many of which were connected with prohormones in DS, the IOC funded a comprehensive study at the Center of Preventive Doping Research in Cologne, Germany that independently analysed 634 DS purchased across 13 different countries (Geyer *et al.*, 2004) (Figure 9.5). This pivotal research confirmed the contamination issue, with 15% of the non-hormonal supplements (e.g. minerals, vitamins, proteins, creatine) being found to contain undeclared anabolic androgenic steroids banned by WADA; 37 products analysed from the UK showed seven products (18.9%) contaminated. Altogether, 289 samples (21% positives) were from companies known to sell steroids/prohormones, but perhaps more worrying 345 samples (9.6% positives) came from companies which did not sell steroid/prohormones. On the basis of the low and varying concentration (0.01–190 μg/g) of the prohormones, the authors interpreted this as cross-contamination and not as intentional administration. Reasons for the cross-contamination were most likely that companies manufacturing prohormones also produced other supplements without sufficient cleaning of production lines, or that the transport containers from raw material suppliers were unclean.

These findings resulted in warnings for athletes and federations on supplement use and the risk of inadvertent doping cases. With the Anabolic Steroid Act 2004, the sale or possession of all prohormones is banned in the US, and the problem of contamination with prohormones has slightly improved.

However the problem has shifted, and results of the IOC Cologne study continue to be confirmed, illustrating that the issues of contamination are still around. Since 2002, DS have been detected which were probably faked with high amounts of classic anabolic steroids or stimulants. For example, the drug sibutramine, classified by WADA as a prohibited substance in competition, has been found in slimming products (e.g. capsules or tea). Not only was the drug not declared on the label, but the products declared only 'natural' ingredients. Furthermore, in addition to sibutramine causing a positive doping test, there are also potential side effects such as increased heart rate or blood pressure. Findings from the laboratory in Cologne show sibutramine metabolites in urine even 50 hours after a single consumption of the tea.

Furthermore, since 2002, DS with high amounts of anabolic steroids (e.g. stanozolol, boldenone, oxandrolone) have been detected. It is likely that these products were intentionally faked with steroids, but not labelled correctly, due to steroids not being allowed in DS. Again not only is the consumption of such products an issue for anti-doping, but the high amounts (>1 mg/g) of steroids found in these products can also result in serious side effects, such as abnormal liver function, menstrual disorders, virilisation, psychological or psychiatric disorders.

As the manufacturers of such products also produce other DS, the risk of cross-contamination is very high. Therefore it is not surprising, that in 2005 vitamin C, multivitamins and magnesium tablets containing methandienone or stanozolol were confiscated, with suggestions that the contamination came through badly cleaned production lines. Again this is not just an issue about anti-doping, but also the potential health risks for young people, females and pregnant women.

Finally, DS have also recently been found with new designer steroids, which are neither listed by WADA nor shown as ingredients in any available medication. Furthermore, little knowledge exists surrounding the effects and side effects of these new steroids. Since manufacturers of these products also produce other DS, cross-contamination with 'new' steroids can be expected, with further potential of detrimental health issues and inadvertent positive doping cases.

The assumption has generally been that the presence of WADA-prohibited substances is the result of inadvertent contamination of raw materials and/or cross-contamination within the manufacturing or packaging process rather than deliberate adulteration of the products in an attempt to increase the supplement's effectiveness. Consequently, the amounts of steroids detected have been extremely variable, even within a single batch, but have generally been very small. However, very low levels of contamination (measured in parts per billion) can still cause positive drug tests in an elite athlete, even though these levels are much lower than acceptable impurity levels (typically around 0.01%) in good manufacturing practice regulations. It is important to note that although this minimal amount of contamination could produce dire consequences for an athlete competing under the WADA code, in most cases this amount is unlikely to cause detrimental health issues for the general consumer. Daily food product

withdrawals and recalls due to mislabelling and undeclared allergens plus issues with impurities and contamination from medicine residues, insects and small pieces of metal and plastic demonstrate that inadvertent contamination is not just an issue for sports nutrition products.

The inadequate regulation of DS means there is no way for consumers to know what many supplements actually contain or how pure the product and its ingredients are. Manufacturers with good quality controls and facilities for testing for banned substance are better able to control the risk. The inception of the WADA code and the implications of strict liability means that athletes are held responsible for whatever is in their bodies irrespective of how it got there. Therefore athletes who compete under the WADA code should be extremely cautious about using supplements and always work with a qualified professional on risk minimisation of supplement use. To help prevent athletes from inadvertent doping, they should use only supplements from low-risk sources. Such sources are established in some countries such as Germany, the Netherlands and the UK, where the databases list DS from companies which perform quality control and screening for WADA substances. However, these databases are still unable to guarantee that the DS is free from risk, but simply offer this minimisation of risk.

Consumers of DS should be aware that if a product offers enormous benefit on performance, increased muscle mass or weight loss, it might be faked or contaminated with a prescriptive drug or even illegal substance, which can cause a positive doping case or serious side effects.

Placebo effect of dietary supplements

Although DS use is widespread in athletes, many do not have an evidence-based proven effect on health or performance. In contrast, athletes explore through their own experience and so it is not surprising that some athletes claim to have success or feel good with certain DS. This leads into two aspects:

(1) athletes respond differently according to the use of DS (responder and non-responder effect);
(2) belief in a product increases performance by teasing performance reserves.

In competition (and training), psychological variables such as motivation or expectancy are important

Table 9.10 Latin square design using four conditions to investigate the placebo effect of drugs/supplements.

1	Inform drug/receive drug
2	Inform drug/receive placebo
3	Inform placebo/receive drug
4	Inform placebo/receive placebo

factors in reaching maximum performance. Since there is an interaction between mind and body, it is not surprising that athletes and coaches sometimes report a positive effect with use of DS. If this effect is based on a 'positive outcome resulting from the belief that a beneficial treatment has been received', it can be classified as a placebo effect. This effect has been acknowledged in medicine for the past 50 years, while systematic research in the field of sports performance is relatively new.

Several authors suggest that investigations on the placebo effect of DS in sports performance should use a so-called Latin square design (Table 9.10).

One of the first placebo studies (Maganaris et al., 2000) was undertaken on 11 weightlifters. They were told they would receive a placebo fast-acting anabolic steroid, which led to a mean improvement of 3.5–5.2% in maximal weight lifted in different tests. In the subsequent second experimental trial, six athletes were correctly informed about the placebo. Those athletes reduced their performance into the range of baseline levels, while the remaining five athletes maintained their improvement.

Another placebo study (Porcari et al., 2006) reported a significant difference on a 5-km run using super-oxygenated water. However, the improvements over baseline levels were higher for the less accomplished runners compared with the experienced runners. Furthermore, the less-experienced runners reported that they felt better and asked where they could buy the product, while the experienced runners did not believe that the product worked. The differences in the appraisals suggest a relationship between performance status and placebo response, which should also be considered when interpreting other studies surrounding the efficacy of DS. Therefore, depending on the research design the interpretation is somewhat limited by the training status of the subjects.

While most studies investigate a positive belief into a treatment, Beedie et al. (2007) found a negative influence on sports performance if subjects were told that the treatment would have a negative effect on sprinting performance. Based on this proposition, the authors speculated that a negative belief about a legitimate supplement might reduce the expected beneficial effects on performance.

In a recent study, Foad et al. (2008) studied the psychological and pharmacological effects of caffeine in cycling performance. The authors supported their data with the ergogenic effect of caffeine use. Surprisingly, the effect was higher when athletes were told that they had not received caffeine compared with telling them that they had received caffeine. Additionally, a negative placebo effect (nocebo) was found in the trial 'inform no treatment/give no treatment'.

In conclusion, studies show that there is a placebo effect surrounding the use of DS on sport performance. However, for better interpretation and further investigations it should be noted that:

- a relationship between performance status and placebo response might exist;
- a positive belief into a product can increase performance while a negative belief can decrease performance;
- the placebo effect observed is different if an active substance is given and belief is manipulated versus a study in which only the belief is manipulated.

Since a placebo effect exists, scientists are required to use double-blind treatments in their research studies. However, some authors speculate that the placebo effect can be seen more within studies than in the real world. A potential reason includes the fact that subjects might not perform at volitional maximum in performance research, but will do so in competition. In turn, this suggests that personality might influence placebo response or that placebo response is different according to personality. Therefore, researchers, athletes and coaches are advised to be cautious in translating observations from the laboratory to the real world, not just from placebo studies.

9.11 Summary

DS use in sport is widespread around the world, with an estimated global market value of more than US$60 billion. DS use is higher for athletes compared with the general population. Surveys show that nearly half of all athletes use supplements, their popularity varying widely between different sports and between athletes of differing ages, performance levels and cultural backgrounds. The most popular DS include multivitamins and some minerals, but product popularity differs vastly between countries. The most common reasons for DS use in the sports and exercise arena are health and performance related.

The list of supplements and ergogenic aids used within the exercise and sporting environment is exhaustive. Supplements also come in many forms and guises. Since it is often unclear which DS might be effective or helpful, the APRID framework provides an example of a ranking system for sports foods, DS and ergogenic aids, based on a risk–benefit analysis of current evidence from both scientific research and clinical dietetic practice.

Supplements classified as 'Acceptable' include sports foods, such as drinks, powders, bars and gels, which are felt to provide a useful, practical, portable and timely source of energy and nutrients and therefore have a genuine role to play in supplementing the diet during both training and competition. A few ergogenic aids (caffeine, creatine and the buffers sodium bicarbonate and sodium citrate) are also ranked in the top 'Acceptable' category, listed under the subheading of 'performance' as substances with substantial evidence for enhanced performance for some athletes in some circumstances.

Athletes should always consider the issues of efficacy, safety and legality/ethics associated with DS products prior to making the decision to use any DS. Unfortunately, all too frequently, specific information is limited. Furthermore, due to poor manufacturing practice, some DS do not contain an adequate dose of the labelled ingredients or contain impurities like glass, lead or animal faeces. Furthermore, the FDA regularly reports on products found to contain effective amounts of prescriptive drugs, which could lead to detrimental side effects.

Another potential health risk is from contamination or fake DS which can cause a positive doping test for those athletes competing under the WADA code. Therefore, athletes competing under the WADA code need to be extremely cautious about using supplements and always work with a qualified professional on risk minimisation of supplement use.

References

Artioli GG, Gualano B, Smith A, Stout J, Lancha AH. Role of β-alanine supplementation on muscle carnosine and exercise performance. Med Sci Sports Exerc 2010; 42: 1162–1173.

Bailey SJ, Winyard P, Vanhatalo A et al. Dietary nitrate supplementation reduces the O_2 cost of low-intensity exercise and enhances tolerance to high-intensity exercise in humans. J Appl Physiol 2009; 107: 1144–1155.

Beedie CJ, Foad AJ. The placebo effect in sports performance. Sports Med 2009; 39: 313–329.

Beedie CJ, Coleman DA, Foad AJ. Positive and negative placebo effects resulting from the deceptive administration of an ergogenic aid. Int J Sport Nutr Exerc Metab 2007; 17: 259–269.

Bergeron MF, Senchina DS, Burke LM, Stear SJ, Castell LM. BJSM reviews: A–Z of nutritional supplements: dietary supplements, sports nutrition foods and ergogenic aids for health and performance Part 13: Electrolytes, Ephedra, Echinacea. Br J Sports Med 2010; 44: 985–986.

Bishop D, Edge J, Davis C, Goodman C. Induced metabolic alkalosis affects muscle metabolism and repeated-sprint ability. Med Sci Sports Exerc 2004; 36: 807–813.

Branch JD. Effect of creatine supplementation on body composition and performance: a meta-analysis. Int J Sport Nutr Exerc Metab 2003; 13: 198–226.

Braun H, Koehler K, Geyer H, Kleinert J, Mester J, Schaenzer W. Dietary supplement use among elite young German athletes. Int J Sport Nutr Exerc Metab 2009; 19: 97–109.

Braun H, Koehler K, Geyer H, Thevis M, Schaenzer W. Dietary supplement use of elite German athletes and knowledge about the contamination problem. In: 14th Annual Congress of the European College of Sport Sciences, Oslo, Norway (Loland S, Bø K, Fasting K, Hallén J, Ommundsen Y, Roberts G, Tsolakidis E, eds). 2009, p 378.

Broad EM, Maughan RJ, Galloway SDR. Effects of L-carnitine L-tartrate ingestion on substrate utilisation during prolonged exercise. Int J Sport Nutr Exerc Metab 2005; 15: 665–679.

Buford BN, Koch AJ. Glycine-arginine-ketoisocaproic acid improves performance of repeated cycling sprints. Med Sci Sports Exerc 2004; 36: 583–587.

Burke L, Pyne D. Bicarbonate loading to enhance training and competitive performance. Int J Sport Physiol Perform 2007; 2: 93–97.

Burke LM, Castell LM, Stear SJ et al. BJSM reviews: A–Z of nutritional supplements: dietary supplements, sports nutrition foods and ergogenic aids for health and performance Part 4: Aspartame, branched chain amino acids, bee pollen, boron, carnitine. Br J Sport Med 2009; 43: 1088–1090.

Burke LM, Castell LM, Stear SJ. BJSM reviews: A–Z of supplements: dietary supplements, sports nutrition foods and ergogenic aids for health and performance Part 1. Br J Sport Med 2009; 43: 728–729.

Burke LM, Castell LM, Stear SJ, Houtkopper L, Manore M, Senchina D. BJSM reviews: A–Z of nutritional supplements: dietary supplements, sports nutrition foods and ergogenic aids for health and performance Part 7: calcium and bone health, Vitamin D, and Chinese herbs. Br J Sport Med 2010; 44: 389–391.

Calder PC, Lindley MR, Burke LM, Stear SJ, Castell LM. BJSM reviews: A–Z of nutritional supplements: dietary supplements, sports nutrition foods and ergogenic aids for health and performance Part 14: Fatty acids and fish oils. Br J Sport Med 2010; 44: 1065–1067.

Castell LM. Glutamine supplementation in vitro and in vivo, in exercise and immunodepression. Sports Med 2003; 33: 1–23.

Castell LM, Burke LM, Stear SJ. BJSM reviews: A–Z of supplements: dietary supplements, sports nutrition foods and ergogenic aids for health and performance Part 2: Amino acids, androstenedione, arginine, asparagine and aspartate. Br J Sport Med 2009; 43: 807–810.

Castell LM, Burke LM, Stear SJ et al. BJSM reviews: A–Z of nutritional supplements: dietary supplements, sports nutrition foods and ergogenic aids for health and performance Part 9: Choline bitartrate plus acetylcholine, chondroitinn/glucosamine, chromium picolinate and cissus quadrangularis. Br J Sport Med 2010; 44: 609–611.

Castell LM, Burke LM, Stear SJ, Maughan RJ. BJSM reviews: A–Z of nutritional supplements: dietary supplements, sports nutrition foods and ergogenic aids for health and performance Part 8: Carbohydrate. Br J Sport Med 2010; 44: 468–470.

Castell LM, Burke LM, Stear SJ, McNaughton LR, Harris RC. BJSM reviews: A–Z of nutritional supplements: dietary supplements, sports nutrition foods and ergogenic aids for health and performance Part 5: Buffers: sodium bicarbonate and sodium citrate; β-alanine and carnosine. Br J Sport Med 2010; 44: 77–78.

Currell K, Syed A, Dziedzic CE et al. BJSM reviews: A–Z of nutritional supplements: dietary supplements, sports nutrition foods and ergogenic aids for health and performance Part 12: cysteine, cystine, cytochrome C, dehydroepiandrosterone, dihydroxyacetone phosphate, pyruvate, dimethylglycine. Br J Sport Med 2010; 44: 905–907.

Davison G, Diment B. Bovine colostrum supplementation attenuates the decrease of salivary lysozyme and enhances the recovery of neutrophil function after prolonged exercise. Br J Nutr 2010; 103: 1425–1432.

Edge J, Bishop D, Goodman C. Effects of chronic nahco3 ingestion during interval training on changes to muscle buffer capacity, metabolism, and short-term endurance performance. J Appl Physiol 2006; 101: 918–925.

EFSA. Tolerable Upper Intake Levels for Vitamins and Minerals, 2006. Available from www.efsa.europa.eu/EFSA/Scientific_Document/upper_level_opinions_full-part33.pdf.

EVM. Safe Upper Levels for Vitamins and Minerals, 2003. Available from http://cot.food.gov.uk/pdfs/vitmin2003.pdf

FNB. Dietary Reference Intakes: A Risk Assessment Model for Establishing Upper Intake Levels for Nutrients. Available from www.nap.edu/openbook.php?isbn=0309063485

Foad AJ, Beedie CJ, Coleman DA. Pharmacological and psychological effects of caffeine ingestion in 40 km cycling performance. Med Sci Sports Exerc 2008; 40: 158–165.

Geyer H, Mareck U, Köhler K, Parr MK, Schänzer W. Cross contaminations of vitamin- and mineral-tablets with metandienone and stanozolol. In: Recent Advances in Doping Analysis (14) (Schanzer W, Geyer H, Gotzmann A, Mareck U, eds). Köln: Sportverlag Strauss, 2006, p 11.

Geyer H, Parr MK, Koehler K, Mareck U, Schänzer W, Thevis M. Nutritional supplements cross-contaminated and faked with doping substances. J Mass Spectrom 2008; 43: 892–902.

Goldfinch J, McNaughton LR, Davies P. Bicarbonate ingestion and its effects upon 400-m. Eur J Appl Physiol Occup Physiol 1988; 57: 45–48.

Graham T. Caffeine and exercise metabolism, endurance and performance. Sports Med 2001; 31: 785–807.

Harris RC, Söderlund K, Hultman E. Elevation of creatine in resting and exercised muscle of normal subjects by creatine supplementation. Clin Sci 1992; 83: 367–374.

Hill CA, Harris RC, Kim HJ et al. Influence of beta-alanine supplementation on skeletal muscle carnosine concentrations and high intensity cycling capacity. Amino Acids 2007; 32: 225–233.

Jager R, Purpura M, Kingsley M. Phospholipids and sports performance. J Int Soc Sports Nutrition 2007; 4: 5.

Lindh AM, Peyrebrune MC, Ingham SA, Bailey DM, Folland JP. Sodium bicarbonate improves swimming performance. Int J Sports Med 2008; 29: 519–523.

Maganaris CN, Collins D, Sharp M. Expectancy effects and strength training: do steroids make a difference? Sport Psychol 2000; 14: 272–278.

Maughan RJ, Depiesse F, Geyer H. The use of dietary supplements by athletes. J Sport Sci 2007; 25: S103–S113.

Mickleborough TD, Ionescu AA, Lindley MR, Fly AD. Protective effect of fish oil supplementation on exercise-induced bronchoconstriction in asthma. Chest 2006; 29: 39–49.

Newsholme E, Blomstrand E. Branch chain amino acids and central fatigue. J Nutr 2006; 136: 274S–276S.

Nieman DC, Williams AS, Shanely RA et al. Quercetin's influence on exercise performance and muscle mitochondrial biogenesis. Med Sci Sports Exerc 2010; 42: 338–345.

Nieper A. Nutritional supplement practices in UK junior national track and field athletes. Br J Sport Med 2005; 39: 645–649.

Penry JT, Manore M. Choline: an important micronutrient for maximal endurance-exercise performance? Int J Sport Nutr Exerc Metab 2008; 18: 191–203.

Petroczi A, Naughton DP. The age-gender-status profile of high performing athletes in the UK taking nutritional supplements: lessons for the future. J Int Soc Sports Nutr 2008; 5: 2.

Poortmans JR, Rawson ES, Burke LM, Stear SJ, Castell LM. BJSM reviews: A–Z of nutritional supplements: dietary supplements, sports nutrition foods and ergogenic aids for health and performance Part 11: Creatine. Br J Sport Med 2010; 44: 765–766.

Porcari JP, Otto J, Felker H, Mikat RP, Foster C. The placebo effect on exercise performance. J Cardiopulmon Rehabil Prev 2006; 26: 269.

Rawson ES, Persky AM. Mechanisms of muscular adaptations to creatine supplementation. Int Sport Med J 2007; 8: 43–53.

Reid M. Free radicals and muscle fatigue: of ROS, canaries, and the IOC. Free Radic Biol Med 2008; 44: 169–179.

Rennie M, Bohe J, Smith K, Wacherhage H, Greenhaff P. Branched-chain amino acids as fuels and anabolic signals in human muscle. J Nutr 2006; 136: 264S–268S.

Requena B, Zabala M, Padial P, Feriche B. Sodium bicarbonate and sodium citrate: ergogenic aids? J Strength Cond Res 2005; 19: 213–224.

Shing CM, Hunter DC, Stevenson LM. Bovine colostrum supplementation and exercise performance potential mechanisms. Sports Med 2009; 39: 1033–1054.

Sims ST, Rehrer NJ, Bell ML, Cotter JD. Preexercise sodium loading aids fluid balance and endurance for women exercising in the heat. J Appl Physiol 2001; 103: 534–541.

Sobal J, Marquart LF. Vitamin/mineral supplement use among athletes: a review of the literature. Int J Sport Nutr 1994; 4: 320–334.

Stear SJ, Whyte GP, Budgett R. Declared dietary supplement usage by British Olympians. Med Sci Sport Exerc 2006; 38: S409.

Stear SJ, Burke LM, Castell LM. BJSM reviews: A–Z of nutritional supplements: dietary supplements, sports nutrition foods and ergogenic aids for health and performance Part 3: Antioxidants and arnica. Br J Sports Med 2009; 43: 890–892.

Stear SJ, Burke LM, Castell LM, Spriet LL. BJSM reviews: A–Z of nutritional supplements: dietary supplements, sports nutrition foods and ergogenic aids for health and performance Part 6: Caffeine. Br J Sports Med 2010; 44: 297–298.

Stear SJ, Castell LM, Burke LM et al. BJSM reviews: A–Z of nutritional supplements: dietary supplements, sports nutrition foods and ergogenic aids for health and performance Part 10: Citrulline, coenzyme Q10, colostrum, conjugated linoleic acid, copper. Br J Sports Med 2010; 44: 688–690.

Stephens FB, Evans CE, Constantin-Teodosiu D, Greenhaff PL. Carbohydrate ingestion augments L-carnitine retention in humans. J Appl Physiol 2007; 102: 1065–1070.

Warren GL, Park ND, Maresca RD, Mckibans KI, Millard-Stafford ML. Effect of caffeine ingestion on muscular strength and endurance: a meta-analysis. Med Sci Sports Exerc 2010; 42: 1375–1387.

Further reading

Burke L, Broad E, Cox G et al. Supplements and sports foods. In: Clinical Sports Nutrition, 4th edn (Burke L, Deakin V, eds). Sydney: McGraw-Hill, 2010, pp 419–500.

Currell K, Jeukendrup AE. Validity, reliability and sensitivity of performance tests. Sports Med 2008; 38: 297–316.

Ebell MH, Siwek J, Weiss BD et al. Strength of recommendation taxonomy (SORT): a patient-centered approach to grading evidence in the medical literature. J Am Board Fam Pract 2004; 17: 59–67.

Geyer H, Parr MK, Mareck U, Reinhart U, Schrader Y, Schänzer W. Analysis of non-hormonal nutritional supplements for anabolic-androgenic steroids: results of an international study. Int J Sports Med 2004; 25: 124–129.

Hopkins WG, Hawley JA, Burke LM. Design and analysis of research on sport performance enhancement. Med Sci Sport Exerc 1991; 31: 472–485.

Jaffer S. Innovations in Sports and Energy Food and Drinks. Business Insights Ltd, May 2008.

Maughan R.J. Contamination of dietary supplements and positive drug tests in sport. J Sports Sci 2005; 23: 883–889.

Maughan RJ, King DS, Lea T. Dietary supplements. J Sports Sci 2004; 22: 95–113.

Maughan RJ, Depiesse F, Geyer H. The use of dietary supplements by athletes. J Sports Sci 2007; 25: S103–S113.

Mintel. Nutrition and Energy Bars. Mintel International Group Ltd, March 2009.

Mintel. Energy Drinks and Energy Shots. Mintel International Group Ltd, July 2009.

Rea P, Ooyen C. Sports Nutrition and Weight Loss Report. Nutrition Business Journal, 2009.

Stear S. Fuelling Fitness for Sports Performance. London: The Sugar Bureau, 2004.

Tallon MS. The Dietary Supplements Market. Business Insights Ltd, October 2007.

Websites

European Food Safety Authority (EFSA): www.efsa.europa.eu
US Food and Drug Administration (FDA): www.fda.gov
Food Standards Agency (FSA): www.food.gov.uk
World Anti-Doping Agency (WADA): www.wada-ama.org

10

Nutrition for Weight and Resistance Training

Stuart M Phillips, Keith Baar and Nathan Lewis

Key messages

- Taking 10 g of essential amino acids, or 20–25 g of protein, results in maximal stimulation of muscle protein synthesis (MPS). Greater protein intake results in an increase in amino acid oxidation, suggesting that greater protein intake has limited effect on MPS and is unnecessary.
- Whey protein, the fast protein component from milk, is high in leucine, rapidly digested and absorbed, and results in the greatest increase in MPS.
- Even though muscle is 'anabolically sensitive' for up to 24 hours after resistance exercise, maximal increases in MPS and muscle size and strength are seen when protein is taken immediately after exercise.
- Both resistance exercise and amino acids activate the mammalian target of rapamycin complex 1 (mTORC1), an important regulator of protein synthesis through its control of translation

initiation and ribosomal biogenesis. mTORC1 activation is required for muscle growth since the mTORC1 inhibitor rapamycin can block the increase in MPS following acute resistance exercise and muscle hypertrophy following training.
- Amino acids activate mTORC1 by activating the RagGTPase proteins and the Ragulator, molecular chaperones that transport mTORC1 to the lysosome where it can be activated by Rheb.
- Resistance exercise increases mTORC1 activity for up to 36 hours. This prolonged increase in mTORC1 activity is necessary for the sustained increase in MPS. Since endurance exercise can turn off mTORC1, partly through activation of the 5 -AMP-activated protein kinase, abstaining from endurance exercise in the period following resistance exercise will maximise MPS from the resistance exercise and nutritional interventions.

10.1 Introduction

Resistance exercise in the presence of proper nutrition is anabolic. The underlying basis for the anabolic state induced by resistance exercise is a pronounced stimulation of muscle protein synthesis (MPS) (Biolo *et al.*, 1995, 1997; Moore *et al.*, 2009a). When MPS exceeds muscle protein breakdown (MPB) then net protein balance (NPB) becomes positive and muscle mass increases (Biolo *et al.*, 1997). Periodic feeding also induces shifts in NPB from negative, during fasting where MPS is less than MPB, to positive, after feeding where MPS is greater than MPB (Tipton *et al.*, 2003). Adequate nutrition therefore assists in the maintenance of muscle protein mass (Tipton *et al.*, 2003; Phillips, 2004). Combining the resistance exercise-induced rise

in MPS with feeding results in an additive effect on MPS and marked increase in NPB (MPS >> MPB) (Biolo *et al.*, 1997; Phillips *et al.*, 2002; Moore *et al.*, 2005, 2009a,b). Repeated bouts of resistance exercise together with feeding therefore results in periodic increases in accretion of proteins over and above that induced by feeding resulting in muscle hypertrophy (Rennie *et al.*, 2004). Figure 10.1 shows a schematic of how a daily protein balance might look in someone consuming protein-containing meals of different sizes at breakfast (07.00), lunch (12.00) and dinner (19.00) throughout the day and the same individual after having performed resistance exercise. The knowledge that allows us to construct this figure comes from a number of acute studies in which the amount of protein, protein type, timing of feeding, and carbohydrate content have all

Sport and Exercise Nutrition, First Edition. Edited by Susan A Lanham-New, Samantha J Stear, Susan M Shirreffs and Adam L Collins.
© 2011 The Nutrition Society. Published 2011 by Blackwell Publishing Ltd.

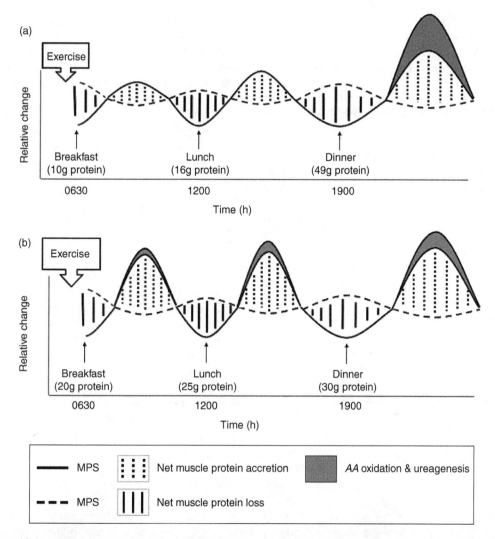

Figure 10.1 (a) Fluctuations in both muscle protein synthesis (MPS) and muscle protein breakdown (MPB) throughout a given day where a person performs a bout of resistance exercise in the overnight fasted state first thing in the morning and proceeds to consume their meals in a typical pattern of breakfast (06.30), lunch (12.00) and dinner (19.00). Note that the protein feeding patterns are consistent with what people typically consume throughout a 'normal' day. (b) An identical pattern of feeding as in (a), but this time with adequate amounts of protein consumed in each meal.

been manipulated with respect to feeding after exercise (Biolo et al., 1995, 1997; Tipton et al., 1999, 2001, 2003; Borsheim et al., 2002, 2004a,b; Bohe et al., 2003). While there are subtleties in the response (see below), as a general starting point Figure 10.1 highlights some fundamental concepts around which we will build. An important point is that the acute measurements of protein synthesis with feeding and after exercise are proposed to be relevant in predicting the long-term change in phenotype (i.e. hypertrophy) that would take place if the acute practice were to be repeated at a

sufficient frequency, intensity and duration. Evidence supporting the fact that acute observations (Wilkinson et al., 2007) are qualitatively predictive of longer-term phenotypic changes (Hartman et al., 2007) has been reported. Another important point is that we focus much of our attention on changes in MPS and not MPB for the main reason that, in a healthy person, changes in MPS are fourfold to sixfold greater than those occurring in MPB (Biolo et al., 1995, 1997; Wilkinson et al., 2007) and as such are of far greater relevance in determining changes in NPB, as Figure 10.1 shows. This chapter covers information on a number of areas, both practical and mechanistic, to allow the reader to gain some fundamental insight into how muscle protein turnover is regulated by resistance exercise and feeding.

10.2 Protein feeding and resistance exercise

Feeding protein results in a substantial hyperaminoacidaemia that promotes a net inward gradient for amino acid transport into muscle (Biolo *et al.*, 1995, 1997). The resulting influx of amino acids (AA) into the free amino pool provides the signal (Anthony *et al.*, 2000, 2002) and building blocks (Biolo *et al.*, 1995, 1997) for a stimulation of MPS. The main AA responsible for the stimulation of MPS is leucine (Anthony *et al.*, 2000, 2002), which is reviewed in greater detail below; however, the relevance of this knowledge gives rise to practical strategies that athletes can employ. Specifically, knowing the leucine content of the food being consumed, the digestion pattern of the protein, along with kinetic measures of protein turnover and their interaction with exercise allows recommendations to be made.

Protein dose

Only two true dose–response studies conducted in humans have been published (Cuthbertson *et al.*, 2005; Moore *et al.*, 2009a). In the first study, Cuthbertson *et al.* reported in young individuals at rest that an oral dose of mixed essential amino acids (EAA) of 10 g resulted in maximal stimulation of MPS. Practically, 10 g of EAA translates into 25 g of high-quality protein such as milk, soy or chicken. However, athletes are not as concerned with doses of protein required to stimulate MPS at rest, but instead after exercise. Moore *et al.* reported that 20 g of isolated egg protein resulted in maximal stimulation of MPS following a bout of intense leg resistance exercise. Consuming an additional 20 g of egg protein (40 g total) resulted in an 11% greater rate of MPS, but a concomitant increase in leucine oxidation over that seen with the 20-g protein dose. Thus, at intakes of protein of 20 g and higher, a greater proportion of the ingested leucine was being oxidised for fuel with minimal further stimulation of MPS (Moore *et al.*, 2009a). An increasing trend toward greater plasma urea nitrogen concentration was also seen, indicating a need to

dispose of excess nitrogen when 40 g of protein was ingested. At lower doses of crystalline AA a similar dose–response phenomenon has been observed when comparing ingestion of 6 g EAA (Borsheim *et al.*, 2002) versus 3 g EAA (Miller *et al.*, 2003).

The fact that 20–25 g of high-quality protein appears to be sufficient to maximally stimulate MPS after exercise supports consuming such a dose at intervals throughout the day. However, a question that remains is how often you can consume such a dose and still get a maximal MPS response. The answer remains unknown at this time; however, the data of Moore et al. (2009b) shed some light on this question. The time course of myofibrillar protein synthesis after a bout of resistance exercise and consumption of 25 g of whey protein shows that myofibrillar protein synthesis remains elevated 5 hours after exercise. The synthesis of non-myofibrillar proteins returned to basal levels by 5 hours. This suggests that in order to maintain non-myofibrillar protein synthesis a second bolus of protein, at somewhere between 4 and 5 hours, is required for a maximal synthetic stimulus.

Protein type

A persistent question is whether proteins are all equal in their capacity to promote MPS. From the standpoint of nitrogen balance the answer would appear to be yes, but nitrogen balance is for the most part reflective of rapid-turnover tissues such as gut, skin and labile proteins (Wayler *et al.*, 1983). As such, balance of nitrogen can be maintained by ingesting varying proteins of generally high quality and no distinction can be drawn between, for example, proteins from plant sources such as soy or those coming from animal sources such as milk or meat (Young *et al.*, 1984a,b). Consequently, an important advance in our understanding of how proteins are different in their capacity to support protein synthesis comes from the work of Boirie and colleagues (Boirie *et al.* 1997; Dangin *et al.*, 2001, 2002) who showed that in so far as milk proteins are concerned there are two different types of proteins, so-called fast and slow proteins (Boirie *et al.* 1997; Dangin *et al.*, 2001). Fast proteins are those from the acid-soluble whey protein fraction that are easily and rapidly digested on ingestion and yield a rapid and relatively transient hyperaminoacidaemia (Boirie *et al.* 1997). By contrast, slow proteins are derived from casein, an acid-insoluble protein that forms a protein 'clump' when exposed to acid. Clumping of casein slows its passage from the stomach and results in slower absorption in the intestine and a prolonged but quantitatively lower aminoacidaemia. Slow absorption means that casein proteins better support the assimilation of AAs in the splanchnic region (Lacroix *et al.*, 2006) and global protein balance than whey (Dangin *et al.*, 2001). In contrast, whey promotes stimulation of protein synthesis in peripheral tissues and a rise in leucine oxidation (Dangin *et al.*, 2001). All these data are, however, at the whole-body level and derived from leucine turnover, which is a measure of protein metabolism that is heavily influenced by the more rapidly turning over proteins in blood and splanchnic tissues and not muscle (Boirie *et al.* 1997; Dangin *et al.*, 2001, 2003). In fact, an often quoted figure is that muscle protein turnover only makes up 25% of whole-body protein synthesis (Nair *et al.*, 1992), but this estimate does not reveal just how inconsistent measures of whole-body protein turnover are with changes in MPS. For example, whole-body protein synthesis, oxidation and flux remain unchanged in young men following a strenuous bout of resistance exercise (Tarnopolsky *et al.*, 1991) and yet we know from multiple studies that this is a time when MPS is substantially elevated (Biolo *et al.*, 1995; Phillips *et al.*, 1997). Thus it is clear that whole-body measures of protein turnover do not correspond with the data from muscle during the acute post-exercise period.

When comparing equivalent amounts of soy and milk protein consumed in the post-exercise period, it is clear that milk proteins promote a much greater NPB and rate of MPS (Wilkinson *et al.*, 2007). Interestingly, the long-term practice of milk consumption versus an isonitrogenous and isoenergetic soy beverage resulted in greater muscle mass accretion measured by dual-energy X-ray absorptiometry and by fibre size increases (Hartman *et al.*, 2007). Hence, as we stated earlier, the short-term changes are reflective and qualitatively predictive of the long-term phenotype. However, it was not known whether there were differing responses in relation to the different sub-protein fractions of milk (i.e. casein and whey). If we use the criteria of the protein-digestibility corrected amino acid score (PDCAAS), then proteins such as casein, whey and soy are all supposedly equivalent (i.e. PDCAAS = 1.0). However, differences in PDCAAS scores do exist if the artificial cap on PDCAAS of 1.0 is lifted and true scores are compared. From this standpoint, casein, whey and soy have PDCAAS scores of 1.23, 1.15 and 1.04, respectively. Perhaps more importantly, despite quite similar EAA contents there are potentially significant differences in leucine content (Tang *et al.*, 2009). The significance of the leucine content of these proteins is not completely understood, but leucine is a key regulatory amino acid in stimulating MPS and as such its influence on responses to a set amount of protein are likely important. For example, the response of both resting-state and post-exercise MPS in response to the ingestion of isoenergetic and isonitrogenous whey, soy and casein showed superior rises in MPS with whey consumption versus both soy and casein (Tang *et al.*, 2009). This may seem somewhat paradoxical based solely on the leucine content of the protein, but an important observation was the rate of digestion of the proteins. As described above, the rate of digestion and absorption differ and as a result the appearance of leucine in the systemic circulation differed markedly between the treatments (Tang *et al.*, 2009). This led us to propose a leucine 'trigger' concept that is dependent not only on the leucine content of the protein but also on the extent to which leucine concentration in the plasma increases (Burd *et al.*, 2009a). The leucine 'threshold' is one at which signalling pathways would be maximally active (see below) and, presumably with the supporting cast of other EAA, allow MPS to proceed maximally. There is obviously a dose–response (i.e. ingested protein–MPS) relationship that is saturable, which may in fact be due to leucine alone. However, this cannot be predicted entirely by the leucine content of the protein but must also take into account the appearance of leucine in the systemic circulation. Obviously if this hypothesis is correct, then anything that changes the appearance of leucine, for example other nutrients in a meal, will affect the response of MPS.

Timing of protein ingestion

Protein ingestion as intact protein or free AA, within close temporal proximity (before, during and after) a resistance exercise bout, has been thoroughly investigated (Phillips, 2004, 2006; Phillips *et al.*, 2005, 2007). Using ingestion of crystalline AA, Tipton *et al.* (2001) showed that 6 g of EAA (equivalent to ~15 g of high-quality milk proteins) and 35 g sucrose before resistance exercise induced

160% greater increase in muscle anabolism compared with post-exercise drink consumption. The only mechanism for this difference was a pre-exercise feeding-induced increase in post-exercise blood flow by almost fourfold over the post-exercise feeding condition that increased in the delivery of amino acids to the muscle. The same group could not subsequently reproduce the results when intact whey proteins were fed immediately before compared with after resistance exercise (Tipton *et al.*, 2006). In a separate study there was no effect of pre-exercise feeding with an EAA plus carbohydrate feeding (Fujita *et al.*, 2009). Thus, recommendations for pre-exercise practice as assistive in promoting anabolism are equivocal at best.

Eating during a bout of resistance exercise or peri-workout nutrition has also been tested. A relevant observation here is that the high energy-consuming process of MPS is not elevated during resistance exercise. Recently, it was reported that co-ingestion of carbohydrate (50% glucose and 50% maltodextrin) and casein protein hydrolysate, which would be close to mimicking whey in terms of the aminoacidaemia it induces, during a combined endurance and whole-body resistance exercise session stimulates MPS even when this exercise bout was performed in the fed state (Beelen *et al.*, 2008). It was speculated that this positive result on MPS during exercise was due to a stimulation of MPS during the rest periods between the exercise sets. Of relevance to athletes, however, is that the accelerated MPS during exercise did not augment protein balance during the subsequent overnight recovery (Beelen *et al.*, 2008). Therefore, there appears to be little benefit to feeding during the resistance exercise in so far as muscle hypertrophy is concerned.

Esmarck et al. (2001) demonstrated the importance of consuming protein within close temporal proximity to the exercise bout. Specifically, elderly men (~74 years) performed resistance training three times a week for 12 weeks and were randomised to receive a protein (skim milk and soy) supplement (10 g protein, 7 g carbohydrate, 3 g fat) immediately after or 2 hours after each training session. Subjects consuming the protein supplement immediately after each training session had significant increases in thigh muscle mass, muscle cross-sectional area, and continued strength increases beyond 5 weeks (the mid-point of the training programme). Delaying the protein consumption by only 2 hours following training resulted in no change in mid-thigh cross-sectional area, no change in fibre area, and no significant increments in dynamic strength beyond week 5 of the programme. These data are difficult to reconcile as increases in muscle mass and strength are hallmark adaptations of resistance exercise, regardless of whether a nutritional intervention is employed in young or the elderly (Frontera *et al.*, 1988; Fiatarone *et al.*, 1990; Hughes *et al.*, 2001; Hunter *et al.*, 2004; Kosek *et al.*, 2006). Furthermore, Verdijk *et al.* (2008) found that in elderly Dutch men who habitually consumed adequate dietary protein by most recommendations (1.1 ± 0.1 g/kg/day), additional protein (i.e. casein hydrolysate) supplementation, 10 g before and 10 g after training, had no additional effect on muscle mass and strength gains compared with the non-supplemented group.

In trained young men who were randomised to consume a protein supplement (whey protein, glucose and creatine) either in the morning before breakfast and late evening before bed or immediately before and after workout, the pre-/post-workout nutrition group experienced greater gains in lean body mass and strength (Cribb & Hayes, 2006). However, in a similar study in which groups consumed their protein supplement (whey and casein) in the morning/evening or before/after workout, no difference in terms of strength gains after a 10-week resistance training programme were observed. However, the authors of the second study noted that the caloric intake (~29 kcal/kg/day) of their subjects, regardless of training group, were below the recommended values for active individuals (Hoffman *et al.*, 2009).

A different effect of protein timing in relation to resistance training has recently been suggested. In a study by Burk *et al.* (2009), young men completed two periods of 8 weeks of defined resistance training where they consumed a protein supplement (~70 g casein) in two stages, half in the morning and half either in the evening (5 hours after training) or immediately before exercise. Even though the increase in strength was the same between groups, the group that consumed the second half of their supplement 5 hours after the training sessions showed greater increases in fat-free mass.

We have reported that in a large cohort ($N = 56$) of young men who consumed either fat-free milk, equivalent soy drink, or carbohydrate immediately after resistance exercise and again 1 hour after exercise that milk induced superior increases in type II fibre size and fat- and bone-free mass (Hartman *et al.*, 2007). While each group showed increments in lean mass, these data illustrate that to maximise the hypertrophic adaptations the intake of a high-quality protein within the first 2 hours following training is important. We have proposed that since resistance exercise is fundamentally anabolic, elevating resting fasted-state MPS for up to 48 hours, feeding and exercise are synergistic, although an early period of post-exercise sensitivity to protein feeding exists (Burd *et al.*, 2009a). That is not to say, however, that feeding at later time points does not offer benefits since it appears that a synergistic relationship between exercise and feeding exists even on the day following resistance exercise. In fact, we have demonstrated that in a group of young subjects who consumed 15 g of whey protein following an acute bout of resistance exercise that the muscle is 'anabolically sensitive' to amino acids for up to 24 hours (Burd *et al.*, 2009b).

While inherent differences in study design, training length, protein type and training status preclude definitive statements regarding timing of protein ingestion, we favour the advice that pre-exercise and peri-exercise protein consumption do not appear as effective in stimulating lean mass gains with resistance training as post-exercise nutrition. Post exercise is a time when the energy status of the cell is returning to resting levels, signalling pathways are still active, the muscle is prone to greater rates of MPS, and all these effects are enhanced with feeding.

There are obviously a number of other variables that will affect the response of MPS with performance of resistance exercise and nutrition, including the nature of the contractile stimulus (load, volume, intensity, duration, etc.), the training state of the individual, and the individual's age, gender and genetic propensity for hypertrophy. However, these are all variables, save for the influence of training status (Tang *et al.*, 2008), on which we have at present very little information and so it is hard if not impossible to review evidence let alone make recommendations.

Mechanisms of action

In order for resistance exercise or nutrition to affect the rate of MPS, one of the three steps of protein synthesis must be altered. These steps – translation initiation, elongation, and termination – determine the rate that new proteins are made from mRNA, translating the genetic code of nucleotides into the functional code of amino acids. Translation initiation is the assembly of the components of the translational machinery: the mRNA that directs the assembly and the ribosome where assembly occurs. Elongation is the process by which amino acid residues are added one at a time to the growing protein. Termination is the process by which the protein is cleaved and released from the ribosome. Under normal conditions, ribosomes are stacked 80–100 nucleotides apart along an mRNA. However, they are capable of stacking much closer, up to 27–29 nucleotides apart (Wolin & Walter, 1988), allowing a threefold increase in protein synthesis without any change in mRNA. Therefore, increasing the rate of initiation is the primary mechanism for accelerating protein synthesis (Gingras *et al.*, 1999). To block protein synthesis, both the rate of initiation and elongation can be used to rapidly stop unwanted or unnecessary translation and conserve energy (Rose *et al.*, 2009). We will not discuss translation in detail here, and for more information on this topic the reader is referred to the following excellent reviews (Kozak, 1989; Hershey, 1991; Gingras *et al.*, 1999).

Translation initiation is controlled by the eukaryotic initiation factor (eIF)2, the initiation factor 4E binding protein (4EBP) and the ribosomal protein S6 kinase (S6K1). All these proteins are in turn controlled by one master regulator of protein synthesis and cell growth, the mammalian target of rapamycin (mTOR), which can exist in two complexes. In the first (mTORC1), mTOR associates with raptor and a number of accessory proteins. This mTOR complex can be turned off with the macrolide antibiotic rapamycin. Raptor is an adapter protein that identifies and binds proteins that contain TOS (TOR signalling) motifs (Schalm *et al.*, 2003) such as 4EBP and S6K1 (Schalm & Blenis, 2002). The second complex (mTORC2) is very similar, consisting of mTOR and many of the same accessory proteins. However, in place of raptor in this complex is rictor, which means that mTORC2 phosphorylates different targets and is rapamycin insensitive (Sarbassov *et al.*, 2005). mTORC2 activates the Rho GTPases (Jacinto *et al.*, 2004), modulates the phosphorylation of protein kinase (PK)C (Sarbassov *et al.*, 2004) and PKB (Sarbassov *et al.*, 2005) and has a role in regulating the cytoskeleton (Jacinto *et al.*, 2004; Sarbassov *et al.*, 2004). In contrast, mTORC1 phosphorylates S6K1, 4EBP, HIF1α and PRAS40 and controls protein synthesis and cell growth (Schalm & Blenis, 2002; Land & Tee, 2007; Oshiro *et al.*, 2007).

The importance of mTORC1 in the development of muscle hypertrophy was first proposed in 1999 when we found that the activity of mTORC1 (as determined by phosphorylation of its target S6K1) 6 hours after a single bout of exercise increased in proportion to the increase in muscle mass following 6 weeks of training (Baar & Esser, 1999). This was confirmed by showing that increasing the activity of mTORC1 (putting an mTORC1 activator into muscle) increases muscle size without exercise and that blocking mTORC1 (with rapamycin) prevented muscle hypertrophy (Bodine *et al.*, 2001). Together, these experiments demonstrate that mTORC1 is activated by resistance exercise and is required for the development of muscle hypertrophy.

As described above, the acute changes in protein synthesis are reflected in the long-term changes in muscle size and strength. Therefore, it is not surprising that the increase in MPS after resistance exercise is completely blocked by the mTORC1 inhibitor rapamycin. Unlike control subjects, subjects given rapamycin before they performed resistance exercise showed no increase in MPS 1–2 hours after they had completed the exercise (Drummond *et al.*, 2009). This shows that mTORC1 is responsible for the acute increase in MPS after resistance exercise.

Like resistance exercise, amino acids, specifically leucine, increase mTORC1 activation. When given an oral supplement containing increasing amounts of leucine, the activity of mTORC1 (determined by the phosphorylation of 4EBP and S6K1) increases in a dose-dependent manner even when there is no change in circulating insulin (Crozier *et al.*, 2005). Even though mTORC1 activity continues to rise with increasing insulin, MPS reaches a plateau at approximately one-third of the maximal activity of mTORC1. This saturation of protein synthesis with amino acid ingestion may underlie the fact that increasing amino acid intake too much has little effect on protein synthesis. Together, this means that mTORC1 is activated by both resistance exercise and amino acid ingestion and increasing mTORC1 is required to increase MPS after resistance exercise.

mTORC1 activation

With this background, understanding the activation of mTORC1 becomes the key to increasing MPS and muscle hypertrophy. Even though we know that mTORC1 is activated by resistance exercise, it is still unclear how this happens. It is clear that the activity of mTORC1 is related to the load on the muscle (Baar & Esser, 1999) and inversely related to the amount of metabolic stress in the muscle (Thomson *et al.*, 2008). This suggests that resistance exercise should be performed against heavy loads over short periods of time to maximise mTORC1 activity, MPS and muscle growth. It is also clear that the activation of mTORC1 by resistance exercise occurs in a manner distinct from its activation by growth factors like insulin growth factor (IGF)-1 (Spangenburg *et al.*, 2008). For example, activation of mTORC1 following resistance exercise occurs independent of the protein kinase B/akt signalling pathway and is independent of the circulating hormone level (West *et al.*, 2009).

In order for amino acids to activate mTORC1, they first must be taken up into the skeletal muscle. The uptake of amino acids into muscle is mediated by a family of transporters known as the solute carriers (SLC). The SLC proteins use gradients established by active transporters such as the sodium/potassium ATPase (Na$^+$/K$^+$-ATPase) to transport amino acids into muscle (Hundal & Taylor, 2009). Following resistance exercise, there is a transient increase in the uptake of amino acids into the working muscle (Biolo *et al.*, 1995). This suggests that membrane permeability for specific amino acids is increased following resistance exercise. Since one of the amino acids taken up at a greater rate is leucine (MacKenzie *et al.*, 2009), the increase in amino acid permeability may play an important role in the synergistic effect of resistance exercise and feeding on mTORC1 activation and MPS. However, it is important to note that the increase in amino acid uptake following resistance exercise is short-lived. Leucine content in muscle increases in the first 90 min after exercise but returns to normal levels by 3 hours (MacKenzie *et al.*, 2009). This might explain the benefit of consuming amino acids immediately following exercise.

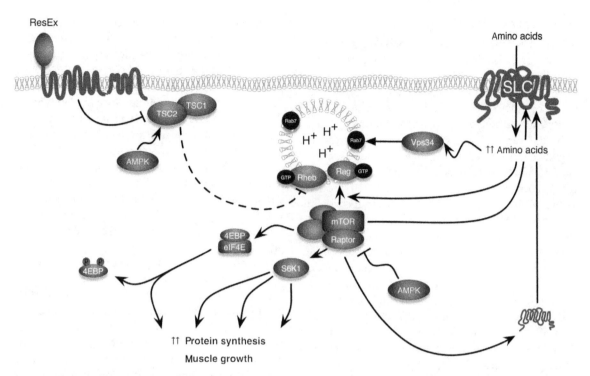

Figure 10.2 A simplified view of mTORC1 activation by resistance exercise and nutrition. Resistance exercise activates a yet to be determined receptor that inhibits the tuberous sclerosis complex (TSC1/2). Inhibition of TSC1/2 relieves the inhibition on the mTORC1 activator Ras homolog enriched in brain (Rheb) on the lysosomal membrane. The subsequent recruitment of mTOR and raptor to the lysosome through their interaction with the Rag-GTPase proteins and Ragulator results in the activation of mTORC1. mTORC1 directly phosphorylates and activates the 70-kDa ribosomal S6 kinase (S6K1) and phosphorylates and inactivates the initiation factor 4E binding protein (4EBP) resulting in increased muscle protein synthesis. mTORC1 simultaneously regulates the production of solute carrier transporters resulting in more amino acid entry into the muscle. The increase in amino acid uptake, specifically of leucine, activates vaculolar protein sorting (Vps)34, the Ragulator, and the Rag-GTPase proteins keeping mTORC1 at the lysosome and prolonging its activation.

Once in the muscle, amino acids activate a primordial shuttling system that is largely unchanged from yeast to human. The key to the activation of mTORC1 by amino acids is its relocation within the cell. In the absence of amino acids, mTOR is spread throughout the cell. In response to amino acids, mTOR associates with a structure called the lysosome, an acid-filled organelle that aids in the intracellular breakdown of protein to amino acids (Sancak *et al.*, 2010). mTORC1 is brought to the lysosomal membrane by proteins called the Rag-GTPases and a three-protein complex called the Ragulator (Sancak *et al.*, 2010). The movement of mTORC1 to the lysosome is facilitated by the primordial kinase Vps34 that increases membrane trafficking (Byfield *et al.*, 2005). Once at the lysosome, mTORC1 can be activated by the small G-protein Rheb (Ras-like protein enriched in brain). The ability of Rheb to activate mTORC1 is normally prevented by the

tuberous sclerosis complex tumour suppressor proteins (TSC1/2). TSC1/2 are inactivated by growth factors and other growth stimuli (Inoki *et al.*, 2002) and their inactivation results in an increase in Rheb activity. In this way, amino acids, through relocation of mTORC1 to the lysosome, combine with the activation of Rheb by growth stimuli, such as resistance exercise, to increase mTORC1 activity (Figure 10.2).

While transient increases in amino acid levels increase MPS, prolonged elevation in amino acid levels might not be beneficial. Prolonged elevation of amino acids can lead to a state of insulin resistance through a feedback mechanism initiated by the mTORC1 target S6K1 (Tremblay & Marette, 2001). Since insulin signalling can decrease protein degradation (Gelfand & Barrett, 1987), this suggests that having continuously high amino acid levels would have a negative effect on NPB in muscle.

Dynamics of mTORC1 signalling

mTORC1 is activated by 30 min following a bout of exercise and remains active for at least 18 hours (MacKenzie *et al.*, 2009). The long duration of mTORC1 activity is likely important for the prolonged increased in MPS following resistance exercise (Phillips *et al.*, 1997). Therefore, it is important to note that mTORC1 can be inactivated by metabolic stress, as would be experienced during long-term aerobic exercise. Metabolic stress inactivates mTORC1 through the 5'-adenosine monophosphate-activated protein kinase (AMPK). AMPK is activated by an increase in the ratio of AMP to ATP within the exercising muscle. When active, AMPK can turn off mTORC1 in two ways (Figure 10.2). First, AMPK can phosphorylate and activate TSC2 (Inoki *et al.*, 2002). Second, AMPK can phosphorylate raptor and disrupt its ability to bind to mTOR (Gwinn *et al.*, 2008). In both these ways, endurance exercise through AMPK can prematurely turn off mTORC1 and MPS (Thomson *et al.*, 2008). Therefore, to maximise MPS endurance exercise should not be performed after resistance exercise.

We have focused on the role of mTORC1 in the control of protein synthesis after resistance exercise since this is an area that has been well studied in the past 10 years. However, this does not mean that other intracellular signalling processes do not play an important role in resistance exercise and amino acid stimulation of MPS and hypertrophy. It is clear that mitogen-activated protein kinase (MAPK/ERK) plays a role in activating MPS (Drummond *et al.*, 2009) and that other proteins like myostatin are important in regulating muscle size (Lee & McPherron, 2001). In the coming years, a role for these and other proteins in amino acid-induced increases in MPS might better develop. Until then, athletes should focus on maximally activating mTORC1 with diet and exercise.

10.3 Practical considerations

What practical advice can be given to athletes, given what has been laid out? It is important to emphasise that these recommendations are based not only on short-term acute studies with increases in NPB as the outcome (due primarily to increased MPS and less often to changes in MPB), but also on long-term training studies in which muscle mass accrual and

strength gains are the main outcomes. What appears critical is to get athletes to consume protein immediately after they complete their workout. The immediate post-workout period is clearly a time when protein ingestion needs to take place to maximise the capacity of the exercise-induced rise in MPS. During this time, exercise and nutrition interact synergistically to promote greater increases in MPS than either protein ingestion or resistance exercise alone (Biolo *et al.*, 1997). In particular, high-quality proteins and EAA in combination with carbohydrate provide a remarkably effective combination of nutrients that will aid in stimulating MPS and suppressing the normal exercise-induced rise in MPB as well as aiding in glycogen repletion.

The dose of protein required to maximally stimulate MPS appears to be 20–25 g, although this study was performed in young men weighing about 86 kg, meaning that a 20-g dose would be distributed over a large volume. The dose of protein that maximally stimulates MPS for lighter persons is probably less and it is most likely that it is determined by the circulating blood leucine concentration. It is unclear at this time whether, for example, a 43-kg person would require only 10 g (i.e. half what an 86-kg person requires) to maximally activate MPS. However, it is safest to assume that this optimal dose of protein is absolute and not relative to body mass and it would therefore be advisable to recommend that athletes consume this dose of protein at each meal to promote optimal adaptation (i.e. increases in MPS that lead to hypertrophy) and possibly tissue repair. The response to this pattern of protein ingestion is shown in Figure 10.1b, highlighting the robust response of MPS with each full meal. This contrasts with the more typical pattern, shown in Figure 10.1a, where suboptimal intake at breakfast and excess intake at dinner lead to decreased MPS and increased amino acid oxidation, respectively. A similar concept has been suggested for older persons in an attempt to slow sarcopenic loss of muscle mass and maintain muscle function (Paddon-Jones & Rasmussen, 2009).

The type of protein to consume after resistance exercise, while still controversial, appears to be high-quality milk proteins, with an advantage of whey protein over soy and casein. Energy definitely factors into the recommendation here, but energy alone is not sufficient to promote optimal gains in muscle mass and must be accompanied by sufficient protein.

The optimal form of energy is carbohydrate, which would aid in replenishment of oxidised glycogen during an exercise bout, but evidence to date is equivocal about whether carbohydrate consumption is advantageous in promoting MPS or suppressing MPB to the extent that would benefit muscle mass and performance in the long run. Nonetheless, there is no question that glycogen is still the preferred fuel for muscular contractions during resistance exercise (MacDougall *et al.*, 1999) and so depletion of glycogen stores may hamper performance. It is also unclear whether athletes in a glycogen-depleted state, even if in energy balance overall, can mount a full and robust MPS response. The suggestion from animal work is that the lower energy charge of the cell, or perhaps reduced glycogen content itself, may impair signalling through mTOR possibly through inhibition by AMPK. Thus athletes attempting to gain full advantage of their resistance exercise workouts should follow the recommendations below.

- Consume protein as soon as possible after exercise in order to take full advantage of the mechanisms put in play by the exercise itself.
- For bigger athletes (≥85 kg) the dose of protein that would maximise MPS appears to be between 20 and 25 g of high-quality protein (eggs, milk, meat).
- Current recommendations for lighter athletes cannot be made at this time, but it is reasonable to assume that they would require something less than 20 g.
- The source of protein appears to be important in determining the phenotypic changes, with milk protein and whey in particular offering some advantage over soy and isolated casein.

- The addition of some carbohydrate to protein after exercise is beneficial in restoring oxidised muscle glycogen, but does not appear to offer a substantive advantage, in terms of stimulating MPS, over protein alone.

10.4 Conclusions and remaining questions

Rather than simply acting as a building block for protein synthesis, protein ingestion modifies the post-exercise signalling response and in doing so eventually modifies the phenotypic adaptation to resistance exercise. As opposed to blithe recommendations to consume excessive quantities of protein, which would promote only amino acid oxidation and ureagenesis, we favour a more measured response where dose and timing of protein ingestion, as well as focusing on high-quality protein ingestion, are more important and relevant to athletes. The emphasis on achieving sufficient protein at each meal and rapidly after exercise without excessive focus on overall protein intake would, at least in our view, be more prudent and would also allow athletes to achieve targets for carbohydrate and micronutrient consumption while consuming a varied diet.

What questions remain to be determined? We are still unaware of what protein doses maximally stimulate MPS in lighter persons, but it seems reasonable to hypothesise that a smaller person would require a smaller dose of protein. What happens to requirements for maximal stimulation of MPS when athletes are in a caloric deficit? A high-protein diet has potential for aiding in weight loss during a hypoenergetic diet period and a hypocaloric/hyperaminoacidaemic diet may 'spare' lean mass and accelerate the change in body composition.

Practice tips: nutrition for weight and resistance training

Nathan Lewis

For the purposes of this chapter, nutrition for weight will refer to increases in weight only, as making weight and weight loss is covered elsewhere. For the practitioner counselling the athlete in relation to nutritional strategies for weight and resistance training, detail and understanding should be sought regarding the following factors.

- *Sport and training*. The athlete's sport, positional role and skill requirements if relevant. Periodisation of the nutritional

strategies in relation to resistance training programme (volume and intensity) unloading and loading phases, and volume and intensity of endurance training as this may undermine gains in lean body mass (LBM). In addition, information on resistance training history and athlete's training age, the timing of resistance training workouts, particularly in relation to endurance training, and seasonal peaking and competitions/matches when other nutritional and training objectives may take priority.

- *Weight*. Athlete's injury and weight history. What is the rationale for weight/body mass (BM) increase, and what are the performance implications? Is the athlete looking to just increase overall BM? If so, any increase in LBM, fat mass (FM), and intracellular and extra-cellular water would be desirable, for example acutely artificially increasing BM through expansion of extracellular and intracellular fluid using sodium, glycerol (now on the WADA list of banned sub-stances) and creatine supplementation. Or is the focus primarily on increasing LBM, while decreasing or minimising increases in FM. What is the time line for the increase in BM? Is the BM increase for a single event, or across the season, and is it realistic? Occasionally targets are set by coaches that are not realistic.

- *Body composition and physical assessments.* How is the increase in BM/LBM to be best quantified? What physical perfor-mance-orientated assessments should be employed alongside body composition assessments, either in the field or the labora-tory to enable successful evaluation of interventions? Which assessment methods are employed will be dictated by costs, accessibility, reliability and specificity, and experience and confidence.
- *Team and staff.* Confirm that the athlete and coach are in agreement with regard to the stated objectives. In addition, seek relevant expertise from colleagues (strength and conditioning coach, physiologist, team doctor if relevant) in relation to the above and give consideration to the perceived and known acute and chronic health and performance implications.

The energy, protein, carbohydrate and supplementation require-ments of athletes have been covered in other chapters, and thus only brief consideration to some additional practical aspects is covered here.

If the goal is to increase the athletes BM (LBM and FM), then a positive energy balance in conjunction with concurrent training through a sustained increase in energy intake is required. If the goal is to increase the athletes LBM whilst decreasing or preventing increases in FM, then an intake of high quality protein is the priority in conjunction with RT to promote sustained periods of positive muscle protein balance. In contrast to a widely held belief, a positive energy balance is not required to increase LBM, and small (1 kg in 8 weeks) increases in LBM, provided the rate of weight loss is not too rapid, can be achieved in the face of a negative energy balance (Garthe *et al.*, 2011). The basis of such a nutrition program is an intake of high quality protein (1.6 g/kg/day) with frequent feedings interspersed throughout the day to augment muscle anabolism to RT. The exact amount of protein per kilogram of body weight across a spectrum of energy intakes, sports and physical demands cannot be stated, and selecting the appropriate intake for the athlete is a combination of experience, science and art, backed-up by appropriate monitoring (blood, urine, body composition, mood state, physical performance) and evaluation. It should be borne in mind, that the degrees of success of such interventions are strongly dictated by the genotype of the athlete.

Estimation of the athlete's energy intake (EI) and energy expenditure (EE) in relation to resistance training allow the practitioner to assess time lines for weight goals, and gain further insight into the athlete's current phenotype. The athlete's daily EE and training session EE can be assessed through a combination of methods, each with limitations. The practitioner is advised to investigate the accuracy of the methods in relation to the sporting environment and athlete population being assessed. Convenient and relatively inexpensive methods for estimating EE include prediction equations and activity records, triaxial accelerometers and heart monitors in combination or separately, and set-up with the athlete's physiological data. Detailed assessments of the athlete's diet using a combination of methods will increase the confidence in the estimates obtained for EI. Methods include a weighed-food intake diary (if feasible and the athlete is motivated), with the numbers of days being recorded needing to be appropriate in terms of the macronutrients being assessed; repeated 24-hour dietary recalls; and asking the athlete to photograph all food and drink against a reference object (a mobile phone camera or digital camera can provide useful additional supportive pictorial information regarding portion sizes and foods consumed). However, it is advisable to select a combination of methods, and use those in which experience and a full understanding of the limitations are known. The type, amount and timing of protein in relation to resistance training have been previously covered in this chapter.

Once estimated, the athlete's daily protein requirements should be spread throughout the day, in the region of five to seven servings, as MPS is only stimulated in the presence of an adequate supply of essential amino acids. With priority given to the serving after resistance training, given the sensitivity of the muscle to protein feeding at this time, the effects of protein feeding and resistance training on MPS are additive. Research to date suggests that to maximally stimulate MPS approximately 20–25 g high-quality protein should be consumed. Therefore total daily protein needs dictating, a similar-sized protein serving at meals and between-meal snacks would be advised, although this may need to be scaled down into smaller divided doses for lighter athletes (e.g. 50-kg female). The interval between protein serves should be in the region of 2.5–3 hours, as MPS will have declined markedly by this time after feeding. It should be borne in mind that feeding protein more frequently is unlikely to confer any additional advantage in terms of MPS, as sustained continuous elevations in the concentrations of essential amino acids in the blood does not lead to sustained elevations in MPS.

When considering the feeding of high-quality protein immediately after resistance training, when appetite may be suppressed as a result of high-intensity training, meat, fish and egg sources are not the most convenient or palatable. The use of milk, yoghurts and protein supplement powders and bars (whey, casein, egg, soya and various combinations) offer athletes a convenient high-quality protein source after resistance training. In addition, powders can provide greater flexibility in tailoring the protein serve to maximise MPS after resistance training. Athletes with high energy and protein requirements (e.g. elite rugby union/league players, Finn sailors), would struggle to meet their daily energy and protein requirements through the use of whole foods only. In addition, athletes would find eating large volumes of whole protein foods immediately after resistance training unpalatable, especially with more than one training session per day, with a resulting rapidly induced satiation. Thus the use of high-protein/energy meal replacement drinks/ powders provides a useful alternative to foods.

When discussing the use of energy/protein supplements with athletes, consideration should be given not only to the risk of contami-nation and need for batch testing, but also to the biological potency of different protein supplements and associated protein fractions, for example colostrum (milk produced by cows in the first days after parturition) and whey proteins vary as a result of differences in the manufacturing process used to derive whey and casein from bovine milk. However, supplements complement the athlete's diet and should not replace good-quality protein sources, for example dairy foods, meats, fish, eggs and combinations of vegetable proteins. Consumption of animal, fish and indeed vegetarian sources of proteins will better enable the athlete to meet his or her broader nutritional requirements. Differences in protein type (whey vs. casein, animal vs. vegetable) have been reported to affect systemic hormone concentrations, namely IGF-1. However, the role of transient changes in systemic anabolic hormones in relation to MPS has recently been questioned.

Consideration should also be given to total daily carbohydrate intake, types of carbohydrate, micronutrient content, and periodisation and timing in relation to training. Intake of carbohydrates after resistance training is not required to achieve positive muscle protein balance and gains in LBM. However, higher carbohydrate intakes may accelerate gains in BM/LBM by (i) reducing fatigue and increasing the intensity and quality of training; (ii) increasing energy availability through attenuation of AMPK inhibition of mTOR; (iii) increasing amino acid availability; (iv) reducing muscle protein breakdown via insulin; and (v) attenuating exercise-induced increases in cortisol (improving muscle protein balance). Removal of carbohydrate in the post-resistance training period may assist in favourably reducing FM. However, sustained severe restriction of carbohydrates (non-periodised) will deplete muscle glycogen stores and negatively alter hormonal balance, mood states and compromise long-term recovery and performance.

No discussion on nutrition for weight and resistance training would be complete without a reference to creatine supplementation (for further information see Chapter 9). A successful outcome in terms of increasing BM and LBM with creatine supplementation depends on the degree to which intramuscular free creatine and phosphocreatine stores change in response to supplementation. Creatine supplementation may lead to an increase in both BM and LBM in conjunction with resistance training through a number of mechanisms: improved cellular hydration; increased testosterone response to resistance training; increased muscle IGF-1; and an increase in satellite cell number and myonuclei, most likely as a result of the athlete's increased ability to generate greater forces and tolerate greater training loads, placing greater stress on the muscle. In addition, advice regarding the timing of creatine supplementation around resistance training may be critical, with supplementation before and after resistance training versus morning and evening, leading to greater increases in LBM, strength, muscle cross-sectional area of type 2 fibres and muscle phosphocreatine and total creatine content. Finally, the use of fish oils may also lead to greater increases in LBM over time by improving muscle protein balance.

References

Anthony JC, Yoshizawa F, Anthony TG, Vary TC, Jefferson LS, Kimball SR. Leucine stimulates translation initiation in skeletal muscle of postabsorptive rats via a rapamycin-sensitive pathway. J Nutr 2000; 130: 2413–2419.

Anthony JC, Reiter AK, Anthony TG et al. Orally administered leucine enhances protein synthesis in skeletal muscle of diabetic rats in the absence of increases in 4E-BP1 or S6K1 phosphorylation. Diabetes 2002; 51: 928–936.

Baar K, Esser K. Phosphorylation of p70(S6k) correlates with increased skeletal muscle mass following resistance exercise. Am J Physiol 1999; 276: C120–C127.

Beelen M, Tieland M, Gijsen AP et al. Coingestion of carbohydrate and protein hydrolysate stimulates muscle protein synthesis during exercise in young men, with no further increase during subsequent overnight recovery. J Nutr 2008; 138: 2198–2204.

Biolo G, Maggi SP, Williams BD, Tipton KD, Wolfe RR. Increased rates of muscle protein turnover and amino acid transport after resistance exercise in humans. Am J Physiol 1995; 268: E514–E520.

Biolo G, Tipton KD, Klein S, Wolfe RR. An abundant supply of amino acids enhances the metabolic effect of exercise on muscle protein. Am J Physiol 1997; 273: E122–E129.

Bodine SC, Stitt TN, Gonzalez M et al. Akt/mTOR pathway is a crucial regulator of skeletal muscle hypertrophy and can prevent muscle atrophy in vivo. Nat Cell Biol 2001; 3: 1014–1019.

Bohe J, Low A, Wolfe RR, Rennie MJ. Human muscle protein synthesis is modulated by extracellular, not intramuscular amino acid availability: a dose–response study. J Physiol 2003; 552: 315–324.

Boirie Y, Dangin M, Gachon P, Vasson MP, Maubois JL, Beaufrere B. Slow and fast dietary proteins differently modulate postprandial protein accretion. Proc Natl Acad Sci USA 1997; 94: 14930–14935.

Borsheim E, Tipton KD, Wolf SE, Wolfe RR. Essential amino acids and muscle protein recovery from resistance exercise. Am J Physiol 2002; 283: E648–E657.

Borsheim E, Aarsland A, Wolfe RR. Effect of an amino acid, protein, and carbohydrate mixture on net muscle protein balance after resistance exercise. Int J Sport Nutr Exerc Metab 2004a; 14: 255–271.

Borsheim E, Cree MG, Tipton KD, Elliott TA, Aarsland A, Wolfe RR. Effect of carbohydrate intake on net muscle protein synthesis during recovery from resistance exercise. J Appl Physiol 2004b; 96: 674–8.

Burd NA, Tang JE, Moore DR, Phillips SM. Exercise training and protein metabolism: influences of contraction, protein intake, and sex-based differences. J Appl Physiol 2009a; 106: 1692–1701.

Burd NA, West DW, Staples AW et al. Stimulation of muscle protein synthesis occurs at lower intensity than previously thought. Med Sci Sports Exerc 2009b; 41: 150.

Burk A, Timpmann S, Medijainen L, Vahi M, Oopik V. Time-divided ingestion pattern of casein-based protein supplement stimulates an increase in fat-free body mass during resistance training in young untrained men. Nutr Res 2009; 29: 405–413.

Byfield MP, Murray JT, Backer JM. hVps34 is a nutrient-regulated lipid kinase required for activation of p70 S6 kinase. J Biol Chem 2005; 280: 33076–33082.

Cribb PJ, Hayes A. Effects of supplement timing and resistance exercise on skeletal muscle hypertrophy. Med Sci Sports Exerc 2006; 38: 1918–1925.

Crozier SJ, Kimball SR, Emmert SW, Anthony JC, Jefferson LS. Oral leucine administration stimulates protein synthesis in rat skeletal muscle. J Nutr 2005; 135: 376–382.

Cuthbertson D, Smith K, Babraj J et al. Anabolic signaling deficits underlie amino acid resistance of wasting, aging muscle. FASEB J 2005; 19: 422–424.

Dangin M, Boirie Y, Garcia-Rodenas C et al. The digestion rate of protein is an independent regulating factor of postprandial protein retention. Am J Physiol 2001; 280: E340–E348.

Dangin M, Boirie Y, Guillet C, Beaufrere B. Influence of the protein digestion rate on protein turnover in young and elderly subjects. J Nutr 2002; 132: 3228S–3233S.

Dangin M, Guillet C, Garcia-Rodenas C et al. The rate of protein digestion affects protein gain differently during aging in humans. J Physiol 2003; 549: 635–644.

Drummond MJ, Fry CS, Glynn EL et al. Rapamycin administration in humans blocks the contraction-induced increase in skeletal muscle protein synthesis. J Physiol 2009; 587: 1535–1546.

Esmarck B, Andersen JL, Olsen S, Richter EA, Mizuno M, Kjaer M. Timing of postexercise protein intake is important for muscle hypertrophy with resistance training in elderly humans. J Physiol 2001; 535: 301–311.

Fiatarone MA, Marks EC, Ryan ND, Meredith CN, Lipsitz LA, Evans WJ. High-intensity strength training in nonagenarians. Effects on skeletal muscle. JAMA 1990; 263: 3029–3034.

Frontera WR, Meredith CN, O'Reilly KP, Knuttgen HG, Evans WJ. Strength conditioning in older men: skeletal muscle hypertrophy and improved function. J Appl Physiol 1988; 64: 1038–1044.

Fujita S, Dreyer HC, Drummond MJ, Glynn EL, Volpi E, Rasmussen BB. Essential amino acid and carbohydrate ingestion before resistance exercise does not enhance postexercise muscle protein synthesis. J Appl Physiol 2009; 106: 1730–1739.

Garthe I, Raastad T, Refsnes P, Kolviste A, Sundgot-Borgen J. Effect of two different weight-loss rates on body composition and strength and power-related performance in elite athletes. Int J Sport Nutr Exerc Metab 2011; 2: 97–104.

Gelfand RA, Barrett EJ. Effect of physiologic hyperinsulinemia on skeletal muscle protein synthesis and breakdown in man. J Clin Invest 1987; 80: 1–6.

Gingras AC, Raught B, Sonenberg N. eIF4 initiation factors: effectors of mRNA recruitment to ribosomes and regulators of translation. Annu Rev Biochem 1999; 68: 913–963.

Gwinn DM, Shackelford DB, Egan DF et al. AMPK phosphorylation of raptor mediates a metabolic checkpoint. Mol Cell 2008; 30: 214–226.

Hartman JW, Tang JE, Wilkinson SB et al. Consumption of fat-free fluid milk after resistance exercise promotes greater lean mass accretion than does consumption of soy or carbohydrate in young, novice, male weightlifters. Am J Clin Nutr 2007; 86: 373–381.

Hershey JW. Translational control in mammalian cells. Annu Rev Biochem 1991; 60: 717–755.

Hoffman JR, Ratamess NA, Tranchina CP, Rashti SL, Kang J, Faigenbaum AD. Effect of protein-supplement timing on strength, power, and body-composition changes in resistance-trained men. Int J Sport Nutr Exerc Metab 2009; 19: 172–185.

Hughes VA, Frontera WR, Wood M et al. Longitudinal muscle strength changes in older adults: influence of muscle mass, physical activity, and health. J Gerontol A Biol Sci Med Sci 2001; 56: B209–B217.

Hundal HS, Taylor PM. Amino acid transceptors: gate keepers of nutrient exchange and regulators of nutrient signaling. Am J Physiol 2009; 296: E603–E613.

Hunter GR, McCarthy JP, Bamman MM. Effects of resistance training on older adults. Sports Med 2004; 34: 329–348.

Inoki K, Li Y, Zhu T, Wu J, Guan KL. TSC2 is phosphorylated and inhibited by Akt and suppresses mTOR signalling. Nat Cell Biol 2002; 4: 648–657.

Jacinto E, Loewith R, Schmidt A et al. Mammalian TOR complex 2 controls the actin cytoskeleton and is rapamycin insensitive. Nat Cell Biol 2004; 6: 1122–1128.

Kosek DJ, Kim JS, Petrella JK, Cross JM, Bamman MM. Efficacy of 3 days/wk resistance training on myofiber hypertrophy and myogenic mechanisms in young vs. older adults. J Appl Physiol 2006; 101: 531–544.

Kozak M. The scanning model for translation: an update. J Cell Biol 1989; 108: 229–241.

Lacroix M, Bos C, Leonil J et al. Compared with casein or total milk protein, digestion of milk soluble proteins is too rapid to sustain the anabolic postprandial amino acid requirement. Am J Clin Nutr 2006; 84: 1070–1079.

Land SC, Tee AR. Hypoxia-inducible factor 1alpha is regulated by the mammalian target of rapamycin (mTOR) via an mTOR signaling motif. J Biol Chem 2007; 282: 20534–20543.

Lee SJ, McPherron AC. Regulation of myostatin activity and muscle growth. Proc Natl Acad Sci USA 2001; 98: 9306–9311.

MacDougall JD, Ray S, Sale DG, McCartney N, Lee P, Garner S. Muscle substrate utilization and lactate production. Can J Appl Physiol 1999; 24: 209–215.

MacKenzie MG, Hamilton DL, Murray JT, Taylor PM, Baar K. mVps34 is activated following high-resistance contractions. J Physiol 2009; 587: 253–260.

Miller SL, Tipton KD, Chinkes DL, Wolf SE, Wolfe RR. Independent and combined effects of amino acids and glucose after resistance exercise. Med Sci Sports Exerc 2003; 35: 449–455.

Moore DR, Phillips SM, Babraj JA, Smith K, Rennie MJ. Myofibrillar and collagen protein synthesis in human skeletal muscle in young men after maximal shortening and lengthening contractions. Am J Physiol 2005; 288: E1153–E1159.

Moore DR, Robinson MJ, Fry JL et al. Ingested protein dose response of muscle and albumin protein synthesis after resistance exercise in young men. Am J Clin Nutr 2009a; 89: 161–168.

Moore DR, Tang JE, Burd NA, Rerecich T, Tarnopolsky MA, Phillips SM. Differential stimulation of myofibrillar and sarcoplasmic protein synthesis with protein ingestion at rest and after resistance exercise. J Physiol 2009b; 597: 897–904.

Nair KS, Schwartz RG, Welle S. Leucine as a regulator of whole body and skeletal muscle protein metabolism in humans. Am J Physiol 1992; 263: E928–E934.

Oshiro N, Takahashi R, Yoshino K et al. The proline-rich Akt substrate of 40kDa (PRAS40) is a physiological substrate of mammalian target of rapamycin complex 1. J Biol Chem 2007; 282: 20329–20339.

Paddon-Jones D, Rasmussen BB. Dietary protein recommendations and the prevention of sarcopenia. Curr Opin Clin Nutr Metab Care 2009; 12: 86–90.

Phillips SM. Protein requirements and supplementation in strength sports. Nutrition 2004; 20: 689–695.

Phillips SM. Dietary protein for athletes: from requirements to metabolic advantage. Appl Physiol Nutr Metab 2006; 31: 647–654.

Phillips SM, Tipton KD, Aarsland A, Wolf SE, Wolfe RR. Mixed muscle protein synthesis and breakdown after resistance exercise in humans. Am J Physiol 1997; 273: E99–E107.

Phillips SM, Parise G, Roy BD, Tipton KD, Wolfe RR, Tarnopolsky MA. Resistance training-induced adaptations in skeletal muscle protein turnover in the fed state. Can J Physiol Pharmacol 2002; 80: 1045–1053.

Phillips SM, Hartman JW, Wilkinson SB. Dietary protein to support anabolism with resistance exercise in young men. J Am Coll Nutr 2005; 24: 134S–139S.

Phillips SM, Moore DR, Tang JE. A critical examination of dietary protein requirements, benefits, and excesses in athletes. Int J Sport Nutr Exerc Metab 2007; 17: S58–S76.

Rennie MJ, Wackerhage H, Spangenburg EE, Booth FW. Control of the size of the human muscle mass. Annu Rev Physiol 2004; 66: 799–828.

Rose AJ, Alsted TJ, Jensen TE et al. A Ca(2+)–calmodulin–eEF2K–eEF2 signalling cascade, but not AMPK, contributes to the suppression of skeletal muscle protein synthesis during contractions. J Physiol 2009; 587: 1547–1563.

Sancak Y, Bar-Peled L, Zoncu R, Markhard AL, Nada S, Sabatini DM. Ragulator–Rag complex targets mTORC1 to the lysosomal surface and is necessary for its activation by amino acids. Cell 2010; 141: 290–303.

Sarbassov DD, Ali SM, Kim DH et al. Rictor, a novel binding partner of mTOR, defines a rapamycin-insensitive and raptor-independent pathway that regulates the cytoskeleton. Curr Biol 2004; 14: 1296–1302.

Sarbassov DD, Guertin DA, Ali SM, Sabatini DM. Phosphorylation and regulation of Akt/PKB by the rictor-mTOR complex. Science 2005; 307: 1098–1101.

Schalm SS, Blenis J. Identification of a conserved motif required for mTOR signaling. Curr Biol 2002; 12: 632–639.

Schalm SS, Fingar DC, Sabatini DM, Blenis J. TOS motif-mediated raptor binding regulates 4E-BP1 multisite phosphorylation and function. Curr Biol 2003; 13: 797–806.

Spangenburg EE, Le RD, Ward CW, Bodine SC. A functional insulin-like growth factor receptor is not necessary for load-induced skeletal muscle hypertrophy. J Physiol 2008; 586: 283–291.

Tang JE, Perco JG, Moore DR, Wilkinson SB, Phillips SM. Resistance training alters the response of fed state mixed muscle protein synthesis in young men. Am J Physiol 2008; 294: R172–R178.

Tang JE, Moore DR, Kujbida GW, Tarnopolsky MA, Phillips SM. Ingestion of whey hydrolysate, casein, or soy protein isolate: effects on mixed muscle protein synthesis at rest and following resistance exercise in young men. J Appl Physiol 2009; 107: 987–992.

Tarnopolsky MA, Atkinson SA, MacDougall JD, Senor BB, Lemon PW, Schwarcz H. Whole body leucine metabolism during and after resistance exercise in fed humans. Med Sci Sports Exerc 1991; 23: 326–333.

Thomson DM, Fick CA, Gordon SE. AMPK activation attenuates S6K1, 4E-BP1, and eEF2 signaling responses to high-frequency electrically stimulated skeletal muscle contractions. J Appl Physiol 2008; 104: 625–632.

Tipton KD, Ferrando AA, Phillips SM, Doyle D Jr, Wolfe RR. Postexercise net protein synthesis in human muscle from orally administered amino acids. Am J Physiol 1999; 276: E628–E634.

Tipton KD, Rasmussen BB, Miller SL et al. Timing of amino acid–carbohydrate ingestion alters anabolic response of muscle to resistance exercise. Am J Physiol 2001; 281: E197–E206.

Tipton KD, Borsheim E, Wolf SE, Sanford AP, Wolfe RR. Acute response of net muscle protein balance reflects 24-h balance after exercise and amino acid ingestion. Am J Physiol 2003; 284: E76–E89.

Tipton KD, Elliott TA, Cree MG, Aarsland AA, Sanford AP, Wolfe RR. Stimulation of net muscle protein synthesis by whey protein ingestion before and after exercise. Am J Physiol 2006; 292: E71–E76.

Tremblay F, Marette A. Amino acid and insulin signaling via the mTOR/p70 S6 kinase pathway. A negative feedback mechanism leading to insulin resistance in skeletal muscle cells. J Biol Chem 2001; 276: 38052–38060.

Verdijk LB, Jonkers RA, Gleeson BG et al. Protein supplementation before and after exercise does not further augment skeletal muscle hypertrophy after resistance training in elderly men. Am J Clin Nutr 2009; 89: 608–616.

Wayler A, Queiroz E, Scrimshaw NS, Steinke FH, Rand WM, Young VR. Nitrogen balance studies in young men to assess the protein quality of an isolated soy protein in relation to meat proteins. J Nutr 1983; 113: 2485–2491.

West DW, Kujbida GW, Moore DR et al. Resistance exercise-induced increases in putative anabolic hormones do not enhance muscle protein synthesis or intracellular signalling in young men. J Physiol 2009; 587: 5239–5247.

Wilkinson SB, Tarnopolsky MA, MacDonald MJ, Macdonald JR, Armstrong D, Phillips SM. Consumption of fluid skim milk promotes greater muscle protein accretion following resistance exercise than an isonitrogenous and isoenergetic soy protein beverage. Am J Clin Nutr 2007; 85: 1031–1040.

Wolin SL, Walter P. Ribosome pausing and stacking during translation of a eukaryotic mRNA. EMBO J 1988; 7: 3559–3569.

Young VR, Wayler A, Garza C et al. A long-term metabolic balance study in young men to assess the nutritional quality of an isolated soy protein and beef proteins. Am J Clin Nutr 1984a; 39: 8–15.

Young VR, Puig M, Queiroz E, Scrimshaw NS, Rand WM. Evaluation of the protein quality of an isolated soy protein in young men: relative nitrogen requirements and effect of methionine supplementation. Am J Clin Nutr 1984b; 39: 16–24.

11
Nutrition for Power and Sprint Training

Nicholas A Burd and Stuart M Phillips

Key messages

- Excessive protein intake for sprint and power athletes is not necessary to maximise muscle hypertrophy, power development, and strength.
- A high-protein diet may confer a metabolic advantage that has important implications for athletes seeking to lose excess body fat but maintain lean body mass.
- The necessity of a high daily carbohydrate intake for sprint and power athletes has never been examined; however, carbohydrate intake is important for glycogen synthesis and ultimate performance benefits.

- Full muscle fibre recruitment during resistance exercise confers a sensitising effect on skeletal muscle to protein feeding for up to 24 hours.
- Creatine monohydrate has been shown to be effective in improving sport performance; however, the beneficial effect of creatine supplementation on enhancing skeletal muscle hypertrophy would be minimal relative to the adaptations seen after a well-designed resistance training programme and adequate nutrition, which includes consuming high-quality proteins at strategic times (i.e. 1–2 hours after exercise) during the course of the day.

11.1 Introduction

Sprint and power training is beneficial for an array of sport activities and/or events. The purpose of power training is similar to that of resistance training: to improve muscle strength and force production. The sport that power training is particularly relevant to is weight-lifting, although other activities also have explosive moments such as throwing sports (e.g. shotput, javelin) and hitting or kicking sports (e.g. tennis, rugby, hockey). The purpose of sprint training is to sustain high power outputs for short periods (i.e. 10–50 s). The sport that sprint training is particularly relevant to is track sprinting (i.e. 100, 200 and 400 m), although other events also include high-intensity sprints such as field and track events (e.g. jumps, hurdles) and middle-distance sports (e.g. cycling, rowing, swimming). Thus many athletes need to undertake power and sprint training to work on their muscle strength, power and/or speed.

Power lifting or Olympic weight-lifting actually involves such exercises as bench press, barbell squats, deadlifts, and various jerk-style lifts (i.e. cleans, snatch) which are performed at maximal loads. Many other athletes will undertake some power and sprint training sessions during their training cycle. Therefore sprint and power athletes engage their muscles in response to a wide variety of contraction stimuli that induce varied effects on muscle protein turnover and ultimately influence skeletal muscle adaptations after a defined training period. However, the ultimate goal of any athlete is to be in a state of net muscle protein balance (NPB) or net protein accretion:

NPB = muscle protein synthesis (MPS) − muscle protein breakdown (MPB)

Exercise and feeding represent two potent anabolic stimuli capable of inducing a chronically positive NBP when synergistically applied to skeletal muscle (Burd *et al.*, 2009). However, other tissues are also stressed with power training, such as tendon and ligaments, which would also require remodelling and repair to adapt to the training stimulus.

Sport and Exercise Nutrition, First Edition. Edited by Susan A Lanham-New, Samantha J Stear, Susan M Shirreffs and Adam L Collins.
© 2011 The Nutrition Society. Published 2011 by Blackwell Publishing Ltd.

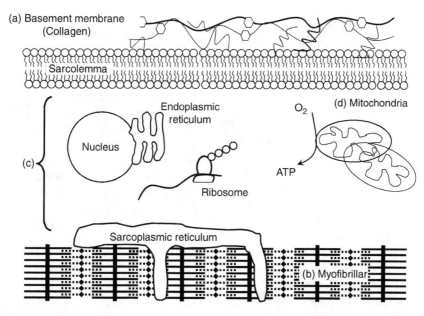

Figure 11.1 A simplified view of human skeletal muscle illustrating the specific muscle protein subfractions. Methods are available to isolate (a) collagen enriched, (b) myofibrillar enriched, (c) non-myofibrillar enriched (i.e. sarcoplasmic) or (d) mitochondrial enriched fractions. Mixed muscle proteins, and their respective synthetic rates, are simply a collective measurement of (a)–(d).

Various methods have been utilised to understand the regulation of MPS in response to different feeding and exercise interventions (Biolo *et al.*, 1997; Phillips *et al.*, 1997; Dreyer *et al.*, 2006; Kumar *et al.*, 2009; Burd *et al.*, 2010a). Some investigators have utilised a model of leg amino acid kinetics based on the arteriovenous difference method, with results heavily influenced by accurate leg blood flow measurements (Biolo *et al.*, 1995a; Tipton *et al.*, 2001). However, other investigators have utilised the precursor-product method to determine the direct incorporation of tracer amino acids into muscle proteins (Phillips *et al.*, 1997; Kumar *et al.*, 2009; Burd *et al.*, 2010a). This method allows the determination of rates of mixed MPS (i.e. a collective measurement of all the proteins within muscle) (Phillips *et al.*, 1997; Dreyer *et al.*, 2006; Burd *et al.*, 2010a,b) or determination of rates of synthesis of specific muscle protein subfractions, such as myofibrillar (Moore *et al.*, 2005, 2009a; Burd *et al.*, 2010a), non-myofibrillar (or sarcoplasmic) (Moore *et al.*, 2009a; Burd *et al.*, 2010a), mitochondrial (Wilkinson *et al.*, 2008), and muscle collagen protein synthesis (Moore *et al.*, 2005) after acute resistance exercise (Figure 11.1). A detailed

discussion of the techniques used to determine muscle protein turnover is beyond the scope of this chapter, but detailed information can be found in a number of reviews (Rennie, 1999; Wagenmakers, 1999; Holm & Kjaer, 2010). It is common among reports to refer to mixed muscle, myofibrillar and leg protein synthesis (LPS) collectively as MPS; however, it will become apparent that under some circumstances, especially when feeding and resistance exercise are superimposed, use of 'MPS' does not capture the true nature of the phenotypic response.

The aim of this chapter is to discuss general nutritional recommendations that will aid the sprint/power athlete in maintaining a net positive muscle balance over the course of the day, which will ultimately translate into a situation of net protein replacement and repair. We also relate our current understanding of the regulation of MPS in response to resistance exercise and feeding, as discussed in Chapter 10, to sprint and power sports and the role of nutrition in these sports. Lastly, we review the role of a commonly consumed supplement, creatine monohydrate, for increasing sprint/power performance.

11.2 General nutritional guidelines for sprint and power-trained athletes

The current scientific literature is deficient in data to construct firm nutritional recommendations for sprint and/or power athletes. This notion is further complicated by the fact that the individual goal of a particular sprint athlete will certainly vary from that of a power athlete. Furthermore, even within a group of power athletes there will be considerable variation in individual goals such that each goal may diverge from that of another based on the type of exercises performed during training. For example, a competitive power lifter commonly performs such lifts as barbell squat, bench press and deadlifts, which are performed at maximal loads and require maximal force development for very few repetitions. On the other hand, an Olympic-style weight-lifter commonly performs exercises requiring a slightly greater skill component, such as snatch, clean, and jerk-style lifts, and which are associated with high muscular power (velocity × mass) production. These fundamental differences in training styles and goals may require nutritional recommendations that are tailored towards each athlete.

Protein requirements

A common characteristic for sprint athletes and power- and weight-lifters is that they all use resistance training as either their primary mode of training or as an adjunct to other forms of training. Thus, it is reasonable to extrapolate data from the resistance training literature to make broad recommendations on protein requirements. Certainly, widespread resistance training dogma would suggest that to build 'serious' muscle it is imperative to construct one's dietary macronutrient intake around protein and this notion does have support in the scientific literature (Tarnopolsky et al., 1988, 1992; Lemon et al., 1992). It would seem, however, that any argument for protein requirements for power athletes, especially those residing in the western hemisphere, would be absurd as most are currently consuming well above the recommended levels, nominally 0.8–0.9 g/kg/day (Phillips, 2004; Institute of Medicine, 2005). Contrary to the view of excessive protein requirements for athletes, another opinion suggests that if the athlete is currently engaged in a strength-training programme,

it may be that protein requirements, as measured by nitrogen balance, are not elevated but actually reduced to some extent (Phillips, 2006; Phillips et al., 2007). This notion is based on the fact that resistance exercise is fundamentally anabolic (Phillips et al., 1997), and a reasonable hypotheses is that resistance training may actually shift the utilisation of dietary amino acids derived from muscle protein degradation toward MPS. Thus, a greater proportion of amino acids, in both the fasted and fed states, are being retained in the largest protein pool, skeletal muscle. Furthermore, it is also important to note that chronic consumption of a high-protein diet (>1.6–1.8 g/kg/day) may actually force the body to adapt and increase the capacity of amino acid catabolism, since excess nitrogen is fundamentally toxic in biological systems, which in turn forces the athlete to continue chronic consumption of high protein loads to avoid excessive amino acid catabolism of small amino acid loads. The current daily recommendation for meeting protein requirements for strength training athletes is 1.6–1.7 g protein/kg/day (e.g. about 128–136 g protein for an 80-kg individual) (Rodriguez et al., 2009), approximately twice that of a sedentary individual (0.8 g protein/kg/day). It is clear that this amount of protein can be easily obtained through normal dietary habits and likely does not require supplemental protein sources. However, it is becoming increasingly evident that one aspect of an athlete's diet that may require special attention is the type/amount of protein consumed and the timing of protein ingestion relative to exercise. Detailed information on these topics can also be found in Chapter 10.

A well-recognised performance advantage for an athlete, where power-to-weight ratio plays an important role, is the maintenance of a high lean body mass to fat mass ratio, which would be a much sought after goal for 100, 200 and 400 m sprinters. In addition, a high lean body mass to fat mass ratio is especially relevant for athletes involved in power lifting and/or Olympic weight-lifting as their competitions are divided by weight classes. Indeed, common acute weight loss strategy among athletes is to restrict food/fluid intake coupled with dehydration strategies prior to competing. It has been suggested that sporting events involving high power outputs and absolute strength are less affected by acute weight loss (Fogelholm, 1994) or dehydration (Cheuvront et al., 2006). In addition, many power and sprint athletes follow a low-residue diet in the last few days leading up to competition to reduce the volume of the faecal contents of the bowel and thereby produce further weight loss (around 300–800 g) (for further information on low-residue diets, see Chapter 20). However, during training performance may be compromised when commencing certain training sessions with low glycogen stores and/or in a dehydrated state. It is worth highlighting that high intakes of dietary protein do appear to confer certain advantages during periods of energy restriction (Mettler et al., 2010). A global finding among studies using higher protein diets is that not only do they result in a greater loss of absolute body weight but a greater amount of that weight loss is accounted for by fat mass, albeit in obese individuals (Parker et al., 2002; Layman et al., 2003, 2005; Noakes et al., 2005). Further, it appears that low-fat dairy is also effective in decreasing fat mass, especially in young women who are relatively low dairy consumers (Josse et al., 2009), which may be related to the interplay between calcium and vitamin D on adipocyte metabolism and inhibition of lipid accretion (Zemel, 2004; Teegarden, 2005).

Effects of protein ingestion on muscle protein synthesis

Pioneering work by Rennie and colleagues demonstrated that feeding a meal doubled the rate at which amino acids are incorporated into muscle proteins (Rennie et al., 1982) and this effect on MPS could be achieved exclusively by the protein component (i.e. amino acids) of food (Bennet et al., 1989). Protein consumption primarily affects MPS through feeding-induced hyperaminoacidaemia, which in turn provides a favourable gradient for inward amino acid transport into the intracellular free amino acid pool within skeletal muscle (Biolo et al., 1997). Interestingly after about 2 hours of constant exposure to mixed amino acids (by infusion), rates of MPS returned to basal levels during the 6-hour infusion (Bohe et al., 2001). Similar effects on rates of myofibrillar and sarcoplasmic protein synthesis has been established after bolus ingestion of 48 g of whey protein (Atherton et al., 2010). It has been suggested that the likely fate of the excess amino acids (those supplied over and above the requirements) is deamination whereby their carbon skeletons are used for fuel or stored as fat (Bohe et al., 2001).

Addition of other macronutrients to protein

It is well established that consuming a bolus dose of protein alone after resistance exercise has a potent stimulatory effect on exercise-mediated rates of MPS (Moore et al., 2009b; Tang et al., 2009; Burd et al., 2010c). A common and relevant question is one related to the value of adding other components of a meal to a protein-containing drink. The primary physiological regulator of insulin secretion is blood glucose concentration and co-ingestion of carbohydrates with dietary protein induces a rapid increase in blood glucose compared with dietary protein alone. There is a great deal of controversy surrounding the role of insulin in regulating muscle anabolism (Volpi et al., 1996; Fujita & Volpi, 2006; Fujita et al., 2006; Rasmussen et al., 2006; Phillips, 2008; Glynn et al., 2010). We and others have proposed that insulin is necessary, but is merely permissive not stimulatory for rates of MPS (Svanberg et al., 1997; Bohe et al., 2003; Cuthbertson et al., 2005; Greenhaff et al., 2008; Wilkes et al., 2009). Specifically, only a small amount (~5 μU/ml) of insulin is necessary to allow a full anabolic response to occur, but any further stimulation of MPS is driven by extracellular amino acid availability. However, muscle NPB is determined by two variables, MPS and MPB, so carbohydrate consumption and the concomitant increase in circulating insulin may have a significant impact on muscle NPB as it appears that hyperinsulinaemia has a potent inhibitory effect on MPB (Pozefsky et al., 1969; Gelfand & Barrett, 1987; Fryburg et al., 1990). Therefore, the question that arises is whether co-ingesting carbohydrate with protein during post-exercise recovery can optimise muscle NPB.

Koopman et al. (2007) demonstrated that following a full body resistance exercise routine, consuming repeated feedings of small aliquots of protein and carbohydrate did not further enhance whole-body protein synthesis or mixed MPS as compared to repeated feedings of protein alone. Furthermore, the co-ingestion of carbohydrate with protein did not further inhibit whole-body protein breakdown. More recently, it was reported that the addition of 90 g or 30 g of carbohydrate to a 20-g essential amino acid drink conferred the same effect on LPS and leg protein breakdown (LPB) (Glynn et al., 2010). However, the researchers failed to include a group which consumed only essential amino acids, precluding their ability to determine the effects of amino acids alone.

We have recently sought to fill this research gap by feeding 25 g of whey protein or 25 g of whey protein plus an additional 50 g of carbohydrate after resistance exercise (Staples *et al.*, 2010). It was demonstrated that consumption of a maximal stimulating dose of whey protein plus carbohydrate had no further stimulatory and/or inhibitory effect on mixed MPS or MPB compared with 25 g of whey protein alone. This is in line with a recent observations that carbohydrate ingestion even beyond a moderate hyperinsulinaemia (~30 μU/ml) has no further effect on LPB (Greenhaff *et al.*, 2008). Therefore, the addition of carbohydrates has no further effect, provided a maximal 25-g dose of whey protein is consumed (Moore *et al.*, 2009b), on mixed MPS or MPB. However, it remains to be seen if carbohydrates are beneficial when a less than optimal dose (<20 g) of high-quality protein is consumed during post-exercise recovery. It is worth highlighting, however, that high-volume leg resistance exercise has been demonstrated to induce an approximately 26% decrease in muscle glycogen (Tesch *et al.*, 1986) and other workers have demonstrated a similar effect on muscle glycogen in bicep muscles after three sets, but not one set, of arm curl exercise (MacDougall *et al.*, 1999). This notion, coupled with the fact that carbohydrate feeding can restore muscle glycogen content after resistance exercise, has important performance implications for sprint and power-training athletes (Pascoe *et al.*, 1993).

A relatively under-studied area is the addition of fat to a protein meal and the subsequent effects on rates of MPS. Indeed, evidence points to a thesis that a large transient 'spike' in hyperaminoacidaemia immediately after exercise is important in maximising exercise-induced rates of MPS. Therefore, it would seem that slowing the absorption of protein, by adding fat, may impact the anabolic response. Indeed, Dangin *et al.* (2001, 2003) provide some support for the concept that consuming other components of a meal (i.e. carbohydrate and fat) has an impact on digestion kinetics and the associated aminoacidaemia. Specifically, it was reported that consuming about 30 g of whey protein alone increased blood leucine concentrations about fourfold (Dangin *et al.*, 2001), whereas in another cohort of young men

consuming about 34 g of whey in combination with about 50 g carbohydrate and about 9 g fat increased blood leucine about threefold (Dangin *et al.*, 2003). Clearly, more research is needed to draw any definite conclusions as to how mixed meal feeding affects exercise-mediated rates of MPS.

Dietary carbohydrate recommendations

Carbohydrate intake to meet training and recovery requirements will largely depend on the number of hours training per day, with current carbohydrate recommendations being in the region of 3–7 g/kg/day when training for 1–2 hours daily (Rodriguez *et al.*, 2009). It has been reported that both interval sprint sessions and an acute bout of resistance exercise can deplete muscle glycogen by about 25–40% (Tesch *et al.*, 1986; Pascoe *et al.*, 1993; MacDougall *et al.*, 1999), and the extent of depletion would largely be dependent on the external work (calculated as the product of repetitions and load) performed during the exercise bout. It has been suggested that female strength athletes may require slightly less carbohydrate than their male counterparts (Volek *et al.*, 2006). This thesis was based on the notion that if a female consumed her daily recommended amount of carbohydrates, this amount could be too large a proportion of her total caloric needs (Volek *et al.*, 2006). Regardless, it remains to be established if habitually high carbohydrate intakes are beneficial for strength training athletes. Furthermore, since total energy intake is a function of total macronutrient intake, it may be advisable that athletes consume carbohydrates at critically important times (i.e. immediately after exercise) and subsequently adjust daily carbohydrate intake on total energy need.

Is there any evidence to suggest that performing resistance exercise in the glycogen-depleted state has detrimental effects on muscular performance and subsequent anabolism? The effects of low glycogen levels on power and strength production during exercise are equivocal. Some studies indicate that glycogen depletion reduces isometric strength, but not isokinetic strength performance (reviewed in Leveritt *et al.*, 1999). Recently, Creer *et al.* (2005) sought to examine the effects of commencing an acute bout of resistance exercise in the glycogen-depleted state. It was found that some of the intramuscular signalling proteins (i.e. Erk1/2, P90RSK, mTOR) shown to be involved in 'turning on' MPS were not affected by low muscle glycogen concentrations; however, an upstream signalling protein, Akt, was only significantly phosphorylated post exercise when glycogen concentrations were not compromised. However, Akt has been reported to be related more to insulin availability rather than directly connected to anabolism (Greenhaff *et al.*, 2008). Therefore, further research is needed to determine the effects of performing resistance exercise with low muscle glycogen concentrations utilising kinetic measurements (i.e. stable isotope methodology).

11.3 Power-type exercises and muscle protein synthesis

Examination of the current literature reveals that few studies have used resistance exercise bouts that resemble a typical power-lifting session to determine exercise-induced increases in rates of MPS. Original research studying resistance exercise and muscle protein turnover utilised high-volume (8–10 sets at 10 repetitions) and high-intensity (~80% of maximal strength) resistance exercise as this was believed to be required to maximise the MPS response (MacDougall *et al.*, 1995; Phillips *et al.*, 1997). Contemporary evidence suggests that lower volumes of exercise can stimulate rates of myofibrillar protein synthesis and as little as three sets of 12–14 repetitions of exercise can stimulate MPS for up to 24 hours (Burd *et al.*, 2010c). We have recently reported, in young men, that an acute bout of resistance exercise performed for four sets of three to five repetitions at near maximal loads (~90% maximal strength) induces an immediate acute rise in myofibrillar protein synthesis but is incapable of maintaining the response during 24–29 hours post-exercise recovery (Burd *et al.*, 2010a). However, it is important to keep in mind that this investigation was performed in the post-absorptive state, which is unlike a typical power athlete's nutritional habits. Interestingly, bolus protein feeding (15 g of whey protein) the day after this type of low-volume and heavy-loading exercise (i.e. four sets of three to five repetitions at 90% maximal strength) potentiated the myofibrillar response to a greater degree than that seen in the absence of preceding contractile activity (i.e. resting conditions) (Burd *et al.*, 2011). The data suggest that maximal fibre activation, induced by the heavy loads, during the exercise bout 'sensitises' skeletal muscle to subsequent protein feeding for up to 24 hours later.

This notion is consistent with resistance exercise being fundamentally anabolic and when combined with adequate nutrition is capable of increasing hypertrophy (Hartman *et al.*, 2007). However, protein feeding immediately after exercise should still be a primary concern of the athlete as this is when MPS is stimulated to the greatest extent (Phillips *et al.*, 1997).

11.4 Sprint-type exercises and muscle protein synthesis

Sprint exercise has been shown to promote endurance-like adaptations (i.e. increased oxidative capacity) (Burgomaster *et al.*, 2005, 2008; Gibala *et al.*, 2006) and increases muscle power; however, a single bout of sprint exercise is of very short duration and performed with maximal or close to maximal efforts, common characteristics of a more growth-promoting stimulus such as resistance exercise. Thus it may be reasoned that a sprint stimulus could create a unique MPS response unlike any response seen after endurance or resistance exercise alone. Unfortunately, our current understanding of muscle protein turnover in response to sprint exercise is, at best, limited.

Examination of the current literature suggests that sprint training can induce some increases (about 4–12%) in muscle size after 6 weeks of sprint training (Allemeier *et al.*, 1994; Harridge *et al.*, 1998) or even significant increases in muscle size after 8 months of training (Cadefau *et al.*, 1990). These gains are astounding considering a well-structured strength training programme may only induce about 10–25% gains in type II fibre size after 12–15 weeks (Hubal *et al.*, 2005; West *et al.*, 2010). However, a prerequisite for hypertrophy is the accretion of myofibrillar proteins, and thus sprint training must be stimulating an increase in rates of myofibrillar protein synthesis during post-exercise recovery. In addition, if sprint training results in increased muscle oxidative potential, then at some point mitochondrial protein synthesis must also be stimulated.

Further support for sprint exercise stimulating acute rises in myofibrillar protein synthesis may be inferred from recent work from our laboratory utilising resistance exercise. We have put forward the thesis that the duration of muscle activation (i.e. time under tension) and type II fibre activation may be a significant contributor in the regulation of rates of MPS after resistance exercise (Burd *et al.*, 2010a,c)

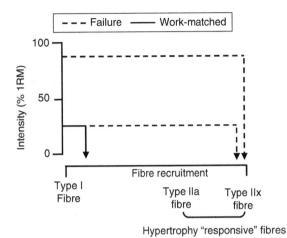

Figure 11.2 A theoretical model depicting the size principle and the orderly recruitment of muscle fibres. Performance of resistance exercise until volitional fatigue (i.e. failure) will necessitate maximal fibre recruitment and culminate in a similar fibre recruitment. However, a low-intensity work-matched condition will require less muscle fibre activation.

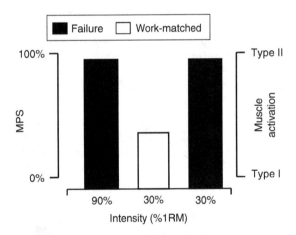

Figure 11.3 Resistance exercise performed until failure, regardless of intensity, will stimulate similar rates of muscle protein synthesis. This effect is likely related to the degree of type II fibre recruitment (Burgomaster et al., 2005).

(Figures 11.2 and 11.3). Thus if our thesis is correct it would appear that acute sprint exercise, and the concomitant recruitment of type II muscle fibres (Mendez-Villanueva et al., 2008), should stimulate an immediate acute rise in myofibrillar protein synthesis; however, the duration of this response may be dependent on the number of sprints performed during the exercise bout (Burd et al., 2010c).

It is well known that resistance exercise and protein feeding enhances rates of MPS greater than the response to either stimuli alone (Biolo et al., 1995b, 1997). Furthermore, it appears that a certain threshold of contractile activity is necessary to maintain this exercise-mediated sensitising effect on skeletal muscle late into recovery (i.e. 24–29 hours later) (Burd et al., 2010c), consistent with the notion that increased contraction volume enhances rates of MPS in the fasted state 24 hours after resistance exercise (Burd et al., 2010a). Feeding during this same 24 hours post-exercise recovery window only potentiates rates of myofibrillar protein synthesis above rested fed rates after exercise performed until exhaustion (i.e. maximal fibre activation) (Burd et al., 2011). Whether sprint exercise also confers this same additive of exercise and feeding in the immediate post-recovery period, or for extended periods (i.e. 24 hours) after the acute bout, remains to be seen, but it would, given the generalisation of our findings, appear likely (Moore et al., 2005).

A noteworthy finding came from Harber et al. (2010), who recently demonstrated that performing cycling exercise for 60 min at about 70% Vo_{2peak} in the fasted or fed states stimulated rates of mixed MPS to a similar extent, suggesting that an additive effect of exercise and feeding was not apparent. Indeed, these data are difficult to reconcile as treadmill walking at approximately 40% Vo_{2peak} for 45 min has been shown to enhance insulin-mediated nutrient delivery and mixed MPS in human skeletal muscle for up to 20 hours in the elderly (Fujita et al., 2007). Alternatively, it may be that younger muscle requires a higher intensity of exercise to confer an additive effect of feeding and exercise during post-exercise recovery, which is in line with our observation from a resistance exercise study which suggests that type II fibre recruitment is important for maximising nutrient sensitivity from exercise. Further, it may simply be that by measuring mixed MPS Harber et al. (2010) missed a stimulation of synthesis occurring in the mitochondrial and/or sarcoplasmic protein subfraction that is not reflected in the mixed protein pool through 'dilution' by a relative lack of stimulation of the myofibrillar protein subfraction.

From the observed stimulation of rates of MPS after different exercise modes, for example cycling (Wilkinson et al., 2008; Harber et al., 2010), treadmill

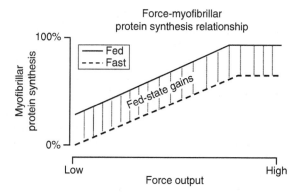

Figure 11.4 A theoretical model illustrating the proposed existence of a myofibrillar–force protein synthetic relationship in skeletal muscle. Increasing the force (i.e. watts) produced during cycling exercise will likely stimulate greater rates of myofibrillar protein synthesis during post-exercise recovery. Feeding during this time will also be additive to the already elevated fasted myofibrillar rate, which is consistent with responses seen in resistance exercise studies.

walking/running (Carraro *et al.*, 1990; Harber *et al.*, 2009), resistance exercise (Phillips *et al.*, 1997; Burd *et al.*, 2010a) or one-legged kicking (Miller *et al.*, 2005), it is apparent that there must be a relationship between myofibrillar protein synthesis and force existing in skeletal muscle. For example, and as Figure 11.4 illustrates, with increasing force output and/or exercise intensity there is a corresponding increase in rates of myofibrillar protein synthesis during exercise recovery, which is largely based on the notion that at higher exercise intensities there would be a greater recruitment of type II fibres. Indeed, there would be a plateau at some point, whereas greater intensities would not further stimulate rates of myofibrillar synthesis. Furthermore, with the well-documented additive effect of feeding and resistance exercise on rates of MPS (Biolo *et al.*, 1997; Wilkinson *et al.*, 2007), it is likely this same phenomenon is apparent after sprint exercise.

11.5 Creatine supplementation

The old adage 'there is no substitute for hard work' holds true for almost any athlete looking to improve performance outcomes in competition. However, at some stage in an athlete's career even small performance gains can be the difference between a gold or silver medal. Creatine has emerged as one of the most popular supplements among all types of

strength and power athlete, from the weekend gym enthusiast to the professional athlete looking to increase performance and/or enhance recovery (Rodriguez *et al.*, 2009). Creatine is naturally found in meat and fish; however, it is commonly supplemented in its synthetic form as creatine monohydrate (Tipton *et al.*, 2007). There are reports demonstrating that considerable variability exists within human muscle in its ability to increase creatine concentrations, which appears to be partly dependent on initial muscle creatine concentrations before supplementation (Harris *et al.*, 1992). Based on this notion, it has been reasoned that vegetarians, a population with low initial muscle creatine content and limited dietary intake, may respond better to creatine supplementation (Burke *et al.*, 2003). What is noteworthy is that creatine supplementation has been associated with increased fluid retention, which may contribute to increased osmotic load in the muscle (Ziegenfuss *et al.*, 1998). Another study by Ziegenfuss *et al.* (2002) has documented a 6.5% increase in thigh muscle volume, as measured by magnetic resonance imaging, after six maximal 10-s cycle sprints coupled with 3 days of creatine supplementation. These gains are assuredly attributed to increased fluid retention and not muscle protein accretion. Regardless, these findings have significance for power and sprint athletes, who have to maintain a certain body weight to remain eligible for their desired weight class or where power-to-weight ratio is beneficial to performance, and thus it may not be advisable to initiate creatine supplementation in the days preceding a competition.

What about performance enhancement? It is unlikely that creatine supplementation would be beneficial during endurance-type activity as normal phosphocreatine (PCr) content is sufficient to maintain ATP during steady-state endurance activities (Balsom *et al.*, 1993). There are reports demonstrating that during non-steady-state exercise such as sprint exercise, where PCr hydrolysis at least accounts for some of total ATP use, creatine supplementation has beneficial effects (Birch *et al.*, 1994; Dawson *et al.*, 1995; Peyrebrune *et al.*, 1998; Preen *et al.*, 2001; Skare *et al.*, 2001); however, others have found no enhanced effect on performance (Febbraio *et al.*, 1995; Cooke & Barnes, 1997; Snow *et al.*, 1998; Glaister *et al.*, 2006). As highlighted in other reviews on this topic (Terjung *et al.*, 2000; Tipton *et al.*, 2007), the discrepancies in the results between the positive effects of creatine on various performance markers may be due to 'responders' versus 'non-responders' among sample populations, which appears to be related to the extent of muscle creatine retention during supplementation (Greenhaff *et al.*, 1993, 1994). Further, the equivocal results among studies may simply relate to the day-to-day inconsistency in subject performance possibly created from variable start reaction times during the different testing visits (Tipton *et al.*, 2007).

Of importance for strength and power athletes, however, are studies demonstrating enhanced resistance exercise-induced adaptations such as strength and hypertrophy after creatine supplementation (Earnest *et al.*, 1995; Volek *et al.*, 1999, 2004; Becque *et al.*, 2000; Rawson & Volek, 2003). The effects of creatine supplementation on muscle protein turnover provide little insight into the mechanisms that may facilitate these potentiated adaptations after resistance training. Indeed, if creatine supplementation permits increased volume of work to be performed during an acute bout of resistance exercise (Earnest *et al.*, 1995; Volek *et al.*, 1999), then it seems likely that it may provide a greater stimulus for myofibrillar accretion (Burd *et al.*, 2010c). However, Phillips *et al.* (2002) found that co-ingestion of creatine with a nutritional beverage during post-exercise recovery had no additional effect on resistance exercise-induced rates of mixed MPS and/or inhibition of MPB compared with the nutritional beverage alone. Further, creatine supplementation in combination with resistance exercise had no effect on rates of myofibrillar protein synthesis or sarcoplasmic protein synthesis over and above that of exercise alone (Louis *et al.*, 2003). Therefore, it appears that the beneficial effect of creatine supplementation, or any supplement for that matter, in enhancing skeletal muscle hypertrophy would be minimal relative to the adaptations seen after a well-designed resistance training programme and adequate nutrition, which includes consuming high-quality proteins at strategic times (i.e. 1–2 hours after exercise) during the course of the day.

11.6 General conclusions

The regulation of skeletal muscle mass is multifaceted and contains a great degree of redundancy (Rennie *et al.*, 2004). Scientific studies are performed under highly controlled laboratory conditions rather than free-living conditions, but serve to provide the obligatory framework on which we build our current understanding and later apply to a 'real world' setting. Even so, it is well established that there are inherent individual differences in so far as the extent of training gains are concerned (responders versus non-responders) (Hubal *et al.*, 2005; Petrella *et al.*, 2008) and thus all findings and subsequent recommendations will not produce the same responses in everyone.

We have provided evidence that an excessive protein intake (>2 g/kg/day) for sprint and power athletes is not a necessary requirement for maximising muscle hypertrophy and strength; however, a high-protein diet may confer a metabolic advantage that has important implications for athletes seeking to lose excess body fat but maintain lean body mass. The necessity of high daily carbohydrate intakes for sprint and power athletes has never been examined; however, carbohydrate intake is important for glycogen synthesis to re-stock glycogen stores used during training. Full muscle fibre recruitment during resistance exercise confers a sensitising effect to protein feeding on skeletal muscle for up to 24 hours. Finally, creatine monohydrate has been shown to be effective in improving sprint and power performance; however, the beneficial effect of creatine supplementation in enhancing skeletal muscle hypertrophy would be minimal relative to the adaptations seen after a well-designed resistance training programme and adequate nutrition, which includes consuming high-quality proteins at strategic times (i.e. 1–2 hours after exercise) during the course of the day.

References

Allemeier CA, Fry AC, Johnson P, Hikida RS, Hagerman FC, Staron RS. Effects of sprint cycle training on human skeletal muscle. J Appl Physiol 1994; 77: 2385–2390.

Atherton PJ, Etheridge T, Watt PW *et al.* Muscle full effect after oral protein: time-dependent concordance and discordance between human muscle protein synthesis and mTORC1 signaling. Am J Clin Nutr 2010; 92: 1080–1088.

Balsom PD, Harridge SD, Soderlund K, Sjodin B, Ekblom B. Creatine supplementation *per se* does not enhance endurance exercise performance. Acta Physiol Scand 1993; 149: 521–523.

Becque MD, Lochmann JD, Melrose DR. Effects of oral creatine supplementation on muscular strength and body composition. Med Sci Sports Exer 2000; 32: 654–658.

Bennet WM, Connacher AA, Scrimgeour CM, Smith K, Rennie MJ. Increase in anterior tibialis muscle protein synthesis in healthy man during mixed amino acid infusion: studies of incorporation of [1-^{13}C]leucine. Clin Sci 1989; 76: 447–454.

Biolo G, Fleming RY, Maggi SP, Wolfe RR. Transmembrane transport and intracellular kinetics of amino acids in human skeletal muscle. Am J Physiol 1995a; 268: E75–E84.

Biolo G, Maggi SP, Williams BD, Tipton KD, Wolfe RR. Increased rates of muscle protein turnover and amino acid transport after resistance exercise in humans. Am J Physiol 1995b; 268: E514–E520.

Biolo G, Tipton KD, Klein S, Wolfe RR. An abundant supply of amino acids enhances the metabolic effect of exercise on muscle protein. Am J Physiol 1997; 273: E122–129.

Birch R, Noble D, Greenhaff PL. The influence of dietary creatine supplementation on performance during repeated bouts of maximal isokinetic cycling in man. Eur J Appl Physiol Occup Physiol 1994; 69: 268–276.

Bohe J, Low JF, Wolfe RR, Rennie MJ. Latency and duration of stimulation of human muscle protein synthesis during continuous infusion of amino acids. J Physiol 2001; 532: 575–579.

Bohe J, Low A, Wolfe RR, Rennie MJ. Human muscle protein synthesis is modulated by extracellular, not intramuscular amino acid availability: a dose–response study. J Physiol 2003; 552: 315–324.

Burd NA, Tang JE, Moore DR, Phillips SM. Exercise training and protein metabolism: influences of contraction, protein intake, and sex-based differences. J Appl Physiol 2009; 106: 1692–1701.

Burd NA, West DW, Staples AW et al. Low-load high volume resistance exercise stimulates muscle protein synthesis more than high-load low volume resistance exercise in young men. PLoS One 2010a; 5(8): e12033.

Burd NA, Dickinson JM, Lemoine JK et al. Effect of a cyclooxygenase-2 inhibitor on postexercise muscle protein synthesis in humans. Am J Physiol 2010b; 298: E354–E361.

Burd NA, Holwerda AM, Selby KC et al. Resistance exercise volume affects myofibrillar protein synthesis and anabolic signalling molecule phosphorylation in young men. J Physiol 2010c; 588: 3119–3130.

Burd NA, West DW, Moore DR et al. Enhanced amino acid sensitivity of myofibrillar protein synthesis persists for up to 24 h after resistance exercise in young men. J Nutr 2011; 14: 568–573.

Burgomaster KA, Hughes SC, Heigenhauser GJ, Bradwell SN, Gibala MJ. Six sessions of sprint interval training increases muscle oxidative potential and cycle endurance capacity in humans. J Appl Physiol 2005; 98: 1985–1990.

Burgomaster KA, Howarth KR, Phillips SM et al. Similar metabolic adaptations during exercise after low volume sprint interval and traditional endurance training in humans. J Physiol 2008; 586: 151–160.

Burke DG, Chilibeck PD, Parise G, Candow DG, Mahoney D, Tarnopolsky M. Effect of creatine and weight training on muscle creatine and performance in vegetarians. Med Sci Sports Exerc 2003; 35: 1946–1955.

Cadefau J, Casademont J, Grau JM et al. Biochemical and histochemical adaptation to sprint training in young athletes. Acta Physiol Scand 1990; 140: 341–351.

Carraro F, Stuart CA, Hartl WH, Rosenblatt J, Wolfe RR. Effect of exercise and recovery on muscle protein synthesis in human subjects. Am J Physiol 1990; 259: E470–E476.

Cheuvront SN, Carter R III, Haymes EM, Sawka MN. No effect of moderate hypohydration or hyperthermia on anaerobic exercise performance. Med Sci Sports Exerc 2006; 38: 1093–1097.

Cooke WH, Barnes WS. The influence of recovery duration on high-intensity exercise performance after oral creatine supplementation. Can J Appl Physiol 1997; 22: 454–467.

Creer A, Gallagher P, Slivka D, Jemiolo B, Fink W, Trappe S. Influence of muscle glycogen availability on ERK1/2 and Akt signaling after resistance exercise in human skeletal muscle. J Appl Physiol 2005; 99: 950–956.

Cuthbertson D, Smith K, Babraj J et al. Anabolic signaling deficits underlie amino acid resistance of wasting, aging muscle. FASEB J 2005; 19: 422–424.

Dangin M, Boirie Y, Garcia-Rodenas C et al. The digestion rate of protein is an independent regulating factor of postprandial protein retention. Am J Physiol 2001; 280: E340–E348.

Dangin M, Guillet C, Garcia-Rodenas C et al. The rate of protein digestion affects protein gain differently during aging in humans. J Physiol 2003; 549: 635–644.

Dawson B, Cutler M, Moody A, Lawrence S, Goodman C, Randall N. Effects of oral creatine loading on single and repeated maximal short sprints. Aust J Sci Med Sport 1995; 27: 56–61.

Dreyer HC, Fujita S, Cadenas JG, Chinkes DL, Volpi E, Rasmussen BB. Resistance exercise increases AMPK activity and reduces 4E-BP1 phosphorylation and protein synthesis in human skeletal muscle. J Physiol 2006; 576: 613–624.

Earnest CP, Snell PG, Rodriguez R, Almada AL, Mitchell TL. The effect of creatine monohydrate ingestion on anaerobic power indices, muscular strength and body composition. Acta Physiol Scand 1995; 153: 207–209.

Febbraio MA, Flanagan TR, Snow RJ, Zhao S, Carey MF. Effect of creatine supplementation on intramuscular TCr, metabolism and performance during intermittent, supramaximal exercise in humans. Acta Physiol Scand 1995; 155: 387–395.

Fogelholm M. Effects of bodyweight reduction on sports performance. Sports Med (Auckland) 1994; 18: 249–267.

Fryburg DA, Barrett EJ, Louard RJ, Gelfand RA. Effect of starvation on human muscle protein metabolism and its response to insulin. Am J Physiol 1990; 259: E477–E482.

Fujita S, Volpi E. Amino acids and muscle loss with aging. J Nutr 2006; 136: 277S–280S.

Fujita S, Rasmussen BB, Cadenas JG, Grady JJ, Volpi E. Effect of insulin on human skeletal muscle protein synthesis is modulated by insulin-induced changes in muscle blood flow and amino acid availability. Am J Physiol 2006; 291: E745–E754.

Fujita S, Rasmussen BB, Cadenas JG et al. Aerobic exercise overcomes the age-related insulin resistance of muscle protein metabolism by improving endothelial function and Akt/mammalian target of rapamycin signaling. Diabetes 2007; 56: 1615–1622.

Gelfand RA, Barrett EJ. Effect of physiologic hyperinsulinaemia on skeletal muscle protein synthesis and breakdown in man. J Clin Invest 1987; 80: 1–6.

Gibala MJ, Little JP, van Essen M et al. Short-term sprint interval versus traditional endurance training: similar initial adaptations in human skeletal muscle and exercise performance. J Physiol 2006; 575: 901–911.

Glaister M, Lockey RA, Abraham CS, Staerck A, Goodwin JE, McInnes G. Creatine supplementation and multiple sprint running performance. Journal of strength and conditioning research/National Strength and Conditioning Association 2006; 20: 273–277.

Glynn EL, Fry CS, Drummond MJ et al. Muscle protein breakdown has a minor role in the protein anabolic response to essential amino acid and carbohydrate intake following resistance exercise. Am J Physiol 2010; 299: R533–R540.

Greenhaff PL, Casey A, Short AH, Harris R, Soderlund K, Hultman E. Influence of oral creatine supplementation of muscle torque during repeated bouts of maximal voluntary exercise in man. Clin Sci 1993; 84: 565–571.

Greenhaff PL, Nevill ME, Soderlund K et al. The metabolic responses of human type I and II muscle fibres during maximal treadmill sprinting. J Physiol 1994; 478: 149–155.

Greenhaff PL, Karagounis LG, Peirce N et al. Disassociation between the effects of amino acids and insulin on signaling, ubiquitin ligases, and protein turnover in human muscle. Am J Physiol 2008; 295: E595–E604.

Harber MP, Crane JD, Dickinson JM et al. Protein synthesis and the expression of growth-related genes are altered by running in human vastus lateralis and soleus muscles. Am J Physiol 2009; 296: R708–R714.

Harber MP, Konopka AR, Jemiolo B, Trappe SW, Trappe TA, Reidy PT. Muscle protein synthesis and gene expression during recovery from aerobic exercise in the fasted and fed states. Am J Physiol 2010; 299: R1254–R1262.

Harridge SD, Bottinelli R, Canepari M et al. Sprint training, in vitro and in vivo muscle function, and myosin heavy chain expression. J Appl Physiol 1998; 84: 442–449.

Harris RC, Soderlund K, Hultman E. Elevation of creatine in resting and exercised muscle of normal subjects by creatine supplementation. Clin Sci 1992; 83: 367–374.

Hartman JW, Tang JE, Wilkinson SB et al. Consumption of fat-free fluid milk after resistance exercise promotes greater lean mass accretion than does consumption of soy or carbohydrate in young, novice, male weightlifters. Am J Clin Nutr 2007; 86: 373–381.

Holm L, Kjaer M. Measuring protein breakdown rate in individual proteins in vivo. Curr Opin Clin Nutr Metab Care 2010; 13: 526–531.

Hubal MJ, Gordish-Dressman H, Thompson PD et al. Variability in muscle size and strength gain after unilateral resistance training. Med Sci Sports Exerc 2005; 37: 964–972.

Institute of Medicine. Dietary Reference Intakes for energy, carbohydrate, fiber, fat, fatty acids, cholesterol, protein, and amino acids. Washington, DC: National Academies Press, 2005.

Josse AR, Tang JE, Tarnopolsky MA, Phillips SM. Body composition and strength changes in women with milk and resistance exercise. Med Sci Sports Exerc 2009; 42: 1122–1130.

Koopman R, Beelen M, Stellingwerff T et al. Coingestion of carbohydrate with protein does not further augment postexercise muscle protein synthesis. Am J Physiol 2007; 293: E833–E842.

Kumar V, Selby A, Rankin D et al. Age-related differences in dose response of muscle protein synthesis to resistance exercise in young and old men. J Physiol 2009; 587: 211–217.

Layman DK, Boileau RA, Erickson DJ et al. A reduced ratio of dietary carbohydrate to protein improves body composition and blood lipid profiles during weight loss in adult women. J Nutr 2003; 133: 411–417.

Layman DK, Evans E, Baum JI, Seyler J, Erickson DJ, Boileau RA. Dietary protein and exercise have additive effects on body composition during weight loss in adult women. J Nutr 2005; 135: 1903–1910.

Lemon PW, Tarnopolsky MA, MacDougall JD, Atkinson SA. Protein requirements and muscle mass/strength changes during intensive training in novice bodybuilders. J Appl Physiol 1992; 73: 767–775.

Leveritt M, Abernethy PJ, Barry BK, Logan PA. Concurrent strength and endurance training. A review. Sports Med (Auckland) 1999; 28: 413–427.

Louis M, Poortmans JR, Francaux M et al. No effect of creatine supplementation on human myofibrillar and sarcoplasmic protein synthesis after resistance exercise. Am J Physiol 2003; 285: E1089–E1094.

MacDougall JD, Gibala MJ, Tarnopolsky MA, MacDonald JR, Interisano SA, Yarasheski KE. The time course for elevated muscle protein synthesis following heavy resistance exercise. Can J Appl Physiol 1995; 20: 480–486.

MacDougall JD, Ray S, Sale DG, McCartney N, Lee P, Garner S. Muscle substrate utilization and lactate production. Can J Appl Physiol 1999; 24: 209–215.

Mendez-Villanueva A, Hamer P, Bishop D. Fatigue in repeated-sprint exercise is related to muscle power factors and reduced neuromuscular activity. Eur J Appl Physiol 2008; 103: 411–419.

Mettler S, Mitchell N, Tipton KD. Increased protein intake reduces lean body mass loss during weight loss in athletes. Med Sci Sports Exerc 2010; 42: 326–337.

Miller BF, Olesen JL, Hansen M et al. Coordinated collagen and muscle protein synthesis in human patella tendon and quadriceps muscle after exercise. J Physiol 2005; 567: 1021–1033.

Moore DR, Phillips SM, Babraj JA, Smith K, Rennie MJ. Myofibrillar and collagen protein synthesis in human skeletal muscle in young men after maximal shortening and lengthening contractions. J Physiol 2005; 288: E1153–E1159.

Moore DR, Tang JE, Burd NA, Rerecich T, Tarnopolsky MA, Phillips SM. Differential stimulation of myofibrillar and sarcoplasmic protein synthesis with protein ingestion at rest and after resistance exercise. J Physiol 2009a; 587: 897–904.

Moore DR, Robinson MJ, Fry JL et al. Ingested protein dose response of muscle and albumin protein synthesis after resistance exercise in young men. Am J Clin Nutr 2009b; 89: 161–168.

Noakes M, Keogh JB, Foster PR, Clifton PM. Effect of an energy-restricted, high-protein, low-fat diet relative to a conventional high-carbohydrate, low-fat diet on weight loss, body composition, nutritional status, and markers of cardiovascular health in obese women. Am J Clin Nutr 2005; 81: 1298–1306.

Parker B, Noakes M, Luscombe N, Clifton P. Effect of a high-protein, high-monounsaturated fat weight loss diet on glycemic control and lipid levels in type 2 diabetes. Diabetes Care 2002; 25: 425–430.

Pascoe DD, Costill DL, Fink WJ, Robergs RA, Zachwieja JJ. Glycogen resynthesis in skeletal muscle following resistive exercise. Med Sci Sports Exerc 1993; 25: 349–354.

Petrella JK, Kim JS, Mayhew DL, Cross JM, Bamman MM. Potent myofiber hypertrophy during resistance training in humans is associated with satellite cell-mediated myonuclear addition: a cluster analysis. J Appl Physiol 2008; 104: 1736–1742.

Peyrebrune MC, Nevill ME, Donaldson FJ, Cosford DJ. The effects of oral creatine supplementation on performance in single and repeated sprint swimming. J Sports Sci 1998; 16: 271–279.

Phillips SM. Protein requirements and supplementation in strength sports. Nutrition 2004; 20: 689–695.

Phillips SM. Dietary protein for athletes: from requirements to metabolic advantage. Appl Physiol Nutr Metab 2006; 31: 647–654.

Phillips SM. Insulin and muscle protein turnover in humans: stimulatory, permissive, inhibitory, or all of the above? Am J Physiol 2008; 295: E731.

Phillips SM, Tipton KD, Aarsland A, Wolf SE, Wolfe RR. Mixed muscle protein synthesis and breakdown after resistance exercise in humans. Am J Physiol 1997; 273: E99–E107.

Phillips SM, Parise G, Roy BD, Tipton KD, Wolfe RR, Tamopolsky MA. Resistance-training-induced adaptations in skeletal muscle protein turnover in the fed state. Can J Physiol Pharmacol 2002; 80: 1045–1053.

Phillips SM, Moore DR, Tang JE. A critical examination of dietary protein requirements, benefits, and excesses in athletes. Int J Sport Nutr Exerc Metab 2007; 17: S58–S76.

Pozefsky T, Felig P, Tobin JD, Soeldner JS, Cahill GF Jr. Amino acid balance across tissues of the forearm in postabsorptive man. Effects of insulin at two dose levels. J Clin Invest 1969; 48: 2273–2282.

Preen D, Dawson B, Goodman C, Lawrence S, Beilby J, Ching S. Effect of creatine loading on long-term sprint exercise performance and metabolism. Med Sci Sport Exerc 2001; 33: 814–821.

Rasmussen BB, Fujita S, Wolfe RR et al. Insulin resistance of muscle protein metabolism in aging. FASEB J 2006; 20: 768–769.

Rawson ES, Volek JS. Effects of creatine supplementation and resistance training on muscle strength and weightlifting performance. Journal of strength and conditioning research/ National Strength and Conditioning Association 2003; 17: 822–831.

Rennie MJ. An introduction to the use of tracers in nutrition and metabolism. Proc Nutr Soc 1999; 58: 935–944.

Rennie MJ, Edwards RH, Halliday D, Matthews DE, Wolman SL, Millward DJ. Muscle protein synthesis measured by stable isotope techniques in man: the effects of feeding and fasting. Clin Sci 1982; 63: 519–523.

Rennie MJ, Wackerhage H, Spangenburg EE, Booth FW. Control of the size of the human muscle mass. Annu Rev Physiol 2004; 66: 799–828.

Rodriguez NR, Di Marco NM, Langley S. American College of Sports Medicine position stand. Nutrition and athletic performance. Med Sci Sport Exerc 2009; 41: 709–731.

Skare OC, Skadberg, Wisnes AR. Creatine supplementation improves sprint performance in male sprinters. Scand J Med Sci Sports 2001; 11: 96–102.

Snow RJ, McKenna MJ, Selig SE, Kemp J, Stathis CG, Zhao S. Effect of creatine supplementation on sprint exercise performance and muscle metabolism. J Appl Physiol 1998; 84: 1667–1673.

Staples AW, Burd NA, West DW et al. Carbohydrates does not augment exercise-induced protein accretion versus protein alone. Med Sci Sports Exerc 2010 [Epub ahead of print].

Svanberg E, Jefferson LS, Lundholm K, Kimball SR. Postprandial stimulation of muscle protein synthesis is independent of changes in insulin. Am J Physiol 1997; 272: E841–E847.

Tang JE, Moore DR, Kujbida GW, Tarnopolsky MA, Phillips SM. Ingestion of whey hydrolysate, casein, or soy protein isolate: effects on mixed muscle protein synthesis at rest and following resistance exercise in young men. J Appl Physiol 2009; 107: 987–992.

Tarnopolsky MA, MacDougall JD, Atkinson SA. Influence of protein intake and training status on nitrogen balance and lean body mass. J Appl Physiol 1988; 64: 187–193.

Tarnopolsky MA, Atkinson SA, MacDougall JD, Chesley A, Phillips S, Schwarcz HP. Evaluation of protein requirements for trained strength athletes. J Appl Physiol 1992; 73: 1986–1995.

Teegarden D. The influence of dairy product consumption on body composition. J Nutr 2005; 135: 2749–2752.

Terjung RL, Clarkson P, Eichner ER et al. American College of Sports Medicine roundtable. The physiological and health effects of oral creatine supplementation. Med Sci Sports Exerc 2000; 32: 706–717.

Tesch PA, Colliander EB, Kaiser P. Muscle metabolism during intense, heavy-resistance exercise. Eur J Appl Physiol Occup Physiol 1986; 55: 362–366.

Tipton KD, Rasmussen BB, Miller SL et al. Timing of amino acid– carbohydrate ingestion alters anabolic response of muscle to resistance exercise. Am J Physiol 2001; 281: E197–E206.

Tipton KD, Jeukendrup AE, Hespel P. Nutrition for the sprinter. J Sports Sci 2007; 25 (Suppl 1): S5–S15.

Volek JS, Duncan ND, Mazzetti SA et al. Performance and muscle fiber adaptations to creatine supplementation and heavy resistance training. Med Sci Sports Exerc 1999; 31: 1147–1156.

Volek JS, Ratamess NA, Rubin MR et al. The effects of creatine supplementation on muscular performance and body composition responses to short-term resistance training overreaching. Eur J Appl Physiol 2004; 91: 628–637.

Volek JS, Forsythe CE, Kraemer WJ. Nutritional aspects of women strength athletes. Br J Sports Med 2006; 40: 742–748.

Volpi E, Lucidi P, Cruciani G et al. Contribution of amino acids and insulin to protein anabolism during meal absorption. Diabetes 1996; 45: 1245–1252.

Wagenmakers AJ. Tracers to investigate protein and amino acid metabolism in human subjects. Proc Nutr Soc 1999; 58: 987–1000.

West DW, Burd NA, Tang JE et al. Elevations in ostensibly anabolic hormones with resistance exercise enhance neither training-induced muscle hypertrophy nor strength of the elbow flexors. J Appl Physiol 2010; 108: 60–67.

Wilkes EA, Selby AL, Atherton PJ et al. Blunting of insulin inhibition of proteolysis in legs of older subjects may contribute to age-related sarcopenia. Am J Clin Nutr 2009; 90: 1343–1350.

Wilkinson SB, Tarnopolsky MA, Macdonald MJ, Macdonald JR, Armstrong D, Phillips SM. Consumption of fluid skim milk promotes greater muscle protein accretion after resistance exercise than does consumption of an isonitrogenous and isoenergetic soy-protein beverage. Am J Clin Nutr 2007; 85: 1031–1040.

Wilkinson SB, Phillips SM, Atherton PJ et al. Differential effects of resistance and endurance exercise in the fed state on signalling molecule phosphorylation and protein synthesis in human muscle. J Physiol 2008; 586: 3701–3717.

Zemel MB. Role of calcium and dairy products in energy partitioning and weight management. Am J Clin Nutr 2004; 79: 907S–912S.

Ziegenfuss TN, Lowery LM, Lemon PW. Acute fluid volume changes in men during three days of creatine supplementation. J Exerc Physiol 1998; 1: 1–14.

Ziegenfuss TN, Rogers M, Lowery L et al. Effect of creatine loading on anaerobic performance and skeletal muscle volume in NCAA Division I athletes. Nutrition 2002; 18: 397–402.

12

Nutrition for Middle-Distance and Speed-Endurance Training

Trent Stellingwerff and Bethanie Allanson

Key messages

- Elite middle-distance athletes undertake a periodised training approach, featuring vastly different training volumes and intensities throughout different times of the year, thus requiring a periodised nutritional approach.
- Dietary carbohydrate (CHO) ingestion should rise progressively from approximately 55 to over 70% of total energy intake (or 7–10 g CHO/kg/day) throughout the yearly periodised training plan.
- Dietary fat intake should gradually decrease from approximately 30% to 20% of total energy intake throughout the yearly periodised training plan.
- Optimising glycogen and protein synthesis is of utmost importance for recovery and is accomplished via the intake of

1.2–1.5 g CHO/kg/hour and about 0.3 g protein/kg over the first few hours of recovery.
- Realising a very low body fat percentage or weight and/or an increased power-to-weight ratio can lead to significant increases in middle-distance performance. Athletes should only aspire to be truly at competition performance weight and body composition for short periods of time throughout the year.
- Supplementation with β-alanine and sodium bicarbonate has been shown to augment intracellular and extracellular buffering capacities, which may lead to a small, but significant, increase in performance.

12.1 Introduction

Events where near-maximal exercise intensity is maintained over exercise durations of approximately 1–8 min are generally considered as middle-distance disciplines. These include track and field (400 m to 1500 m), individual track cycling time trial and cycling pursuit (500 m to 4000 m), swimming (100 m to 400 m), rowing/kayak and speed skating (500 m to 5000 m). For simplicity, throughout the rest of this chapter, the athletets who participate in this group of events will simply be referred to as middle-distance athletes.

Given the considerable contribution of both the aerobic and anaerobic energy systems to providing the required energy, middle-distance athletes could be described as being at the cross-roads of metabolism. Accordingly, all elite middle-distance athletes undertake a periodised training approach, featuring

vastly different training volumes and intensities throughout different times of the year. Indeed, when examining the training of elite middle-distance athletes, the volume of training in the aerobic development phase rivals that of a long-distance athlete (e.g. marathoner), while the intensity, quality and speed of training during the competition season is similar to that of a sprinter.

This chapter provides relevant information on nutrition recommendations linked to acute and chronic periodised training situations and competitive events for middle-distance athletes. Body composition is a product of training energy expenditure coupled with nutritional energy intake, and is also described within a yearly periodised approach. Several nutritional supplements relevant to middle-distance athletes, as well as emerging future nutritional research directions, are also discussed.

Sport and Exercise Nutrition, First Edition. Edited by Susan A Lanham-New, Samantha J Stear, Susan M Shirreffs and Adam L Collins.
© 2011 The Nutrition Society. Published 2011 by Blackwell Publishing Ltd.

Table 12.1 Differences in energy source provision in anaerobic-based sporting events.

Event time range	Event example	Approximate percent Vo_{2max}	Percent energy contribution		
			CP	Anaerobic	Aerobic
0.5–1 min	400 m running; individual cycling TT (500 m or 1 km); 500 m speed skating; 100 m swimming disciplines	~150	~10	~47–60	~30–43
1.5–2 min	800 m running; 1500 m speed skating; 200 m swimming disciplines	113–130	~5	~29–45	~50–66
3.5–5 min	1500 m running; individual cycling pursuit (3 or 4 km); 3000 m speed skating; 400 m swimming disciplines	103–115	~2	~14–28	~70–84
6–8 min	3000 m running; 5000 m speed skating	98–102	<1	~10–12	~88–90

Source: data adapted from Gastin (2001).

12.2 Energy systems in middle-distance athletes

Chapters 2 and 3 provide an in-depth discussion on the metabolic regulation and biochemistry of fuel metabolism during exercise. However, given that middle-distance athletes are at the cross-roads of metabolism (utilising nearly an equal contribution of aerobic and anaerobic metabolism), some further discussion on energy systems is warranted. Table 12.1 outlines the percentage energy contribution across a range of event lengths for the three primary energy systems that provide adenosine triphosphate (ATP), namely creatine phosphate (CP), anaerobic glycolysis (also named substrate-level phosphorylation), and aerobic metabolism (also named oxidative phosphorylation). Carbohydrate (CHO) is the primary fuel for exercise intensities greater than about 75% Vo_{2max}, while the bulk of fuel provided by aerobic metabolism at lower exercise intensities is from endogenous fat stores. However, during exercise situations with increasing intensity, ATP production from aerobic metabolism cannot match the rate of ATP utilisation, and the shortfall in energy supply is made up by anaerobic metabolism. Anaerobic metabolism provides energy through both the CP system and by the breakdown of glycogen, via glycogenolysis, with lactate formation. However, the high rate of energy demand results in excessive pyruvate production, which exceeds the rate at which it can be aerobically oxidised by pyruvate dehydrogenase in the mitochondria. This leads to the extreme levels of lactate production associated with all middle-distance races and some training situations. Impressively, middle-distance events that last about 4 min (Table 12.1) are conducted at about 20 times resting Vo_{2max} values, with resultant blood lactate concentrations approaching approximately 25 mmol/l.

12.3 Periodised nutrition to match periodised training programmes

Periodisation is defined as the purposeful sequencing of different training units (long-duration, medium-duration and short-term training cycles and sessions) so that athletes can attain the desired physiological readiness for optimal targeted performances on demand. Traditional periodisation sequences training into the four main distinct macrocycles or phases: (i) general preparation phase; (ii) specific preparation phase; (iii) competition phase; and (iv) transition phase (or rest and recovery phase; Figure 12.1). The exercise training stimuli during these different phases can differ drastically in terms of intensity, volume and duration, and therefore so do the types of fuels (CHO vs. fat) and the amount of energy (kilocalories) that are used to generate the required ATP (see section 12.2). An appreciation of the vastly different energy systems and required fuels to produce ATP must be taken into consideration when recommending both acute and seasonal nutrition intakes to optimise training adaptations and race performance in middle-distance athletes. However, currently this concept of nutritional and physiological periodisation throughout the year is a research area that is very underdeveloped and ripe

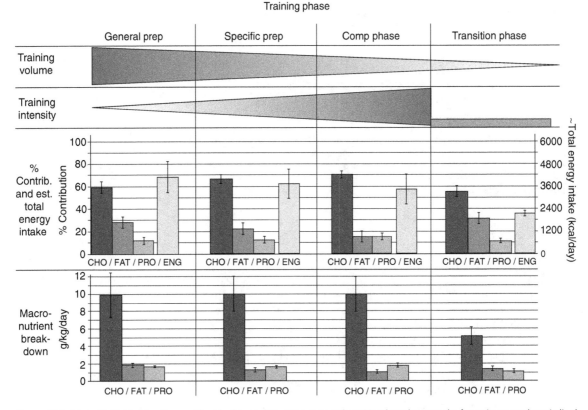

Figure 12.1 Schematic highlighting the considerable changes between energy and nutritional needs across the four primary yearly periodised training phases for a 70-kg middle-distance athlete. Nutrition recommendations adapted from Tarnopolsky *et al.* and Burke *et al.* Prep, preparation; Comp, competition; CHO, carbohydrate; FAT, fat; PRO, protein; ENG, energy; Est, estimated; Total energy intake reported in kcal, nutritional calories.

for scientific examination (for review see Stellingwerff *et al.*, 2007).

Accordingly, Figure 12.1 outlines a contemporary approach to nutritional periodisation, which takes into account acute and seasonal nutrition needs induced by specific training loads. The top bars of the figure provide a context for the general emphasis on training volume and intensity. Generally there are large training volumes of lower intensity during the general preparation phase, with an inverse relationship found during the competition phase. The next section of the figure highlights the approximate percentage contribution of each of the three major macronutrients, while highlighting the total daily energy intake. Finally, the bottom section gives an overview of the approximate number of grams per kilogram body weight per day that are needed for each of the three macronutrients, again across the four different periodised training phases. Throughout

Figure 12.1, the error bars represent the large degree of individual variability in caloric and macronutrient intake. Specific nutrition recommendations are further highlighted below for each of the three major macronutrients.

General energy intake and macronutrient recommendations

Total energy intake

During the bulk of the training season, adequate energy must be consumed to support the intensive training load. Dietary intake studies have demonstrated that female endurance athletes report much lower values for mean energy intake per kilogram body weight compared with male athletes (170 kJ/kg/ day for females vs. 230 kJ/kg/day for males). Hence, there needs to be a greater emphasis on helping females meet their daily recommended energy intake needs, which is more a sociological than physiological factor. Unfortunately, many athletes aspire to be at target body weight or body composition all year round, which is both physiologically and psychologically challenging (see section 12.5).

Generally, during the championship racing season energy expenditure is diminished compared with the previous training phases. Therefore, total caloric intake must also be appropriately decreased. However, *ad libitum* caloric intake is not immediately matched with reduced energy expenditure, as found during the competition phase. Therefore, athletes need to make conscious decisions about limiting their total energy intake during this phase, instead of adhering to their habitual diet, in order to maintain an ideal peak body composition. Finally, during the transition (or rest and recovery periods), most athletes take a period of rest for both mental and physical recovery in which training is generally very low. Some weight gain during this phase is natural, and because of the diminished training, nutritional energy intake during this phase must be reduced. Accordingly, the macronutrient and energy recommendations are the same as for the general public.

Dietary carbohydrate intake recommendations

The amount of CHO that is oxidised during exercise is very dependent on exercise intensity, with considerable CHO oxidation when exercising above 75% Vo_{2max}. Therefore, since much of middle-distance training is at or above 75% Vo_{2max}, and this dependency on CHO-based ATP provision increases throughout the phasing of the yearly training towards a championship peak, CHO-rich foods must provide the majority of the energy provision. When examining all the studies that have published dietary data on endurance athletes, males consume between 8.4 and 9.1 g CHO/kg/day, which is within the recommended range (see review by Burke *et al.*, 2001). These data are supported by the fact that the diet of African world-class runners comprises predominantly CHO, with less fats and proteins. Conversely, female endurance athletes report much lower relative daily CHO intakes (5.5 g/kg/day) compared with male athletes.

A high-CHO diet leads to augmented glycogen stores, translating into an increased time to exhaustion, compared with low-CHO diets. Conversely, extremely low CHO diets (3–15% CHO) have uniformly been shown to impair both high-intensity and endurance-based performance. Recent evidence suggests there might be some training advantages to periodically cycling glycogen stores, so that some training is undertaken with low glycogen availability (see section 12.7). However, competition should always be undertaken with high muscle glycogen content. In support of this, longitudinal training studies have failed to show superior training outcomes with subjects consuming a very high CHO diet compared with subjects consuming a moderate CHO diet (for review see Burke *et al.*, 2001). Therefore, to maintain immune function, recover glycogen stores and reduce over-training, a habitually high CHO diet (7–10 g CHO/kg/day) is recommended.

Dietary fat intake recommendations

Although the majority of dietary fuel for middle-distance athletes is in the form of CHO, fat also serves many important roles and is a vital fuel source during endurance-based training. Skeletal muscle stores a significant amount of fat in the form of intramuscular triacylglyceride (IMTG) that, due to its energy density, represents about 70–100% of the energy stored as glycogen. There is now a general consensus that IMTG is a viable fuel source in both males and females during prolonged moderate-intensity exercise up to about 85% Vo_{2max}. The general preparation phase features considerable amounts of prolonged endurance training where endogenous fat sources are a significant fuel source. The amount of ingested dietary fat required for daily IMTG repletion has been estimated at about 2 g/kg/day, and intake beyond this level may compromise muscle glycogen recovery and muscle tissue repair. During other training phases, some dietary fat is needed, but not at the levels needed during high-volume training phases.

For long-term health benefits, an adequate intake of polyunsaturated fatty acids, especially the ω-3 subclass, is advised. Sources of ω-3 fatty acids include cold water fish, such as salmon, mackerel, sardines and tuna. Other unsaturated choices for fats include olive oil, peanut oil, avocados, almonds and peanuts. Conversely, saturated fats, including *trans*-fatty acids or hydrogenated fats, should be limited in the overall diet. Fat intake should be limited, but is still a very important component of a healthy diet, for reasons such as providing fuel during training, for aiding the absorption of fat-soluble vitamins A, D, E and K, to provide substrate for hormones and cellular and myelin sheath integrity.

Dietary protein intake recommendations

During endurance exercise, protein oxidation accounts for only 2–5% of total energy expenditure. However, this proportion of amino acid oxidation can increase when training at higher intensities, during longer exercise durations, or when CHO stores are depleted (for review see Tarnopolsky, 1999). It is with this underlying rationale that the 2000 American College of Sports Medicine (ACSM) consensus statement concluded that endurance athletes should consume more protein (~1.2–1.4 g/kg/day) than the current Dietary Reference Intake (DRI) for sedentary individuals (0.8 g/kg/day). Since protein intake greater than 1.7 g/kg/day has been shown to be oxidised or result in positive nitrogen balance, Tarnopolsky has estimated that highly trained endurance athletes who undertake a large and intense training load should ideally aim for a protein intake of 1.5–1.7 g/kg/day. Dietary studies in endurance athletes from Western countries have consistently shown that with current dietary practices, hard training athletes who consume over 3000 kcal/day generally already consume more protein than any elevated dietary recommendation.

12.4 Post-training nutritional recovery

Given the diversity of training and competition that middle-distance athletes undertake, an individualised post-training nutritional recovery approach needs to be implemented. Accordingly, Table 12.2 illustrates the different training and competition situations that will elicit different specific nutrition recovery needs and, consequently, different macronutrient recommendations. For information on post-exercise rehydration recommendations, see Chapter 7. Recovery nutrition regimens emphasise the re-synthesis of CHO energy stores (primarily glycogen) and the synthesis of new proteins through the consumption of dietary protein. The sections below highlight the type of specific macronutrients and timing to maximise these recovery processes. Although fat consumption plays a fundamentally important role in the general daily diet (section 12.3), it plays a lesser role during acute post-exercise

recovery. Therefore, during the first 2 hours after long aerobic endurance training (training associated with high energy expenditures), it is suggested that a reasonable intake of fat (0.2–0.3 g/kg) will be sufficient to initiate the re-synthesis of IMTG. A daily total fat target of upwards of 2 g/kg may be required during very heavy training phases if IMTG replenishment in one day is needed (see Figure 12.1) (see Further reading section for recent reviews on post-exercise recovery).

Glycogen re-synthesis

Muscle glycogen is the primary fuel for middle-distance athletes. Therefore, glycogen is of utmost importance with regard to optimising its re-synthesis. The highest rates of muscle glycogen synthesis occur during the first hour immediately after exercise. When the time for glycogen recovery is very short (<4 hours), such as between training bouts, contemporary studies suggest utilising immediate and frequent smaller CHO doses (i.e. 20–30 g CHO every 20–30 min) for an overall intake rate of 1.2–1.5 g/kg/hour for the first several hours of recovery (Table 12.2). During short-term recovery (<4 hours), high levels of fat and protein intake should also be avoided as they delay gastric emptying and can also potentially cause gastrointestinal upset for the subsequent exercise bout. Furthermore, the immediate post-exercise consumption of CHO intake is very important, as delaying the intake of CHO until 2 hours after exercise has a significant negative effect on muscle glycogen re-synthesis for up to 8 hours. Conversely, when recovery periods are long (~24 hours), immediate post-exercise consumption of CHO is not required to maximise muscle glycogen content for the following day, as long as the total daily required CHO needs are met.

The majority of studies have found no further enhancement of glycogen re-synthesis with the addition of amino acids or protein in combination with CHO and protein mixtures. However, during situations of prolonged recovery (>4 hours), then protein must also be consumed during recovery to optimise post-exercise muscle protein synthesis and whole-body protein balance.

Protein synthesis

Beyond current daily protein recommendations, strong emerging evidence suggests that the timing and periodisation of this protein throughout the day,

Table 12.2 Recommendations for acute (first several hours after exercise) recovery nutrition across different training and competition situations.

	Specific type of training			
	Long aerobic/endurance training	Intense short duration or prolonged resistance circuit training	Technical drills/ short-duration resistance training	Situations of short recovery (<4 hours)
Exercise characteristics	• Prolonged aerobic exercise (>1 hour) of easier intensity • Primarily aerobic metabolism (fat and CHO)	• High-intensity training of shorter durations (~20–40 min) • Primarily anaerobic metabolism (primarily CHO)	• Low volume of explosive movements • Primarily anaerobic metabolism (PCr + CHO)	• Multiple races or training sessions on the same day
Specific recovery needs	• Energy replacement (fat and CHO) • Carbohydrate intake of primary importance for glycogen re-synthesis • Protein needed for muscle recovery and remodelling	• Energy replacement (primarily CHO) • Carbohydrate intake of primary importance for glycogen re-synthesis • Protein needed for muscle recovery and remodelling	• Energy needs are low • Lower carbohydrate intake needs (some glycogen re-synthesis needed) • Protein needed for muscle recovery and remodelling	• Some energy replacement (primarily CHO) • Carbohydrate intake of primary importance for glycogen re-synthesis • Focus on foods that are GI tolerable for subsequent exercise (minimise fat and protein intakes)
Macronutrient recommendations (within first 2 hours)	• CHO: ~1.2–1.5 g/kg • PRO: ~0.3 g/kg • Fat: ~0.2–0.3 g/kg	• CHO: ~1.2–1.5 g/kg • PRO: ~0.3 g/kg • Fat: minimal requirements	• CHO: ~0.5–1.0 g/kg • PRO: ~0.3 g/kg • Fat: minimal requirements	• CHO: ~1.2–1.5 g/kg • PRO: minimal requirements • Fat: minimal requirements
Practical example for 70-kg athlete	• 750 ml CHO sports drink, with protein recovery bar, and ~300 ml milk	• Individual mini-veggie and meat pizza, ~300 ml juice and 1 piece of fruit	• Fruit smoothie (~300 ml: skim milk, yoghurt, fruit + PRO powder) and 1 piece of fruit	• 750 ml CHO sports drink *and/or* high-CHO food snacks (e.g. sports bar, crackers, cookies)

CHO, carbohydrate; GI, gastrointestinal; PCr, phosphocreatine; PRO, protein.
Nutrition recommendations adapted from Moore *et al.* (2009), Tipton & Wolfe (2004) and Burke *et al.* (2004).

and the type and amount of protein, has a great impact on the efficacy of the protein to increase protein synthesis and optimise post-exercise recovery.

Type of protein
It appears that an essential element in optimising protein synthesis is the macronutrient protein, and several studies have indirectly elucidated that only essential amino acids are needed to stimulate protein synthesis. Further, the combined effects of exercise and post-exercise protein intake can result in additive effects for improving protein synthesis. Most recent evidence has also shown that in order to optimise

muscle protein synthesis (not whole-body or splanchnic protein turnover), whey protein appears to be superior to either soy or casein.

Amount of protein
Despite the fact that body-builders have long believed in very large post-exercise protein intakes (>40 g) to maximise the anabolic effect, recent data suggest otherwise. A very well conducted dose–response study was recently published by Moore *et al.* (2009), which examined the effects of five increasing doses of dietary protein on muscle protein synthesis after resistance exercise. This study clearly showed that there appears

to be a maximal effective dose of about 20 g of dietary protein for stimulating muscle anabolism after resistance exercise. Although no studies have yet clearly established whether more or less protein is needed to optimise acute protein synthesis for athletes of varying body weights, when examining the totality of acute studies, a body weight-corrected protein dose of about 0.3 g/kg appears to provide an optimal dose (Table 12.2).

Timing of protein ingestion

There is a paucity of scientific studies examining the timing of protein ingestion around exercise to maximise the protein synthesis response. The few studies that have examined nutritional timing show mixed results when testing whether the immediate intake of protein either before or after exercise is optimal. Although the muscle appears sensitive to protein even 24 hours after exercise, analogous to glycogen re-synthesis, the delayed intake of protein also appears to diminish the post-exercise protein synthesis response. Accordingly, immediate post-exercise protein intake resulted in significantly greater leg protein uptake versus delayed protein intake 3 hours later. More studies are needed to examine nutritional timing of macronutrients throughout the day, and in particular around exercise, to better elucidate the optimal timing for recovery and adaptation. Nevertheless, it can currently be concluded that protein and CHO should be ingested in close temporal proximity to the exercise bout to maximise the anabolic response of training.

12.5 Specific body composition requirements

Chapters 17 and 18 fully discuss body composition outcomes and common pitfalls. However, further discussion specific to middle-distance athletes is highlighted below. For middle-distance athletes, realising a very low body fat percentage, weight and/or an increased power-to-weight ratio can all lead to significant performance increases, but various approaches can be undertaken. For example, despite the fact that 2000-m rowers (less weight dependent) and 1500-m runners (fully weight dependent) could both be considered middle-distance athletes, the types of body composition that dictate success are fundamentally different between these sports.

Optimising body composition focuses on losing body fat, while concurrently maintaining or minimising the loss of lean muscle mass. Accordingly, an approximate healthy target percentage body fat for an elite track and field middle-distance athlete might be 5–10% fat for males and 8–15% fat for females.

Achieving extremely low body fat is less important in less weight dependent anaerobic sports, such as rowing or track cycling, where maximal power outputs are more important. Nevertheless, beyond this 'ideal' height, weight and body composition, there are always athletes that excel who do not exactly fit within this mould. A number of athletes (primarily female) are over-mindful of the benefit that low body weight brings to performance, and many believe that more weight loss is better. In many circumstances, further weight loss in already lean athletes can actually cause loss of muscular power and strength, increased risk of stress fractures, decreased immune function and circumstances leading to the Female Athlete Triad, which all lead to a decrease in performance and compromised health. Like training and nutrition, body composition should also be periodised over the training year, and athletes should only aspire to be truly at competition performance weight and body composition for short periods of time throughout the year. Some athletes aspire to be at competition weight year-round by not taking in enough calories, but this approach can be both physically and emotionally difficult and can lead to risk of injury, sickness and health issues.

There is a real lack of strong scientific research looking at how best to approach common questions about changing and optimising body composition in elite athletes while concurrently undertaking extreme training loads in relation to performance outcomes. Most studies show that when individuals are in negative energy balance, they will lose both body fat and muscle mass. However, recent data by Mettler et al. in trained subjects suggests that through aggressive exercise and dietary protein periodisation, muscle mass can actually be 100% maintained while losing total body weight during a 2-week period of a large 40% negative energy balance. In this study, subjects utilised a higher daily protein diet (~2.3 g/kg/day), with resistance exercise, to lose significant weight (~1.5 kg), of which nearly 100% was fat loss not muscle loss. Therefore, a combined approach of slightly decreasing energy intake (~500 kcal) plus either a maintenance of training load or slightly increased energy expenditure is the best approach to optimising body composition over a 3–6 week period prior to the targeted competitive season. During these periods of negative energy balance in elite training athletes aspiring to lose weight, it has been suggested that daily protein intake be raised to about 2.3 g/kg/day and utilisation of protein maximised by optimising recovery routines.

12.6 Supplements for the middle-distance athlete

The cause of fatigue during exercise is not singular in nature, but instead involves complex and multi-factorial mechanisms. However, the primary causes of fatigue during maximal exercise lasting from about 1 to 10 min involves limitations imposed by anaerobic glycolysis as well as negative consequences resulting from the associated muscular acidosis caused by declining muscle pH. Intense exercise can cause significant decreases in muscle pH, from resting values of about 7.1 down to 6.3–6.5, via the formation and accumulation of hydrogen ions. This drop in muscle pH has been shown to negatively affect metabolic processes, inhibiting the re-synthesis of phosphorylcreatine and inhibiting glycolysis and the muscle contraction process itself. Accordingly, a higher buffering capacity in humans has been directly associated with improved performance in sprint exercise and cycling endurance performance. There are two primary supplements that middle-distance athletes can potentially utilise to augment buffering capacity and potentially improve performance: (i) prolonged supplementation with β-alanine to increase muscle carnosine content to enhance intracellular (inside muscle) buffering; and (ii) acute supplementation with sodium citrate or sodium bicarbonate can be used to enhance extracellular (outside muscle) buffering (Figure 12.2). As of 2010, all these substances are not on the World Anti-Doping Agencies (WADA) Prohibited Substances List.

Intracellular buffering

Carnosine (β-alanyl-L-histidine) is a cytoplasmic dipeptide found at high concentrations in skeletal muscle and most predominantly in type II (fast twitch)

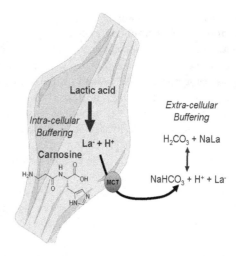

Figure 12.2 Schematic showing the biochemistry of the two primary intracellular and extracellular buffering systems involving carnosine and sodium bicarbonate, respectively. H_2CO_3, carbonic acid; MCT, monocarboxylate transporter; $NaHCO_3$, sodium bicarbonate; H^+, hydrogen cation; La^-, lactate anion.

muscle (for review see Derave et al., 2010). Since the 1930s, carnosine has been recognised as a potent intramuscular buffer due to its nitrogen-containing imidazole ring, which can directly buffer H^+ ions at a pK_a of 6.83 (Figure 12.2); the pK_a is the acid dissociation constant, and when the pK_a is within the physiological pH range of muscle (6.5–7.1), it can act as a hydrogen ion proton acceptor. The contribution of muscle carnosine to total intracellular muscle buffering capacity has been calculated to reach about 15%.

Prolonged β-alanine supplementation leads to increased muscle carnosine content

A prolonged β-alanine supplementation period is needed to increase muscle carnosine content. All studies to date that have measured muscle carnosine following β-alanine supplementation have shown a significant increase in muscle carnosine levels when using 3–6 g of β-alanine every day over 4–8 weeks. On average, this has led to a significant 40% increase in muscle carnosine (or an increase of approximately 10–15 mmol/kg d.w. of muscle carnosine). The elimination of augmented skeletal muscle carnosine after the termination of β-alanine supplementation is very slow, with an estimated washout time of 14–15 weeks after a 50% increase in muscle carnosine.

Increase in muscle carnosine leading to anaerobic performance benefits

As with most novel supplements there is an initial period where studies need to elucidate the best circumstances for use, which depend on many factors: (i) type of subject (trained vs. untrained); (ii) length of supplementation and total amount of supplementation; (iii) amount of 'active' ingredient needed in the muscle for an effect (e.g. carnosine); and (iv) the type of performance test to show an effect. Although some studies have not found enhanced performance resulting from augmented muscle carnosine content, several well-performed studies have shown that prolonged β-alanine supplementation can result in significant anaerobic performance benefits (for review see Derave et al., 2010). The studies not demonstrating positive performance effects are most likely due to inadequate β-alanine dosing protocols, studies not using well-trained subjects, being underpowered and/or inappropriately designed performance tests. Performance tests that allow for the best use of augmented muscle carnosine need to be implemented specifically in terms of intramuscular H^+ buffering found during very intense exercise lasting from about 1 to 10 min. Overall, the emerging data are starting to reveal that when subjects consume about 3–6 g β-alanine daily over 4–8 weeks (total β-alanine intake >120 g), an increase in muscle carnosine of about 40–50% (up to about 30–35 mmol/kg d.w.) can be achieved, which will lead to positive anaerobic performance outcomes. At this point, whether prolonged β-alanine supplementation can also lead to significantly enhanced weight training, or sprint (<15 s) and endurance (>20 min) performance, remains to be further established.

Extracellular buffering

During intense anaerobic exercise, intracellular buffering mechanisms can become overwhelmed and is insufficient to buffer the excess of H^+ ions, resulting in metabolic acidosis. Accordingly, lactate anions (La^-) and H^+ can be transported via monocarboxylate transporters to the extracellular spaces (see Figure 12.2). H^+ cations are transported against a concentration gradient, and therefore any mechanism to increase the rate of H^+ efflux from the muscle will maintain muscle pH and delay fatigue during intense exercise. One such mechanism is the blood bicarbonate pool (HCO_3^-), which combines with H^+ to form H_2CO_3,

which immediately dissociates to form CO_2 and H_2O (see Figure 12.2). Since the 1930s, it has been shown that metabolic alkalosis can be induced by artificially raising the blood's buffering capacity through supplementation with sodium bicarbonate ($NaHCO_3$) or sodium citrate ($Na_3C_6H_5O_7 \cdot 2H_2O$), which leads to increased muscle buffering by improving the rate of H^+ efflux from active skeletal muscle. However, studies of whether sodium bicarbonate supplementation can significantly delay fatigue and improve performance have been mixed (for review see McNaughton, 2000).

The normal protocol for inducing metabolic alkalosis, and improving the blood's buffering capacity, is by large (~300 mg/kg) acute supplementation with either sodium bicarbonate or sodium citrate in solution 1–3 hours before an anaerobic-based competition. However, the performance results are very mixed, with some studies showing a performance benefit and others showing no effect compared with placebo (for review see Maston & Tran, 1993). Additionally, some of these studies did not use either an optimal performance test or bicarbonate dose, or had a limited number of subjects, and therefore were drastically under-powered.

A 1993 meta-analysis by Matson and Tran on the performance effects of sodium bicarbonate found that, on average, bicarbonate supplementation resulted in a performance effect that was 0.44 standard deviations (SD) better than the control trial, with most studies featuring relatively untrained subjects. An improvement of 0.44 of the SD would result in a modest 0.8-s improvement over a race lasting 1 min 45 s, which for world-class athletes is within a worthwhile range of improvement. Recent publications since 2000 support this meta-analysis and appear to show a clearer performance benefit, albeit in laboratory settings, and have also shown benefits in swimming, judo and repeated sprint performance.

When supplemented properly, there appears to be a small but significant effect of sodium bicarbonate in improving intense exercise performance in events lasting from about 1 to 5 min or with repeated sprints, with less pronounced effects on single sprints (<50 s) or longer exercise (>5 min). However, there is a high degree of individual tolerance and variability, as sodium bicarbonate can cause significant gastrointestinal upset (e.g. stomach upset, diarrhoea) in about 50% of individuals. Therefore, as with any new intervention, athletes and coaches need to thoroughly experiment with sodium bicarbonate in practice and low-key competitions to ascertain individual water retention and gastrointestinal effects, before implementation into major targeted championships.

12.7 Perspectives on future research directions

It has been established that with a highly specific and regular exercise stimulus (e.g. either resistance vs. endurance training) skeletal muscle is highly plastic and adaptable, from a genetic and molecular perspective, leading to functional outcomes such as muscle growth or improved endurance. However, as previously discussed, middle-distance athletes have an incredibly diverse training programme that often utilises concurrent training, which is 'the concomitant integration of both endurance and resistance training in a periodised training plan' (for review see Coffey & Hawley, 2007). Recent data have suggested that there are several emerging scientific directions for further enhancing nutrition and exercise adaptations involving the periodic application of training in an energy depleted state (either low exogenous or endogenous CHO availability).

Effects of carbohydrate availability on endurance training adaptation

Traditionally, most experts recommend that athletes should endeavour to replenish muscle glycogen stores after exercise to ensure subsequent training bouts are conducted in a glycogen-compensated state. However, reports from professional cyclists and East African distance runners indicate that some of these athletes purposely and periodically undertake training in a glycogen-depleted state, or a fasted/water-only state, in an attempt to 'force the muscle to adapt to the next level'. Accordingly, a recent training study by Hansen *et al.* (2005) reported increased endurance adaptation and performance when half of endurance training sessions (5 days/week over 10 weeks, in previously untrained males) were undertaken in a muscle glycogen-depleted state (training twice per day, so the second training bout was glycogen depleted), as compared with 100% of training conducted in a glycogen-loaded state. Several follow-up studies have also confirmed enhanced training adaptations

with low energy availability training (either low muscle glycogen or low exogenous CHO availability via overnight fasted training), including elevations in resting muscle glycogen content, increased maximal activity of several key β-oxidation pathway enzymes, elevated skeletal muscle fatty acid protein transporters, and higher rates of whole-body fat oxidation. However, contrary to the findings of Hansen *et al.*, a significantly greater post-training performance enhancement with low-energy training, as compared to training with ample energy availability, has not consistently been shown.

In summary, these scientific results have caused a degree of uncertainty with the idea that athletes should always strive to endurance train with ample exogenous and endogenous CHO availability. Despite the fact that this type of low-energy training is both physiologically and psychologically challenging, perhaps athletes may need to periodically cycle glycogen stores and undertake fasted training to maximise the full benefits of their training. However, whether this nutrition cycling clearly leads to a significant training-induced performance benefit, compared with standard training regimes, remains to be established.

Effects of carbohydrate availability on strength training adaptation

Contrary to the emerging data that periodic low-energy training may further enhance aerobic training adaptation, opposing results have been found when examining the net protein balance, or skeletal muscle protein turnover rate, for optimising resistance exercise. Protein synthesis is an energetically costly process and directly associated with energy availability. Therefore, it appears that to optimise the effects of resistance training, training sessions should always be commenced with full muscle glycogen stores. Overall, data would suggest that middle-distance athletes undertaking both endurance and resistance types of training should phase their daily exercise with at least several hours of recovery (rest and nutrition) between the two differing stimuli, and always attempt to undertake resistance training in an energy replete and recovered state. However, much more research is needed to better characterise the adaptations induced by concurrent training on divergent responses in molecular signalling, leading to functional protein synthesis.

12.8 Conclusion

The remarkable variety in both acute training sessions and yearly periodised training programmes with middle-distance athletes results in considerable challenges and planning to optimise the nutritional impact of general recovery and supplement nutrition interventions. Furthermore, no two athlete's physiology, training programme, body composition and nutritional responses are alike. Thus, the interactions between training, competition and nutrition need to be approached on an individual basis and be continually adjusted and adapted. Both intracellular and extracellular buffering agents can be considered to enhance performance, but more research needs to be undertaken to examine the long-term impact that these buffering agents may have on training adaptation. New insights into low-energy training suggest that there may be unique nutritional and training periodisation to optimise training adaptations, which may be different than the nutritional intakes that an athlete would implement during competition season. Nevertheless, since the training and competition physiology of middle-distance athletes spans the entire continuum of energy systems, these athletes provide a unique opportunity in which many different nutrition approaches can be considered.

Practice tips: Middle distance and speed endurance training

Bethanie Allanson

- Large variations in energy expenditure and the contribution of macronutrients as energy substrates exist across training phases and the competitive season. To optimise performance in each training phase and in competition, nutrition strategies for energy intake, fuelling and recovery should be modified with each training phase to complement the change in training load and intensity.
- Athletes should be monitored and encouraged to maintain carbohydrate and energy intakes that are sufficient to support training loads. Monitoring dietary intake and body composition (e.g. anthropometry, DEXA) throughout a season (and over a number of seasons) can help determine an appropriate weight and body composition for competition as well as ensuring that body fat levels are adequate during heavy training phases.
- Athletes should only maintain their competition weight for a short period of time. Some athletes and coaches may strive for a low body weight all year round so it is important to provide education on the role of nutrition in optimising strength and power, and preventing illness and injury. Additionally, it may provide a psychological advantage for athletes to know there is potential for improvement coming into their main competitions. Following these key events, athletes should aim to increase body weight and body fat levels steadily back to out-of-competition levels.
- During the competition phase, athletes should be aware of their reduced energy requirements and advised on how to alter their diet to ensure that while energy intake is decreased, the nutrient quality of the diet remains high. It is important to maintain an adequate intake of a number of key nutrient and non-nutrient components of food including carbohydrate, protein, calcium, iron, magnesium and antioxidants that can all affect performance if dietary intake is insufficient. A multivitamin may be necessary for energy intakes below 1500 kcal.
- Nutritional recovery after training is vital in the short term for an athlete to make optimal gains from one training session and to restore glycogen, fluid and electrolytes for the next workout. In the long term, nutritional recovery is critical to ensure optimal adaptation. Recovery needs will vary with different training stimuli (e.g. resistance session versus technique-based session) so recovery strategies should be modified accordingly. In times of reduced energy intake, it is critical that an athlete's recovery is not compromised, and training sessions are supported with nutrition.
- Fat has a vital role as a fuel source, in the absorption of fat-soluble vitamins and in maintaining the integrity of cell membranes. Some athletes follow a very low fat diet in an attempt to modify body composition or maintain a low body weight, while others will have an excessive intake of fat in their diet (often saturated fat) that will make it hard to achieve desired body composition. It is important for athletes to understand the role of fat in the diet, and for performance. Encourage an appropriate fat intake from monounsaturated and polyunsaturated fat sources, for example olive oil, peanut oil, nuts, seeds, avocados, and oily fish rich in ω-3 fatty acids such as tuna, salmon, sardine and mackerel, which are beneficial for athletes due to their anti-inflammatory properties.
- Dehydration is associated with reduced cognitive function, immune suppression and the premature onset of fatigue. Athletes should focus on hydration, ensuring that they replace fluid losses from one training session to the next. Fluid balance studies or assessing the specific gravity of the first urine sample of the day can provide athletes with valuable information regarding the adequacy of their rehydration strategies.
- Because of the potential side effects associated with buffers, athletes should experiment with supplement regimens during training and minor competitions. Given that most major championships will involve heats and finals, it is important for athletes using sodium bicarbonate or sodium citrate to simulate the scenario of competition racing to determine whether they will load for each race (this may involve loading multiple times in a relatively short time frame) or for finals only.

Further reading

Burd NA, Tang JE, Moore DR, Phillips SM. Exercise training and protein metabolism: influences of contraction, protein intake, and sex-based differences. J Appl Physiol 2009; 106: 1692–1701.

Burke LM, Cox GR, Culmmings NK, Desbrow B. Guidelines for daily carbohydrate intake: do athletes achieve them? Sports Med 2001; 31: 267–299.

Burke LM, Kiens B, Ivy JL. Carbohydrates and fat for training and recovery. J Sports Sci 2004; 22: 15–30.

Coffey VG, Hawley JA. The molecular bases of training adaptation. Sports Med 2007; 37: 737–763.

Derave W, Everaert I, Beeckman S, Baguet A. Muscle carnosine metabolism and beta-alanine supplementation in relation to exercise and training. Sports Med 2010; 40: 247–263.

Gastin PB. Energy system interaction and relative contribution during maximal exercise. Sports Med 2001; 31: 725–741.

Hansen AK, Fischer CP, Plomgaard P, Andersen JL, Saltin B, Pedersen BK. Skeletal muscle adaptation: training twice every second day vs. training once daily. J Appl Physiol 2005; 98: 93–99.

Jentjens R, Jeukendrup A. Determinants of post-exercise glycogen synthesis during short-term recovery. Sports Med 2003; 33: 117–144.

McNaughton LR. Bicarbonate and citrate. In: Nutrition in Sport (Maughan RJ, ed.). Oxford: Blackwell Science, 2000, pp 393–404.

Matson LG, Tran ZV. Effects of sodium bicarbonate ingestion on anaerobic performance: a meta-analytic review. Int J Sport Nutr 1993; 3: 2–28.

Mettler S, Mitchell N, Tipton KD. Increased protein intake reduces lean body mass loss during weight loss in athletes. Med Sci Sports Exerc 2010; 42: 326–337.

Moore DR, Robinson MJ, Fry JL et al. Ingested protein dose response of muscle and albumin protein synthesis after resistance exercise in young men. Am J Clin Nutr 2009; 89: 161–168.

Stellingwerff T, Boit MK, Res P. Nutritional strategies to optimize training and racing in middle-distance athletes. J Sports Sci 2007; 25 (Suppl 1): S17–S28.

Tarnopolsky MA. Protein metabolism in strength and endurance activities. In: Perspectives in Exercise Science and Sports Medicine: The Metabolic Basis of Performance in Exercise and Sport (Lamb DR, Murray R, eds). Carmel, IN: Cooper Publishing Group, 1999, pp 125–164.

Tipton KD, Wolfe RR. Protein and amino acids for athletes. J Sports Sci 2004; 22: 65–79.

13
Nutrition for Endurance and Ultra-Endurance Training

Andrew Bosch and Karlien M Smit

Key messages

- Training for endurance and ultra-endurance events presents specific challenges for the athlete, e.g. high training load and short recovery periods. Low body fat levels may benefit performance and are often pursued obsessively by endurance athletes. However, severe restriction of energy intake and dietary variety can lead to fatigue, nutritional deficiencies, hormonal imbalances and disordered eating.
- Athletes participating in a daily training programme should aim to:
  - optimise repletion of muscle glycogen stores by consuming a diet high in carbohydrate;
  - optimise recovery by ingesting a carbohydrate and protein mixture soon after completion of training;
  - adapt dietary recommendations to individual goals, and responses to various strategies, which may involve adjusting timing, type and amount of carbohydrate ingestion before and during exercise.
- More research is needed on strategies such as fat loading to improve performance in endurance and ultra-endurance events. However, supplements such as carbohydrate gels and sports drinks containing carbohydrate offer enhanced performance during racing.

13.1 Introduction

With the increased popularity of participation in endurance and ultra-endurance events, there has been a growing interest and need for more research into the nutritional requirements of these sports, as well as a demand for information on products and supplements available on the market, that may be beneficial to the athlete.

Events in question range from endurance events (e.g. 42.2-km marathon races that elite athletes complete in just over 2 hours) to ultra-endurance (>4 hours), adventure racing and extreme events (e.g. mountain climbing) (Table 13.1). This chapter discusses the various nutritional challenges involved and provides evidence-based practical recommendations to support and optimise training for participation in these events.

13.2 Energy systems for endurance and ultra-endurance training and events

Endurance and ultra-endurance events continue for a number of hours. During such exercise, muscle glycogen is the main source of fuel for the first 90–120 min, together with blood glucose and fat from stores both from within the muscle as well as from elsewhere in the body. As exercise duration increases, the muscle glycogen stores become depleted and fat oxidation provides a higher relative proportion of the energy needs. While the fat supply is large and could fuel the body for days, the limitation lies in the rate at which energy can be released from fat. Thus, increasing muscle glycogen stores to the highest possible concentration prior to the commencement of endurance exercise, and the intake of exogenous sources of carbohydrate during such events, are critical for optimal performance.

Sport and Exercise Nutrition, First Edition. Edited by Susan A Lanham-New, Samantha J Stear, Susan M Shirreffs and Adam L Collins.
© 2011 The Nutrition Society. Published 2011 by Blackwell Publishing Ltd.

Table 13.1 Examples of endurance and ultra-endurance events.

Sport	Discipline	Examples of international events
Running	Road running (marathons and ultra-marathons)	New York marathon, Berlin marathon, Comrades ultra-marathon, London to Brighton ultra-marathon
	Trail running	
Cycling (single and multi-day events)	Mountain biking	Cape Epic
	Road cycling	Gira de Italia, Tour de France
Aquatic events	Open water long distance swimming	Rottness canal swim
	Canoeing/kayaking	Devizes–Westminster, Duzi marathon
	Open water sailing	Cape to Rio yacht race
Nordic skiing	Cross country ski-ing	Engadin Ski Marathon
Multidisciplinary	Biathlon, triathlon, pentathlon	Ironman, 70.3, Olympic, Sprint triathlons
Extreme and adventure events	Running, cycling, hiking	Augrabies extreme marathon, Pikes Peak marathon

The energy demand of daily training for endurance and ultra-endurance events can, in itself, be demanding, from the point of view of providing sufficient energy. Specifically, the muscle glycogen reserves can become depleted after successive days of heavy training if appropriate attention is not given to dietary carbohydrate intake.

13.3 Common nutritional issues and challenges

Training for endurance and ultra-endurance events can lead to various nutritional issues and challenges.

Challenges regarding physique and health issues

In many endurance sports, achieving low body fat and weight enhances performance, as it improves the power-to-weight relationship. This can result in the following.

- Risk of disordered eating.
- Menstrual disturbances in females.
- Vitamin and mineral deficiency, e.g. iron deficiency in certain at-risk groups such as those on a restricted energy intake and vegetarians.
- Decreased immune function after prolonged exercise.

Challenges regarding training load

- Maintaining high carbohydrate and energy requirements to meet heavy training demands.
- Strategies to cope with short recovery periods between training sessions, e.g. optimising recovery

- Provision of adequate fuel and fluid intake during training sessions, including practice of race-day situations.
- Achieving appropriate carbohydrate, protein and micronutrient intake, when energy intake is restricted, to achieve body composition goals.
- Gastrointestinal disturbances and discomfort during prolonged or high-intensity running sessions.

13.4 Nutritional strategies to optimise endurance or ultra-endurance training

Carbohydrate loading

Carbohydrate loading is a dietary technique used prior to an endurance race to enhance performance. To achieve carbohydrate loading, high-carbohydrate foods or drinks, or both, are ingested on the days before an event to increase the stores of carbohydrate (muscle glycogen) in the muscles.

The carbohydrate-loading diet was first popularised in the late 1960s after it had been found by researchers at that time, particularly Ahlborg *et al.* (1967) and Bergstrom *et al.* (1967), that muscle glycogen stores could be increased by ingesting a high (70%) carbohydrate diet for 3 days or more, subsequent to depletion of the muscle glycogen stores. Specifically, glycogen depletion was achieved by a prolonged bout of exercise and by subsequently ingesting a diet low in carbohydrate for a number of days. Muscle glycogen concentrations in some of the initial studies were as low as 35 mmol/kg w.w. muscle after such an exercise bout followed by 3 days of a low-carbohydrate diet. With these low muscle glycogen concentrations at the start of exercise, the average exercise time before exhaustion was only 57 min. After ingestion of a high-carbohydrate diet (~600 g of carbohydrate daily) for a number of days, average muscle glycogen concentrations increased to 184 mmol/kg w.w. and exercise time increased to 167 min before exhaustion occurred.

Importantly, the original research was done with relatively untrained people participating in the experiments. It was later demonstrated that the depletion phase, consisting of a prolonged bout of exercise followed by a low-carbohydrate diet for a number of days, is unnecessary in trained athletes. Specifically, it was found that trained people need only to eat a high-carbohydrate diet for 3 days (500–600 g of carbohydrate daily, or 7–10 g/kg/day) which, combined with a reduction in training, results in similar glycogen concentrations as when the original loading regimen is followed. The reason for the difference between trained and untrained people lies in an enzyme involved in the storage of muscle glycogen – glycogen synthase – which is activated in untrained individuals by the depletion phase of the carbohydrate-loading regimen. In trained people, this enzyme is already maximally activated as a result of daily training partially depleting the muscle glycogen reserves each day. No further activation occurs following a period of low carbohydrate intake and thus the depletion phase is unnecessary in people who regularly engage in prolonged training.

More recently, it has been shown that in highly trained athletes even 3 days of carbohydrate loading is longer than needed to maximise muscle glycogen stores. By ingesting 10 g/kg/day of carbohydrate, maximal muscle glycogen concentrations can be attained within just 24–36 hours in trained athletes. Thus it is clear that the muscle of trained individuals has the capacity to rapidly synthesise glycogen, when carbohydrate intake is high and training load is reduced.

As early as 1980, however, it was well established that performance was enhanced by high muscle glycogen concentrations and impaired by low muscle glycogen concentration, that training could substantially lower muscle glycogen, but that a high-carbohydrate diet could rapidly raise muscle glycogen concentration to optimal levels. Thus, Costill and Miller (1980) speculated that endurance athletes

could become progressively muscle glycogen depleted over successive days of hard training, but that this could conceivably be reversed if a high-carbohydrate diet was ingested each day. This led to a study by Costill et al. (1981) which indeed showed that muscle glycogen could effectively be replenished after each day of training, provided that sufficient carbohydrate was ingested. Specifically, runners in the study ingested a low-carbohydrate diet, a mixed diet or a high-carbohydrate diet after exercise, which consisted of a 16.1-km run at 80% Vo_{2max}, followed immediately by five 1-min sprint runs, with a 3-min rest interval between each. This protocol effectively lowered muscle glycogen stores (55 mmol/kg w.w.), incurring the same results as would a hard training session. When the high-carbohydrate diet was ingested (648 g in 24 hours), muscle glycogen concentrations were measured at a normal resting level for trained runners, e.g. approximately 130 mmol/kg w.w. 24 hours after the previous training session. This was not achieved in the case of the low-carbohydrate and mixed diets. Thus, the high carbohydrate consumption successfully restored muscle glycogen within 24 hours of strenuous training, where muscle glycogen stores had been substantially reduced. Although there was no improvement in a subsequent performance trial, the runners with high muscle glycogen content had a lower rating of perceived exertion (RPE) than runners with low muscle glycogen concentration. Although improvement over such a short distance might not be expected as a result of higher starting muscle glycogen concentration, this is an important observation in light of the findings in a later experiment by Sherman et al. (1981). This study found that while runners and cyclists who ingested carbohydrate 10 g/kg/day during a period of 7 days of hard training maintained muscle glycogen concentrations, neither training capacity nor exercise performance was affected in those cyclists and runners who did not ingest a high-carbohydrate diet and had lower muscle glycogen stores. This therefore raised the question as to whether the ingestion of a high-carbohydrate diet had any importance in maintaining high muscle glycogen concentrations. However, RPE had not been measured in this study, but was based on the results of the study by Costill et al. (1981); it is conceivable that the RPE would have been lower in those runners and cyclists who had higher muscle glycogen concentrations.

Glycaemic index of carbohydrate for optimising muscle glycogen storage

Various studies have been conducted to determine whether the glycaemic index of the carbohydrate used, when attempting to optimise muscle glycogen stores, has any effect on the rate of muscle glycogen re-synthesis. Although Chen *et al.* (2008) showed that carbohydrate loading with high glycaemic index carbohydrate foods did not result in superior performance compared with low glycaemic index foods in a 10-km run preceded by a 1-hour run at 70% Vo_{2max}, it cannot be assumed that the high glycaemic index foods did not result in higher initial muscle glycogen concentrations due to the fact that muscle glycogen concentration was not measured in the study and that the total exercise performed was probably not long or severe enough to deplete muscle glycogen stores.. Indeed, a number of other studies have shown the contrary: improved muscle glycogen storage when the carbohydrate ingested has been of a high glycaemic index. Importantly, it should be noted that the participants referred to in the previous study, where it was shown that maximal muscle glycogen stores could be attained within 24 hours of ingesting a high-carbohydrate diet, had ingested high glycaemic index carbohydrates. Nevertheless, the effect of glycaemic index on rate of muscle glycogen storage needs further research. Nevertheless, there appears to be sufficient evidence to justify inclusion of at least some high glycaemic index carbohydrates as part of the carbohydrate intake when attempting to optimise the rate of muscle glycogen synthesis.

Types of carbohydrate for optimal muscle glycogen restoration

Besides consideration of the glycaemic index of the carbohydrate foods used, when attempting to optimise the rate of muscle glycogen synthesis by carbohydrate loading, any high-carbohydrate low-fat food or drink can be used as part of a high-carbohydrate diet. The same applies to the specific case of rapid restoration of muscle glycogen in daily training. Among suitable food items are bread, rice, pasta and potatoes. Potatoes have a high glycaemic index, making them an ideal food type to include in a diet aimed at rapidly restoring muscle glycogen used in daily training, as this would take advantage of the apparently higher muscle glycogen concentrations achieved from ingestion of high glycaemic index foods.

Effect of carbohydrate on cortisol concentrations

While carbohydrate ingestion has been promoted as an important post-exercise recovery food to restore muscle glycogen, less well known is its potential effect on reducing post-exercise cortisol concentrations. This was shown by Bird *et al.* (2006), although these findings have not been consistently reported. A reduction in post-exercise cortisol concentration would be beneficial, as high cortisol concentrations have been postulated to have a catabolic effect on muscle, as discussed under the later section on protein supplementation and enhanced recovery.

High-carbohydrate diet to support daily training: summary

In addition to specific carbohydrate loading prior to endurance events, athletes should aim to have a high carbohydrate intake as part of their normal diet in order to meet the fuel requirements of their training programme and to optimise restoration of muscle glycogen stores between workouts (Table 13.2). This helps to replenish glycogen stores from one day of training to the next, so that training intensity can be optimised. To achieve this, nutrient-rich carbohydrate foods should be chosen and added to other foods in order to provide a good source of protein and other nutrients, such as minerals and vitamins. These nutrients may assist in the overall recovery processes from training and, in the case of protein, may promote additional glycogen restoration, when carbohydrate intake is suboptimal. Table 13.2 indicates appropriate amounts of carbohydrate to be ingested under different conditions and also provides a general target that must be fine-tuned according to the athlete's nutritional goals and feedback. Poor training performance, unexpected fatigue, frequent illness, or failure to achieve expected outcomes from a specific training session may be indirect signs that the athlete's carbohydrate intake is inadequate. These recommendations may not be feasible for athletes (mainly females) whose focus on low body mass and body fat levels requires moderate energy restriction and therefore a lower carbohydrate intake. This may be solved by periodising nutritional goals and carbohydrate intake. For example, lower carbohydrate intake to optimise weight loss may be the priority for out-of-competition training periods, whereas

Table 13.2 Carbohydrate requirements during endurance and ultra-endurance training.

Training condition	Recommended carbohydrate intake
Daily refuelling requirements for training programmes < 60–90 min per day or low-intensity exercise	Daily intake of 5–7 g/kg
Daily refuelling for training programmes > 90–120 min per day	Daily intake of 7–10 g/kg
Carbohydrate loading for endurance and ultra-endurance events	Daily intake of 7–10 g/kg
Carbohydrate intake during training sessions and competition events greater than 1 hour	1 g/min or 45–60 g/hour
Rapid recovery after training session or multi-day competition, especially when there is less than 8 hours until next session	Intake of 1–1.5 g/kg every hour in the early stages of recovery after exercise, contributing to a total intake of 6–10 g/kg over 24 hours

Table 13.3 Practical ways to increase carbohydrate intake.

- Increase the number of meals and snacks throughout the day. Plan ahead so that snacks are always available during the day
- Make carbohydrate-rich foods the basis of each meal and snack, e.g. bread, pasta, couscous, noodles, potato, rice, crackers, fruit
- Time your intake around training. Include a recovery snack containing carbohydrate shortly after the training session and, in addition, have a meal approximately an hour later
- Reduce foods that are high volume and may be limiting your appetite. This may mean replacing some wholegrain foods with lower fibre alternatives. Dried fruit or puréed fruit can be added to cereal and porridges
- Include carbohydrate/energy-rich fluids. Ensure that all fluids contribute energy (replace diet drinks and large volumes of water with sports drinks, juices, fruit smoothies or low-fat dairy drinks)
- Include condiments, e.g. jam, honey and sugar, to increase energy intake without adding volume

carbohydrate intake should be increased during competition preparation and during recovery to optimise glycogen stores.

Table 13.3 suggests practical ways to meet these suggested high carbohydrate requirements.

Individualising carbohydrate ingestion

While an argument has been presented that post-training ingestion of carbohydrate may optimise recovery and that ingestion of large amounts of carbohydrate, on a daily basis and as part of a high-carbohydrate diet, will enhance muscle glycogen re-synthesis, there are certain circumstances where this recommendation may not be optimal. For someone who is particularly interested in optimising fat loss rather than performance, ingesting such large amounts of carbohydrate may be contraindicated. Similarly, ingestion of carbohydrate or a small high-carbohydrate breakfast 2–3 hours prior to training

may be indicated for someone with a high training regimen, such as a cyclist, who may spend many hours on the bike, or a triathlete, who may spend a number of hours training on the bike to be followed later in the day by a run and/or swim session. Such athletes may not have sufficient time to adequately replace carbohydrate, unless pre-training carbohydrate is ingested, as well as carbohydrate during the training session. On the other hand, such a regimen may not enhance metabolic adaptation to fat burning. Many runners, for example, typically start their morning training session in an overnight fasted state, which would ensure metabolic adaptation to optimise fat oxidation. This may not be too dissimilar to the current experimental condition referred to as 'train low, compete high', in which athletes deliberately train in a carbohydrate-depleted state with a view to enhancing fat oxidation. However, such runners would be advised that on at least some occasions they should follow the regimen they would utilise on race day, e.g. to have a small breakfast some hours before training and to ingest carbohydrate during the session, so as to determine any adverse effects (see Table 13.4 for carbohydrate options to ingest during training).

Each type of endurance and ultra-endurance discipline will present a unique set of nutritional challenges, with regard to rehydrating and refuelling, during training. This is due to a wide range of variables, such as environment (e.g. hot and humid temperatures versus cold/freezing temperatures), intensity, length and type of exercise, availability of additional aids (e.g. shops) en route, as well as type of clothing and gear (e.g. the availability of pockets, hydration bladders, bags and bottle cages on bikes). Since individual taste preferences vary and change

Table 13.4 Carbohydrate-dense options containing 45–60 g of carbohydrates per portion (during exercise).

600–800 ml commercial carbohydrate drink (6–8% carbohydrate)

500 ml soft drink (10% carbohydrate, e.g. Coke)

300–400 ml of carbohydrate drink + 1 energy or breakfast bar (~30 g of carbohydrate)

300–400 ml of carbohydrate drink + 1 large banana

300–400 ml carbohydrate drink + 4–5 gums or jelly sweets (gelatine-based chewy candy)

300–400 ml carbohydrate drink + 1 carbohydrate gel sachet (~20 g of carbohydrate)

300–400 ml carbohydrate drink + ~50 g chocolate bar or 30 g nougat

250 ml soft drink + 3–4 baby potatoes

250 ml soft drink + 1 sandwich (2 slices bread) or roll

If only drinking water

1 carbohydrate gel (~20 g carbohydrate) + 1 energy or breakfast bar (~30 g of carbohydrate)

3 baby boiled potatoes + 1 carbohydrate gel (~20 g)

4–5 jelly sweets + 1 large banana

Medium muffin (~120 g) or 2 slices fruit cake

Table 13.5 Examples of a pre-exercise meal/snack options.

A	Cup of oats or cereal with low-fat milk or yoghurt (sugar or honey optional)
B	Crumpets or pancakes drizzled with honey and yoghurt and served with fruit salad
C	Couple of slices of toast with scrambled egg and a glass of fruit juice
D	Liquid meal replacement containing at least 30 g of carbohydrate[a]
E	A sports bar (low fibre and low fat) + a cup of fruit juice or energy drink[a]

[a] Good choices for those who cannot tolerate solid food or have a low appetite.

during prolonged exercise, it is important to experiment with different flavours of carbohydrate drinks and food options.

If a small breakfast is to be ingested prior to a race, it is important that the athlete experiments with the time at which the breakfast is ingested (see Table 13.5 for examples of pre-exercise meals and snacks). Although some studies have shown no ill effect as a result of ingesting carbohydrate a short while before the start of exercise, others have shown a resultant reactive hypoglycaemia. Free fatty acids, too, may be suppressed for some time following a carbohydrate-containing breakfast, and it is highly probable that fatty acid oxidation may be impaired as a result, which would increase the reliance on muscle glycogen utilisation as a fuel substrate.

A pre-exercise meal should contain sufficient fluid to maintain hydration, be relatively low in fat and fibre to facilitate gastric emptying and minimise gastrointestinal distress, be high in carbohydrate to maintain blood glucose and maximise glycogen stores, contain a moderate amount of protein, and be familiar to the athlete. The size and timing of the pre-exercise meal are interrelated. Accounting for gastric emptying, smaller meals can be consumed in closer proximity to the event than larger meals, which should be consumed only when more time is available before exercise or

competition. Amounts of carbohydrate that have been shown to enhance performance have ranged from approximately 200 to 300 g for meals consumed 3–4 hours before exercise. Data are equivocal about whether the glycaemic index of carbohydrate in such pre-exercise meals affects performance.

Protein requirements during training

Protein is a key nutritional component for those involved in endurance training, although the nature of that importance is still not unquestionably proven. Evidence suggests that endurance athletes need more protein than the Recommended Dietary Allowance. However, research into the efficacy of increased protein or amino acid intake, as well as optimal daily requirements of elite athletes, has yet to be determined. Nevertheless, current recommendations for daily protein intake during hard endurance training are 1.2–1.7 g/kg/day, with the higher value during periods of increased training load. Thus, these targets for protein intake must take into account the individual's requirements, goals and training programme.

Generally, protein requirements can easily be met through a healthy balanced diet. Adding lean protein (e.g. skinless chicken, fish, lean meat, legumes, eggs, low-fat dairy) to meals and snacks will ensure that optimal protein intake is achieved. Skimmed milk powder can also be used to enrich milk, porridges and soups. Examples of foods containing 10 g of protein are:

- 40–50 g lean meat, skinless chicken *or* fish *or* low-fat cheese *or* nuts (high in fat and should be limited if calorie intake is to be limited);
- 2 eggs;

- 300 ml low-fat milk/yoghurt;
- ½ to ¾ cup dried beans, lentils or split peas.

It is important that protein intake does not replace carbohydrate intake. There appears to be no reason for protein intakes to be above 2 g/kg/day in endurance athletes.

Effect of protein ingestion on protein synthesis activation, exercise performance and post-exercise recovery

One of the challenges in sports nutrition is optimising performance, and recovery after exercise. While restoration of muscle glycogen concentration may be important in this regard, ingestion of protein or protein hydrolysates, particularly those containing the branched-chain amino acid (BCAA) leucine, may further improve performance or the rate of recovery, or both. There is some research evidence, such as that of Elliot *et al.* (2006), which suggests that whole milk can also increase muscle protein synthesis and increase strength gains, a role traditionally ascribed to whole protein isolates.

In addition, various studies have shown that both protein and protein hydrolysate, ingested together with carbohydrate are effective in increasing the rate of muscle glycogen re-synthesis under certain circumstances, such as when carbohydrate intake alone is not high enough. Whey, casein and soy protein, and to a lesser degree protein hydrolysate, are supplemental protein sources often used by athletes. More studies are appearing in literature showing an increase in protein synthesis following ingestion of such proteins, thus providing a potential mechanism for improved recovery.

Effect on insulin concentration

The co-ingestion of protein, or protein hydrolysate, and carbohydrate has been shown to increase plasma insulin concentrations (van Loon *et al.*, 2000a; Bird *et al.*, 2006). This is potentially important, as in addition to stimulating the uptake of glucose by skeletal muscle, insulin is also known to increase glycogen synthase activity and, in this way, the rate of muscle glycogen re-synthesis may be accelerated in a post-exercise environment. Indeed, higher glycogen synthesis rates have been demonstrated following the addition of intact protein, protein hydrolysate, free leucine and free phenylalanine to carbohydrate recovery drinks

(van Loon *et al.*, 2000b). However, this appears to be primarily when carbohydrate ingestion is suboptimal.

Effect on cortisol concentration

Ingestion of carbohydrate and amino acids causes a reduction in cortisol concentration during exercise (Bird *et al.*, 2006). Such an effect is desirable as in addition to inducing breakdown of proteins, glucocorticoids such as cortisol have been shown to prevent the (desirable) BCAA-induced anabolic shift in protein balance and inhibit their action on the phosphorylation of proteins in the pathway, leading to increased muscle protein synthesis (Bird *et al.*, 2006). Therefore a reduction in the plasma cortisol response may simultaneously lessen the catabolic effect typically observed during prolonged exercise and allow greater potential for leucine-stimulated protein synthesis.

Effect on protein synthesis

There is a growing body of evidence that certain proteins, protein hydrolysate and BCAAs all exert an anabolic effect on protein metabolism. Leucine, in particular, has been shown to promote protein synthesis via activation of the mammalian target of rapamycin (mTOR), p70 S6 kinase and the eukaryotic initiation factor 4E-binding protein-1 pathways. This cascade of phosphorylation has the potential to cause an increase in protein synthesis, and indeed this has been confirmed in studies using tracer techniques. Increases in protein synthesis following protein ingestion have been shown in a number of studies (Beelen *et al.*, 2008), in which increased rates of synthesis were shown after the ingestion of protein hydrolysate. Interestingly, Elliot *et al.* (2006) have reported increased muscle protein synthesis rates in resistance-trained study participants when milk was ingested as a protein source. It is noteworthy that this is not the only study which has shown a positive effect following ingestion of milk, particularly chocolate-flavoured milk (which has a higher carbohydrate content).

Ingestion of protein before exercise

One example of the potential net anabolic effect of BCAA ingestion was provided by, amongst others, Shimomura *et al.* (2006) who reported a reduction in delayed-onset muscle soreness and enhanced recovery following ingestion of 5 g of BCAAs before exercise. The authors postulated that BCAAs may attenuate exercise-induced protein catabolism, and that leucine may stimulate muscle protein synthesis, resulting in the observed reduction in delayed-onset muscle soreness. It should be noted, however, that although BCAAs may stimulate protein synthesis, the other amino acids are also needed to complete the process of protein synthesis, thereby making the case that the optimal option is the ingestion of complete protein or protein hydrolysate rather than single amino acids or BCAAs.

Ingestion of protein during exercise

Ivy et al. (2003) were among the first to show an improvement in cycling time to fatigue when protein (whey) was ingested during exercise. More recently, Saunders et al. (2009) showed an improvement in cycling time trial performance, late in exercise, when protein hydrolysate was ingested during a prolonged (60-km) ride.

Enhanced performance, as shown by Ivy et al., may be due to reduced muscle damage. Studies by Luden et al. (2007), Romano-Ely et al. (2006) and Saunders et al. (2004, 2007) are amongst those that have shown reduced creatine kinase concentrations (a marker of muscle damage) in cyclists, runners and football players after ingestion of a mixture of carbohydrate and protein.

Ingestion of protein after exercise

Numerous studies in the scientific literature have investigated the effect of both protein and protein hydrolysate ingestion on post-exercise recovery. The majority of studies have shown a positive effect, especially with regard to the reduction in delayed-onset muscle soreness. Although not a study on endurance exercise, Buckley et al. (2010) showed an intriguing effect in a comparison of different protein types (whey and casein), and protein hydrolysate, when ingested after muscle-damaging exercise. After first measuring force output on an isokinetic ergometer, muscle damage was then induced in the study participants, after which the different protein types were ingested. Interestingly, the most rapid return to initial muscle force output occurred in the group who had ingested protein hydrolysate.

Conflicting scientific evidence

Despite many studies that have shown a positive effect as a result of ingestion of protein, findings from research studies have not been consistent, with a significant number showing no positive effect. This may be partly attributed to the number of variables involved. Specifically, protein can be ingested prior to training, during training or after training; the protein can be in the form of whey, casein, soy or protein hydrolysate; the type of exercise can be running, cycling or resistance training; and the level of athlete participating in the studies vary from untrained, moderately trained to highly trained. Finally, the assessment of efficacy has itself varied from time trial, time to fatigue, indicators of enhanced recovery, to measures of muscle damage. All these factors have the potential to explain conflicting results in experiments. For example, two apparently identical studies may obtain different results depending on whether the participants are trained or untrained, or whether the performance measure used is a time trial or time to fatigue.

Conclusion: carbohydrate and protein ingestion to optimise training

Despite the growing body of research data, definitive answers nevertheless remain elusive, with some studies showing a positive effect on performance or recovery, or both, as a consequence of protein or protein hydrolysate ingestion prior to, during or after exercise, while others have not.

It is currently unclear whether proteins from different sources may induce different degrees of anabolic response in muscle protein synthesis after training. Nevertheless, ingestion of a protein hydrolysate, whole milk or whey protein isolate together with carbohydrate after prolonged exercise potentially offers a threefold effect for enhanced recovery.

(1) A reduction in cortisol concentration and concomitant reduction in the associated catabolic effect.
(2) An increased rate of post-exercise muscle glycogen synthesis, possibly mediated via the higher insulin concentrations when carbohydrate and protein are co-ingested.
(3) Stimulation of muscle protein synthesis via the mTOR and related pathways, leading to downstream enhanced muscle protein synthesis and thereby improving rate of recovery.

Collectively, it appears that studies where protein hydrolysate, rather than whole protein, has been ingested have more consistently resulted in a positive outcome. Nevertheless, endurance athletes may have

Table 13.6 Recovery snacks.

250–350 ml carbohydrate energy drink + 250 ml liquid meal
   supplement (containing >10 g of protein per serving)
250–350 ml smoothie (made with fruit, low-fat yoghurt plus honey)
250–350 ml milkshake or flavoured milk drink
250 ml fat-free/low-fat fruit yoghurt or 350 ml drinking yoghurt
Sandwich with lean protein filling (e.g. reduced fat cheese/egg/
   chicken) + 1 fruit
1½ cups of cereal with low-fat/fat-free milk
1 high protein bar (>10 g protein) with a cup of fruit juice
500–750 ml carbohydrate energy drink or cold drink or fruit juice +
   protein hydrolysate providing ~10 g of protein

an improved rate of recovery by ingesting either protein hydrolysate or another protein supplement, together with carbohydrate, soon (within 1 hour) after completion of training. Many studies have utilised 0.8 g/kg of carbohydrate ingested with 0.2–0.4 g/kg of protein or protein hydrolysate. Alternatively, there have been a number of studies, such as that of Elliot *et al.* (2006), which have shown positive effects when chocolate-flavoured milk has been ingested after exercise. In addition to specific post-exercise beverages containing protein and carbohydrate, other types of protein-containing snacks may also be ingested. Table 13.6 provides examples of post-exercise 'recovery' snacks providing about 50 g of carbohydrate plus more than 10 g of protein.

13.5 Achieving low body fat mass (Table 13.7)

Achieving low body fat is an important goal for endurance athletes. However, the pursuit of an extremely low body fat mass can potentially increase the risk of a variety of problems related to the athlete's current and long-term health, performance and psychological well-being. This is discussed in more detail elsewhere.

Adopting a balanced long-term weight loss strategy is crucial for the endurance athlete wanting to lower body fat and weight. If large losses are needed, this should be planned well in advance, preferably during the 'off-season' and not close to important events. The main aim of dietary intervention is to promote a moderate energy deficit whilst maintaining adequate intakes of nutrient-dense carbohydrate, lean protein and essential micronutrients to maintain optimal

performance and health. Consulting with a registered sports dietitian may be helpful in developing a practical and individualised plan.

Sensible weight loss goals in athletes are about 0.5–1 kg body fat per week; this can be related to a maximum of around a 5-mm reduction in total skinfolds per week over seven or eight sites, achieved by an energy deficit of around 500–1000 kcal/day. Such a daily energy deficit can be achieved by making changes to existing eating habits, following a prescribed quantified eating plan, increasing energy expenditure, or a combination of these strategies. For any weight management plan to be successful, it needs to be sustainable. The eating plan therefore needs to be practical and easy to follow in all situations: at home, travelling and when eating out.

It is generally recommended that for females, energy intake should not be lower than 30–35 kcal/day per kilogram fat-free mass plus the energy cost of training. Care should be taken with low-calorie eating plans (<1500 kcal or 6300 kJ/day) due to the risk of insufficient micronutrients. Very low energy diets that provide 1600–2400 kJ (400–600 kcal) and less than 100 g of carbohydrate per day are not recommended for athletes and include side effects such as dehydration, glycogen depletion, nausea, headaches, light-headedness and loss of lean body mass.

Carbohydrate intake at 3–5 g/kg for light and moderate training is recommended, increasing to 6–8 g/kg during heavy training. During this time, it is important to give priority to nutrient-dense carbohydrates (e.g. wholegrain cereals, porridges, breads, rice, pasta, potatoes and starchy vegetables, fruit and low-fat dairy products) rather than energy-dense carbohydrates (e.g. cold drinks, sports drinks, energy bars, sugar, jam, sweets).

Protein recommendations range from 1.4 to 1.7 g/kg, aiming for the upper level if there is a substantial energy restriction. This may assist in the maintenance of lean body mass and helps promote satiety at meal times.

Fat is needed for insulation and protection, as well as for fat-soluble vitamins and essential fatty acids and should therefore not be totally excluded from the diet. However, it is energy dense (1 g = 9 kcal/38 kJ) and should therefore be limited to 1–1.5 g/kg/day (<30% of total energy intake) (see Chapter 17 for further information on weight management).

Table 13.7 Practical dietary strategies to lower body fat.

Plan ahead

Plan regular meals and snacks in advance to encourage healthy eating habits

Use meals (e.g. breakfast or dinner) as a post-recovery meal instead of adding additional calories in the form of an additional snack or meal

Manage appropriate portion sizes

Eat regularly: this helps to keep blood sugar levels stable and helps to prevent over-compensation at meal times or snacking on 'unhealthy' food

Educate yourself on ideal portion sizes. Buy pre-portioned snacks to prevent over-eating

Keep unhealthy foods and snacks out of sight. If they are visible, consumption is more likely

Once food is plated, store leftovers in plastic containers out of sight. If desirable, ask someone to portion the food

Increase your fibre intake by choosing whole wheat grains, breads and cereals, legumes and bulking up on 'free vegetables', e.g. lettuce, cucumber, tomato, broccoli, cauliflower, peppers. This adds volume to meals, providing a feeling of fullness, without adding too many calories

Include lower glycaemic index carbohydrates, e.g. sweet potato instead of regular potato, for a fuller stomach for longer

Eat mixed meals (combining protein and a small amount of fat with meals)

Eat slowly: try putting knife and fork down between mouthfuls

Ensure portion sizes are reduced appropriately when tapering training

Keep fat intake in check

Choose healthier cooking methods, e.g. baking, steaming, grilling, and boiling. Avoid food that has been fried, deep-fried or grilled in a lot of butter/oil

Change to low-fat or fat-free (skimmed) dairy products

Adapt recipes and use reduced-fat ingredients, e.g. low fat evaporated milk/yoghurt instead of cream

Choose low-fat sauces, e.g. tomato-based sauces instead of mayonnaise-based sauces and dressings

Choose lean protein sources. Trim the visible fat off meat and remove the skin of chicken before cooking

Choose snacks with <5 g of fat per 30 g of carbohydrate

Limit calorie-dense foods and drinks

Drink mainly water to satisfy fluid requirements

Dilute fruit juices and cordials with water

Limit refined carbohydrate, e.g. soft drinks, sports drinks, gels or sweets for training purposes only

Limit alcohol to 1 unit (females) to 2 units (males) per occasion. Stretch alcohol intake by adding ice, water or soda to drinks, e.g. spritzers or choose light alcoholic options

Manage social activities

Choose restaurants that provide healthier options

Order smaller options, e.g. order half portions or two starters as a main meal

Start meals with a salad or a non-creamy soup

Make healthier choices by avoiding creamy foods and order dressing on the side

Optimising fat burning after training

Fat burning can be increased by avoiding food/drink for up to 90 min after exercise, as this takes maximal advantage of the increase in metabolic rate after exercise. Unfortunately this will decrease post-exercise recovery rate

13.6 Nutrition to enhance immunity

There is strong evidence that there is depression of the immune system (especially after acute high-intensity exercise) lasting from 3 to 72 hours after training (depending on how immune function is measured). During this time, there is an increased risk of contracting minor illnesses or infections, the most common being upper respiratory tract infections (URTIs). This may cause interruptions to training or under-performance in competition. Post-exercise immune depression seems to be most pronounced after continuous, prolonged (>90 min)

exercise at moderate to high intensity (55–75% Vo_{2peak}), especially when no food (carbohydrate) is ingested after exercise.

The athletes at risk of nutrition-related immune system disturbances include:

- those restricting their energy intake or following weight-loss diets;
- those with restricted intake (e.g. vegan);
- those consuming large quantities of supplements and therefore displacing micronutrient intake;
- those with poor nutritional practices or unbalanced diets (e.g. fat exclusion diets).

Table 13.8 Potential nutritional strategies to support the immune system.

Nutritional strategy	Mechanism
Sufficient energy and protein intake	Although extreme malnutrition in athletes is unlikely, moderate protein deficiency causes some impairment of host defence mechanisms
	Protein and/or energy malnutrition is often accompanied by deficiencies in micronutrients
Sufficient carbohydrate intake	Sufficient carbohydrate intake decreases the cortisol concentration, resulting in fewer disturbances in blood immune cell counts
Sufficient fat intake	Fat intake of <15% of total energy is not recommended due to the loss of micronutrients
	The ω-3 fatty acids might play a beneficial role because they counteract the production of prostaglandin hormones and subsequent suppression of the cellular immune system
Appropriate vitamins and minerals	Deficiencies of vitamins (e.g. A, E, B_6, B_{12}, C) and minerals (iron, zinc, magnesium, selenium, copper, manganese) have been shown to impair immune function and decrease the body's resistance to infection
	Isolated deficiencies of magnesium, manganese, selenium and copper are rare
	Excessive intakes of iron, zinc and vitamin E can impair immune function
Ingest carbohydrates during exercise	Evidence suggests that carbohydrate intake during marathon running may decrease the incidence of post-marathon URTIs
Prevent excessive dehydration during exercise	Dehydration will elevate catecholamines and cortisol which can lead to immunosuppression
	Fluid replacement improves saliva flow rate during exercise, thus maintaining the supply of several proteins (e.g. IgA, lysozyme) that have microbial properties

Table 13.9 General recommendations to decrease risk of illness in athletes.

Keep life stresses to a minimum
Avoid over-training and chronic fatigue
Ensure enough sleep and a consistent sleep pattern
Eat a well-balanced diet to avoid deficiencies and ensure adequate intake of carbohydrate, protein, fluid and micronutrients (especially iron, zinc, and vitamins B_6, B_{12}, C and E)
Avoid a dry mouth, both during training and at rest
Before important race events, avoid sick people and large crowds whenever possible
Ensure adequate carbohydrate intake (45–60 g/hour) during prolonged (>90 min) or high-intensity exercise sessions
Take a broad-range multivitamin and mineral supplement to support a restricted intake, such as during weight loss regimens, when travelling, or when availability or variety of fresh fruit and vegetables is limited
Possibly supplement with probiotics when travelling; iron supplements should not be taken during periods of infection
Practice good hygienic principles, e.g. wash hands regularly, do not share water bottles, cutlery and towels. Clean bottles and hydration packs well after each use
Avoid rapid weight loss (has been related to adverse immune changes)

Some nutritional strategies that have been shown to help maintain an effective immune system are provided in Table 13.8 and further information can be found in Chapter 21.

Furthermore, there has been research on immune-enhancing supplements in athletes, for example zinc, ω-3 fatty acids, plant sterols, antioxidants (e.g. vitamins C and E, β-carotene, N-acetylcysteine and butylated hydroxyanisole), glutamine, bovine colostrum, and carbohydrate. More recent studies have included quercetin, isoquercetin, epigallocatechin 3-gallate (EGCG), β-glucan, and other plant polyphenols. Such studies have shown that there may be a decreased incidence of URTIs when taking these supplements (see Chapter 21 for further information). Table 13.9 lists general recommendations for decreasing the risk of illness in athletes.

Antioxidant supplements

Acute physical exercise induces reactive oxygen species (ROS) in the muscle and in other organs, causing damage to the cell and mitochondrial cell membrane, deterioration of the immune system, ageing, cancer and atherosclerosis. It has been generally accepted that increasing the concentrations of antioxidants within a muscle cell should provide greater protection against these oxidising agents and should therefore reduce fatigue. However, the functional significance of exercise-induced oxidative stress is open to discussion. Specifically, results from several studies indicate that ROS are signal molecules that serve to upregulate the expression of a number of genes. Thus, ROS can exert favourable effects and can be involved in the process of training adaptation.

It seems that antioxidant supplementation may decrease training efficiency because it prevents optimal cellular adaptations to exercise. In addition, there is evidence to show that antioxidants may minimise the health benefits of exercise, such as loss of the exercise-induced decrease in insulin resistance.

13.7 Gastrointestinal problems

Gastrointestinal symptoms commonly observed in endurance athletes include bowel urgency, stomach cramps, diarrhoea, heartburn and nausea. Various circumstances seem to play a role, for example the type of exercise, the intensity and duration of the training session or race, medication, hydration status, the type and volume of food consumed before and during exercise, as well as underlying medical conditions such as irritable bowel syndrome or inflammatory bowel disease.

Some recommended strategies include establishing a routine of emptying the bowel before physical activity, training and racing on an empty stomach, avoiding solid food, or following a low-fibre and low-residue diet before competition (see Chapter 20 for further information).

13.8 Iron deficiency

It is commonly believed that endurance athletes, particularly female endurance runners and vegetarians, have an increased risk of iron deficiency. This is supported by target levels for iron status measures, for example serum ferritin is often set well above the normal population standards to provide a margin of safety for athletes. An important risk factor is the low-energy or low-iron diet. Females, vegetarian eaters, and those following diets with restricted quantity and variety are at highest risk.

The true prevalence of iron-deficiency anaemia in endurance athletes is probably no greater than that in the general population. However, when a reduced iron status occurs, it may be problematic for performance or adaptation to training, particularly when training at altitude. The literature is unclear (mostly due to methodological concerns) as to whether iron depletion, in the absence of anaemia, actually impairs exercise performance.

Dietary interventions to reverse or prevent a decline in iron status involve strategies to increase total iron intake as well as to increase the bioavailability of iron. Self-medicating with iron supplements in the absence of a confirmed iron status may have negative side effects (e.g. haemosiderosis or iron overload) and is therefore strongly not advised (see Chapter 8 for more detailed information on iron).

13.9 Key supplements for endurance and ultra-endurance training/events (Table 13.10)

Broad-spectrum multivitamin and mineral supplement

- Offers support for those following a low-energy or weight-loss diet (<1900 kcal for females or 2300 kcal for males), with restricted variety or an unreliable food supply (e.g. when travelling).
- If no deficiency is present, it may not improve performance.

Single-nutrient supplements (e.g. calcium, vitamin B$_{12}$, iron)

- Will not correct poor diet.
- Recommended only if diet cannot supply the Dietary Reference Intakes (DRIs) or if a deficiency has been established.
- Calcium supplementation may be recommended for treating or preventing osteoporosis or bone stress injuries. However, calcium without adequate oestrogen/progesterone status cannot guarantee bone status improvement.
- Supplementation with certain vitamins or minerals may cause side effects, e.g. constipation.
- Excessive intakes of some vitamins may impair the absorption of other nutrients.
- Some vitamins at high intakes can be toxic.

Liquid meal replacements

- Are convenient and low in bulk and can be used for a pre-event meal, post-exercise recovery or to supplement a high-energy diet in situations where athletes lack appetite or suffer from gastrointestinal disturbances.
- Lactose-free options are available for those with lactose intolerance.
- Over-reliance may lead to displacement of whole foods.

Table 13.10 Key supplements for endurance and ultra-endurance training/events.

Product	Rationale for use	Concerns/side effects/safety
Broad-spectrum multivitamin and mineral supplement	Support for low-energy/fat loss diets (<1900 kcal for females or 2300 kcal for males) or restricted variety diets or unreliable food supply (e.g. travel)	If no deficiency exists, may not improve performance
Single-nutrient supplements (e.g. calcium, vitamin B_{12}, iron)	If diet cannot supply the DRIs or if deficiency has been established. To improve performance Calcium to treat or prevent osteoporosis or bone stress injuries	Will not correct poor diet. Excessive intakes of some vitamins may impair the absorption of other nutrients; some vitamins at high intakes can be toxic May cause side effects, e.g. constipation Calcium without adequate oestrogen/progesterone status cannot guarantee bone status improvement
Liquid meal replacements	Easily prepared meal replacement for lack of appetite or high energy requirements. Low bulk pre-event meals, post-exercise recovery and travel	Expensive Over-reliance may lead to displacement of whole foods Lactose-free options available for lactose intolerance
High-carbohydrate supplements, e.g. sports drinks, high-carbohydrate sports drinks, soda drinks, powders, sport bars, cereal or breakfast bars, sport gels	High-carbohydrate requirements, e.g. heavy training or carbohydrate loading, before, during and after exercise Lack of appetite Convenience	Overuse may lead to weight gain or disturb macronutrients
High-protein supplements, e.g. protein powders, protein hydrolysate, skimmed milk powder, higher protein sports bars	For athletes not able to meet protein requirements, e.g. vegetarians, or for athletes with additional protein requirements, e.g. growth spurt To add to carbohydrate sources for recovery Skimmed milk powder is economical and ideal for fortifying food and drink for recovery or lack of appetite	Expensive May inappropriately displace whole foods or carbohydrate Protein overload may lead to excess body fat storage
Prebiotics and probiotics	Immune and gut benefits (e.g. for athletes with traveller's diarrhoea or IBS or in those taking antibiotics)	Immune benefits not confirmed
Caffeine	Caffeine ingestion prior to exercise may have performance-enhancing effects in endurance athletes, by possibly decreasing perception of effort and fatigue and increasing utilisation of free fatty acids during exercise. New evidence show maximal benefits of caffeine at small to moderate doses (1–3 mg/kg) Foods and drinks that may contain caffeine include coffee, tea, soft drinks, chocolate, energy drinks, sport supplements and chewing gum	Further research and individual testing by athletes are needed to define the range of caffeine protocols At high doses, caffeine can cause nausea, trembling, nervousness, headaches, insomnia and diarrhoea

DRI, Dietary Reference Intake; IBS, irritable bowel syndrome.
Table adapted from Kohler *et al.*, South African Journal of Sports Medicine, 2005.

- Risk of contamination with banned substances needs to be considered.

High-carbohydrate supplements
For example, sports drinks, high-carbohydrate sports drinks, soda drinks, powders, sport bars, cereal or breakfast bars, sport gels.

- Can help meet high carbohydrate requirements, for example during periods of heavy training or carbohydrate loading, before, during and after exercise, or in cases where the athlete lacks appetite.
- Overuse may lead to weight gain or disturb macronutrients.

High-protein supplements

For example, protein powders, protein hydrolysate, skimmed milk powder, higher protein sports bars.

- Recommended for athletes not able to meet protein requirements (e.g. vegetarians), or for athletes with additional protein requirements (e.g. growth spurt with a lack of appetite).
- When added to carbohydrate sources it can be used for recovery.
- May be expensive. Skimmed milk powder is an economical alternative and ideal for fortifying food and drink for recovery, or when athlete lacks appetite.
- May inappropriately displace whole foods or carbohydrate.
- Protein overload may lead to excess body fat storage.

Prebiotics and probiotics

- Promote gastrointestinal function and have benefits for athletes with traveller's diarrhoea, irritable bowel syndrome or those taking antibiotics.
- The immune benefits are not yet established.

Caffeine

- Caffeine ingestion prior to exercise may have performance-enhancing effects in endurance athletes, by possibly decreasing perception of effort and fatigue and increasing utilisation of free fatty acids during exercise. New evidence shows maximal benefits of caffeine at small to moderate doses (1–3 mg/kg).
- Further research and individual testing by athletes are needed to define the range of caffeine protocols.
- Foods and drinks that may contain caffeine include coffee, tea, soft drinks, chocolate, energy drinks, sport supplements and chewing gum.
- At high doses, caffeine can cause nausea, trembling, nervousness, headaches, insomnia and diarrhoea.

13.10 Future research areas and conclusions

While it is clear that to maintain optimal training for endurance events a diet high in carbohydrate foods should be ingested to maintain muscle glycogen, and while research has shown clear benefits from carbohydrate loading prior to such events and carbohydrate ingestion during them, the situation is not as clear-cut with protein ingestion. Although the body of scientific evidence is fairly strong that post-exercise protein ingestion activates protein synthesis, the exact effect of different types of whole protein and protein hydrolysates remains equivocal. Further research is therefore needed to clarify the specific advantages or disadvantages of different types of protein, when ingested as a post-exercise recovery beverage. More controversial is the effect of protein and protein hydrolysates ingested either prior to or during exercise: a number of studies have shown a positive effect on performance, while others have failed to demonstrate any benefit at all. Future studies should therefore attempt to clarify the contradictory results obtained in research evidence to date, particularly investigating such questions regarding the effect of training status, type and duration of exercise, and type of protein ingested at outcome.

References

Ahlborg B, Bergstrom J, Brohult J, Ekelund LG, Hultman E, Maschio G. Human muscle glycogen content and capacity for prolonged exercise after different diets. Forvarsmedicin 1967; 3: 85–99.

Beelen M, Tieland M, Gijsen AP et al. Coingestion of carbohydrate and protein hydrolysate stimulates muscle protein synthesis during exercise in young men, with no further increase during subsequent overnight recovery. J Nutr 2008; 138: 2198–2204.

Bergstrom J, Hermansen L, Hultman E, Saltin B. Diet, muscle glycogen and physical performance. Acta Physiol Scand 1967; 71: 140–150.

Bird SP, Tarpenning KM, Marino FE. Effects of liquid carbohydrate/essential amino acid ingestion on acute hormonal response during a single bout of resistance exercise in untrained men. J Nutr 2006; 22: 367–375.

Buckley JD, Thomson RL, Coates AM, Howe PR, DeNichilo MO, Rowney MK. Supplementation with a whey protein hydrolysate enhances recovery of muscle force-generating capacity following eccentric exercise. J Sci Med Sport 2010; 13: 178–181.

Chen YJ, Wong SH, Wong CK, Lam CW, Huang YJ, Siu PM. Effect of pre-exercise meals with different glycemic indices and loads on metabolic responses and endurance running. Int J Sport Nutr Exerc Metab 2008; 18: 281–300.

Costill DL, Miller JM. Nutrition for endurance sport: carbohydrate and fluid balance. Int J Sport Nutr 1980; 1: 2–14.

Costill DL, Sherman WM, Fink WJ, Maresh C, Witten M, Miller JM. The role of dietary carbohydrates in muscle glycogen resynthesis after strenuous running. Am J Clin Nutr 1981; 34: 1831–1836.

Elliot TA, Cree MG, Sanford AP, Wolfe RR, Tipton KD. Milk ingestion stimulates net muscle protein synthesis following resistance exercise. Med Sci Sports Exerc 2006; 38: 667–674.

Ivy JL, Res PT, Sprague RC, Widzer MO. Effect of a carbohydrate-protein supplement on endurance performance during exercise of varying intensity. Int J Sport Nutr Exerc Metab 2003; 13: 382–395.

Kohler R, Meltzer S, Jakoet I, Noakes T. A practical guide to the use of nutritional supplements in South Africa. South African Journal of Sports Medicine 2005; 17: 48–52.

Luden ND, Saunders MJ, Todd MK. Post-exercise carbohydrate–protein–antioxidant ingestion decreases plasma creatine kinase and muscle soreness. Int J Sport Nutr Exerc Metab 2007; 17: 109–123.

Romano-Ely BC, Todd MK, Saunders MJ, Laurent TS. Effect of an isocaloric carbohydrate–protein–antioxidant drink on cycling performance. Med Sci Sports Exerc 2006; 38: 1608–1616.

Saunders MJ, Kane MD, Todd MK. Effects of a carbohydrate–protein beverage on cycling endurance and muscle damage. Med Sci Sports Exerc 2004; 36: 1233–1238.

Saunders MJ, Luden ND, Herrick JE. Consumption of an oral carbohydrate–protein gel improves cycling endurance and prevents post-exercise muscle damage. J Strength Cond Res 2007; 21: 678–684.

Saunders MJ, Moore RW, Kies AK, Luden ND, Pratt CA. Carbohydrate and protein hydrolysate co-ingestions: improvement of late-exercise time-trial performance. Int J Sport Nutr Exerc Metab 2009; 19: 136–149.

Sherman WM, Costill DL, Fink WJ, Miller JM. Effect of exercise-diet manipulation on muscle glycogen and its subsequent utilisation during performance. Int J Sports Med 1981; 2: 114–118.

Shimomura Y, Yamamoto Y, Bajotto G et al. Neutraceutical effects of branched-chain amino acids on skeletal muscle. J Nutr 2006; 136: 529–532.

van Loon LJ, Kruijshoop M, Verhagen H, Saris WH, Wagenmakers AJ. Ingestion of protein hydrolysate and amino acid–carbohydrate mixtures increase post-exercise plasma insulin responses in men. J Nutr 2000a; 130: 2508–2513.

van Loon LJ, Saris WH, Kruijshoop M, Wagenmakers AJ. Maximising post-exercise muscle glycogen synthesis: carbohydrate supplementation and the application of amino acid or protein hydrolysate mixtures. Am J Clin Nutr 2000b; 72: 106–111.

Further reading

Burke L, Deakin V. Clinical Sports Nutrition, 3rd edn. Syudney: McGraw-Hill Australia, 2006.

International Journal of Sport Nutrition and Exercise Metabolism 2007; 17 (Suppl).

Koopman R, Wagenmakers AJ, Manders RJ et al. Combined ingestion of protein and free leucine with carbohydrate increases post-exercise muscle protein synthesis in vivo in male subjects. Am J Physiol 2005; 288: E645–E653.

Nieman DC. Immunosupport for athletes. Nutr Rev 2008; 66: 310–320.

Nimmo MA, Ekblom B. Fatigue and illness in athletes. J Sport Sci 2007; 25 (Suppl 1): S93–S102.

Position Statement of the American Dietetic Association, Dieticians of Canada, and the American College of Sports Medicine: Nutrition and athletic performance. J Am Diet Assoc 2009; 109: 509–527.

14
Nutrition for Technical and Skill-Based Training

Shelly Meltzer and Neil Hopkins

Key messages

- Nutrition and training strategies that enhance cognitive skills and fatigue resistance are paramount to success in a wide range of team and individual technical and skill-based sports.
- A variety of adaptation techniques involving psychological, theoretical and tactical training are useful in preparing athletes for successful competition.
- Nutrition may trigger training adaptations on a physiological and on a practical level. A good nutrition plan can help build confidence and reduce stress at competition.
- Dietary strategies that may impact on arousal, anxiety, fatigue and skills include manipulation of body composition and optimisation of the overall diet, specifically the type, timing and amounts of carbohydrate, fluid and caffeine, as well as ensuring an adequate intake of micronutrients.
- The effect of protein on skill and technique is unclear. There is also limited or no evidence to support the use of herbals for improving cognition, skills or technique.

- Dietary strategies should be individualised and periodised. This requires matching dietary intakes to the different phases of training (macro-, micro- and meso-cycles) and taking into account factors unique to each athlete (e.g. age, gender, level of play, position of play, body composition and goals, as well as cultural and socio-economic factors) and also, in the case of a team sport, any dynamics that may impact on nutrition.
- Ongoing monitoring and feedback is essential to systematically fine-tune interventions.
- A multilateral and practical approach is important to ensure implementation of dietary advice. This involves establishing lines of communication with all role players: the athlete, the relevant sports science and coaching staff and food service providers.

14.1 Introduction

All sports require varying degrees of skill and technical ability. Each athlete has a built-in set of visual, perceptual and cognitive skills that will determine the level of success. Some of these skills can also be developed and enhanced through sport specific training. Cognitive training is very important for technical and skill-based sports as they require a higher amount of cognitive thought and processing. In many sports the mastery of skill and technique is in fact essential for success.

It is difficult to separate skill and technique without considering factors such as speed, control, flexibility, tactics, pacing ability, power or experience. Many of these factors are influenced by an athlete's personal circumstance and socio-demographic factors like financial constraints, training facilities, place and type of abode, accessibility to coaching support and science. In other words, performance is multidisciplinary and is determined by a complex mixture of physical fitness and mental skills and the art of successful intervention requires practical interpretation of sports science.

This chapter focuses on dietary strategies to enhance the cognitive and sporting performance of athletes taking part in either individual or team-based sports. There is a large continuum of technical and

---

Sport and Exercise Nutrition, First Edition. Edited by Susan A Lanham-New, Samantha J Stear, Susan M Shirreffs and Adam L Collins.
© 2011 The Nutrition Society. Published 2011 by Blackwell Publishing Ltd.

skill-based sports. At one end are the sports like pistol shooting, archery and Formula 1 car racing that require large involvement of the central nervous system and where the demand for mental stamina outweighs the contributions from the other systems. At the opposite end of the continuum are sports such as squash or football that are anaerobic–aerobic activities with large metabolic demands requiring the muscular, technical and central nervous systems to work optimally at the same time. Paramount to success in these sports is the integration of cognitive function, mental readiness, reaction response and motor control. The brain plays a vital role in these sports as it is the governor that controls the body for all tasks, whether it is focusing on a set target such as with archery or pistol shooting, or remembering a line-out call in rugby.

Successful performance in technical and skill-based sports, whether individual or team-based, involves fatigue resistance as well as optimal cognitive function for decision-making and proper execution of complex skills. Thus performance is determined by a complex mixture of physical fitness and mental skills. In a football match, players may have to run quickly to the ball or scene of play, perform manoeuvres involving strength, and execute skills involving cognitive function and fine motor control. If careful planning and adequate nutrition strategies are not followed, then the brain will not receive the nutrients it needs and the body will fatigue as a result. The knock-on effect is that performance will deteriorate as concentration wanes and fatigue sets in.

It is important that all individual requirements are taken into account when planning any nutrition strategy. Factors such as age, gender, level of play, skills, and individual goals have to be considered. The athlete will then need to be monitored to see how he or she responds and adapts to each intervention within the different periods of training. This will always be individual, or case specific, and not necessarily sport-specific. This is evident when considering that two evenly matched squash players will expend more energy in a competitive match than an elite squash player competing against a novice. This difference in energy expenditure during squash has previously been reported to be as much as 2083 kJ/hour.

It is also important to remember that even in a team sport like football there is a high degree of inter- and intra-individual variability in work rates between

players, and every player is unique with factors such as position of play, genetics, body composition, age, growth, gender as well as cultural and socio-economic differences impacting on nutritional demands and requirements. As is the case for individual sports, some general principles will apply but, in addition, team dynamics will come into play, and so individualised intervention within the team setting is optimal.

The first half of this chapter identifies nutrients and strategies including training strategies that impact on skill and technique (i.e. the science) and the second half shows how to integrate nutrition into various periods of training (i.e. the practice). Practical strategies based on current evidence (and experience) for both individual sports (squash) and team sports (football) are provided to highlight some unique differences in these situations. This chapter uses a periodised programme for squash to explain the basic concepts of nutrition and training. This plan can be used as a template for other technical/skill-based sports, although further adjustments will need to be made if it is to become athlete or sport specific.

14.2 Optimising skill and technique and the concept of adaptation

Adaptation takes place after repetitive exposure to a specific task. The greater the amount of adaptation, the better the athlete's performance will be. The time required for adaptation will depend on the volume and intensity of the stimulus as well as the complexity of the sport. Each sport has its own unique needs and it is for this reason that athletes and coaches need to follow a multilateral approach when establishing a sport-specific plan.

Studies have looked at how different nutrition strategies may trigger training adaptations through nutrient–gene interactions (nutrigenomics) involved with training. An example of a strategy would be the 'train-low, compete-high' regimen which has become popular even in some team sports and is based on the premise that by training with low muscle glycogen stores (achieved by a low-carbohydrate diet, training or manipulating timing of training) subsequent training adaptations will be improved. However, more conclusive results from longer-term studies conducted on trained athletes 'in the field' are needed before global practical recommendations can be made. Should athletes wish to experiment with this approach, it would be prudent to do this early in the season/pre-season.

Training for the technical aspects of sport involves many hours of focused mastery of specific tasks. The athlete can spend hours perfecting technique and economy of movement. The technical training can begin in more 'clinical' or familiar environments and progress into more unfamiliar settings. Training under unusual circumstances can prepare the athlete or team for any eventuality (weather, noise, lighting, pitch condition, equipment, etc.). This will ensure that the athlete can focus on the task at hand rather than the distraction of external stimuli.

Sports such as football and squash require a large amount of anticipation. These sports require the athlete to play a mental game of chess while pushing the body to perform at the same time. Training tactical factors allows the athlete and coach to prepare situational probabilities and strategies for each game or each opponent. Sound theoretical knowledge of the sport and the laws of the sport will also enhance performance. The more psychological, theoretical and tactical training that takes place before the competition, the less situational stress will be endured during the competition itself.

From a nutritional perspective, it is also vitally important that an athlete, or team, plans for all situations and eventualities. Leaving nothing to chance will go a long way to building overall confidence and reducing unnecessary stress during competition.

Motor learning, cognitive training and skills development

Classroom tactical sessions are commonplace in technical or skilled-based sports. These classroom sessions are essential in the planning process and require exam-like concentration. It is important to recognise that eating plans should be strategised for these sessions as well. Pangs of hunger or low blood sugar levels have the potential to derail the learning process for the athlete.

Training for a technical or skill-based sport is not all about getting the heart rate up, hustle and bustle, or sprinting from here to there. Quieter sessions are also required. Professional athletes will often set aside time for visualisation sessions. This internal form of meditation requires a deep peace but also an unrivalled amount of concentration. For this internal meditation it is important that adequate dietary practices are implemented to ensure that athletes do not lose focus and shift attention onto the next meal they are craving. It is also important to make sure that the food is the correct food that does not cause bloating or gastrointestinal discomfort, which may become a distraction.

It is important for athletes to train the way they wish to play. The athlete and coach have to strategise the training programme to ensure that physical and mental preparation closely mimics match/game situations. It is therefore important to challenge the athlete's cognitive ability under fatigue circumstances likely to be encountered during competition situations. However, it is unwise to tamper with the athlete's diet or sleeping patterns to achieve this fatigue-like state. Strategies like this have been used successfully for elite Special Forces units to condition them for the extreme situations and possible death they may encounter while on duty. The requirements of an athlete and an elite soldier differ remarkably and the coaching team needs to realise this before embarking on a 'tough-love' approach.

However, there are other strategies that can be used to challenge the athlete mentally. These strategies include 'pre-fatiguing' the athlete in a normal training session or match-like session and then using a cognitive drill either related to the sport or a drill aimed at challenging the athlete mentally. The following are examples of some motor learning/cognitive drills currently in use: situational probabilities; anticipation and memory recall; reaction ball (erratic bounce ball); letter ball (ball with random letters/numbers); colour beacons; numbers; directions; agility ladders; electronic resources (Stroop test); and many more. The only limit to resources such as these is the level of the coaching team's creativity.

Nutrition strategies

There are several nutrition strategies that may impact on arousal, anxiety, fatigue and skills, but this needs to be considered in conjunction with environmental, psychological and practical factors as in practice this is what may determine food availability, appetite and choices.

Body composition, skill and technique

Body composition may affect skill and technique. In squash, having excessively high body fat levels may reduce agility and speed as well as heat tolerance, whilst having excessively low body fat levels may mean an athlete lacks endurance or is not consuming adequate nutrients for training and competition demands. In golf, there is no scientific evidence to show that overweight golfers will improve their game with weight loss; however, there are other benefits such as improved heat tolerance, endurance and fitness that may help prevent fatigue and affect skill and concentration.

Practice tips

- Work with the individual athlete to determine appropriate body composition goals and calculate a practical programme that ties in with training (see section on preparation phase, p. 182).
- Monitor all changes, which may need to be gradual as this may also require adjustments to technique.

Carbohydrate

Carbohydrate is recognised as an important ergogenic aid affecting peripheral mechanisms (muscle), and also immune and central nervous function. Inadequate carbohydrate intakes will have a negative impact on performance resulting in fatigue and/or reduced work capacity across a whole range of sports, from single or repeated high-intensity bouts of exercise to sports of moderate intensity but longer duration. The brain is reliant on glucose for its fuel and even subtle reductions in blood glucose concentrations or carbohydrate availability to the brain can result in central fatigue. Thus symptoms related to inadequate carbohydrate intakes range from hypoglycaemia with overt signs of fatigue, to disorientation and impaired work capacity (reductions in pacing strategies or muscle fibre recruitment) to impairments of skill, concentration and tactical decision-making.

Some specific benefits that have been shown to be associated with feeding carbohydrate during exercise (e.g. in football studies) include faster sprint times, higher jump heights (in fourth quarter of team game), reduced force sensation, enhanced and preserved motor skills (like dribbling ability and shooting), and improved mood late in exercise.

Some recent and intriguing research has shown that even just rinsing the mouth with carbohydrate (sweet or maltodextrin) during exercise may postpone or attenuate central fatigue development. The researchers suggest that the caloric content of the carbohydrate activates brain regions that were possibly inactive or inhibited and through this mechanism mediates a neural response. Mouth rinsing may be a useful ergogenic method for athletes needing to manage their calorie intake or for athletes who for situational reasons cannot tolerate ingesting large volumes of food/fluid (exercise of greater than 1 hour duration). More research is needed on athletes in competition situations and in a fed state.

Glycaemic index and glycaemic load

It is not entirely clear whether the glycaemic index (GI) (ranking of individual carbohydrates according to overall effects on blood glucose levels) or the glycaemic load (also considers amount of carbohydrate) offers the athlete a clear performance advantage. Some studies have shown that carbohydrate ingestion during endurance exercise negates the effect of the consumption of pre-exercise GI meals while other investigations have shown that when nutritional strategies incorporating GI are applied to multiple meals, there is no clear advantage to the athlete in terms of exercise performance and capacity.

Practice tips

- Carbohydrate intake goals are athlete and sports specific. Moreover, for an individual athlete, absolute amounts of carbohydrate required may vary according to specific training and competition schedules (see p. 185 and Table 14.6). Total daily carbohydrate intake goals may be anywhere in the range 3–12 g/kg/day, depending on the type of training, level of competition, and goals of the athlete.
- Timing of carbohydrate proximate to training can impact on performance and recovery: 1–4 g/kg carbohydrate should be consumed 1–4 hours before training/competing; during exercise, if the session is 1 hour, mouth rinsing with carbohydrate may suffice, but beyond 90 min of exercise a carbohydrate intake of 0.5–1.0 g/kg/hour is advised and this increases to ~1.5–1.8 g/kg/min if exercise extends beyond 4 hours.
- Athletes who are especially susceptible to hunger and/or dips in blood sugar, concentration and focus during an event need to ensure an adequate intake of carbohydrate, before, during and after an event, including low GI foods (and foods low in fibre and residue for gut comfort) before the event and then select moderate to high GI foods during and after exercise.

Protein

The effect of protein on skill and technique is unclear. Theoretically, the rationale of ingesting branched-chain amino acids (BCAAs) during prolonged exercise would be to improve the psychological perception of fatigue (i.e. central fatigue by decreasing serotonin) but studies using this strategy have shown mixed results. In fact taking BCAAs during exercise may cause ammonia to be produced and this may cause fatigue. There are some studies which report that when inadequate amounts of carbohydrate are ingested during exercise, and glucose availability is compromised, endurance time to fatigue may be extended by adding protein to sports drinks. However, the mechanism for this is not clear and may just be an energy effect.

Fluid

The impact of hypohydration on performance in team sport and sports involving skill and technique is not as extensive as that seen during endurance exercise. Interpretation of studies is also complicated by different protocols, for example the techniques used to achieve hypohydration (sweating, diuretics, exercise, energy restriction) and/or rehydration (volume and type of fluid and rate of ingestion). In team sports, research is complicated by the high degree of inter- and intra-individual variability in work rates between players that are often unpredictable and random. There is very large inter-individual variation in sweating, and dehydration also affects individuals differently and may be influenced by the type and mode of exercise and temperature outside. Moreover, a cognitive skill may deteriorate with dehydration in a laboratory setting, but psychological arousal in a competition may compensate for the deficit. A lower body mass may make some skills or activities easier, like sprinting or jumping (if muscle force or power is not reduced) and bowling speed in cricket. However, the decrease in physiological demand and subsequent improved performance may mask any other potential negative effects of hypohydration (such as bowling accuracy in cricket and withstanding tackles). Current evidence can be summarised as follows.

- Hypohydration, if of a sufficient level, can affect physical and cognitive performance, but not all hypohydration negatively affects performance.

- The environmental conditions experienced by an individual can influence both the hydration status, by means of influencing sweat loss, and the physiological responses to that hydration status.
- Athletes who do not drink anything during exercise will perform less well than they would if they drank ad libitum (according to thirst).
- If players are more than 2.5–3% dehydrated and thirsty in warm to hot conditions, cognitive function, mood and mental readiness may be impaired.

A number of factors come into play when advising individuals or teams on fluid. Other roles that fluid has on performance need to be considered. Fluid can also be a practical source of nutrients such as carbohydrate (and protein if needed) and electrolytes. By increasing the production of saliva, which has antimicrobial properties, fluid may impact on immune function and help fight infections. Fluid in the recovery period is important, since players continue to lose fluid by sweating or urinating and drinks are a practical way of taking in carbohydrate (and even a little protein), needed for recovery and anabolic processes, when appetite is reduced.

Understanding the individual (e.g. heavier players may require more fluid), the impact of the environment (e.g. in a colder environment, the carbohydrate to fluid ratio of a drink may be higher), the rules of the sport (opportunities to drink), and the influence of uniforms/protective gear is important when developing fluid strategies. In a sport like Formula 1 racing, the environmental constraints (fireproof outfits and helmet, cabin conditions) and racing conditions impact heavily on fluid demands and delivery. Using practical systems like Camel Packs and specialised in-car drinking systems, and providing fluids with sodium, should be considered. Sodium improves fluid absorption and retention and decreases urine output. Opportunities to drink fluid may vary (informal breaks and stoppages in a team sport), the demand for fluid and fuel may vary (e.g. more mobile football players may require more fluid and carbohydrate; a squash player may become dehydrated at temperatures of 25°C after less than 30 min), and in many sports the length of a game may be unpredictable.

Practice tips

- Athletes should always take personally labelled drinks to practices, see that they are accessible and familiarise themselves with their own fluid requirements in different environmental conditions.
- Body weight can only be used as a *general* guideline and to encourage an increased awareness of individual fluid requirements. Players should be weighed before and after exercise in minimal clothing, taking into account urine losses and drink volume.
- Athletes should start games and training well hydrated and utilise every opportunity (e.g. stoppages/half time) to drink sufficient fluid. Players need to continue to replace fluid losses in the recovery period and fluid should also be provided at meal/snack times to encourage further intake.
- More is not better: athletes should not drink at rates greater than sweat losses so that they gain weight during training or matches.
- Fluid absorption is best if the stomach is kept partially filled during exercise. In a football match for example, this can be achieved by drinking 250–500 ml immediately before running onto the field and then topping this up during the match.
- Sports drinks are practical as they provide carbohydrate and electrolytes such as sodium as well as fluid.
- Having access to cool and flavoured fluids may encourage intake and help with cooling in hot humid environments.
- Other cooling strategies are very important to prevent heat stroke in hot conditions. These include staying in the shade during breaks and removing warm jerseys, using cold-water ice packs and side-line fans.

Dehydration, over-hydration and cognitive skills

Both dehydration and over-hydration can impact on cognitive skills and performance. Early signs of dehydration include headache, fatigue, loss of appetite, flushed skin, heat intolerance, light-headedness, dry mouth and eyes, and dark urine with a strong odour. Advanced signs require urgent medical intervention and include difficulty in swallowing, clumsiness, shrivelled skin, sunken eyes and dim vision, painful urination, numb skin, muscle spasms, 'abnormal behaviour' and delirium.

Over-drinking, even in team sports, has been reported: American football players, in an attempt to prevent heat cramps, over-hydrated by drinking too much water. Signs of over-hydration include nausea, vomiting, extreme fatigue, respiratory distress, dizziness, confusion, disorientation, oedema (rings, shoes, watches may feel tight), coma, seizures, and even death if left untreated.

Alcohol

Alcohol, by impacting on metabolic, cardiovascular, thermoregulatory and neuromuscular systems, can have profound negative effects on performance. Skill and behavioural changes like reduced reaction time and poor judgements, impaired balance, accuracy, hand–eye coordination, strength, power and endurance are associated with alcohol intake. Athletes celebrating or commiserating after a game with alcohol may be distracted from sound recovery strategies, injury treatment and sleep. Drinking alcohol after a match interferes with the recovery of the body's carbohydrate stores, and by increasing urinary fluid losses delays rehydration. Alcohol also has a vasodilatory effect, which can increase bleeding and swelling, thus delaying or slowing recovery of soft-tissue damage and rehabilitation from injury.

For an athlete needing to manage weight, it is important to consider the significant calories contributed by alcohol (29 kJ/g, 7 kcal/g) and its potential to increase endogenous fat.

Practice tips

- Adhere to the 24-hour rule, i.e. avoid alcohol in the 24 hours before a match and in the 24 hours after a match, if any soft-tissue injuries or bruising have occurred. Some teams may have a ban on alcohol intake!
- Ensure that plenty of non-alcoholic drinks are available after training or a match. Those players who choose to drink alcohol should first see that they are adequately rehydrated and refuelled with carbohydrates and fluid before drinking alcoholic drinks, which in any case should be limited.

Caffeine

One of caffeine's primary sites of action is the central nervous system and it has been shown to affect cognitive performance in different modes of exercise (endurance, high-intensity intermittent and strength–power). Studies have shown that moderate doses of caffeine can result in several advantageous improvements important for team sports like football, field hockey and rugby, including a 10% improvement in ball-passing accuracy with a caffeine intake of 6 mg/kg, and maintenance of sprint times.

However, caffeine can be a double-edged sword. It may increase arousal, but as a central nervous stimulant it can be counter-productive by also increasing nervousness and anxiety and may cause palpitations, headaches, visual disturbances and dehydration. Some individuals are more sensitive to the effects of caffeine; this may be related to habitual intake, gender, type of exercise, level of training, and body weight. More is also not necessarily better. Several studies have shown that significant improvements in performance can be achieved with doses as low as 2–3 mg/kg and it has been suggested that at higher doses caffeine may stimulate the central nervous system to the point at which the usually positive ergogenic responses are overridden.

Vitamins, minerals and herbals

Deficiencies of certain minerals (e.g. iron) and vitamins may directly or indirectly impact on fatigue and performance, and athletes who eat restricted diets or limit food choices are generally advised to take a low-dose multivitamin and multimineral supplement. Deficiency of vitamin A is strongly associated with night blindness and reduced ability to adjust to changes in darkness and light thus impacting on visual skills. Supplements of vitamins B_1, B_6 and B_{12} (which are rapidly depleted in times of tension or stress) have been found to improve firing accuracy in pistol shooting, but other well-conducted studies to prove the efficacy of the many supplements, including herbals, marketed to improve mental strength or a calming effect in athletes are limited.

There are additional ergogenic aids that may benefit some athletes participating in technical or skill-based sports. Ergogenic aids such as creatine, β-alanine and other buffers may have added benefits for technical or skill-based athletes, though not on a cognitive level. These are discussed in Chapter 9, and the athlete is always reminded of the health and legal risks associated with some supplements. According to the World Anti-Doping Agency (WADA) rules, athletes are liable and responsible for any and all substances appearing in their urine and blood, should they test positive for any banned substances.

14.3 Principles of periodisation

Definition/terminologies

The most important concept in any sport, team or individual, is periodisation. It is what sets the good teams apart from the average teams. Being successful in sport is all about planning. In business there is strategy, in sport there is periodisation. The term 'periodisation' originates from the word 'period' and describes when the phases of training are broken down into smaller time periods that are easier to manage and plan for. These phases are designed to culminate in peak championship performance. There are no hard and fast rules about periodisation because it is an art rather than a science. Periodisation requires careful planning and fine-tuning from day to day, week to week, month to month, and year to year. This planning process differs from sport to sport and team to team according to what the sport-specific outcomes are, for example which energy pathways, muscle fibre types, neuromuscular systems need to be developed. The annual plan will also be directly linked to the level of competition (club, provincial, or national).

Super-compensation

A central tenant of exercise is the super-compensation cycle. It illustrates the importance of recovery following a bout of exercise. If the duration and frequency of training are planned correctly and if the athlete's body is allowed the optimal amount of recovery between sessions, then the body will rebound, or super-compensate. This super-compensation level is a higher level of physical ability than at the point of the initial bout of exercise. If there is failure to plan the correct volume and intensity of training, then the athlete's body and performance will go into decline (Figures 14.1 and 14.2).

Recovery for the mind is just as important as recovery for the body, especially in technical sports. Planning is essential to ensure adequate recovery between sessions, between competitions and in the

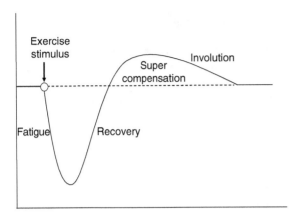

Figure 14.1 Super-compensation cycle. (Adapted with permission from Bompa T, Haff GG. Periodization: Theory and Methodology of Training, 5th edn. Champaign, IL: Human Kinetics, 2009. Modified from Yakovlev N. Sports Biochemistry. Leipzig: Deutche Hochschule für Körpekultur, 1967.)

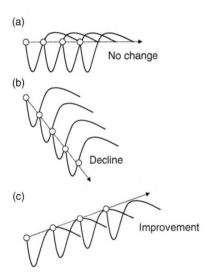

Figure 14.2 Practical example of the importance of the super-compensation cycle: (a) no change; (b) decline in performance; (c) improvement in performance. (Part b adapted with permission from Bompa T, Haff GG. Periodization: Theory and Methodology of Training, 5th edn. Champaign, IL: Human Kinetics, 2009.)

Table 14.1 Hypothetical training diary for a squash player, used to monitor training volume and load to avoid over-training.

Variable	Description	Value
Training	Morning session 　Duration 　RPE (1–10) Mid session 　Duration 　RPE (1–10) Afternoon session 　Duration 　RPE (1–10) Total hours of training Total hours of rest Difficulty for the day (RPE 1–10)	
Sleep	Hours of sleep Quality of sleep 　Poor 　Average 　Good Waking mood 　Tired 　Refreshed	
Heart rate Diet	Resting heart rate Number of meals Number of snacks and recovery snacks Quality of diet 　Poor 　Adequate 　Good Units of alcohol Caffeine intake Supplements Weight (morning)	
Psychology	Enthusiasm (1–10) Mood 　Negative 　Neutral 　Positive	

wtransition phase. Rest on its own is not sufficient. The body needs assisted recovery to speed up the process. Assisted recovery includes diet, massage (physiotherapy), hydrotherapy (pool-based recovery), active rest (light movement or exercise), cross-training, sports psychology, meditation, visualisation, as well as other forms of rest. The correct diet during recovery will ensure that the athlete returns to exercise with a fully recharged system. In a technical and skill-based sport resting the mind and eating appropriately during the recovery phase will have visible results. If the athlete has not been rested mentally or psychologically and not eaten appropriately, then performance will deteriorate rapidly. According to the super-compensation model, fatigue will set in sooner if there is inadequate preparation or rest. Using a training diary is a good way of monitoring training load and is a vital piece in the puzzle if

Table 14.2 Hypothetical year planner for a squash player.

January	February	March	April
Transition phase	*Transition phase/ preparation phase*	*Preparation phase*	*Preparation phase/ competition phase*
In-depth dietary assessment and planning with multidisciplinary management team	Calculating dietary requirements and advising on practical implementation	Liaising and coordinating travel and competition nutrition arrangements Continuing monitoring Reassessment	Ensuring contingency nutrition plans in place; travel nutrition supplements and supplies Continuing monitoring Reassessment
May	**June**	**July**	**August**
Competition phase Continuing monitoring, reassessment and fine-tuning	*Competition phase* Continuing monitoring, reassessment and fine-tuning	*Competition phase* Continuing monitoring, reassessment and fine-tuning	*Competition phase* Continuing monitoring, reassessment and fine-tuning
September	**October**	**November**	**December**
Competition phase Continuing monitoring, reassessment and fine-tuning	*Competition phase* Continuing monitoring, reassessment and fine-tuning	*Competition phase* Continuing monitoring, reassessment and fine-tuning	*Competition phase/transition phase* Debrief and reassessment

over-training is to be avoided. A simple version of a training diary is shown in Table 14.1.

Influence of periodisation on training and nutrition strategies

Training cycles

The macro-cycle is the 'big' picture. It is the planning for the entire year. The annual plan can be broken down into three phases: preparation, competition and transition. The preparation phase begins with general preparation and conditioning, and progresses to more sport-specific conditioning. The competition phase begins with pre-competition training where the athlete will start actual match or game situation training. The meso-cycle is one step down from the macro-cycle. It is monthly periodisation aimed at peak-performance at the desired time. Careful planning of meso-cycles will result in optimal conditioning (super-compensation) at the time of competition. The micro-cycle is the smallest unit of the 'athletic plan'. It is a day-to-day or weekly periodisation. Training stimuli may vary considerably during the different phases in terms of intensity, volume and duration and will influence and determine dietary requirements.

For example, energy requirements can be increased by 3000 kJ/hour during match play for squash and a football match can increase requirements by approximately 6700 kJ (for a typical 75-kg player).

The macro-cycle: training and nutrition

As can be seen from the year planner (Table 14.2), the competition phase, which may involve travel, can take up most of the year and this has huge physiological, practical and even psychological implications. Athletes often have to juggle these demands with work or study commitments.

Using the example of the squash player, the transition phase (December and January) is used to give the body a welcome rest from athletic training. It is also a period where athletes can spend time working on aspects of their physical conditioning in the gym building up strength, on the pitch/court working on agility/plyometrics/speed, or doing cross-training for cardiovascular endurance. The athlete can also spend time working on mental conditioning during this period.

The *transition phase* is an important phase from a dietary perspective, and the dietary approach will depend on expected outcomes. If the goal is rest, and the intensity and volume of training has been significantly reduced, the athlete needs to cut back on energy intake to prevent unnecessary weight gain.

This may be a challenge over the 'holiday period' when alcohol and parties may be the norm and athletes may require additional creative ideas and plans so as not to let go completely.

For the sports dietitian or nutritionist, working with the athlete in the transition and early preparation phase there is an opportunity to assess dietary requirements and gather information including athlete-specific information: socio-demographic, dietary, medical and biomedical information; supplement regimens; food preferences; weight history and goals; training and competition demands and schedules; and logistical information with regard to travel and competition. It is an opportunity to meet with relevant role players in the sports science and coaching team and to establish and outline roles and responsibilities to ensure consistent messages.

In the *preparation phase* there is an increased volume or amount of training with a decreased intensity. This could be as a result of more sport-specific training, more gym work, or more additional training such as cross-training (where a different modality or sport is used to condition the body). This increased volume can be attained through an increase in the frequency of the training sessions or the duration of the training session. As the competition phase approaches the intensity of training will increase, simulating match/game situations, and the volume will decrease. The preparation phase can be broken down into general preparation and sport-specific preparation. The general preparation involves conditioning for strength, power and cardiovascular endurance. The sport-specific preparation includes functional strength training, explosive power and sport-specific endurance.

Specific body composition goals should be identified early (i.e. in the transition or early preparation phase) and timed so that desired changes can be achieved well in advance of competition, so as not to compromise performance and immunity (see Chapter 17 for further information on weight management and weight making). The preparation phase is also an important opportunity to experiment, log and review specific strategies (e.g. types of foods, supplements, timing of intake, competition-specific action plan).

In the preparation phase, nutrition plans for competition need to be outlined and strategised, as even the best training plans cannot be optimised if the food is limited or not available at competition, resulting in a wasted opportunity. This may involve liaising with airlines, hotels, restaurants and caterers at match venues and at functions to discover all foods and drinks available, timing of meals, etc. Approaches may vary depending on the athlete, the sport, the team and logistics. For a smaller team who are self-responsible for food preparation, menus, recipes, shopping lists and restaurant guides may be provided, whereas for bigger teams staying in hotels it may be important to send menus and guidelines to hotels and event caterers.

With a good preparation plan, nothing is left to chance in the *competition phase*. It is useful to use a check-list with all travel requirements: supplements, food, contact details of suppliers and caterers, and other individual specific information. In this phase it is important to keep to practised strategies and to check (ahead of time) that appropriate pre- and post-match food and drink options are available for all scenarios, for example should athletes suffer from travellers' diarrhoea or lack appetite. If all plans are in place, only fine-tuning should be needed in the competition phase. Eating regimens before and after competition will depend on the athlete, the sport and the situation. A golden rule is not to be influenced by others or be under pressure to try anything new. At the end of the competition phase it is important to debrief and to gather information for future planning.

The meso- and micro-cycles: training and nutrition

To illustrate how to match and calculate dietary requirements to the different training demands, it is important to know the training details of the meso- and micro-cycles (Tables 14.3–14.5) and to use this as a starting point. Nutritional guidelines can then be calculated in terms of absolute amounts of carbohydrate, protein and fat. It is important to relate this back to energy requirements and then to monitor each athlete's response, bearing in mind that goals will be individual and responses may also be individual.

The following example of the squash player (and in Table 14.6) shows how dietary interventions can be periodised to match training phases so as to optimise performance.

Table 14.3 Hypothetical month planner for a squash player.

January	February	March	April
Rest	Rest	Cross-training	Conditioning (gym)
Cross-training	Cross-training	Conditioning (gym)	Conditioning (sport)
Conditioning (gym)	Conditioning (gym)	Conditioning (sport)	Conditioning (match)
	Conditioning (sport)		Compete (easy)
May	**June**	**July**	**August**
Conditioning (sport)	Conditioning (sport)	Conditioning (sport)	Conditioning (sport)
Conditioning (match)	Conditioning (match)	Conditioning (match)	Conditioning (match)
Compete (easy)	Compete (hard)	Compete (hard)	Compete (hard)
September	**October**	**November**	**December**
Conditioning (sport)	Conditioning (sport)	Conditioning (sport)	Conditioning (sport)
Conditioning (match)	Conditioning (match)	Conditioning (match)	Conditioning (match)
Compete (hard)	Compete (hard)	Compete (hard)	Compete (hard)
			Rest

Table 14.4 Hypothetical week planner for a squash player.

January	February	March	April
Light week	Light week	Hard gym week	Hard squash week
Light week	Light week	Hard gym week	Hard squash week
Light week	Easy squash week	Hard squash week	Taper
Light week	Easy gym week	Hard gym week	Compete[a]
May	**June**	**July**	**August**
Recovery	Recovery	Hard squash week	Recovery
Hard squash week	Hard gym week	Hard squash week	Easy squash week
Taper	Hard gym week	Taper	Taper
Compete[a]	Hard squash week	Compete[a]	Compete[a]
September	**October**	**November**	**December**
Recovery	Recovery	Hard squash week	Recovery
Easy squash week	Hard gym week	Hard squash week	Taper
Taper	Hard gym week	Taper	Compete[a]
Compete[a]	Hard squash week	Compete[a]	Recovery

[a] Compete: squash tournament minimum of three matches in preliminary rounds and maximum of eight matches.

Light week

Physical requirements The light week is designed to give the body 'active rest' in the transition phase. The athlete should perform low-intensity exercise rather than resting completely. Low-intensity exercise includes light gym, walking, hiking, swimming, easy jogging, etc. There is no need to include exercise related to the athlete's sport. The easy week is designed for cross-training and possibly recreation.

Dietary requirements Energy intake requirements decrease to match the decrease in physical activity. Daily nutrient goals are in the range of 3–5 g/kg for

Table 14.5 Hypothetical day planner for a squash player.

	Monday	Tuesday	Wednesday	Thursday	Friday	Saturday	Sunday
Light week	Cardio	Rest	Rest	Cardio	Rest	Rest	Rest
	Rest	Cardio	Rest	Rest	Cardio	Rest	Rest
	Core	Rest	Rest	Core	Rest	Rest	Rest
	Monday	Tuesday	Wednesday	Thursday	Friday	Saturday	Sunday
Easy squash	Squash	Gym	Squash	Gym	Squash	Rest	Rest
	Rest	Rest	Rest	Rest	Rest	Rest	Rest
	Cardio	Squash	Rest	Squash	Cardio	Rest	Rest
	Monday	Tuesday	Wednesday	Thursday	Friday	Saturday	Sunday
Easy gym	Gym	Squash	Gym	Squash	Gym	Rest	Rest
	Rest	Rest	Rest	Rest	Rest	Rest	Rest
	Cardio	Gym	Core	Gym	Cardio	Rest	Rest
	Monday	Tuesday	Wednesday	Thursday	Friday	Saturday	Sunday
Hard gym	Gym	Gym	Gym	Gym	Gym	Gym	Rest
	Squash	Rest	Squash	Rest	Squash	Rest	Rest
	Cardio	Squash	Rest	Squash	Cardio	Cardio	Rest
	Monday	Tuesday	Wednesday	Thursday	Friday	Saturday	Sunday
Hard squash	Squash	Gym	Squash	Gym	Squash	Squash	Rest
	Rest	Skills	Rest	Skills	Rest	Skills	Rest
	Squash	Squash	Squash	Squash	Squash	Rest	Rest
	Monday	Tuesday	Wednesday	Thursday	Friday	Saturday	Sunday
Taper	Squash	Squash	Squash	Skills	Cardio	Rest	Rest
	Rest	Rest	Rest	Rest	Rest	Rest	Rest
	Hydro	Massage	Hydro	Massage	Rest	Rest	Rest
	Monday	Tuesday	Wednesday	Thursday	Friday	Saturday	Sunday
Recovery	Rest	Rest	Cardio	Skills	Squash	Squash	Rest
	Rest	Rest	Rest	Rest	Rest	Rest	Rest
	Hydro	Massage	Hydro	Massage	Rest	Rest	Rest
	Monday	Tuesday	Wednesday	Thursday	Friday	Saturday	Sunday
Compete	Match	Match	Match	Match	Match	Match	Match
	Hydro	Hydro	Hydro	Hydro	Hydro	Hydro	Hydro
	Massage	Massage	Massage	Massage	Massage	Massage	Massage

carbohydrate, 1–1.5 g/kg for protein and 1–1.5 g/kg for fat. If weight loss or a decrease in fat mass is a goal, the athlete should keep to the lower range of carbohydrate and fat recommendations, with higher protein intakes to promote satiety. The emphasis should also be on selecting foods rich in fibre and low in energy density. High calorie-concentrated snacks and sports-specific products like carbohydrate drinks and bars should be replaced with lower calorie fluid options and low-fat high-fibre snacks.

Easy squash week

Physical requirements   In the easy squash week the emphasis is on returning to squash after a short period of no sport-specific training or after recovery. The gym sessions are of lighter intensity and focus on light cardiovascular exercise and flexibility. Each gym session will last between 30 and 60 min. The squash sessions are longer in duration, 60–90 min, and focus on squash technique, drills and situational probabilities. The intensity of each squash session is low.

Table 14.6 Energy and macronutrient intake requirements for a 70-kg squash player, periodised according to the phases of training.

Physical requirements	Dietary requirements
Light week	Total kJ/day 9437 CHO 280 g/day Protein 87.5 g/day Fat 87.5 g/day
Easy squash/easy gym	Total kJ/day 12 553 CHO 420 g/day Protein 94.5 g/day Fat 105 g/day
Hard squash/hard gym	Total kJ/day 14 791 CHO 490 g/day Protein 119 g/day Fat 122.5 g/day
Taper/recovery	Total kJ/day 8456 CHO 280 g/day Protein 84 g/day Fat 63 g/day
Competition	Total kJ/day 13 664 CHO 590 g/day Protein 84 g/day Fat 77 g/day

Dietary requirements With the increase in training, total energy requirements increase. Although the training is of lighter intensity, there are days where total duration of training may be as much as 150 min. Daily carbohydrate requirements therefore increase to 5–7 g/kg, protein to 1.2–1.5 g/kg and fat can increase to 1.5 g/kg. The exact amount will depend on many factors such as dietary and weight history, anthropometric goals, gender (e.g. females may require less protein), age (adolescents or growing athletes require more protein per kilogram body weight) and even environmental factors like altitude.

Distribution of energy intake and timing of food intake proximate to training is important. To promote recovery, 1–1.2 g/kg of high-GI carbohydrate-rich foods should be consumed immediately after training sessions. If appetite is limited, a small amount of protein can replace some of the carbohydrate so that the ratio of carbohydrate to protein of the recovery snack is 3–4:1 Adding some protein may also promote better carbohydrate storage and result in faster repair and recovery of muscles as well as the synthesis of new protein.

For training sessions longer than 1 hour, carbohydrate consumption during exercise is recommended.

This should be in the range 0.5–1.0 g/kg/hour, with the lower range of carbohydrate sufficing if the intensity of training is low. For athletes needing to lose or manage weight, less concentrated sports drinks can be used but still ensuring the provision of 30 g carbohydrate per hour. Alternatively, the athlete can experiment with rinsing the mouth with carbohydrate if the session is less than an hour, and over and above this meeting fluid requirements with water or a sports water.

It is important that the athlete brings portable snacks and drinks to training, particularly since training venues often have limited or inappropriate options available. In team situations, it may be useful to develop practical recovery nutrition strategies for the whole team, for example setting up a fridge with options in the recovery area and organising the purchasing and replenishment of supplies.

Easy gym week
Physical requirements In the easy gym week the emphasis is on preparing for the strength training to follow. Easy gym weeks can be used to cover gym technique and familiarise the body to the strength training routine. The gym sessions are of low intensity and last for 30–60 min. They include basic resistance training with light weights (50–60% of 1RM), flexibility and cardiovascular conditioning.

Dietary requirements Same principles as for the easy squash week.

Hard gym week
Physical requirements In the hard gym week the emphasis is on building a solid base of strength specific for squash. The hard gym week will mainly involve isotonic resistance training but will also include plyometrics, agility and power-lifting drills. The intensity of the gym training can be achieved through the loading, the duration or the frequency of the sessions. The hard gym week requires the intensity of squash to taper off to avoid overloading the athlete. There should be a higher ratio of strength training to squash. The duration of the gym sessions is 60–90 min and the loading is moderate to heavy depending on the muscle group or exercise (60–80% of 1RM).

Dietary requirements With the intensity, duration or frequency of gym sessions increasing, nutritional requirements increase. Daily carbohydrate requirements may increase significantly to 7–10 g/kg, protein to ≥1.7 g/kg and fat to 1.5–2 g/kg. Only modest increases in protein are required; this is because with training, adaptations will have occurred which 'spare' protein and the increased carbohydrate intakes will also be protein-sparing.

On occasions where there are three training sessions in a day, recovery nutrition strategies are imperative. Small frequent meals and compact forms of carbohydrate such as fluid (also beneficial for hydration) and sugar-rich special sport supplements are usually well tolerated. The latter options should be added as a supplement (rather than as a substitute) to the basic nutrient-rich diet so as not to crowd out essential nutrients. Liquid meal supplements can be a convenient source of both carbohydrate and protein as well as micronutrients. Athletes can also use liquid meal supplements to help control energy (kJ/kcal) intake when trying to gain or lose weight, selecting products to match their individual goals (calcium-rich dairy options may help with weight/fat loss), tolerance (soy-based products offer an alternative for lactose-intolerant athletes and whey protein contains virtually no lactose), or preference.

Hard squash week

Physical requirements   The emphasis in the hard squash week is on squash. There can still be strength training and other sessions, but the ratio is in favour of squash. The intensity of the other sessions is kept low and within the time frame of a squash match. This means that if the squash match is expected to last 40–80 min, then the training sessions should not be longer than 80 min. The hard squash week should simulate what the athlete is likely to expect in the competition phase. The intensity of the squash can be achieved through the loading, the duration or the frequency of the squash sessions. The number of practice matches and game situations can be increased. Smaller, league or friendly, matches are an ideal way of achieving this.

Dietary requirements   Same principles as for the hard gym week.

Taper

Physical requirements   The taper phase is designed to rest the body. It is aimed at recovery for the body and mind before the competition phase. The strength training and gym sessions fall away and the general intensity of squash is low. There are fewer exercise sessions and more recovery and tactical/skill sessions. Towards the end of the taper week there is no squash.

Dietary requirements/notes   To avoid unnecessary weight gain before competition, and with the decrease in energy expenditure, it is important that athletes make a concerted effort to reduce their calorie intake. This is best achieved by reducing daily carbohydrate intake to 3–5 g/kg (cutting back on all added concentrated carbohydrate-rich options), protein to 1.2 g/kg and fat to 0.8–1.0 g/kg. The focus should be on nutrient-rich foods and all practical strategies to ensure accessibility to suitable options need to be explored and implemented.

Competition

Physical requirements   The competition week is focused primarily on producing optimal performance during a match situation. The athlete will compete at the highest possible intensity with one match per day. The duration of each match varies depending on the level of the competition and the opposition. The rest of the time is spent recovering for the next day and the next match in the tournament.

Dietary requirements/notes   With the variable and unpredictable nature of the match and tournament, squash players need to be prepared for all scenarios. The intensity and duration of each match can significantly increase nutrient requirements. Carbohydrate needs may be as high as 8–10 g/kg/day, with protein intake of 1.2 g/kg/day and fat 1–1.2 g/kg/day contributing the balance of energy. Players need to begin a tournament optimally fuelled, refuelling and topping up reserves as soon as possible after the match to promote rapid recovery. Having access to palatable sports drinks is critical and players need to be encouraged to ensure adequate hydration. Should stress or anxiety impact on appetite, low-residue calorie concentrated foods and meal replacements can be used to help meet nutrient demands. All drinks, foods and supplements should have been tried and tested in training.

Recovery

Physical requirements   The recovery phase is designed to rest the body. It is aimed at recovery for the body and mind following the competition phase.

There is only light exercise aimed at active recovery. There is no strength training in the recovery phase and squash is only resumed towards the end of the week.

Dietary requirements/notes   Absolute nutrient and energy requirements will be very similar to those in the taper phase. The athlete may need additional encouragement and ideas so as not to 'let go' completely and resort to inappropriate food and drink and alcohol but to keep to the general prudent principles.

Further reading

Ali A, Williams C, Nicholas CW, Foskett A. The influence of carbohydrate–electrolyte ingestion on soccer skill performance. Med Sci Sports Exerc 2007; 39: 1969–1976.

Below PR, Mora-Rodriguez R, Gonzalez-Alonso J, Coyle EF. Fluid and carbohydrate ingestion independently improve performance during 1 h of intense exercise. Med Sci Sports Exerc 1995; 27: 200–210.

Bompa T. Periodization. Theory and Methodology of Training. Champaign, IL: Human Kinetics, 1999.

Bonke D, Nickel B. Improvement of fine motoric movement control by elevated dosages of vitamin B1, B6, and B12 in target shooting. Int J Vitam Nutr Res Suppl 1989; 30: 198–204.

Burke LM. Fluid guidelines for sport: interview with Professor Tim Noakes. Int J Sport Nutr Exerc Metab 2006; 16: 644–653.

Burke LM. Caffeine and sports performance. Appl Physiol Nutr Metab 2008; 33: 1319–1334.

Burke LM, Hawley JA. Fluid balance in team sports: guidelines for optimal practices. Sports Med 1997; 24: 38–54.

Castell LM, Burke LM, Stear SJ, Maughan RJ. BJSM reviews: A–Z of nutritional supplements, sports nutrition foods and ergogenic aids for health and performance Part 8. Br J Sports Med 2010; 44: 468–470.

Chambers ES, Bridge MW, Jones DA. Carbohydrate sensing in the human mouth: effects on exercise performance and brain activity. J Physiol 2009; 587: 1779–1794.

Currell K, Conway S, Jeukendrup AE. Carbohydrate ingestion improves performance of a new reliable test of soccer performance. Int J Sport Nutr Exerc Metab 2009; 19: 34–46.

Edwards AM, Mann ME, Marfell-Jones MJ et al. The influence of moderate dehydration on soccer performance: physiological responses to 45-min of outdoors match-play and the immediate subsequent performance of sport-specific and mental concentration tests. Br J Sports Med 2007; 41: 385–391.

Foskett A, Ali A, Gant N. Caffeine enhances cognitive function and skill performance during simulated soccer activity. Int J Sport Nutr Exerc Metab 2009; 19: 410–423.

Fredholm BB, Battig K, Holmen J, Nehlig A, Zvartau EE. Actions of caffeine in the brain with special reference to factors that contribute to its widespread use. Pharmacol Rev 1999; 51: 83–133.

Girard O, Chevalier R, Habrard M, Sciberras P, Hot P, Millet GP. Game analysis and energy requirements of elite squash. J Strength Cond Res 2007; 21: 909–914.

Graham TE. Caffeine and exercise: metabolism, endurance and performance. Sports Med 2001; 31: 785–807.

Graham TE, Spriet LL. Catecholamine, and exercise performance responses to various doses of caffeine. J Appl Physiol 1995; 78: 867–874.

Goldstein ER, Ziegenfuss T, Kalman D et al. International Society of Sports Nutrition position stand: caffeine and performance J Int Soc Sports Nutr 2010; 7: 5.

Hawley JA, Gibala M, Bermon S. Innovations in athletic preparation: role of substrate availability to modify training adaptation and performance. J Sports Sci 2007; 25 (Suppl 1): S115–S124.

Kreider RB, Wilborn CD, Taylor L et al. ISSN Exercise and Sport Nutrition Review: research and recommendations. J Int Soc Sports Nutr 2010; 7: 7.

Lees A. Science and the major racket sports: a review. J Sports Sci 2003; 21: 701–732.

McGregor SJ, Nicholas CW, Lakomy HK, Williams C. The influence of intermittent high-intensity shuttle running and fluid ingestion on the performance of a soccer skill. J Sports Sci 1999; 17: 895–903.

Meltzer ST, Fuller C. Eating for Sport. London: New Holland Publishers, 2005.

Meltzer ST, Fuller C. Practical Nutrition for Rugby. www.sarugby.co.za/boksmart/Default.aspx?contentId=18731

Monpetit RR. Sports medicine. Sports Med 1990; 10: 31–41.

Noakes TD. Drinking guidelines for exercise: what evidence is there that athletes should drink 'as much as tolerable', 'to replace the weight lost during exercise' or 'ad libitum'? J Sports Sci 2007; 25: 781–796.

O'Connor H, Caterson I. Weight loss and the athlete. In: Clinical Sports Nutrition, 3rd edn (Burke L, Deakin V, eds). Sydney, Australia: McGraw-Hill, 2006, pp 135–165.

Rodríguez NR, Dimarco NM, Langley S. American College of Sports Medicine position stand. Nutrition and athletic performance. Med Sci Sports Exerc 2009; 41: 709–731.

Sawka MN, Burke LM, Eichner ER, Maughan RJ, Montain SJ, Stachenfeld NS. American College of Sports Medicine position stand. Exercise and fluid replacement. Med Sci Sports Exerc 2007; 39: 377–390.

Schneiker KT, Bishop D, Dawson B, Hackett LP. Effects of caffeine on prolonged intermittent-sprint ability in team-sport athletes. Med Sci Sports Exerc 2006; 38: 578–585.

Stuart GR, Hopkins WG, Cook C, Cairns SP. Multiple effects of caffeine on simulated high-intensity team-sport performance. Med Sci Sports Exerc 2005; 37: 1998–2005.

Tarnopolsky M. Protein and amino acid needs for training and bulking up. In: Clinical Sports Nutrition, 3rd edn (Burke L, Deakin V, eds). Sydney, Australia: McGraw-Hill, 2006, pp 73–103.

Tarnopolsky MA, Bosman M, Macdonald JR, Vandeputte D, Martin J, Roy BD. Post-exercise protein–carbohydrate and carbohydrate supplements increase muscle glycogen in men and women. J Appl Physiol 1997; 83: 1877–1883.

Tipton KD, Wolfe RR. Protein and amino acids for athletes. J Sports Sci 2004; 22: 65–79.

Tipton KD, Rasmussen BB, Miller SI et al. Timing of amino acid–carbohydrate ingestion alters anabolic response of muscle to resistance exercise. Am J Physiol 2001; 281: E197–E206.

Winnick JJ, Davis JM, Welsh RS, Carmichael MD, Murphy EA, Blackmon JA. Carbohydrate feedings during team sport exercise preserve physical and CNS function. Med Sci Sports Exerc 2005; 37: 306–315.

Zawadski KM, Yaspelkis BB, Ivy JL. Carbohydrate–protein complex increases the rate of muscle glycogen storage after exercise. J Appl Physiol 1992; 72: 1854–1859.

Zemel MB. Role of calcium and dairy products in energy portioning and weight management. Am J Clin Nutr 2004; 79: 907S–912S.

15
Nutrition for Disability Athletes

Jeanette Crosland and Elizabeth Broad

Key messages

- There is limited research available on athletes with disabilities.
- Athletes with a disability should be considered to have the same sports nutrition demands as able-bodied athletes; however, the application of nutrition recommendations may require some modification.
- Individual assessment of each athlete is vital.
- It is important for the sports nutrition practitioner to spend time understanding the specific disability classifications, rules of sport, and the physiological and medical implications of an athlete's disability.

15.1 Introduction

The focus of most sports nutrition research and texts is on able-bodied athletes. The number of sports and events in which disability athletes are given the opportunity to compete is expanding, the number of athletes within a class is increasing, and hence disability sport continues to become more competitive. The exposure of these athletes to exercise science and nutrition education has lagged behind that of their able-bodied counterparts, with the focus often being more on their underlying medical conditions rather than 'performance'. This is exacerbated by the fact that the range of disabilities and the variations in functionality between, and even within, a class make publishing research on disability athletes in peer-reviewed journals difficult due to relatively small subject numbers in each group.

Readers are encouraged to begin by considering disability athletes to be the same as their able-bodied counterparts when it comes to the physiological demands of their sport and the specific nutrition issues which need to be considered for training and competition. This chapter aims to describe the unique physiological and medical aspects of athletes in disability sport, highlighting the primary differences which practitioners need to consider when working with disability athletes compared with able-bodied

athletes. In many instances the challenges lie more in the practical nature of sports nutrition delivery, whereas in others the challenge will be in the assessment of physiological demand. Either way, working with these athletes can be challenging, but is equally rewarding.

15.2 Disability sport

Disability sport began as part of the rehabilitation process and Dr Ludwig Guttmann began the original move into the competitive arena when he established the first ever 'disability' games in 1948 at Stoke Mandeville Hospital in the UK, inviting sporting clubs and other hospitals to take part. In 1984 the first Paralympic Games (meaning the Parallel Games, as it was planned to run in parallel with the Olympics) were held in Stoke Mandeville and also in New York. In 1988 the Paralympic Games joined the Olympic timetable with athletes competing in Seoul. In 1976 the first Paralympic Winter Games were held in Ornskoldsvick in Sweden, again joining the Olympic cycle in 1994 at Lillehammer in Norway. Now, the Paralympic Winter and Summer Games are held 2 weeks following the Olympics, in the same city and same venues. Paralympic events are also integrated into many individual sports' world championships and a limited range of classes/events

---

Sport and Exercise Nutrition, First Edition. Edited by Susan A Lanham-New, Samantha J Stear, Susan M Shirreffs and Adam L Collins.
© 2011 The Nutrition Society. Published 2011 by Blackwell Publishing Ltd.

Table 15.1 Sports currently included in Paralympic competition.

Summer sports
Archery
Athletics
Basketball
Boccia
Cycling
Equestrian
Fencing
Football 5-a-side
Football 7-a-side
Goalball
Judo
Powerlifting
Rowing
Rugby
Sailing
Shooting
Swimming
Table tennis
Tennis
Volleyball

Winter sports
Alpine skiing
Nordic skiing
Ice sledge hockey
Wheelchair curling

are included within major events such as the Commonwealth Games.

Athletes now train and compete at an elite level and Table 15.1 shows the current summer and winter sports which are included in the Paralympic Games. This list continues to expand. For example, wheelchair dance is now included as an International Paralympic Committee (IPC) sport but is not included in the Games, and paratriathlon and paracanoeing are likely to be introduced into the Paralympic Games in 2016 (www.paralympic.org).

15.3 Classification in disability sport

There are a number of sporting categories where disability athletes can compete, even though not all categories are represented in the Paralympic Games. These include the following.

- *Athletes with cerebral palsy (CP).* There are a range of categories within this grouping where athletes display permanent disabling symptoms, primarily affecting voluntary control of musculature, and this group also includes individuals who have suffered a stroke or head injury. At one end of the spectrum athletes have minimal disability and, whilst able to compete in a running event, may suffer from balance and coordination problems. More severely affected athletes will be able to walk, although their legs and/or arms may be unable to perform a normal range of movements with complete control. Some athletes use wheelchairs for daily life, or just to compete. At the most severely affected end of the spectrum, athletes have movement problems that affect the entire body and are unable to propel a manual wheelchair. They would normally live and compete in an electric wheelchair and will often have difficulty with hand movement control.

- *Athletes who use wheelchairs.* This includes those with spinal cord lesions, spina bifida and polio. Athletes in this category are defined by the point and completeness of injury on the spinal column and the effect this has on the functionality of the individual (Figure 15.1). Athletes with other medical conditions may compete in a wheelchair even if they do not use one on a regular basis.

- *Athletes with amputations, dwarfism or 'les autres' conditions.* This category accommodates athletes with physical disabilities not covered by other sports organisations and classification systems, including Friedreich's ataxia, multiple sclerosis, severe burns, muscular dystrophies, and lower-limb deformities.

- *Athletes who are visually impaired.* This impairment can range from partial visual impairment to total blindness. Competitors in this category will normally compete with a 'buddy' or companion/guide.

- *Athletes who are deaf.* This is defined as those who have lost at least 55 decibels in the better hearing ear. There are specific sporting events organised for the deaf but they do not currently compete in the Paralympic Games.

- *Athletes with cognitive or intellectual disabilities.* This category has proven to be difficult to truly assess in the past, and the category was removed from the Paralympic Games after 2000. Improved guidelines for classification were called for, and at present this category is likely to be reintroduced. It includes a range of clinical disorders, including Down's syndrome, but three key factors must be complied with: IQ less than 75, age of onset under 18 years, and limitations in adaptive behaviour.

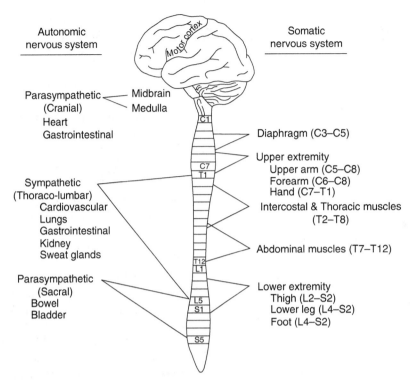

Figure 15.1 Diagrammatic illustration of the central nervous system and the outflow levels for the somatic and autonomic nervous system neurones. General innervations from each spinal cord level are indicated. (Reproduced from Glaser 1985, with permission from Wolters Kluwer Health.)

There are classification systems which group athletes together in order that they can fairly compete against each other. The classification is based on functional ability of the athlete and therefore athletes with different physical disabilities may compete in the same sport. For example, wheelchair basketball may include those with spinal cord injury, amputation or 'les autres' (other) conditions. Each athlete must compete seated in a wheelchair and individual players are allocated a classification point based on their functional ability. Each wheelchair basketball team can only have a set number of total points on the court at any time, which effectively means a minimum number of low classification players. In contrast, goalball is a sport in which only visually impaired athletes can compete. In some cases, the rules governing a disability sport are different to those of the able-bodied sport (e.g. rowing distances are 1000 m rather than 2000 m). These rules can change rapidly as the sports governing bodies move to greater equality, so practitioners are encouraged to familiarise themselves with the rules and current

'performance' standards when working with disability athletes. Further information about the rules governing each sport and classification can be obtained from the IPC website (www.paralympic.org).

15.4 Energy requirements

Energy requirements are well understood in able-bodied sport; however in disability sport there is little scientific evidence on which to base the assessments of individuals. Earlier chapters in this book examined the differences in energy and nutritional requirements with respect to the type of sport being undertaken and in broad terms these principles hold true in disability sport. However, within the umbrella of disability sport there is a wide range of energy requirements based on the physiology of the sport and functional capabilities of the individual athlete. Unfortunately few researchers have quantified values for energy intake, resting energy expenditure, or the energy expenditure of activity in disability athletes.

Much of the work that has been carried out on energy expenditure has focused on athletes with spinal cord injury (SCI) (i.e. paraplegic and tetraplegic/quadriplegic individuals). Other information can be gleaned from research carried out with non-athletic populations with SCI. Where a spinal cord lesion has occurred, there is a reduced muscle mass below the lesion and the athlete also has a reduced maximal heart rate. Lowered resting metabolic rates have been recorded, and thus total daily energy expenditure has also been shown to be lower. Consequently, the energy requirements of athletes with SCI are likely to be lower than those expected for able-bodied athletes. Where the facility to measure energy expenditure exists there is little problem in matching intake to expenditure, but in many cases energy requirements are calculated based on equations. The information currently available would suggest that energy requirements could be up to 30% lower in wheelchair athletes with SCI when compared with calculations made using standard prediction equations, and the deficit increases the higher the level of SC lesion. One recent paper outlines the estimated energy expenditure of activities (including exercise) in SCI individuals, based on measures undertaken in a non-athlete sample (Collins et al., 2010). This represents the most comprehensive activity-related data to date on this group, and whilst it is likely to be a useful resource it must be noted that many of the figures provided are based on very small sample sizes (two to three individuals), especially for females. The diet of wheelchair athletes therefore needs to focus on nutrient-dense foods and appropriate energy and macronutrient intakes, as an excessive energy intake will result in increased body fat which can hinder wheelchair propulsion. Some wheelchair users may be prone to pressure sores, and it may be necessary at times to increase energy intake to assist with the healing process.

Athletes who are visually impaired or deaf or who have cognitive disabilities will have functional and physiological capabilities that are generally the same as able-bodied athletes and therefore are likely to have comparable energy requirements. However, practical factors such as access to shopping, cooking facilities, feeding difficulties and social activity may have an effect on the types of food contained in the daily diet, and the amount of energy consumed and expended on a daily basis. This may impact on the body mass and composition of the individual, necessitating dietary management to either lose body fat or gain muscle mass.

Athletes with CP will have varying energy needs depending on their mode of ambulation. Some athletes with CP have minimal disruption to physical capabilities and therefore will exhibit similar energy expenditures to able-bodied individuals. Those who use a wheelchair may have lowered energy requirements, and some athletes in, for example, field athletics or boccia may use an electric wheelchair, thereby possibly reducing energy expenditure even further. In contrast, many athletes with CP have athetosis: muscle spasm that results in irregular jerky movements. Whilst these uncontrolled spasms can increase the energy expenditure of the individual, they can also limit the voluntary activity of the individual thereby negating the increase in energy expended. Furthermore, some athletes may have physical feeding difficulties that may limit energy intake and it may be necessary to consider supplemental feeding. Each athlete will need to be assessed on an individual basis and regular assessment of body composition/body mass and training capability may assist in ascertaining energy requirements.

Athletes with amputations and a number of those athletes classified as 'les autres' will have an altered gait when walking, which can increase their energy requirement. However this altered gait may also limit the amount of 'free' activity within a day. In amputee athletes there is also a reduced lean muscle mass which may reduce resting energy expenditure. Hence the net result may be an energy requirement which is not elevated above that of a sedentary able-bodied individual of similar body size.

Together with the lack of research on energy expenditure in disability athletes, there is also a lack of reported dietary intakes in this athlete population. Many disability athletes take up sport as part of their rehabilitation process, suggesting that their original framework will have been a rehabilitation-based one. It is vital for the practitioner to consider the stage of recovery from trauma of the individual. There will have been a progression in nutritional terms, starting with a high energy intake to support the initial recovery, usually followed by energy restriction to assist the loss of body fat. The sports nutritionist or dietitian meeting these individuals as athletes may feel that they are under-reporting their intake. An inadequate energy intake can compromise the ability to gain muscle mass, restrict training capability, and may increase their risk of illness and injury. Conversely, the difficulty in estimating energy expenditure can result in the practitioner over-estimating energy requirements, which can result in prescription of a dietary intake that results in body fat gain and subsequent restriction of mobility. In these situations, a stepwise progression of dietary intake towards more 'optimal' levels could be undertaken with frequent reviews to determine the response, considering not only body composition (more so than body mass) changes along with training responses.

In summary, while future research into energy intakes and expenditure would make the process simpler, each athlete must be individually assessed in terms of their energy requirements. It is important for practitioners to recognise where the limitations lie in using equations to estimate energy expenditure in the disability sport population, as well as understanding not only the physiological demands of their sport but also the nature of their non-exercise-related activity. Applying a flexible approach in providing nutritional advice, with regular assessment of body composition changes and training responses, is crucial. Practitioners should allocate time to observe athletes in their sporting environment and discuss progress with coaches and other support staff in order to better understand the impact of dietary changes. Practitioners are encouraged to report their findings wherever possible in order to add to the literature available.

15.5 Carbohydrate requirements

Very little research has been undertaken on carbohydrate (CHO) requirements of disability athletes. Therefore, assessing the CHO needs of this group of athletes requires an understanding of the physiological demands of exercise and the basis upon which CHO recommendations for athletes are made (see Chapter 4). Whilst it might be reasonable to assume CHO requirements will be the same as for able-bodied athletes undertaking the same type of events, there remain a number of crucial questions which have not yet been answered. Most of these relate to assessing the relative intensity of effort performed.

Wheelchair users, regardless of the cause of their disability, use upper body musculature in the trunk and arms for mobility. There is growing evidence in the literature on physiological aspects of wheelchair performance (e.g. with regard to percentage of $V_{O_{2max}}$ or peak power output) which will enable a reasonable estimate of likely CHO usage to be made. Indications are that the proportional use of CHO and fat as fuel sources in trained SCI athletes is similar to that of trained able-bodied athletes at the same relative exercise intensity. The primary question is whether the storage capacity for glycogen is the same in upper body musculature as it is for the lower body. The only report available regarding muscle glycogen usage of wheelchair athletes provided evidence that the rate of glycogen usage during exercise was similar to the rate of glycogen usage in able-bodied athletes, although the total glycogen store available at the start of exercise was lower. If this is the case, the reliance on exogenous CHO sources in endurance exercise is likely to be higher in wheelchair athletes.

While there is no physiological difference within the active muscles of visually impaired athletes compared with their able-bodied counterparts, the speed or pace of performance tends to decrease with increasing visual impairment. For example, the world record at present for the T11 (greatest visual impairment) category 5-km track event is 15 min 11.07 s compared with 12 min 37.00 s for able-bodied males. In some activities, the slower pace will potentially result in a reduced demand on CHO as a fuel source. Hence, it becomes important to understand the intensity of effort relative to the individual athlete's maximal capacity, along with the duration of the event and the training state as these are all known to influence CHO requirements, especially in events where CHO availability may limit performance. Some visually impaired athletes may also have diabetes, so consideration should be made as to the distribution of CHO at each meal and snack with their diabetes management. It is important that athletes with diabetes consume sufficient CHO to support their training.

Dietary CHO recommendations for athletes with disabilities will also need to be considered in relationship to total energy requirements. It may be necessary to set a CHO intake at the lower end of recommended intakes in order to allow room for sufficient protein and some dietary fat if energy budgets are restricted. In a similar way to estimating energy requirements, there will need to be some 'trial and error' involved in recommending appropriate CHO intakes in disability athletes.

15.6 Protein and amino acid requirements

Whilst protein requirements are continually a subject of research in the sporting world, there is a dearth of information regarding the protein requirements of disability athletes. The principles of requirement will most likely be the same for disability athletes as for able-bodied athletes, and the need to ensure adequate total daily intake plus protein intake for optimal post-exercise recovery remains important.

It should be remembered that in disability sport there may be athletes with medical conditions having renal involvement. It is important that those working in this field undertake a good medical history as part of an initial assessment of an athlete and check whether there are any renal issues to consider.

One area of particular note is with visually impaired athletes, where the visual impairment may be a result of diabetes, indicating that the individual is already presenting with macular degeneration. Where diabetes exists, the recommendations for protein intake for other potential complications of diabetes should be considered before the requirement for exercise. This is one area where health may override sport in terms of requirements, and it may be necessary to prescribe protein intakes at the lower end of the range recommended for athletes (see Chapter 5). When working with athletes who have diabetes it is important that practitioners ensure that they have all the necessary medical information available, while non-clinical practitioners should seek advice from the medical team working with the athlete, remembering to obtain the athlete's permission first. The website www.runsweet.com is a useful source of information about diabetes and sport.

15.7 Fat

As with dietary protein, there have been no studies published in disability athletes regarding dietary fat requirements. In balancing energy intake with energy expenditure, dietary fat may be one macronutrient which could be manipulated to ensure that sufficient CHO and protein are consumed. Further, considering some potential medical complications of disability (e.g. wound healing and coexisting diabetes), the consumption of unsaturated and ω-3 fats may be more important to emphasise in this athlete population. The consideration of potential interactions with medication (such as warfarin) must also be made.

15.8 Fluid and electrolytes

All athletes should be aware of their own sweat rate and should plan their fluid intakes accordingly during and after exercise. Assessment of hydration status and/or sweat rates can be undertaken as discussed in Chapter 7, although assessment of hydration status from visual scales of urine colour can be influenced by medications, inducing a mismatch between colour and hydration status. Those using catheters and bags will also see a change in the colour of urine so, where possible, urine specific gravity (USG) of a single morning urine sample is the preferred method. It is important to note that many wheelchair-bound athletes will deliberately induce a degree of dehydration overnight in order to manage toileting needs. This must be clarified with individuals and should not be deemed an inappropriate course of action, although some improvements in fluid intake and timing may be possible in order to prevent severe dehydration. A check should be made to ensure the athlete has regained euhydration prior to exercise, wherever possible using USG, bearing in mind the likely effect of a recent bolus of fluid on USG and colour readings (see Chapter 7). Where regular testing of USG is not possible, an initial comparison of urine colour to USG will allow individual athletes to recognise which colours they should relate to on a colour chart, and therefore target, to achieve euhydration.

When considering the fluid needs of disability athletes the group which generally requires the greatest attention are wheelchair users who have SCI. Athletes with a SCI down the spine will have some use of the sympathetic nervous system, especially if the lesion is incomplete. Those with higher lesions will have a more limited capacity to utilise this system. The sympathetic nervous system is involved in the rate of blood flow to the skin and also in the sweat rate of an individual. Therefore those with SCI will have a reduced sweat rate and the rate of sweat loss will be proportional to the area of skin able to produce sweat (i.e. the area of skin with remaining neural innervation). There is some evidence that sweat rates above the lesion may actually be increased in order to aid temperature control. Hence, in practice, whilst the sweat rate of an individual athlete can be quite consistent session to session, sweat rates vary substantially between individuals with SCI even when they have similar levels of cord lesion, highlighting the importance of individual assessments and fluid intake recommendations. Regardless of sweating capacity, SCI athletes are generally considered to be compromised in terms of their thermal regulation and hence at greater risk of heat exhaustion, with the risk increasing in higher levels of spinal cord lesion. Other factors may also impair thermoregulation in wheelchair users, such as anticholinergic drugs used to control muscle spasm and the positioning of the athlete's body and style of movement within the wheelchair. Thermal regulation may be an issue in less active sports, such as shooting, archery and field athletics, where exposure to sun and heat can result in heat gain from the environment even without physical exertion. Consequently, some athletes will use cooling strategies such as cooling vests or hand cooling to help maintain appropriate body temperatures before, during or after competition. Simple measures such as the use of shade, water sprays or cold wet towels to the head and neck have also proven to be effective in helping this process. However, it should be remembered that the effect of cooling may result in athletes drinking a reduced fluid volume as their perceived exertion is reduced, as can be the desire to drink. Conversely, in cool environmental conditions, SCI athletes may require active heating due to their impaired ability to constrict peripheral blood vessels to promote heat retention.

The practical issue of toilet access will influence the athlete's desire to take fluid on board. In certain sports, such as alpine skiing, toilet access can be very difficult and in others such as wheelchair tennis some players have their racket taped to their hand. Similarly, some disability athletes may have had gastrointestinal surgery resulting in colostomy or ileostomy use. Intakes of large volumes of fluid at one time should be avoided due to the risk of 'dumping' from the stoma, especially for ileostomies. Balancing good hydration with practical issues can therefore be challenging. Fluids used for sport will be similar to those used by able-bodied athletes but hydration monitoring is key to ensuring appropriate intake, which may be lower.

Autonomic dysreflexia (AD) is an issue for athletes with SCI at a level of T6 and above. AD is a potentially life-threatening condition which occurs as a result of uncontrolled reflex sympathetic activity resulting in a significant rise in blood pressure. If untreated, it can result in seizures and intracranial haemorrhage. It occurs as the result of a trauma such as a blocked catheter, over-distension of the bladder, urinary tract infection, constipation, pressure sores or an injury due to poor lifting and movement. Susceptible individuals normally carry medication to treat the condition but in terms of hydration strategies, the sudden intake of large volumes of fluid causing distension to the bladder should be avoided, as should constipation causing extra pressure on the bowel.

Electrolyte intakes assist in the absorption of fluid, and the principles of adding electrolytes to fluids consumed around exercise are the same as for able-bodied athletes. Athletes with raised blood pressure may be reluctant to use sports drinks with added sodium. There is, to date, no research on this issue, but the use of sports drinks at specific times to help optimise hydration, and fuelling, may be advantageous even in individuals with raised blood pressure. It may be advisable to discuss this issue with the athlete's doctor.

Other groups of disability athletes are likely to have fluid requirements which are similar to those of able-bodied athletes. Athletes with CP, who experience frequent athetosis or muscle spasm, may have raised sweat rates. As with able-bodied athletes, individual assessment of sweat losses and fluid intakes are encouraged, and the physical and practical issues of accessing fluids in all groups should be remembered.

15.9 Micronutrients and other nutrients

As Chapter 8 outlines, the micronutrient needs of athletes are generally considered to be no different to those of the general population, other than iron. Furthermore, it is generally believed that the higher energy intakes of athletes (if attained through a range of nutritious foods) will meet any greater micronutrient needs. This may not be an accurate assumption to make in disability athletes, particularly where energy requirements are relatively low. It is therefore important to also consider nutrient density when prescribing diets for disability athletes.

The bone density of individuals with SCI is known to be lower below the level of the spinal cord lesion compared with able-bodied controls. Similarly to other athletes, however, the bone density of the primary 'movers', or limbs which take the largest load in movement, are higher than sedentary controls. Lower bone density is also common in athletes with CP whose mobility is reduced. Therefore, it is difficult to ascertain whether calcium requirements are different to those of the general population.

Since many athletes train indoors, and some disability athletes may have restricted mobility which limits their daily outdoor exposure, the nutrient requiring greater consideration in this group may be vitamin D. Vitamin D is an essential nutrient for optimising bone density, but has also been shown to be important in inflammation and immune and muscle function. Vitamin D status has been shown to be declining in many countries, and is exacerbated by the wearing of clothing that covers most of the body (e.g. the lower limbs of wheelchair-dependent athletes), a reduced total surface area which can be exposed to sunlight (as in amputees), and/or the use of certain medications. If increasing exposure to sunlight (e.g. 5–30 min/day on face, hands, arms and back without sunscreen depending on latitude, season and skin pigmentation, avoiding the middle of the day) is not viable, it is important to ensure adequate dietary vitamin D intake or supplementation with vitamin D ($1000–2000\,IU/day$ vitamin D_3) is necessary. Foods rich in vitamin D include cod liver oil and oily fish, although many countries allow fortification of milk and margarines, so it is necessary to check food labels.

Iron requirements of athletes with a disability are unknown. In many instances, it could be assumed that dietary iron requirements are similar to those of able-bodied counterparts. However, there may also be many athletes whose dietary requirements are not elevated above the sedentary population due to their mode of mobilisation (e.g. wheelchair athletes) since the 'impact' damage to red blood cells is reduced.

Finally, dietary fibre may require greater consideration in disability athletes. Restricted mobility can influence bowel motility, as can injuries involving the gastrointestinal tract. Bowel function may therefore be altered, especially in athletes with SCI. Constipation, and the use of stool softeners, is common in SCI. Furthermore, bowel movements may need to be well controlled in these athletes so that they occur at a convenient time when access to a bathroom is easy. Athletes who undertake manual evacuation need to allow sufficient time for this process and early-morning activities may mean a very early start for these athletes. Therefore, any consideration of a change in fibre intake should be discussed with the athlete and/or carer.

15.10 Supplements and ergogenic aids

As with able-bodied athletes, although there are many athletes who will not require, nor benefit from, a nutritional supplement or ergogenic aid, there may be occasions where consideration for this is warranted. As outlined in Chapter 9, the decision to use a supplement should be made on an individual basis, be evidence-based, and must ensure that safe sources are used.

Sports drinks are likely to be useful for disability athletes who are training or performing over prolonged periods or in the heat. Athletes who need to restrict calories may find water, with a calorie-free flavouring and added salt, a better alternative to use routinely, saving sports drinks for specific occasions. Similarly, sports gels, bars and liquid meal supplements may provide a useful adjunct to food in athletes with a disability and should be considered according to nutrient and energy needs, timing and practicality.

There may be some individuals where nutritional intake is restricted either for body fat reduction or due to feeding difficulties. In these athletes a broad-spectrum vitamin and mineral supplement may be beneficial.

Although no research has been undertaken on ergogenic aids in disability athletes, their potential use should only be considered once an athlete has achieved a consistently high level of training and competition and displayed appropriate dietary management. For example, powerlifters may benefit from creatine supplementation, whilst middle-distance track and swimming athletes may benefit from products which enhance buffering capabilities. As with energy and CHO requirements, consideration of the suitability of an ergogenic aid requires a complete understanding of the physiological demands of the event/sport and the individual athlete. In the case of disability athletes, medical backgrounds should also be considered.

There are a small number of occasions where caution may be required when considering supplementation.

- Athletes with renal impairment should not use creatine or protein-based supplements.
- Athletes with diabetes may have a higher risk of renal impairment and it may be useful to involve the medical team in discussion concerning supplementation if it is being considered by a squad.
- Athletes with diabetes may use sports drinks during their training and competition but it is important to ensure that the quantities are being controlled in a way that is appropriate to the type of diabetes and treatment of the individual.
- Individuals who have cardiac arrhythmias or palpitations should speak to their physician before using any form of caffeine. Similarly, individuals with some medical conditions may be prone to hyperactivity and caffeine could potentially have an adverse effect on performance.
- Individuals whose medication may interact with any particular supplement. An understanding of medications is important.

15.11 Body composition assessment

The assessment of body composition changes over time is a useful adjunct in determining effectiveness of training prescription and its interaction with dietary intake. This is equally important in an athlete with a disability as it is in the able-bodied athlete population, and is particularly important when the suitability of dietary changes are being evaluated. As outlined in Chapter 17, there are several techniques which can be used to assess body composition in athletes.

The interpretation of body mass and simple body composition evaluations such as body mass index (BMI) in a disability group can be problematic. SCI and spina bifida result in muscle atrophy and bone resorption, both of which influence absolute mass. Similarly, since methods involving estimation of body density (such as underwater weighing and densitometry) assume a constant density of all tissues, many of these assumptions are violated in situations where muscle atrophy or bone resorption are present. Stretch stature can also be difficult to accurately estimate in athletes with CP, SCI and spina bifida, which limits the appropriateness of bioelectrical impedance. This is exacerbated by the fact that there is evidence that the composition and resistivity of the fat-free mass alters following SCI. Waist girth correlates strongly with body fat (assessed by dual X-ray absorptiometry or DEXA) in individuals with SCI. The use of DEXA has been shown to be valid for assessing body composition changes in athletes with SCI by some researchers, although the positioning of some wheelchair users needs further investigation as it may affect the validity of repeat assessments. Whilst becoming more common, it remains an expensive and often difficult-to-access tool. The validity of using DEXA for body composition assessment in amputees and dwarfs has not been assessed.

Many body composition assessment methods rely on assumptions and/or regression equations based on data taken from able-bodied individuals, and hence may not be valid in a disabled athlete group. Skinfold results should always be reported as a sum of skinfolds, rather than attempting to convert to a percentage body fat through the use of regression equations. Similarly, certain techniques are not appropriate, or may require modification, in a disabled athlete population. For example, a sum of seven skinfolds cannot be obtained from a bilateral leg amputee, and may not be appropriate in an individual with SCI and substantial muscle atrophy in the lower limbs. Similarly, skinfolds can be difficult to obtain in athletes with burns. In athletes with muscle atrophy (SCI, some CP, and spina bifida), taking skinfold measures can be problematic as it can be more difficult to differentiate the fat component of the skinfolds. Hence, it is more appropriate to use limbs where muscle atrophy is less substantial (e.g. use the alternate side of the body in an athlete with unilateral atrophy), or to reduce the number of sites from which skinfolds are taken (sum of four sites: bicep, tricep, subscapular and abdominal) in a wheelchair-bound athlete.

Dwarfs can exhibit very different body shapes, and with this comes a different body composition with higher fat levels, the alteration of which may prove to be difficult. Standard body composition data cannot be used for comparison.

Finally, very little has been published in this athlete population to use as normative data for physique traits or to consider in relation to performance. It is recognised that bone density and muscle mass is higher, and body fat lower, in the upper body of athletes with SCI than their sedentary counterparts. Hence, the effective use of body composition assessment in a disability athlete is essential and the valid interpretation of results relies on an understanding of the underlying assumptions and limitations of the technique used. Recording time since onset of injury, the specific nature of disability (e.g. level of spinal cord lesion, complete or incomplete lesion, amputee compared with congenital malformation) and competitive classification of the athlete is important when undertaking body composition assessments in athletes with a disability so that, over time, the potential to pool data for analysis is possible.

15.12 Practical aspects

When starting work with a disability athlete or squad, practitioners should take the time to get to know the sport. Observing training and competition, familiarising with the physiology, and checking the rules (they may be different to the able-bodied version of the sport) will help the practitioner understand the athletes' needs. A medical assessment of each player is essential for ascertaining any problems which may relate to nutrition, and non-clinically trained staff must be aware of professional boundaries.

If the disability of the athlete is acquired and relatively new, the individual may be working with psychological support to overcome issues, some of which may relate to nutrition. Communication with coaches and other practitioners working with the athlete can be invaluable.

It is important to ask athletes about their disability and how they cope with a range of issues such as accessing food, toilet facilities, catheterisation (for SCI), independence in daily life, whether they have spasms, medications, medical complications, etc. Some athletes may want other individuals, who are heavily involved in the daily care or living habits of the athlete, to be present at consultations.

15.13 Daily life

There are a number of disability groups where shopping and feeding may need extra consideration. Families, partners, carers or other significant individuals may need to be included in advice concerning food intake and it should be established how the athlete will cope with shopping and cooking issues. Internet-based ordering and home delivery of groceries can be a useful tool in athletes with limited mobility. Practical cookery sessions may help and when planning such a session, a few checks will help things go smoothly, such as the following.

- For wheelchair users ensure that the work surface to be used is at a suitable height. Similarly it is important that the sink/cooker/microwave are accessible from chair height.
- For visually impaired athletes discuss how to maintain a safe environment with regard to pans, hot dishes, knives, etc. Using ready prepared or frozen vegetables, for example, can be much safer and easier than peeling and preparing vegetables. Visually impaired individuals are generally familiar with using a clock system for direction, which can be a useful tool in setting up a kitchen or serving a meal.
- Athletes with leg amputations may be able to stand and cook but may need a stool or chair of an appropriate height to rest occasionally. Practical shopping sessions should be kept to less than 1 hour to prevent fatigue in these individuals.
- Athletes with CP and those with compromised arms (amputees, malformations) may require modified recipes to simplify the process of meal preparation, especially with regard to cutting and peeling. These athletes should be carefully observed during practical cooking sessions and support equipment may be required to improve safety. It is also important to recognise that food preparation can take longer for these athletes, since tasks like chopping can be more time-consuming. It is important to develop a range of meal options which involve less preparation time yet retain the nutritional value.

Some athletes may employ methods of eating which are unusual to you. For example those with no hands may use their feet to eat, and visually impaired individuals may use a clock system to identify where their food is on the plate and will need someone to describe that position. Visually impaired athletes will also require assistance in familiarising themselves to a new food environment, especially where buffet service is involved, in order to locate food items. Wheelchair users may need assistance to serve food in a self-service situation and to carry trays to their seat. Athletes with learning disabilities may have unusual reactions or apparent 'fear' of eating some foods. This can be very challenging to overcome and will take time and patience to ensure adequate nutrition is achieved. Occasionally supplementary feeding may be required.

15.14 Travel

When travelling with a squad of disability athletes, an advance visit to the hotel and training complex is very useful. It will help to identify any issues with wheelchair access and provide an insight into any potential issues relating to food as well as other aspects of daily life. If this is not possible, details should be actively sought from the team manager and/or other key staff to assist with the planning of meals, training snacks, fluids and other activities. Athletes should consider the implications of travel.

- Wheelchair athletes undertaking flights will commonly restrict their fluid intake prior to and during the flight. Despite requesting aisle seats with the best toilet access, the limited width of aisles, manoeuvrability, and size of toilets can be a significant deterrent to wheelchair-bound athletes. Athletes who intermittently catheterise may have a more comfortable journey if they use a bag for flights.
- Athletes who use catheters should carry sufficient equipment to last the journey, and some may find it useful to carry other equipment such as raised toilet seats.
- Remind athletes to keep their drinks bottle with them on the flight. Storing it in the luggage compartment will make life difficult for many disability athletes.
- Athletes who take medication for a medical condition should carry a letter from their doctor confirming the need to use the medication and it is advisable to check that the medications are legal in the country to be visited.
- When organising insurance, any existing medical conditions must be declared or insurance will be invalid.

Practice tips

- Become familiar with the rules of play and physiology of disability sport before working with the athletes.
- Each athlete must be assessed individually in terms of their nutritional needs. The techniques used to assess nutrient requirements may be the same as for able-bodied athletes, but for disability athletes there are a number of additional questions that need addressing. It is important to gather information regarding the duration, type and cause of disability, mobility, medications, feeding issues and medical considerations.
- Practice similar assessments as you would an able-bodied athlete in terms of determining requirements before, during and after training and the demands of their training and competition loads.
- Assessment of body composition change over time is as equally important in disability athletes as it is in able-bodied athletes. However, limitations of techniques must be understood and the appropriate techniques may require some modification.
- Make sure that you are familiar with any pre-existing medical issues, along with any that may arise during the course of your involvement with the athlete. If you are not clinically qualified seek appropriate help.
- Consider the practical issues involved in shopping, cooking and eating for the athletes you are working with.
- It is extremely important to include support personnel and carers in any nutritional education sessions.
- The energy requirements of some disability athletes may be very different to the normal standards for able-bodied athletes. The consumption of nutrient-dense foods is a high priority for maintaining nutritional quality in those with energy-restricted diets. Athletes with disabilities who travel or eat out frequently may need extra guidance. Small changes in energy intake can have a larger impact on body fat and mass in this population, and in some subgroups making small changes can have a fairly major psychological impact. Conversely, some individuals have high energy requirements, and may require energy supplements in addition to high-energy foods and fluids.
- When advising about fluid intake, ask athletes how they manage their bladder control and the likely effects of increasing fluid intake. Be willing to trial strategies in conjunction with the athlete to come up with the best scenario and look at additional cooling methods for those with SCI.
- When assessing hydration status, wherever possible encourage measurement of USG rather than just using a visual assessment.
- If working as part of a team, or in an unfamiliar environment for the athletes, you may be required to provide some assistance. For example, visually impaired athletes will generally require assistance in orientation and locating food and utensils at a dining hall when they first arrive. If operating from self-contained units, it is best to room them with sighted athletes who understand how to explain the presentation of food on a plate (such as the clock system). Depending on the disability, assistance with carrying food to the table and cutting up food may be required.

Further reading

Abel T, Platen P, Rojas Vega S, Schneider S, Struder HK. Energy expenditure in ball games for wheelchair users. Spinal Cord 2008; 46: 785–790.

Broad EM. The effects of heat on performance in wheelchair shooters. Masters thesis, University of Canberra, Canberra, 1997.

Bulbulian R, Johnson RE, Gruber JJ, Darabos B. Body composition in paraplegic male athletes. Med Sci Sports Exerc 1997; 19: 195–201.

Collins EG, Gater D, Kiratli J, Butler J, Hanson K, Langbein WE. Energy cost of physical activities in persons with spinal cord injury. Med Sci Sports Exerc 2010; 42: 691–700.

Genin JJ, Bastien GJ, Franck B, Detrembleur C, Willems PA. Effect of speed on the energy cost of walking in unilateral traumatic lower limb amputees. Eur J Appl Physiol 2008; 103: 655–663.

Glaser RM. Exercise and locomotion for the spinal cord injured. Exerc Sports Sci Rev 1985; 13: 263–303.

Goosey-Tolfrey VL, Crosland J. Nutritional practices of competitive British wheelchair games players. Adapt Phys Activ Q 2010; 27: 47–59.

Goosey-Tolfrey VL, Diaper NJ, Crosland J, Tolfrey K. Fluid intake during wheelchair exercise in the heat: effect of localized cooling garments. Int J Sports Physiol Perform 2008; 3: 145–156.

Johnson RK, Hildreth HG, Contompasis SH, Goran MI. Total energy expenditure in adults with cerebral palsy as assessed by doubly-labeled water. J Am Diet Assoc 1997; 97: 966–970.

Jones LM, Goulding A, Gerrard DF. DXA: a practical and accurate tool to demonstrate total and regional bone loss, lean tissue loss and fat mass gain in paraplegia. Spinal Cord 1998; 36: 637–640.

Knechtle B, Muller G, Willmann F, Eser P, Knecht H. Fat oxidation at different intensities in wheelchair racing. Spinal Cord 2004; 42: 24–28.

Kocina P. Body composition of spinal cord injured adults. Sports Med 1997; 23: 48–60.

Mollinger LA, Spurr GB. Daily energy expenditure and basal metabolic rates of patients with spinal cord injury. Arch Phys Med Rehabil 1985; 66: 420–426.

Monroe MB, Tataranni PA, Pratley R. Lower daily energy expenditure as measured by a respiratory chamber in subjects with spinal cord injury compared with control subjects. Am J Clin Nutr 1998; 68: 1223–1227.

Price MJ. Thermoregulation during exercise in individuals with spinal cord injury. Sports Med 2006; 36: 863–879.

Price MJ, Campbell IG. Effects of spinal cord lesion level upon thermoregulation during exercise in the heat. Med Sci Sports Exerc 2003; 35: 1100–1107.

Skrinar GS, Evans WJ, Ornstein LJ, Brown DA. Glycogen utilisation in wheelchair-dependent athletes. Int J Sports Med 1982; 3: 215–219.

Sutton L, Wallace J, Goosey-Tolfrey V, Scott M, Reilly T. Body composition of female wheelchair athletes. Int J Sports Med 2009; 30: 259–265.

Ward KH, Meyers MC. Exercise performance of lower-extremity amputees. Sports Med 1995; 20: 207–214.

Webborn N, Price MJ, Castle PC, Goosey-Tolfrey VL. Effects of two cooling strategies on thermoregulatory responses of tetraplegic athletes during repeated intermittent exercise in the heat. J Appl Physiol 2005; 98: 2101–2107.

Willis KS, Peterson NJ, Larson-Meyer DE. Should we be concerned about the Vitamin D status of athletes? Int J Sport Nutr Exerc Metab 2008; 18: 204–224.

16
Competition Nutrition

Louise M Burke

Key messages

- Sporting competitions are undertaken in many formats and the nutrition strategies that should be practised will differ between events and even between athletes in the same event.
- The common goal of sports nutrition is to assist the athlete to perform at his or her best using strategies before, during and between events that reduce or delay the onset of factors that would otherwise reduce performance. These factors include inadequate fluid and fuel status, and gastrointestinal problems.
- For events lasting an hour or longer, the athlete should aim to optimise body carbohydrate stores by consuming carbohydrate-rich foods in the hours and day(s) prior to their event. Carbohydrate intake during competition lasting 1 hour or more can enhance performance. Even small amounts can be of benefit

- in shorter events in this range, but as the duration of the event increases, so does the amount of carbohydrate needed to optimise performance.
- Athletes should start competition well hydrated, and consume fluids during the event to minimise the fluid deficit incurred through sweating, especially in hot conditions.
- When an athlete is required to compete in several events in a short period, strategies to enhance recovery of fluid and fuel are important.
- All dietary strategies intended for competition day should be practised in training to develop and fine-tune a personalised approach.

16.1 Introduction

Athletes prepare for weeks, years and even a whole career for a specific competitive event. Sporting competitions vary according to a multitude of factors: the intensity, duration and type of event, the environment in which it is performed, the number and frequency of times the athlete must compete to decide the eventual winner, and whether it is an individual event or a team effort. In some sports, these factors are more or less the same from one competition to the next, while in other sports each competition is literally a new ball game. Despite the diversity of features, competition involves a common theme: athletes desire to perform at their best or at least better than their rivals. This chapter reviews competition eating strategies that can provide an important contribution to achieving this goal. Given the complex range of competition settings and requirements in the world of sport, we will

see that practical solutions to overcome logistical challenges in the field are just as important as the science that provides the evidence base for these strategies.

16.2 Nutrition and fatigue during competition

During most sports there are periods – sometimes intermittently throughout, but particularly towards the end of the event – in which there is a reduction in exercise outputs such as speed, power, time spent in high-intensity activities or skill. Fatigue is the common term used to describe this failure to maintain a desired or optimal sporting output and we might expect the winners of competitive events or athletes who achieve a personal best to be those who fatigue least or less. There are a variety of ways in which exercise fatigue can occur, with nutrition playing a role in many of these (Table 16.1). The

Sport and Exercise Nutrition, First Edition. Edited by Susan A Lanham-New, Samantha J Stear, Susan M Shirreffs and Adam L Collins.
© 2011 The Nutrition Society. Published 2011 by Blackwell Publishing Ltd.

Table 16.1 Factors related to nutrition that could produce fatigue or suboptimal performance during sports competition.

Factor	Description	Examples of high risk/common occurrence in sports
Dehydration	Failure to drink enough fluid to replace sweat losses during an event. May be exacerbated if the athlete begins the event in fluid deficit	Events undertaken in hot conditions, particularly for athletes with high-intensity activity patterns and/or heavy protective garments. Repeated competitions (e.g. tournaments) may increase risk of compounding dehydration from one event to the next
Muscle glycogen depletion	Depletion of important muscle fuel due to high utilisation in a single event and/or poor recovery of stores from previous activity/event. Generally thought to occur in events longer than 90 min	Well known in endurance events such as marathon and distance running, road cycling and Ironman triathlons. May occur in some team sports in 'running' players with large total distances covered at high intensities (e.g. midfield players in football, backs in rugby). Repeated competitions (e.g. tournament) may increase risk of poor refuelling from one match to the next
Hypoglycaemia and failure of blood glucose to provide alternative source of carbohydrate for glycogen-depleted muscle	Mismatch between blood glucose appearance, muscle glucose uptake and muscle requirement for exogenous carbohydrate fuel. New research shows that even in the absence of low blood glucose concentrations or additional muscle carbohydrate demand, carbohydrate intake can enhance performance	May occur in athletes who fail to consume carbohydrate during prolonged events with high carbohydrate demands. Even shorter events of 45–75 min duration may benefit from the carbohydrate intake to promote a 'happy brain' which will choose a faster pacing strategy. This includes half marathon, 40-km time trial and many team games
Disturbance of muscle acid–base balance	High rates of H^+ production via anaerobic glycolytic power system	Prolonged high-intensity activities lasting 1–8 min, e.g. rowing events, middle-distance running, 200–800 m swimming, track cycling team pursuit. May also occur in events with repeated sustained periods of high-intensity activity, perhaps in some team games and racquet sports
Depletion of phosphocreatine stores	Inadequate recovery of phosphocreatine system of power production leading to gradual decline in power output in subsequent efforts	Occurs in events with repeated efforts of high-intensity activity with short recovery internals, perhaps in some team games and racquet sports
Gastrointestinal disturbances	Disturbances such as vomiting and diarrhoea may directly reduce performance as well as interfere with nutritional strategies aimed at managing fluid and fuel status	Poorly chosen intake of food and fluid before and/or during event. Risks included consuming a large amount of fat or fibre in pre-event meal, consuming excessive amounts of single carbohydrates during the event or becoming significantly dehydrated
Salt depletion (?)	Inadequate replacement of sodium lost in sweat. There is anecdotal evidence that salt depletion may increase the risk of a specific type of whole-body muscle cramp	Salty sweaters: individuals with high sweat rates and high sweat sodium concentrations that may acutely or chronically deplete exchangeable sodium pools
Water intoxication/hyponatraemia (low blood sodium)	Excessive intake of fluids can lead to hyponatraemia, ranging from mild (often asymptomatic) to severe (can be fatal). While this problem is more of a medical concern than a cause of fatigue, symptoms can include headache and disorientation, which can be mistaken as signs of dehydration	Athletes with low sweat losses (e.g. low-intensity exercise in cool weather) who over-zealously consume fluid before and during the event. This has most often been seen during marathons, ultra-endurance sports and hiking

risk of these occurring in an event depends on factors such as the duration and intensity of the exercise involved, environmental conditions (e.g. temperature and humidity), how well trained the athlete is, individual characteristics of the athlete, and success of nutrition strategies before and during the event.

It is relatively easy to investigate the physiological factors causing fatigue in simple exercise tasks such as running or cycling, particularly when undertaken in a laboratory under controlled conditions. With care, the knowledge gained from laboratory simulations of simple competitive events may be transferred to the real-life performances of athletes. Even so, it would be useful to have more field studies of race performance and how well various nutrition interventions can enhance outcomes in the real world of sport. It is more complicated to measure or predict factors limiting the performance of complex sporting events, particularly ball games and racquet sports in which competition demands differ between athletes and change from game to game. Whatever the sport or event, scientists try to pinpoint the likely risk that various factors will cause fatigue, based on the available applied sports research, as well as accounts of the past competition experiences of the athletes involved. With this knowledge, athletes can then be guided to undertake specific competition nutrition strategies that will minimise or delay the onset of these problems.

The range of competition strategies available to athletes include practices of fluid and food intake before, during and in the interval between events, as well as the acute or chronic use of supplements with ergogenic effects such as caffeine, creatine and the buffering agents (i.e. extracellular buffering with bicarbonate supplementation, intracellular buffering with β-alanine supplementation). Since the role of ergogenic aids is covered in other areas of this text (see Chapter 9 on supplements, plus a separate commentary on buffering agents in Chapter 12), we concentrate here on issues of dietary practices around the event. Although these strategies will form the basis of competition eating, they could also be implemented around training sessions. This will allow the athlete to experiment and fine-tune their personalised competition plan, including learning the habits or gastrointestinal tolerance needed to carry it out

successfully. These strategies may also help to support the training sessions and allow the athlete to train well.

16.3 Pre-competition fuelling

A goal of pre-competition eating is to prepare the body's carbohydrate stores in anticipation of the fuel needs of the event. In events of less than 90-min duration, the athlete's increased capacity to store muscle glycogen will generally be adequate to meet competition fuel demands. Unless there is muscle damage, the athlete should be able to restore muscle glycogen content with as little as a day's intake of a carbohydrate-rich diet in combination with rest or light training. The carbohydrate targets needed to restore glycogen will vary according to the level of depletion, but somewhere in the range of 6–10 g/kg will generally suit most athletes.

The fuel demands of some events are even greater than the muscle's normal glycogen stores. Marathons, road cycling races and Ironman triathlons are all sports in which competitors can feel the fatigue – often called 'hitting the wall' – associated with glycogen depletion. However, it may also happen to players in mobile positions in lengthy team sports, such as mid-fielders in football or backs in rugby, because of their requirement to complete many repetitions of sprinting at high intensity. Where possible, such athletes should try to 'carbohydrate load' or super-compensate glycogen stores prior to the event. The evolution of carbohydrate-loading strategies provides an example of a common story in sports nutrition. The first protocols were developed in the 1960s when exercise scientists used muscle biopsy techniques to examine the storage and utilisation of muscle fuels during exercise in active but untrained men. A doubling of glycogen stores was achieved with a week-long technique involving a 3-day depletion phase (low carbohydrate plus training) followed by a 3-day loading phase (taper plus high carbohydrate intake). This was quickly adopted by athletes when it was found to prolong the time that race pace could be sustained, delaying fatigue or producing a faster race time. A modification to the protocol was developed two decades later, when further investigations on well-trained individuals found that glycogen super-compensation

Table 16.2 A 48-hour carbohydrate-loading menu providing a daily carbohydrate intakes of ~10 g/kg for a 50-kg female athlete and 65-kg male athlete.[a]

Day	50-kg female runner (~500 g/day carbohydrate)	65-kg male runner (~650 g/day carbohydrate)
Day 1 Note 1: the menu focuses on the carbohydrate-rich foods; other foods can be added to balance the meal. An exercise taper should accompany this menu to optimise muscle glycogen storage. It is possible that glycogen super-compensation can be achieved by 2 days of such a diet, at least in well-trained athletes who can arrange a suitable exercise taper	Breakfast: 2 cups of flake cereal + cup milk + banana, 250 ml of sweetened juice Snack: 500 ml bottle soft drink Lunch: 1 large bread roll with fillings, 200 g of flavoured yoghurt Snack: 2 slices of toast + jam, 250 ml of sweetened fruit juice Dinner: 2 cups of cooked pasta + ½ cup sauce, 2 cups of jelly Snack: 250 ml of sweetened fruit juice + 2 crumpets and honey	Breakfast: 2 cups of flake cereal + cup milk + banana, 250 ml of sweetened fruit juice Snack: 500 ml bottle soft drink, 2 slices of thick toast + jam Lunch: 2 large bread rolls with fillings, 200 g of flavoured yoghurt Snack: coffee scroll or muffin, 250 ml of sweetened fruit juice Dinner: 3 cups of cooked pasta + ¾ cup sauce, 2 cups of jelly Snack: 2 crumpets and honey + 250 ml of sweetened fruit juice
Day 2 Note 2: a low-residue version of this diet can allow the athlete to reduce gut contents in preparation for the race. To achieve this, the athlete should consume only 'white' versions of cereal and grain foods, and avoid fruit and vegetables other than well-cooked or puréed versions	Breakfast: 2 cups of flake cereal + cup milk + cup sweetened canned fruit, 250 ml of sweetened fruit juice Snack: 500 ml fruit smoothie Lunch: 2 stack pancake + syrup + 2 scoops ice cream, 500 ml soft drink Snack: 50 g of dried fruit, 250 ml of sweetened fruit juice Dinner: 2 cups of rice dish (e.g. fried rice, risotto) Snack: 1 cup of fruit salad + scoop ice cream	Breakfast: 2 cups of flake cereal + cup milk + cup of sweetened canned fruit, 250 ml of sweetened fruit juice Snack: 500 ml fruit smoothie Lunch: 3 stack pancake + syrup + 2 scoops ice cream, 500 ml soft drink Snack: 100 g of dried fruit, 250 ml of sweetened fruit juice Dinner: 3 cups of rice dish (e.g. fried rice, risotto) Snack: 2 cups of fruit salad + 2 scoops of ice cream

[a] Athletes of differing sizes should scale this intake up or down according to their body mass.

could be achieved without the need for the depletion phase. These findings not only shortened the carbohydrate-loading protocol, but eliminated the need for the effort and discomfort involved in trying to exercise on an extreme diet.

Most recently, sports scientists have found that a well-trained muscle is able to maximise glycogen stores with as little as 24–36 hours of high carbohydrate intake/rest. Thus, carbohydrate loading is now a practical option for a large range of athletes who compete in fuel-demanding events. Examples of a dietary plan that provides the requirements of 10 g/kg are summarised in Table 16.2. For some athletes this may require additional focus on carbohydrate-rich foods and drinks, and a higher energy intake than normal, while for others it may be as

simple as tapering the training load to allow fuel to be stored. A final twist is that some athletes like to combine carbohydrate loading with a low-residue/low-fibre dietary plan that reduces gastrointestinal contents over the day(s) before competition while achieving muscle fuel goals. This provides the advantage of reducing body mass by 0.5–2 kg (providing a small but useful advantage in sports where the athlete carries his or her own body mass over distances) or removing the likelihood for a bowel movement on the day of the event (sometimes impractical in the field of play).

A final consideration in competition preparation is the effect and the environment of the competition taper. In many sports, the achievement of a competition peak is preceded by a distinct training taper, in which the volume of training is dramatically reduced for a period of 1–3 weeks. This reduces the athlete's energy expenditure, but paradoxically also increases their leisure time which encourages 'boredom eating'. Another factor that can lead to a mismatch in energy intake is the food environment often encountered in the competition phase. Athletes may be travelling away from home and dietary supervision, or being exposed to 'all you can eat' catering in athlete villages or hotels. Unless the athlete is sufficiently knowledgeable and committed, it can be easy to overeat. Many athletes (and their coaches) have been dismayed to find that they have gained significant body fat over a competition period that could have been prevented by an eating plan tailored to their real energy needs and changed access to food.

16.4 The pre-event meal

Foods and drinks consumed in the 4 hours before an event have a role in fine-tuning competition preparation in the following ways.

- To enhance muscle glycogen stores if they have not been fully restored or loaded since the last exercise session. This is often an issue in sports where the athlete competes in heats and finals, or several matches in a tournament.
- For events undertaken in the morning, to restore liver glycogen stores after an overnight fast.
- To ensure that the athlete is well hydrated, especially where a fluid deficit is likely to occur during the event and/or the athlete may be dehydrated from a hot environment or previous exercise.
- To achieve gut comfort throughout the event, neither letting the athlete become hungry nor suffer gastrointestinal distress or upset.
- To include foods and eating practices that are important to the athlete's psychology or superstition.

The array of events, environments, timetables and food facilities in which competition is undertaken makes it impossible to suggest a set routine that will work for all athletes. Instead, each athlete should develop an eating plan that works for that individual, based on personal preferences and past experiences. Some general principles include the consumption of substantial amounts of carbohydrate-rich foods or drinks prior to endurance events, and the avoidance of large amounts of fibre or fat by athletes who are at risk of gut problems. Pre-event hydration should involve drinking a comfortable amount of fluid sufficiently ahead of the event so that there is time for the urination of excess fluids. Table 16.3 provides some examples of carbohydrate-rich food choices that may suit different situations. In team sports, it is often customary to eat the pre-event meal as a group meal to promote bonding or the sharing of game plans. In such a case, a variety of foods should be provided buffet-style to allow each player to select the amount and type of food of their choice. Where athletes suffer from pre-event nerves or when an event scheduled in the early morning creates difficulty in eating a substantial amount of food beforehand, it can often be useful to choose a liquid version of the pre-event meal. Specially formulated liquid replacement meals are available but athletes can also make their own version using sweetened dairy foods as a base.

Special attention has been focused on the possible disadvantages of consuming carbohydrate in the hours prior to exercise. Although it can enhance body carbohydrate stores, it also increases the rate at which carbohydrate is utilised as a fuel during subsequent exercise due to alterations in prevailing hormone (i.e. insulin) concentrations. Early sports nutrition guidelines warned against the intake of carbohydrate in the hour before exercise in case it impaired performance via an increased utilisation and earlier fatigue of body carbohydrate stores. This may be the case for some individual athletes, especially in situations where the amount of carbohydrate consumed before the event is small and unable to counter the increase in exercise carbohydrate use. Several options are able to minimise the problems: consuming adequate pre-exercise carbohydrate (>1 g/kg) to offset the increased reliance on carbohydrate fuel use and choosing carbohydrate-rich sources that are lower in glycaemic index and cause less perturbation to the hormonal adjustment to their intake. However, the most effective strategy to maintain carbohydrate availability during the event is to continue to consume it throughout exercise. This offers a number of benefits to the muscle and central nervous system that will be subsequently discussed.

Table 16.3 Carbohydrate-rich foods and fluids suited to special needs of competition.

Pre-event meals
Breakfast choices
Breakfast cereal + low-fat milk + fresh or canned fruit
Muffins or crumpets + jam or honey
Pancakes + syrup
Toast + baked beans (this is a high-fibre choice)

Lunch or dinner choices
Rolls or sandwiches
Fruit salad + low-fat fruit yoghurt
Spaghetti with tomato or low-fat sauce
Baked potatoes with low-fat filling
Creamed rice

Easily digested choices
Liquid meal replacement
Fruit smoothie (low-fat milk + fruit + yoghurt or ice cream)

Recovery snacks providing carbohydrate and protein
250–350 ml of liquid meal replacement, milk shake or fruit smoothie
500 ml of flavoured low-fat milk
60 g (1.5–2 cups) of breakfast cereal with ½ cup of milk
1 round of sandwiches with cheese, meat or chicken filling, and 1 large piece of fruit or 300 ml of sport drink
1 cup of fruit salad with 200 g of fruit-flavoured yogurt or custard
200 g of fruit-flavoured yoghurt or 300 ml of flavoured milk and 30–35 g cereal bar
250 g (large) baked potato with grated cheese filling
150 g thick-crust pizza with lean meat and cheese topping

Fuelling during the event
60 g carbohydrate is provided by:
600–800 ml of sport drink
3 sachets of sport gel
1.5 sport bars
2–3 cereal bars or granola bars
Large bread roll filled with jam or honey
2 large bananas or 4 medium pieces of other fruit
90 g of jelly confectionery or sports confectionary
550 ml of cola drinks
120 g of fruit bread or cake
95 g dried fruit or 1400 g of trail mix
Note that when high rates of carbohydrate intake are required (60–90 g/hour), special sports products made with a 2:1 ratio of glucose to
    fructose will enhance intestinal absorption of carbohydrate

Portable carbohydrate-rich foods suitable for the travelling athlete
Breakfast cereal (and skim milk powder)
Cereal bars, granola bars
Dried fruit, trail mixes
Rice crackers, dry biscuits
Spreads: jam, honey
Sport bars
Liquid meal replacements: powder and ready-to-drink forms

16.5 Fluid intake during exercise

In events lasting longer than about 45 min there may be opportunities and advantages to consuming fuel and fluids during the session. Fluid intake can help to offset the dehydration incurred through the loss of sweat. Sweat is lost during exercise as a means to dissipate the heat generated by muscular work or absorbed from the environment, and when it can be evaporated it provides an effective strategy to maintain body temperature within its homeostatic range. As the resulting fluid deficit increases, however, it gradually increases the stress associated with exercise, for example increases in heart rate or the perception of effort, and can reduce performance. The point at which this becomes noticeable or significant will depend on the individual, the environment (effects are greater in the heat or at altitude) and perhaps the focus of the exercise (recreational exercisers may stop exercising if it becomes uncomfortable; elite athletes may be prepared to tolerate greater discomfort but equally may have a greater incentive to perform well given the small margins between winning and losing).

In general, we suggest that athletes use the opportunities specific to their sport to replace as much of their sweat loss as is practical during the event, and particularly to keep the fluid deficit below 2% of body mass in stressful environments. Depending on the event, there may be opportunities to drink during breaks in play (i.e. half time, substitutions or time-outs in team games) or during the exercise itself (from aid stations, handlers or self-carried supplies). Table 16.4 summarises the main issues with fluid intake across a range of sports. Athletes can get a feel for their typical sweat losses during an event by conducting periodic checks of hydration during training sessions or events as is practical. Checking body mass before and after the session, then accounting for the weight of drinks and foods consumed during the session, will allow the athlete to calculate sweat rates, rates of fluid replacement and the total sweat deficit over the session. Across a range of sports, sweat losses can vary from 500 ml to 2 l per hour depending on the intensity and duration of exercise, the prevailing environment, the athlete's degree of acclimatisation and the need to wear heat-retaining clothing or protective equipment.

Fluid mismatches during competitive events mostly err on the side of a fluid deficit, which athletes may then judge as being tolerable or as needing to be addressed within the logistics of their sport and the availability of fluids. However, it is possible for some athletes to over-hydrate if they drink excessively during events in which sweat rates are actually low. This situation is generally unnecessary and may even be dangerous if it leads to the potentially fatal condition of hyponatraemia (low blood sodium concentration, often known as water intoxication). Good drink choices will depend on the sport and on other nutritional goals that might be important. Clearly,

a fluid needs to be palatable and available to encourage intake. However, other characteristics include temperature, which can be manipulated both to enhance palatability in the specific environment and to contribute to body temperature regulation (cold fluids and ice slurries can reduce core temperature in hot conditions while warm fluids may increase body temperature losses in cold environments). Sports drinks formulated to meet a range of needs in sport generally contain electrolytes (to encourage fluid intake by maintaining thirst, and possibly to replace large sweat sodium losses in salty sweaters) and carbohydrates (to provide an additional fuel source during the event).

16.6 Fuel intake during competition

The muscle and central nervous system can both benefit from the intake of carbohydrate during exercise. A range of mechanisms is possible and may occur singly or in combination according to the intensity and duration of the event and the athlete's nutritional preparation. Until recently, guidelines for the intake of carbohydrate during exercise stated that it would only be valuable during events longer than 1 hour in duration and recommended an intake of 30–60 g/hour, fine-tuned with individual experience. The intake of a sports drink in volumes of 400–800 ml/hour would typically allow such targets to be met. Again, the specific characteristics of a sport, such as the scheduling of breaks, competition rules, logistics and culture, will determine the opportunities for consuming a sports drink or other carbohydrate-containing source during the event (see Table 16.4). Some new research has suggested ways in which fuelling guidelines need to be updated for shorter sustained-intensity events, and for longer or ultra-endurance sports.

In longer events such as Ironman triathlons or stage races in road cycling, it has been curious to observe that top athletes self-select carbohydrate intakes that are much higher than recommended by sports nutrition guidelines, often around 80–90 g/hour. This poses the question of who is wrong: the guidelines or the athletes? The answer has been answered in several ways. The first piece of information is emerging evidence of a dose–response relationship between carbohydrate intake and performance in sports lasting

Table 16.4 Summary of key issues involved in developing individual hydration and fuelling plans for various types of sporting activities.

Type of sports	Key issues to consider in devising specific plan for competition fluid/fuel replacement
Continuous endurance events, e.g. distance running, road cycling, triathlon	Fluids and foods must be consumed during the race while athlete is on the move
	Access to supplies is enhanced in events where drinks are provided by aid stations or handlers
	Access to drinks/foods is reduced in events where athlete must carry their own supplies
	Opportunity to drink/eat is limited by consideration of the time lost in obtaining and consuming fluid
	Opportunity to drink/eat is limited by gastrointestinal discomfort associated with drinking while exercising
	Ability to consume fluid/foods during races may be enhanced by practising during training to develop gastrointestinal tolerance and the skills that allow drinking on the move
	Creative devices such as fluid back-packs and spill-proof bottles may enhance access to fluid and the ease of drinking on the move
Team and racquet sports, e.g. football codes, tennis, basketball	Fluids/foods can be consumed during breaks in game or pauses in play that are specific to the sport (e.g. timeouts, change of ends, half-time, substitutions)
	Opportunities to drink/eat are increased in sports in which there are a number of formal and informal breaks, and where there is free player rotation
	Access to fluid is increased by having a team drink supply close to the field of play and, where rules permit, having trainers take drinks to players
	Access to fluid is reduced in sports in which rules prevent carriage of fluid onto field of play
	In some team sports there is a culture that dehydration during training can 'toughen' players
	Individual drink bottles may enhance hydration practices by increasing awareness of total fluid intake
Sprint, strength and power events (brief high-intensity sports), e.g. track and field events	No need or opportunity to hydrate/fuel during brief events, but athletes may need to rehydrate/refuel between events especially in multiple event competition
Weight-making sports, e.g. wrestling, boxing, martial arts, lightweight rowing, weightlifting	Education is needed to minimise reliance on dehydration to make weight for competition
	Weight-making practices may also involve poor fuelling in the days leading into the event
	Depending on the rules of the competition, the recovery period between weigh-in and competition can vary from an hour to a day. Aggressive refuelling and rehydration may be needed, but caution may be needed to reduce risk of gut upsets during the event
Skill sports, e.g. golf, shooting, archery	*Access* to fluid is reduced when sessions are undertaken in a remote environment
Aquatic sports, e.g. swimming, water polo	Fluid needs are likely to be lower than equivalent land-based sports activities due to opportunity to dissipate heat through convection/conduction in water rather than sweating
	Drink bottles on pool deck are suitable for water polo
	Race rules in open water swimming dictate the access to feed stations or handlers
Winter sports, e.g. alpine and Nordic skiing, skating	*Access* to fluid is reduced when session is undertaken in remote environment, or sub-zero temperatures (drinks freeze)
	Fluid needs (sweat losses) altered by cold environment or altitude
	Voluntary fluid intake may be enhanced by provision of warm fluids

3 hours or more; in other words, the greater the carbohydrate dose, the better the performance (up to a point, of course). It appears that as events get longer and beyond the fuelling capacity of muscle glycogen stores, good performance requires an alternative carbohydrate source to be supplied. The limiting factor is the amount of carbohydrate that can be absorbed from the gut. However, the second new piece of

information is that gut absorption can be enhanced if the athlete consumes a blend of different types of carbohydrates that are transported across the intestine in different ways. The maximum absorption of glucose appears to be about 60 g/hour, but if a blend of glucose and fructose is consumed it can be increased to 90 g/hour. This has led to the production of new sports products (drinks, bars, gels, etc) with special carbohydrate blends. These will not provide extra benefits for endurance events of 1–2 hours where 30–60 g of carbohydrate intake is adequate, but will allow larger amounts to be consumed in longer events where it can contribute to the special fuel needs. It appears also that the gut can be 'trained' to increase its absorption rates of carbohydrate by regularly training with carbohydrate intake.

The new insight into carbohydrate intake during events of intermittent or sustained high intensity lasting about 1 hour is just as intriguing. In such events, muscle glycogen stores are adequate for fuel needs so theoretically there should be no advantage to consuming carbohydrate during the event. Yet a number of studies involving continuous cycling or running have recorded benefits. Incredibly, the benefits occur even if the carbohydrate is not actually consumed: even swilling a carbohydrate drink around the mouth and spitting it out allows the athlete to perform better. The emerging theory is that there are receptors in the mouth that sense the presence of carbohydrate, allowing the brain to feel energised and pace at a higher level. This means that athletes in shorter events should also consider the benefits of consuming or tasting even a small amount of carbohydrate at regular intervals throughout the event. However, it also reminds us that the brain plays a role in determining performance that should be further investigated.

16.7 Recovery between events

The final siren or finish line is not necessarily the end of the athlete's competition nutrition plan. In many sports, competition involves a series of events or games before the final winner is decided, and the athlete will need to bounce back as quickly or as effectively as possible for the next round. Despite the best nutrition practices during the first session, it is likely that the athlete will need to restore fluid and fuel levels, and to try to repair any damage that has occurred. The same recovery guidelines practised in training in terms of rehydration (Chapter 7), refuelling (Chapter 4) and replacement/adaptation involving protein synthesis (Chapter 5) will all be part of the process. The recovery period between events may be less than an hour (e.g. races in a swimming programme or track meet), 3–4 hours (e.g. singles and doubles matches on the same day of a tennis tournament) or 1–2 days (e.g. team sports in a tournament format). This period may not allow full recovery, and there may be challenges in terms of access to appropriate supplies of foods and fluids in the competition environment. However, with good planning, the athlete should aim to recover as well as possible, and better than his or her competitors.

Alcohol

One post-competition nutritional practice that merits special mention is excessive intake of alcohol. This is often part of the culture of team sports, but can also be found in other sports with the justification of 'team bonding', 'celebrating' or 'commiserating'. The downside of excessive intake may be a direct interference with many of the processes of recovery: alcohol may increase diuresis and impair rehydration, as well as impair protein synthesis and glycogen storage. However, the major effect is likely to be indirect: when excessive alcohol is consumed, athletes are likely to be distracted and unlikely to follow sensible nutrition eating practices. High-risk behaviour of many sorts can also interfere with the athlete's health and reputation.

16.8 Summary

Competing at an optimal level requires a dedicated and personalised nutrition plan aimed at reducing or delaying the onset of factors that would otherwise reduce performance. These factors are specific to the event and to the individual. A plan practised in training will allow the athlete to feel confident and ready to perform at his or her best.

Further reading

Balsom PD, Wood K, Olsson, P, Ekblom B. Carbohydrate intake and multiple sprint sports: with special reference to football (soccer). Int J Sports Med 1999; 20: 48–52.

Burdon CA, O'Connor HT, Gifford JA, Shirreffs SM. Influence of beverage temperature on exercise performance in the heat: a systematic review. Int J Sport Nutr Exerc Metab 2010; 20: 166–174.

Burke L. Practical Sports Nutrition. Champaign, IL: Human Kinetics, 2007.

Burke LM, Pyne DB. Bicarbonate loading to enhance training and competitive performance. Int J Sports Physiol Perform 2007; 2: 93–97.

Burke LM, Claassen A, Hawley JA, Noakes TD. Carbohydrate intake during prolonged cycling minimizes effect of glycemic index of pre-exercise meal. J Appl Physiol 1998; 85: 2220–2226.

Bussau VA, Fairchild TJ, Rao A, Steele PD, Fournier PA. Carbohydrate loading in human muscle: an improved 1 day protocol. Eur J Appl Physiol 2002; 87: 290–295.

Carter JM, Jeukendrup AE, Jones DA. The effect of carbohydrate mouth rinse on 1-h cycle time trial performance. Med Sci Sport Exerc 2004; 36: 2107–2111.

Carter J, Jeukendrup AE, Jones DA. The effect of sweetness on the efficacy of carbohydrate supplementation during exercise in the heat. Can J Appl Physiol 2005; 30: 379–391.

Casa DJ, Stearns RL, Lopez RM et al. Influence of hydration on physiological function and performance during trail running in the heat. J Athl Training 2010; 45: 147–156.

Currell K, Jeukendrup AE. Superior endurance performance with ingestion of multiple transportable carbohydrates. Med Sci Sport Exerc 2008; 40: 275–281.

Derave W, Everaert I, Beeckman S, Baguet A. Muscle carnosine metabolism and beta-alanine supplementation in relation to exercise and training. Sports Med 2010; 40: 247–263.

Dougherty KA, Baker LB, Chow M, Kenney WL. Two percent dehydration impairs and six percent carbohydrate drink improves boys basketball skills. Med Sci Sport Exerc 2006; 38: 1650–1658.

Dugas JP, Oosthuizen U, Tucker R, Noakes TD. Rates of fluid ingestion alter pacing but not thermoregulatory responses during prolonged exercise in hot and humid conditions with appropriate convective cooling. Eur J Appl Physiol 2009; 105: 69–80.

Ebert TR, Martin DT, Bullock N et al. Influence of hydration status on thermoregulation and cycling hill climbing. Med Sci Sport Exerc 2007; 39: 323–329.

Gonzalez RR, Cheuvront SN, Montain SJ et al. Expanded prediction equations of human sweat loss and water needs. J Appl Physiol 2009; 107: 379–388.

Hawley JA, Schabort EJ, Noakes TD, Dennis SC. Carbohydrate-loading and exercise performance: an update. Sports Med 1997; 24: 73–81.

Jentjens RL, Achten J, Jeukendrup AE. High oxidation rates from combined carbohydrates ingested during exercise. Med Sci Sport Exerc 2004; 36: 1551–1558.

Jeukendrup AE. Carbohydrate and exercise performance: the role of multiple transportable carbohydrates. Curr Opin Clin Nutr Metab Care 2010; 13: 452–457.

Jeukendrup AE, Chambers ES. Oral carbohydrate sensing and exercise performance. Curr Opin Clin Nutr Metab Care 2010; 13: 447–451.

Karelis AD, Smith JW, Passe DH, Peronnet F. Carbohydrate administration and exercise performance: what are the potential mechanisms involved? Sports Med 2010; 40: 747–763.

Karlsson J, Saltin B. Diet, muscle glycogen, and endurance performance. J Appl Physiol 1971; 31: 203–206.

Kirkendall DT, Foster C, Dean JA, Grogan J, Thompson NN. Effect of glucose polymer supplementation on peformance of soccer players. In: Science and Football: Proceedings of the 1st World Congress of Science and Football, Liverpool, 13–17 April 1987 (Reilly T, Lees A, Davids K, Murphy WJ, eds). London: E. & F.N. Spon, 1988, pp 33–41.

Kuipers H, Fransen EJ, Keizer H. A. Pre-exercise ingestion of carbohydrate and transient hypoglycemia during exercise. Int J Sports Med 1999; 20: 227–231.

Lanspa S, O'Brien J. Fluid tolerance while running: effect of repeated trials. Int J Sports Med 2008; 29: 878–882.

Moseley L, Lancaster GI, Jeukendrup AE. Effects of timing of pre-exercise ingestion of carbohydrate on subsequent metabolism and cycling performance. Eur J Appl Physiol 2003; 88: 453–458.

O'Reilly J, Wong SH, Chen Y. Glycaemic index, glycaemic load and exercise performance. Sports Med 2010; 40: 27–39.

Pahnke MD, Trinity JD, Zachwieja JJ, Stofan JR, Hiller WD, Coyle EF. Serum sodium concentration changes are related to fluid balance and sweat sodium loss. Med Sci Sport Exerc 2010; 42: 1669–1674.

Rodriguez NR, Di Marco NM, Langley S. American College of Sports Medicine position stand. Nutrition and athletic performance. Med Sci Sport Exerc 2009; 41: 709–731.

Sawka MN, Burke LM, Eichner ER, Maughan RJ, Montain SJ, Stachenfeld NS. American College of Sports Medicine position stand. Exercise and fluid replacement. Med Sci Sports Exerc 2007; 39: 377–390.

Sherman WM, Costill DL, Fink WJ, Miller JM. Effect of exercise–diet manipulation on muscle glycogen and its subsequent utilisation during performance. Int J Sports Med 1981; 2: 114–118.

Shirreffs SM, Maughan RJ. The effect of alcohol on athletic performance. Curr Sports Med Rep 2006; 5: 192–196.

Simard C, Tremblay A, Jobin M. Effects of carbohydrate intake before and during an ice hockey game on blood and muscle energy substrates. Res Q Exerc Sport 1988; 59: 144–147.

17
Losing, Gaining and Making Weight for Athletes

Helen O'Connor and Gary Slater

Key messages

- Physique or body morphology contributes to athletic success for a range of reasons, including a size advantage, greater 'power to weight', lower energy cost of locomotion, superior thermoregulation or 'artistic impression'.
- Plasticity of weight, lean and fat mass is limited by genetic predisposition. Some athletes engage in extreme diet and training regimens to strive for what are sometimes genetically unattainable physique goals.
- Dietary restriction increases the risk for nutrient and energy deficiency, endocrine and immune function disturbance, osteopenia and disordered eating. Athletes without adequate professional support to manage physique goals often fall victim to 'fad' diets and unsafe weight loss/making practices that are inadequate for their special needs.

- The identification of a suitable weight category is critical for athletes competing in weight category sports. While remaining competitive is important, so too is the ability of the athlete to achieve a specified weight without adversely impacting health or performance.
- Gaining muscle size and strength are common goals of many athletes. A successful muscle hypertrophy programme demands consideration of the overall training programme as well as nutritional support. The latter includes an energy-dense meal plan, with adequate carbohydrate to support training plus small serves of high-quality protein at meals and snacks.
- The monitoring of body composition enables diet and training to be adjusted to optimise results. Preferred techniques should be reliable and sensitive to small but important changes while also being cost-effective, accessible and safe.

17.1 Introduction

Although many factors ranging from skill, metabolic capacity through to psychological attributes contribute to athletic success, physical morphology or physique, including body mass or composition, size and shape are important for optimising athletic performance for most athletes. The impact of physique varies across sports and competition levels but specific, often extreme morphological characteristics are critical to success at the elite level in some sports (e.g. professional body-builders, sumo wrestlers), whereas a wider variety of morphologies are acceptable in others (e.g. netball, softball). This can often be explained by playing role or position in team sports (e.g. prop forward or linemen versus a winger or quarterback in rugby or American football) or a competition rule in others (e.g. weight category sports such as lightweight rowing or boxing or jockeys). However, in individual sports where physique attributes are diverse (e.g. archery, golf, lawn or ten-pin bowling), success may be more closely linked to skill or psychological attributes than anthropometric characteristics.

Support for the contribution that specific physique characteristics make to athletic success is often difficult to justify from the scientific literature. This is mostly because it is challenging to recruit sufficient numbers of high-calibre athletes and design studies sensitive and powerful enough to evaluate the impact of subtle physique changes on sports performance, especially when competition success is decided by incredibly small margins. However, there are a number of lines of evidence demonstrating how and why

Sport and Exercise Nutrition, First Edition. Edited by Susan A Lanham-New, Samantha J Stear, Susan M Shirreffs and Adam L Collins.
© 2011 The Nutrition Society. Published 2011 by Blackwell Publishing Ltd.

physique matters to athletic performance. Some of this evidence comes from longitudinal data on groups of successful athletes, including competition gradients revealing selection of more extreme and homogeneous morphologies at the elite level. Comparison of athletes to the source population from which they were derived often also demonstrates how they possess unique physique characteristics as a group and that these remain almost unchanged despite strong secular trends in the opposing direction (e.g. marathon runners and professional jockeys remain short and light despite secular increases in height and mass). Physiology, particularly the influence of body size on the energy cost of movement, heat production and thermoregulation, also explains why athletes with high energy expenditures and heat exposure (e.g. endurance runners, triathletes) tend to be smaller and lighter.

This chapter describes a range of issues relating to losing, gaining and making weight for athletes. It investigates why athletes are often driven to extreme lengths to attain a particular physique and outlines the strengths, limitations and risks associated with various strategies used to manipulate physique, with a particular focus on dietary intervention. It also briefly summarises the effectiveness of dietary supplements/sports foods, which are often used to facilitate weight or fat loss or gain. However, for a more extensive coverage of sports supplements refer to Chapter 9.

17.2 Sports-specific evidence linking physique attributes to athletic performance

Sports vary widely in the specific challenges they present to athletes. In endurance sports (e.g. marathon, triathlon), body weight is carried over a distance and this results in a significant energy cost and increased heat production. Low body mass, the result of low body fat, smaller stature and lean mass is a distinct advantage for endurance sports such as distance running as it reduces the energy cost of locomotion and minimises heat production. From a thermoregulatory viewpoint, low body fat and a higher body surface area to mass ratio promotes superior heat loss (O'Connor & Olds, 2007). Longitudinal data on elite marathon runners throughout the twentieth century

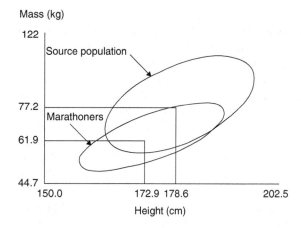

Figure 17.1 Bivariate distributions of height (cm) and mass (kg) for elite marathoners and the source population. The ellipses are 90% density ellipses for both marathoners and the source population. Mass values are plotted on a log scale. (Reproduced from O'Connor H, Olds T, Maughan R. Physique and performance for track and field events. J Sports Sci 2007; 25 (Suppl 1): S49–S60, Routledge 2007, reprinted with permission from Taylor & Francis Group.)

(Figure 17.1) demonstrate that low body mass and stature are characteristics which have remained static over many decades, indicating they are critical to performance success at the elite level and that this is unlikely to change significantly in the future.

Conversely, in sports such as gridiron, rugby union football or throwing disciplines (e.g. shot put, discus and hammer), high body mass relative to stature (or mesomorphy) is a desired trait and athletes in these sports typically have a body mass index (BMI) greater than 30 kg/m². This is in the obese range for European Caucasian populations, although the elevated BMI in athletes reflects high muscular development not excessive fatness. Data from elite throwers between the late 1920s and 1990s indicates an accelerated rate of body mass increase, between threefold and sevenfold greater than the source population (approximately 3–7 kg per decade) (Norton & Olds, 2001). Unlike marathon running, where body mass remains static and apparently optimised for this activity, the extreme changes in mass in throwing sports provides an example of open-ended optimisation, where further increases in lean mass would still be expected to be beneficial.

In sports such as basketball and high jump, a high degree of ectomorphy (tallness without excessive lean or fat mass) is important. In fact, the value of stature to high jump performance was demonstrated by the dramatic 10-cm increase in the height of elite high jump competitors over the two Olympiads after the 'Fosbury flop' (rather than the straddle) technique helped snare a gold medal at the 1968 games (Stepnicka, 1986). Analysis of high jump performance by Khosla and McBroom (1988) reported that a female jumper would be 191 times more likely to make an Olympic final if she were ≥1.8 m compared with ≤1.51 m tall. Greater stature (and indeed wider arm span) is also important for other sports including rowing due to improved oar leverage which enhances propulsion through the water. Although not able to be modified by diet or training, a wide range of different statures, limb lengths and skeletal ratios are important across sports (reviewed by O'Connor & Olds, 2007).

Optimising power through an increase in lean and minimising 'dead' or fat mass, known as increasing the power-to-weight ratio, is important in many sports (e.g. jumping, cycling, gymnastics, rowing or kayaking), especially those where body mass must be moved further or rapidly through space, overcoming gravitational, wind or water resistance. As lean and fat mass can be influenced by diet and training, athletes and coaches are keen to manipulate these, often using anthropometric, diet and training information from current champions to guide their approach. While lean and fat mass are adaptable compared with stature, limb lengths and breadths, which are not, genetics still limits the potential for body composition changes. These limits are sometimes not well understood by athletes and coaches who relentlessly pursue specific and often elusive body composition goals using extreme diet and training strategies that risk athlete health (reviewed by O'Connor & Caterson, 2010).

Specific physique characteristics are sometimes required for aesthetic reasons and coaches and athletes are aware that failure to attain the right appearance will result in lower scores for artistic impression (e.g. rhythmic gymnastics, figure skating and diving). These scores come down to the 'trained eye' of the judge who likely experienced similar evaluation during their own athletic careers. Sometimes the extreme leanness (e.g. rhythmic gymnastics, ballet dancing) desired is driven largely by appearance rather than performance enhancement but opinion and culture within the sport are often entrenched

and difficult to change. In recent years, the need for athletes to appear physically attractive is also driven by sponsorship opportunities which help to fund if not completely outstrip the financial rewards of successful competition. The desired physique may be dictated by societal attractiveness rather than athletic performance (O'Connor & Caterson, 2010).

Finally, in weight category sports (e.g. professional jockeys, lightweight rowing and combat sports such as boxing, taekwondo, judo, wrestling) achieving a designated weight is the competition rule and athletes are unable to participate if they do not 'make weight'. In the combat sports, greater stature and lean mass is usually an advantage and as competition success is decided by defeating a specific series of opponents within a category, athletes are enticed by the option of weighing in at a lower weight so they have a size advantage. In this case, the competition weight is typically achieved with at least some degree of acute weight loss via dehydration and often severe food/fluid restriction. Following weigh-in, athletes have a defined period (which varies between sports) to re-establish hydration and energy stores. Apart from professional boxing/wrestling, where competitors may get up to 24 hours after weigh-in before competing, the time allocated to recover is usually inadequate to completely restore hydration and energy reserves. During a competitive season, athletes may need to make weight often and, for some events, many times over successive days. In the case of professional jockeys, riders do this day in and day out for their entire career and unlike all other weight-making sports, they must remain at the target weight during each ride with no opportunity to recover (reviewed by Wallberg-Rankin, 2010).

Although there is an undisputed advantage of size when competing in combat sports and of greater stature and lean mass in lightweight rowing, the degree of dehydration and food restriction may negate the size benefit, especially if there is too much acute weight loss. A number of athletes have died as a result of unsafe, acute weight-making practises and over time health risks associated with the chronic use of inappropriate weight making is also significant (see pp. 224–225).

Clearly, physique characteristics impact performance and this is more important for some sports than others. Characteristics such as stature and skeletal lengths and breadths are not able to be manipulated but body weight and lean and fat mass are more plastic and are able to be changed. Athletes can employ effective strategies to move towards their physique goals but need to be aware that genetic potential limits the capacity for change. Strategies used need to be both safe and effective.

17.3 Challenges for optimising physique

Genetic factors

Estimates of the heritability of body composition vary, with data from twin studies the highest (~80% heritable) and adoption studies the lowest (~10–30%). An overall estimate of 25–40% for the heritability of human fatness has been proposed but this may increase to 70% in some environments. Well-controlled twin studies have shown that the increase in body weight and fat in response to positive energy balance via over-feeding is three times greater within twin pairs than between (reviewed by O'Rahilly et al., 2003). Similar findings have been reported for gains in lean mass and under-feeding resulting in weight loss. The identification of a genetic profile which may predispose an individual to lean mass gain and success in strength power sports has become an area of recent research interest As with body fatness, it is likely that a series of genes or a polygenic profile may better describe the predisposition to high lean mass and success in strength/power sports. Together, these findings demonstrate that genes not only have a strong influence on natural physique but also modify the responsiveness to strategies such as diet and/or exercise to influence characteristics such as fat and lean mass.

Genes potentially influence physique at a number of levels through energy storage and mobilisation, fuel oxidation at rest and during physical activity through to taste and food preference, appetite and inclination to be physically active. A number of susceptibility genes have been identified as influencing physique, increasing the likelihood of a particular phenotype but not necessarily its expression, which is also influenced by environmental factors (Bray et al., 2009). An in-depth discussion on the influence of genes and physique is beyond the scope of this chapter but the recommended reading identifies relevant literature for the interested reader. Research

into the generic determinants of body composition enhances our understanding of mechanisms underpinning the differences in human physique and provides evidence supporting why some athletes respond more favourably or rapidly to diet or exercise interventions than others. However, the key variables in physique manipulation remain with diet, training or both.

Challenges of the athlete environment

Athletes typically have hectic schedules which accommodate training in addition to work or study, family and social life. In some sports, athletes are well supported financially and circumstances including proximity of training, flexibility of study or work result in attainment of sport–life balance. Other athletes may have substantial and inflexible travel, study or workload commitments. This can limit the time and resources needed for food preparation, and for those living in dormitory settings, meal provision may not suit sports-specific needs. Younger athletes who move away from home to access high performance training and competition experience may find their cooking, shopping and/or budgeting skills are inadequate (Heaney et al., 2008).

Travelling to competition also interferes with dietary goals as finding appropriate choices at competition venues, airport lounges or selecting unfamiliar foods in foreign countries may be difficult with suitable choices limited. Although competition dining halls typically have a wide choice of appropriate foods, the temptation of unlimited portions and many highly palatable options can derail pre-planned weight management strategies.

Athletes in Western countries are also surrounded by an obesogenic environment where a healthy diet is not necessarily followed by immediate family or peers. To optimise performance and achieve an ideal physique, athletes usually need to eat differently to those in their immediate circle. Misinformation in the mass media, especially the internet, that promotes rapid and easy weight/fat loss or lean gain spreads quickly though athlete networks. Often the results of these strategies are exaggerated and negative side effects under-reported. Safe and effective approaches to physique optimisation are needed to navigate this list of environmental challenges and be sensitive to the specific and varied needs of athletes.

Growth and pubertal changes

During puberty, the physique changes and there is a significant increase in stature and body mass. In boys there is an increase in lean mass while in girls greater deposition of body fat prevails. Some of the pubertal physique changes may be beneficial immediately (e.g. increases in stature, total and lean mass) while others may be detrimental (e.g. increases in total body mass, especially if fat). In many cases, the influence of puberty depends on the sport and the individual athlete. Increases in stature may initially be detrimental for coordination and agility but eventually beneficial in many sports such as tennis, high and long jump, basketball and heavyweight rowing. Some increase in stature or lean mass may be beneficial but not if the changes are too great (e.g. in gymnastics, substantial increases in stature may decrease capacity to tumble effectively). Athletes may not reap the benefit of the physique changes that occur in puberty for a number of years until technique catches up with new body dimensions and strength fully develops. Pubertal changes commence and develop at different rates. Some children enter puberty early and this is often an advantage for sports where greater stature, lean mass and strength are important (e.g. football or swimming). Early pubertal development may be a disadvantage especially for girls in aesthetic sports (e.g. rhythmic gymnastics or ballet dancing) if there is a substantial and rapid increase in body fat. Clearly, puberty and adolescence is a time when physique changes will usually have some influence on athletic performance and chronological age fails to establish a level playing field.

Physique management can also be more challenging with adolescent athletes gaining independence and experiencing social pressure to eat out, usually at more affordable establishments such as fast food outlets. Research on adolescent eating patterns highlights a preference for energy-dense high-fat/sugar foods, and during this life phase the onset of alcohol intake usually occurs. In some sports, alcohol intake can be excessive and used as a team-bonding strategy. Restrictive and disordered eating may be an issue for other athletes and this is often triggered by the physique changes (e.g. increased adiposity particularly in girls) that commence in puberty. Energy restriction and weight loss may impact growth, maturation, health and performance in young athletes (see Chapter 23).

The challenges of training

Variability and interruption to training

The amount of energy expended by athletes is influenced by a wide range of factors including training intensity, duration, frequency and modality (e.g. swimming stroke, player position). Expenditure also increases with body mass, especially in weight-bearing (e.g. running) versus weight-supported (e.g. swimming, cycling, rowing) activities. Well-trained athletes become skilful and more efficient, using less energy than the untrained when the same training is performed. Periodisation (programmed blocks of variation in training intensity, duration and frequency), which varies energy expenditure, often quite widely from week to week, can also make it difficult for athletes to consume an appropriate amount of energy to support training needs and simultaneously manage physique goals (O'Connor & Caterson, 2010). Athletes may also compensate for high training energy expenditures by extending nocturnal sleep and/or increased sedentary periods or naps throughout the day. In younger developing athletes, participation in other sporting activities or school physical education programmes further elevates daily energy expenditure. Interruption to habitual expenditure due to illness, injury, seasonality of sport or competition taper also challenges the maintenance of energy balance. Although training energy expenditure is generally advantageous for maintaining a lean physique, the interplay of these factors can complicate dietary management.

Clinically, estimation of individual energy requirements over a wide range of daily expenditures is complex and is usually best managed by progressive modification of the athlete's habitual diet. Planning that attempts to rely solely on theoretical estimates (see p. 215) rather than individualised athlete-centred energy prescription is unlikely to be successful. Practically, athletes often find it useful to have a core eating plan which covers daily requirements for a non-training day and then a range of eating strategies to address the additional expenditure for the suite of training sessions they undertake. These fuelling strategies can be incorporated when a session is included and omitted when it is not. This approach can also be used to address different nutrient needs such as incorporating carbohydrate and/or protein before and/or after resistance training sessions or carbohydrate during and immediately after high-intensity endurance sessions. The approach helps to educate the athlete on adapting dietary intake for the kinds of training they engage in and helps avoid habitual over-consumption when training is interrupted (e.g. during off-season, competition tapers and periods of illness and injury). Meals are also easier to plan and monitor from the practitioner perspective. An important consideration for those athletes who are aiming to significantly increase lean mass is a gradual increase in energy intake to account for elevation in both resting and overall daily energy costs due to greater resting and locomotion energy expenditure.

Training and appetite

Exercise is generally accepted as stimulating an increase in overall appetite to promote the restoration of fuels and maintenance of body weight. Unfortunately, relatively few studies have investigated the impact of exercise on appetite and even fewer in athletic populations (King et al., 1994). Factors reported as influencing post-exercise energy intake include the intensity, duration and modality of exercise and studies have demonstrated that post-exercise intake can result in partial, complete and even over-compensation of the energy expended. Evidence suggests a weak coupling between energy intake and expenditure in the short term and that some individuals are better able to match energy intake with exercise expenditure. Differential appetite-related compensatory responses can therefore make it easier or more difficult for particular individuals to reduce weight/fat through exercise.

Although additional research is required, studies suggest that higher intensity exercise blunts short-term appetite compared with lower intensity, even when total work performed is identical (King et al., 1994). Mechanisms are unclear but may relate to differences in metabolites or appetite-related hormones (e.g. lactate, adrenaline, leptin, ghrelin) or change in body temperature. Surprisingly, anecdotal evidence for a greater appetite after swimming has not been evaluated but there is evidence from at least one study suggesting exercise in cold versus neutral water temperature stimulates greater post-exercise energy intake. This effect of temperature needs further confirmation. Some studies also report an influence of gender, with evidence of greater compensation of energy after exercise in women than men. The impor-

tance of maintaining energy reserves in women for reproductive purposes has been proposed as an explanation of these differences but the impact of gender on exercise-related appetite remains largely unexplored and requires further research.

In addition to energy intake, exercise may also alter macronutrient selection, specifically driving the appetite for carbohydrate which may eventually be satisfied in Western environments with additional and passive over-consumption of fat (i.e. palatable meal/snack options containing carbohydrate also provide significant amounts of fat). A case has been made for the influence of the fuel mix oxidised during exercise such that individuals with higher respiratory exchange ratios (R or RER) (evidence of higher carbohydrate oxidation) would have greater appetite for carbohydrate after exercise than those with ratios in the fat oxidation range (Tremblay et al., 1985). Additional research is required to confirm this. However, evidence of more sensitive regulation of energy intake has been reported in habitual exercisers but this has not been studied in athlete groups, where periodised programmes may challenge the consistency of exercise. Practically, the impact of appetite should be assessed in athletes presenting for physique management support as there are a number of dietary strategies that may assist 'hungry athletes' at risk of over-compensating energy intake after exercise (see p. 218) and also strategies for athletes who struggle to consume adequate energy to promote weight gain (see p. 225).

17.4 Strategies to promote weight and fat loss

Manipulation of energy intake

Total energy intake and expenditure are accepted as the most influential environmental factors regulating body mass. Consumption of energy above daily requirements results in gains of body mass and inadequate energy intake results in loss. Although energy requirements can be assessed directly by measuring body heat production or estimated via a number of indirect methods including calorimetry (oxygen cost measurement), the wide variation in energy requirements, even at rest, make accurate prediction of individual energy needs challenging. Energy expenditure at rest is strongly and positively correlated with lean mass (higher lean mass, higher energy expenditure) but is also influenced by age, gender and individual metabolic factors that are under genetic control. Resting metabolic rate (RMR) can be estimated via a number of prediction equations (e.g. Harris–Benedict, Schofield, Cunningham equations) which are sometimes used to investigate the plausibility of reported energy intake in the clinical setting. Most of these equations have not been validated in elite athletes and may not accurately reflect RMR in this population (Manore & Thompson, 2010). Dietary energy recommendations such as the Recommended Dietary Allowances (or Intakes) make use of these equations and also empirical data in the published literature to set appropriate energy intake levels for the population ranging from sedentary though to heavy work situations.

In athletes, estimation of total daily energy requirements is complicated by the variability in the duration and intensity of training and a wide range of other factors including environmental conditions (temperature, humidity, wind, etc.), athlete body mass/composition, age, gender and skill. When undertaking the same activity, children typically have a higher energy cost relative to body mass than adults as they are less skilful and efficient than a well-trained adult. Women typically have a lower energy cost at rest and during activity than men due to lower total body and lean mass. While the energy cost of activity is difficult to predict accurately, a number of regression equations and published resources exist which assist estimation (Manore & Thompson, 2010) and can be used as a general guide to the appropriateness of energy intake in athletic populations.

To achieve weight or fat loss, athletes must be in mild to moderate energy deficit (~10–20% reduction from intake required to achieve energy balance). Severe deficits more likely compromise intake of important macronutrients and micronutrients and are associated with fatigue and delayed recovery and increase the risk of energy deficiency and overtraining syndrome. Some athletes who only require minor weight or fat loss can achieve the required energy deficit by small simple dietary changes, primarily a focus on reduction in dietary fat (which is energy dense and often over-consumed in Western diets), which creates a sufficient deficit to promote adequate weight loss. This approach is less restrictive, avoids systematic energy restriction and optimises micronutrient intake. Unfortunately, *ad libitum* low-fat eating may not produce an energy deficit sufficient to promote substantial fat loss. When planned energy restriction is required, careful dietary design is necessary to optimise nutrient intake and prevent insufficient energy availability. Initially, gradual energy reduction (~10 or 20%) may prevent the athlete from feeling too hungry and help with identification of the minimum restriction needed to obtain desired results (American College of Sports Medicine, 2009). Erratic restrictive dieting or repeated weight cycling should be avoided as it is associated with adverse health risks including obesity in later life (see p. 224).

Most athletes are protected from fat gain due to higher energy expenditure than sedentary individuals and biological adaptation, particularly associated with aerobic training including increased skeletal muscle oxygen delivery (through improved capillarisation), greater mitochondrial density and elevated concentrations of enzymes required for fat metabolism. Athletes participating in skill/aesthetic-based sports (e.g. gymnastics, diving, figure skating) do not adapt 'fat burning' machinery to the same extent and despite many hours of exercise, expend substantially less energy. These athletes more often struggle with physique management. Selective survival of those with the genetic propensity to be light and/or lean operates at the elite level of these sports. However, even these athletes usually need to control and limit energy consumption to achieve the desired levels of leanness, especially women where desired adiposity is often well below what is biologically natural. In these athletes there can be a serious risk of energy deficiency and other health problems including disordered eating (see p. 224).

Manipulation of macronutrient intake and energy density

Dietary energy is provided by the macronutrients, with each delivering a different amount of energy (known as the Atwater factors) per gram: protein 17 kJ/g; fat 37 kJ/g; carbohydrate 16 kJ/g; alcohol 29 kJ/g. Until the 1990s it was unconditionally accepted that each kilojoule consumed had the same value regardless of which macronutrient it came from (i.e. a kilojoule from carbohydrate was equal to one from fat or protein). Excess consumption above daily energy and immediate nutrient storage needs (e.g. carbohydrate as glycogen and protein to maintain amino acid turnover pools) would then be deposited as fat in adipose tissue via the process of *de novo* lipogenesis. Scientific opinion particularly in the 1990s challenged this view, claiming *de novo* lipogenesis was an expensive process and only occurred in situations of forced over-feeding, not when food, particularly carbohydrate, was ingested *ad libitum*. Carbohydrate intake was also thought to be tightly regulated as body stores are limited and ingestion linked to their replenishment. This, combined with the greater energy density of fat and epidemiological research associating obesity prevalence to an increase in fat as opposed to carbohydrate or energy intake, supported the case for fat as a central driver of weight and fat gain.

These ideas were rapidly disseminated to the community with the general message that it was more difficult to gain weight from a high-carbohydrate compared with a high-fat diet, even if carbohydrate was unrestricted. A plethora of low-fat diets, fat counters and low-fat (but often sweetened) food products emerged, encouraging a focus on tight control of total fat intake and liberal unrestricted carbohydrate intake. Despite the exciting promise of achieving weight loss by adoption of a low-fat, *ad libitum* carbohydrate diet, the results were disappointing and obesity prevalence continued to rise worldwide. Athletes too were influenced by this low-fat eating style and given the well-documented importance of carbohydrate for sports performance (Chapter 4), this approach seemed ideal for those who needed to reduce body weight or fat but still maintain high training loads and optimal competition results. Like the general population, however, athletes also became disillusioned with low-fat high-carbohydrate diets. Concern over the type of carbohydrate, particularly high fructose corn syrup used in many of the low-fat products (and athlete sports foods), has also been raised in the scientific literature. Carbohydrate from high fructose corn syrup may be metabolised differently in the liver and more likely result in fat storage. The impact and mechanism of action underpinning the link with obesity is controversial and requires additional research. Unfortunately, the general community and athletes are often unaware of the energy density (number of kilojoules per gram food) of high-fat and some low-fat products and that high energy density is linked

with passive over-consumption and fat gain. Sports foods by design are energy dense to provide a convenient and compact source of energy to consume when energy/nutrient needs are difficult to meet from usual meals, possibly resulting in failure to adequately moderate intake of these within the daily energy budget.

The optimal macronutrient distribution required to promote weight loss is still controversial and many research studies are now dedicated to understanding the potential influence and benefits of macronutrient manipulation. The pendulum has swung towards research on lower carbohydrate, higher protein, moderate fat diets for weight management in the general population. Athletes are also experimenting with this approach and there is evidence of them adopting moderate (e.g. the Zone diet) through to extremely low-carbohydrate diets (e.g. Atkins diets) to reduce weight and fat (see p. 218). Athletes often turn immediately to popular diets to achieve instant results and by virtue of their higher energy expenditure and because these diets are almost always low in kilojoules, pleasing and rapid results are often achieved in the short term. However, athletes risk both short-term and longer-term performance decline in addition to a range of negative health consequences (see section 17.6) if they adopt these diet strategies.

Emerging evidence under what is known as the 'protein leverage hypothesis' (PLH) suggests that protein, a nutrient somewhat forgotten in weight management throughout the 1990s, has an important role to play. Central to PLH is that protein, not carbohydrate, is the most tightly regulated nutrient. Evidence in humans and in other vertebrates suggests that when faced with a wide variety of foods, ingestion of protein is a priority and food will continue to be consumed until obligatory protein requirements are met. In the Western diet, highly palatable, protein-poor, high-fat/carbohydrate foods, which are easily available and inexpensive, may be passively over-consumed before protein needs are achieved. As protein typically provides a significantly lower proportion of dietary energy than either carbohydrate or fat, a small decrease in the percentage of dietary protein drives additional food intake until protein requirements are satisfied, the so-called protein leverage effect. It is theoretically possible that increased protein needs of athletes magnify this leverage but at this stage additional research is required to confirm its existence (Simpson & Raubenheimer, 2005).

Reduced carbohydrate diets

Reduced carbohydrate diets (e.g. Atkins, Zone and South Beach diets) are currently popular in the general community and with athletes. The mechanism underpinning the proposed efficacy of these plans is based on the reduction of glycaemic load, decreased insulin secretion and, for Atkins, the induction of ketosis stimulated by severe restriction of dietary carbohydrate. A number of studies have now evaluated the efficacy of reduced carbohydrate diets, most notably the Dr Atkins programme (low carbohydrate, high protein and fat) on weight and fat loss. Evidence suggests that there is a greater weight/fat loss in the short term (up to 3 months) and medium term (up to 6 months) compared with more traditional diets. However, these early results are not maintained and in the longer term (6–12 months), weight is regained (Sacks et al., 2009). Furthermore, weight loss is not superior to programmes which include professional support and behaviour modification (Wadden & Foster, 2000). Early weight (as opposed to fat) loss on Atkins results from glycogen depletion and associated water loss. Additional weight loss has been attributed to the satiating effects of a higher protein intake, which results in lower total energy consumption, not ketosis as originally proposed (Sacks et al., 2009). Short-term success on Atkins has also been associated with adherence and this likely stems from the novelty, simplicity and monotony (limited food variety) of this style of eating. Studies specifically designed to evaluate the impact of food variety indicate that energy intake increases with the number of available foods (Stubbs et al., 2001).

Despite the media hype, Atkins and other reduced carbohydrate programmes such as the Zone diet are no better at maintaining weight/fat loss than balanced macronutrient diets in the longer term. In addition, there are some concerns regarding longer-term safety as ketosis is potentially harmful (associated with hyperlipidaemia, optic neuropathy, osteoporosis and altered cognitive function) and nutrient inadequacy (especially for fibre, vitamins B_1, B_2 and C and minerals calcium and magnesium) primarily due to the limitation of fruit, starchy vege-

tables, grains and dairy foods increases the risk for deficiency and reduced intake of key phytochemicals associated with positive health benefits. In athletes, inadequate carbohydrate intake decreases muscle glycogen stores and has been shown to impair high-intensity training, immune function and recovery (see Chapter 4). The impact on lean mass is unclear (reviewed by O'Connor & Caterson, 2010). Early performance enhancement following weight or fat loss from these diets needs to be countered with the longer-term detrimental effects and the likelihood of weight regain. In practice, athletes attempting to reduce body mass more often adopt certain aspects of reduced carbohydrate diet programmes, typically an increase in protein and a modest reduction in carbohydrate intake and glycaemic index rather than extreme carbohydrate restriction. Unfortunately, popular diet trends travel rapidly through athlete networks and pose a significant risk to younger athletes or those with inadequate support to manage weight and fat loss via more appropriate strategies.

Low glycaemic index and high-fibre diets

Low glycaemic index (GI) diets may enhance satiety (reviewed by McMillan-Price & Brand-Miller, 2006) and a recent systematic review of their use in obesity management suggests this approach has a small positive effect in promoting weight loss (Thomas et al., 2007). Unlike carbohydrate restriction, low-GI diets are associated with positive rather than negative health consequences, although the impact on glycogen stores and athlete performance from chronic use has not been evaluated. As with low-GI diets, high-fibre diets are also associated with enhanced satiety and positive health benefits. In many (but not all) cases high-fibre foods are also low in GI. Use of a high-fibre low-GI meal plan is likely helpful to athletes who need to reduce energy intake, especially to combat hunger and provide greater meal volume. Strategic use of higher fibre snacks between meals may also be beneficial in reducing the build-up of hunger at main meals.

Dairy and higher calcium diets

Evidence from a number of large population studies (reviewed by Major et al., 2008) supports an inverse association between diary intake and BMI. Some (but not all) clinical trials have also demonstrated a positive role for dairy intake (calcium >800 mg/day) in supporting greater weight/fat loss in obese individuals. Plausible biological mechanisms, including the impact of calcium/dairy foods on appetite reduction in addition to a role for intracellular calcium in the regulation of adipocyte lipid metabolism and triglyceride storage, have been proposed. High intake of dairy calcium is also reported to result in about a 2.5-fold increase in faecal fat excretion, which is a small but useful energy loss (~350 kJ) (reviewed by Major *et al.*, 2008). However, increased faecal fat excretion fails to explain the magnitude of the observed weight/fat loss in recent clinical trials suggesting other mechanisms are also at play. Interestingly, positive results are associated with the intake of dairy foods (usually reduced fat milk/yoghurt) not calcium supplements. Reduced fat dairy foods are therefore a nutritious and prudent inclusion in meal plans for weight/fat loss.

Popular diets, meal replacements and commercial weight loss programmes

Clearly, there are numerous 'popular' or 'fad' dietary programmes and examination of all is beyond the scope of this chapter. While any strategy reducing energy intake below expenditure will result in weight loss, the aim for most athletes is to promote fat reduction while maintaining lean mass and optimising performance. Most popular diets fail to provide sufficient energy to support athlete training programmes and are inadequate in key micronutrients (reviewed by Williams & Williams, 2003).

Meal replacement diets work on the basis of energy reduction through meal substitution with commercially supplied meals/beverages designed to provide adequate micronutrients in a lower energy, compact, convenient form. These can be attractive as they appear to take the guesswork out of energy restriction and claim to be palatable and satiating. These replacements can only be used in the short term as they become boring and repetitive. As they are designed for obese sedentary individuals, they fail to provide sufficient energy and macronutrients for athletes. The extreme version of these very low energy diets are suited only to the very obese under medical supervision and are definitely not recommended for use in athletes.

Commercial weight loss programmes (e.g. Weight Watchers, Jenny Craig) are also designed for overweight sedentary individuals not elite athletes. Some

of these programmes may offer adapted guidance for active persons but typically support staff possess inadequate sports nutrition/dietetic expertise to tailor eating programmes for elite athletes. One benefit of some of the commercial programmes and individual counselling with trained professionals (e.g. dietitians, psychologists) includes the incorporation of behaviour modification techniques, which have been clearly shown to enhance weight/fat loss in both the short and long term (reviewed by O'Connor & Caterson, 2010).

Exercise-related strategies to promote weight and fat loss

Exercise intensity and mode of cross-training

Maintenance of exercise training is important to promote and sustain fat loss and optimal physique in athletes. Cross-training is used in many sports not only to develop or extend physiological attributes but also to assist with fat loss or lean mass gain. Traditionally, lower-intensity, longer-duration endurance exercise has been used as the main prescription for promoting additional fat loss, as in addition to increasing energy expenditure it is known to promote adaptations that enhance fat oxidation (see Chapter 6). While the proportion of fat oxidised is greater at low to moderate exercise intensities, well-trained athletes oxidise substantial proportions of fat at moderate to higher intensities providing exercise is below the anaerobic threshold. As more energy is used at higher intensities, a greater total amount of fat can be utilised in less time using this strategy. There also appear to be benefits to appetite reduction (see p. 215) and a number of studies have reported on unexpectedly greater fat loss after higher intensity exercise (Knechtlet *et al.*, 2008; Trapp *et al.*, 2008), even when the energy expended was approximately half of a comparison group undergoing endurance training (Tremblay *et al.*, 1994). The potential benefit of higher-intensity exercise is worth consideration.

Cross-training strategies should be carefully selected and programmed to avoid over-training and injury and need to be tailored to the needs of individual athletes. Although there is anecdotal evidence that some exercise modalities (e.g. running) are more effective for fat loss than others (e.g. swimming), this has not been established in the scientific literature. Prescription of high-impact weight-bearing activities such as running in non-running-trained athletes needs to take into consideration the potential increased risk of injury.

Fat adaptation, 'train low' strategies

Although not typically employed to induce fat loss, chronic fat adaptation strategies and the more recently introduced 'train low' approach (programming training under glycogen replete or deplete states) (see Chapter 6) both drive cellular adaptations upregulating fat oxidation. Enhanced fat oxidation is an obvious benefit for achieving a lean physique, although the training required to achieve these adaptations is more suited to endurance athletes. Some athletes attempt to achieve improved fat oxidation though 'fasted exercise' (typically first session of the day before breakfast) and recently this has also been shown to enhance fat oxidation (Stannard *et al.*, 2010), again in endurance-trained athletes. Thus far, the benefit of these types of strategies on weight or fat reduction has not been evaluated and if beneficial would likely only translate to athletes undergoing substantial endurance training.

17.5 Making weight

Rationale for competition weight limits and 'making weight'

Establishment of weight categories within specific sports promotes fairness and safety amongst competitors, ensuring only athletes of similar size compete against each other. However, the option of competing in a weight category below that normally maintained in training to achieve a potential size and leverage advantage over smaller opponents is an enticing option to many athletes. Weight loss prior to competition is typically achieved by a combination of chronic body composition adjustments and/or acute loss, the latter known as 'making weight' or 'weight cutting', in the hours or days immediately prior to competition. This practice is most widespread in sports where the loss required to move from one division to the next tends to be smaller. Details of all Olympic weight category sports are provided in Table 17.1, including body mass limits and rules governing weigh-in procedures.

Body mass losses within the range of 3–4 kg over 3–4 days or less have been reported amongst athletes in weight category sports with strategies such as fluid and energy restriction, fasting and increased exercise common. Other more extreme weight loss methods have also been reported, including the promotion of passive and active sweat loss and, in some cases, vomiting plus the use of pharmacological agents including laxatives and diuretics (Steen & Brownell, 1990), the latter in breach of the World Anti-Doping Code. Given the methods undertaken and rates of weight loss achieved, body fat contributes little to acute loss, with most achieved via a reduction in body water, glycogen and potentially muscle mass.

Performance and health implications associated with 'making weight'

The performance decrement associated with acute weight loss will depend on the sport and the balance between the degree of weight loss and any potential advantages gained from competing in a lower weight category against smaller, less powerful opponents. While activities demanding high power output and absolute strength are less likely to be influenced by acute weight loss (e.g. competitive weight-lifting) performance is typically compromised in sports requiring a significant contribution from aerobic and/or anaerobic energy metabolism (Fogelholm, 1994). Impairment may be offset when a recovery period is afforded between weigh-in and competition, as occurs for all Olympic weight category sports. In wrestling, an acute loss of body mass prior to competition has, on occasion, been associated with greater competitive success, most likely because athletes with greater muscle mass have an advantage in relative strength and power over smaller opponents (Wroble & Moxley, 1998). Muscular strength and power advantages are probably less salient in sports like lightweight rowing because of the greater aerobic demands, although lightweight rowers who win medals at world championships have greater muscle mass than non-medallists.

Any potential performance benefit of weight making needs to be evaluated against the serious health implications of aggressive, acute weight loss. Recognising this, the American College of Sports Medicine (ACSM) have published two position statements addressing the safety and impact of weight making (Oppliger *et al.*, 1996). These endorse an alternative to acute weight loss, promoting the manipulation of training and diet to create a small energy deficit that induces a gradual reduction in

Table 17.1 Olympic weight category sports, including weight categories and competition weigh-in rules.

Sport	Gender	Weight category	Timing of weigh-in	Frequency of weigh-in
Rowing	Male	Boat average 70 kg, maximum of 72.5 kg (lightweight) Unrestricted (heavyweight)	2 hours prior to scheduled race start, for 1 hour	Before *all* races throughout competition
	Female	Boat average 57 kg, maximum of 59 kg (lightweight) Unrestricted (heavyweight)		
Judo	Male	<60 kg 60–66 kg 66–73 kg 73–81 kg 81–90 kg 90–100 kg +100 kg	At least 2 hours prior to the scheduled start time	Once, on the day of competition for the specified weight category
	Female	<48 kg 48–52 kg 52–57 kg 57–63 kg 63–70 kg 70–78 kg +78 kg		
Taekwondo	Male	<58 kg 58–68 kg 68–80 kg +80 kg	The day before competition for 2 hours at a time to be decided by organising committee	Once, on the day of competition for the specified weight category
	Female	<49 kg 49–57 kg 57–67 kg +67 kg		
Boxing	Male	<48 kg 48–51 kg 51–54 kg 54–57 kg 57–60 kg 60–64 kg 64–69 kg 69–75 kg 75–81 kg 81–91 kg	Morning of first day of competition, at least 6 hours before first scheduled bout. At least 3 hours before first scheduled bout on all subsequent days in which athlete competes	Before *all* bouts throughout competition
Weight-lifting	Male	<56 kg 56–62 kg 62–69 kg 69–77 kg 77–85 kg 85–94 kg 94–105 kg +105 kg	2 hours prior to the start of competition, for 1 hour	Once, on the day of competition for the specified weight category
	Female	<48 kg 48–53 kg 53–58 kg 58–63 kg 63–69 kg 69–75 kg +75 kg		

(Continued)

Table 17.1 (*Cont'd*)

Sport	Gender	Weight category	Timing of weigh-in	Frequency of weigh-in
Wrestling (Greco-Roman, Freestyle)	Male	<55 kg 55–60 kg 60–66 kg 66–74 kg 74–84 kg 84–96 kg 96–120 kg	Weigh-in the day before scheduled competition for specified weight division	Once, on the day of competition for the specified weight category
	Female	<48 kg 48–55 kg 55–63 kg 63–72 kg		

Table 17.2 American College of Sports Medicine recommendations for weight management in wrestling.

Educate coaches and athletes about the adverse consequences of prolonged fasting and dehydration on physical performance and physical health

Discourage the use of thermally stressful environments like saunas, sweat-promoting suits plus the use of laxatives and diuretics for 'making weight'

National governing bodies of sport to adopt legislation that schedules weigh-ins immediately prior to competition, eliminating the potential of recovery after weigh-in

Encourage the monitoring of body mass during training to monitor hydration practices of athletes and the prescription of fluid intake after training to support rehydration

Assess the body composition of athletes during the pre-season to assist in the identification of an appropriate weight category, directed by a minimum allowable body fat level for both males (5–7%) and females (12–14 %)

Maintain adequate dietary intake to support training, including a minimum daily energy intake (>7100 kJ/day or 1700 kcal/day) rich in carbohydrate, adequate protein and low fat

total mass, with an emphasis on decrements in body fat. While prepared specifically for wrestling, the recommendations are relevant to other weight category sports (Table 17.2). The position statements emphasise coach and athlete education on sound nutrition and weight control behaviours to curtail weight cutting, as athletes often seek weight management guidance from coaches or other athletes rather than health/sport science professionals.

Successful interventions such as the Wisconsin Wrestling Minimum Weight Project aimed to reduce unhealthy weight-making practices via three key strategies: determination of an individual athlete minimum competitive weight (based on a body fat level of 7%), limiting weekly weight loss (no more than 3 pounds or 1.4 kg) and nutrition education to assist in achieving specified goals (Oppliger *et al.*, 1998). However, there is evidence of continued use of extreme weight-making practices. The hyperthermia-related death of three young wrestlers attempting to reduce

weight by 7–9% via rigorous diet and fluid restriction, together with intense exercise in the heat wearing sweat-promoting suits, demonstrates the dire consequences resulting from aggressive weight-making strategies. This tragic incident prompted sport governing bodies, including the National Collegiate Athletic Association (NCAA), to implement individual weight certification programmes similar to that in Wisconsin.

Pre-competition body mass management guidelines

Competition preparation must begin with identification of an appropriate weight category, one which maximises the athlete's potential for success by ensuring he or she is competing against athletes of equal or lesser size and strength/power while also being achievable with strategic training and nutrition support. Establishing a physique profile on an athlete over a number of years helps to identify a body composition that each individual athlete is capable of achieving. If body fat levels are above those identified as optimal for that individual athlete, adequate time should be allocated to support a reduction with regular assessment of body mass and body composition critical. Dietary adjustments should aim to create a modest (up to ~2000 kJ/day) negative energy balance to promote a weight loss of no more than 0.5–1.0 kg/week. Faster loss likely impairs training quality and may promote greater rates of lean body mass loss, ultimately impairing performance. Consideration may also need to be given to recovery weeks where training quality is a prioritised over fat loss and nutrition support adjusted to accommodate this. Euhydration should be encouraged during the weeks prior to competition to support optimal training quality.

Athletes should aim to be within 2–3% of their competition weight in the last 1–2 weeks prior to competition. A physique assessment during this time can then identify whether the final adjustments in body mass should come from further fat loss and/or strategic use of acute weight loss 24–48 hours before weigh-in. This may include the use of a low-residue low-volume meal plan to assist in reducing faecal bulk and thus body mass as well as moderation of fluid intake. This approach in combination can induce a 2–3% body mass loss without the health risks associated with strategies such as sweat loss in thermally stressful environments. As with any pre-competition strategy, this approach should be trialled in training with the support of suitably qualified health/sports science professionals to assess both tolerance and the amount of weight loss achieved. Similarly, if a traditional pre-competition training taper is to be implemented, energy intake will need to be adjusted accordingly to prevent weight gain. If fluid intake is moderated in the last 24–48 hours before weigh-in, nutritional recovery strategies to be implemented in the time frame between weigh-in and competition must also be trialled in training to assess effectiveness and tolerance.

Recovery following weigh-in

Athletes are encouraged to pay particular attention to dietary intake in the days and hours before competition, under the assumption that pre-competition nutritional strategies can influence competitive outcomes. For athletes competing in weight category sports, the pre-

competition meal also offers an opportunity to recover, at least partially, from the physiological effects of any acute weight loss strategies undertaken prior to weigh-in. The intake of fluid, electrolytes and carbohydrate are particularly important during this time, although the specific nutritional recovery strategies implemented may vary depending on the method of acute weight loss implemented. Thus, recovery practices between weigh-in and competition should be prioritised, and a structured individualised nutritional plan implemented.

Consumption of a drink volume approximating 150–200% of the existing fluid deficit is required to acutely restore fluid balance (i.e. within 6 hours), accounting for obligatory urinary, sweat, respiratory and metabolic losses that persist after exercise. However, replacement of 100% of fluid losses incurred during exercise may be sufficient for full restoration of plasma volume within 90 min provided adequate sodium is co-ingested and the fluid deficit is not large, i.e. 3% or less. A sodium intake within the range 50–60 mmol/l is recommended for optimal rehydration and can be derived from both food and drinks (Maughan & Leiper, 1995).

Rates of gastric emptying at rest and during exercise may decrease by as much as 20–25%, and the risk of gastrointestinal symptoms exacerbated, while in a hypohydrated state. Despite this, gastric emptying rates within the range 900–1000 ml/hour are possible when aggressive rehydration strategies are employed in the first 2 hours after exercise-induced hypohydration. Ingesting additional fluid above this volume may be contraindicated, offering no additional benefit and potentially increasing the risk of gastrointestinal distress.

The ergogenic potential of pre-exercise carbohydrate intake on endurance performance has been well researched. However, the performance implications of carbohydrate ingestion in the few hours prior to brief high-intensity exercise has been less widely investigated, especially among athletes in weight category sports who routinely undertake acute energy restriction prior to competition that is capable of reducing muscle glycogen stores by 30–50%. In an effort to address this issue, Walberg-Rankin et al. (1996) provided wrestlers with a high (75%) carbohydrate beverage following 3 days of energy restriction that resulted in a 3.3% body mass loss. While this restored anaerobic performance, an energy-matched, moderate (47%) carbohydrate intake did not, suggesting that sufficient carbohydrate intake following weigh-in may be important in maintaining performance. Maximal rates of muscle glycogen restoration are achieved with a carbohydrate intake of approximately 1.2 g/kg/hour, with preference for high glycaemic index choices.

Sport-specific considerations for making weight

Practitioners require thorough sports-specific knowledge when counselling athletes in weight category sports, including competition regulations (weight classifications, frequency of weigh-in, recovery period following weigh-in) and the metabolic demands of both training and competition. Recognition that variation in weight-making regulations for specific events influences body mass management goals and practices as well as nutritional recovery strategies is also critical. For example, the eight weight classifications normally contested in taekwondo are consolidated into four at Olympic competition. Similarly, international wrestling competition permits upwards of a day between weigh-in and competition, while the US collegiate system only allows 1–2 hours. Appreciation of the anomalies and nuances of weight category sports enables the practitioner to be more effective in assisting athletes to optimise performance in a manner which does not adversely affect health in the short or long term.

17.6 Risks of weight/fat loss and making weight

Energy deficiency, endocrine dysfunction, osteopenia and disordered eating

The recommendation to undertake weight or fat loss in athletes is a serious decision. Dieting increases the risk for inadequate nutrient intake, especially when energy restriction is severe. The onset of dieting can commence the journey towards disordered eating. This can even be the case when an athlete is provided with professional advice that is sensible and evidence based. Athletes presenting for weight or fat loss are not at health risk of excess fat; rather the intervention is specifically for performance or aesthetic reasons. Risks are likely greater for younger athletes who are

still growing and who may be struggling with many other issues that can be exacerbated by elite level training pressures and body image concerns.

Energy restriction increases the risk for energy deficiency and this may result in menstrual dysfunction and osteopenia in female athletes. Osteopenia considerably increases the risk for stress fractures (particularly pelvic and tibia), which at the very least will result in a modest degree of training interruption or, at worst, will recur and may be career ending. Re-establishment of bone integrity may not be possible and predisposes the athlete to osteoporosis in later life (see Chapter 19). Although the mass media, coaches or other athletes may casually discuss implementing dietary restriction, it is not low risk even when professionally supported. Recommending an athlete to reduce weight or fat without facilitating professional support should be avoided and places the athlete at an unacceptable risk. Unfortunately, problems may not be immediately apparent and early positive results can mask underlying issues and emerging deficiencies that eventually become larger unresolvable problems. Professional and empathic support is necessary and careful expert navigation of pubertal changes, especially in girls, is critical (see Chapter 23).

In elite athletes, where there is clearly a benefit of lower body weight and fat for competition, this can often be periodised to minimise the time and extent of restriction. Delaying the recommendation to achieve extreme levels of leanness in younger developing athletes is also advocated to postpone dietary restriction until after puberty and the athlete has moved closer to peak bone mass, is more mature and is better able to cope, understand and navigate the risks.

Reduction of lean mass, resting metabolic rate and impact of 'weight cycling'

Severe energy restriction results in lean mass reduction that lowers RMR, making subsequent weight loss more difficult. Although exercise promotes gains in lean mass, this is lost with dieting, even when combined with resistance training. Repeated cycles of weight loss and gain or 'weight cycling' may also exacerbate the loss of lean mass and reduction in RMR, although evidence suggests that this can be restored once dieting is ceased. Weight cycling has been proposed to increase the risk for early mortality, although this has not been clearly established. A study of retired athletes suggests that weight cycling increases the risk for weight gain and obesity in later life (Saarni et al., 2006), but additional studies in athletes are required to confirm this.

Illness and immunity

Dieting has been associated with increased illness and reduced immunity. This may be mediated by inadequate carbohydrate intake, which is known to help attenuate elevated cortisol levels associated with exercise. Inadequate nutrient intake, particularly antioxidants and ω-3 fatty acids, may also compromise immune function (see Chapter 21).

17.7 Strategies for weight gain

The desire to increase muscle mass is common for athletes in sports where strength/power attributes are critical to competitive success. Gaining muscle mass demands consideration of a range of issues, including the overall training programme, training status or 'training age' of the individual, as well as their genetic profile and dietary intake. Whether an athlete loses or gains muscle mass is a result of the chronic balance between skeletal muscle protein synthesis and breakdown. If the balance is positive (i.e. synthesis exceeds breakdown), skeletal muscle hypertrophy will result, whereas skeletal muscle atrophy occurs when chronic protein degradation exceeds synthesis. Protein turnover is influenced by a number of stimuli, the most powerful of which are nutrient intake and exercise. While both of these factors influence skeletal muscle breakdown, the primary determinant of net muscle protein balance in response to both exercise and nutrition is change in muscle protein synthesis.

Training to optimise lean mass gain

Preparation for most sports includes a combination of sport-specific and other conditioning training. When strength/power traits or larger body size is advantageous, conditioning will almost certainly include a structured resistance or strength training programme. When concurrent strength and endurance training are undertaken, resistance

training adaptations are compromised, presumably because of the associated fatigue and muscle damage, catabolic endocrine response, possible fibre type transformations, substrate depletion and increased energy expenditure. If skeletal muscle hypertrophy is a priority, a 'hypertrophy phase' needs to be incorporated into the athlete's annual training cycle. The off-season or early pre-season may be opportune times to focus on gains in muscle size and strength, where an emphasis can be placed on resistance training and less on sport-specific conditioning.

Muscle protein synthesis is increased in response to both resistance and endurance exercise, as is muscle protein breakdown, though to a lesser extent. As a consequence, muscle protein balance improves in response to exercise but does not become positive without protein intake or, more specifically, essential amino acid ingestion. This elevation in protein synthesis and degradation is maintained for upwards of 24–48 hours following exercise, highlighting a critical period in which optimisation of dietary intake is paramount if gains in muscle mass are to be maximised. The synergistic interaction between resistance exercise and diet has been the source of significant research investigation in recent years, the results having application within the sports context but also in the treatment of clinical conditions like sarcopenia.

Protein intake and lean mass gain

Understanding of the critical role played by diet in optimising resistance training adaptations has rapidly expanded in recent years (Burd et al., 2009). While debate continues on the need for additional protein, guidelines for athletes undertaking strength training recommend a protein intake approximately twice current recommendations for sedentary counterparts or as much as 1.6–1.7 g/kg/day. Given the wide distribution of protein in the food supply and increased energy intake of athletes, most strength-trained athletes easily achieve these increased protein needs. Exceeding the upper range of protein intake guidelines offers no further benefit and merely promotes protein oxidation. A period of resistance training also reduces protein turnover and improves net protein retention, effectively reducing dietary protein requirements of experienced resistance-trained athletes.

Simply contrasting an athlete's daily protein consumption against guidelines does not address if intake has been optimised to promote gains in muscle mass. Consideration of other dietary factors, including the source and daily distribution of intake and the proximity to training, is also important (Tang & Phillips, 2009). Athletes typically consume the majority of daily protein intake at main meals, with less consumed in between or in snacks before and after training. Dietary protein ingestion elevates muscle protein synthesis, with a concomitant minor suppression in muscle protein breakdown, resulting in a positive net balance. When consumed in close temporal proximity to resistance exercise, the protein synthetic response to ingestion is exacerbated. The ingestion of just 20 g of high biological value protein (equivalent to about 9 g of essential amino acids) after resistance exercise appears to be sufficient to maximally stimulate muscle protein synthesis, with amounts in excess of this oxidised (Moore et al., 2009). Less is known about optimal protein distribution outside of training but inclusion of at least small amounts in all meals and snacks may be beneficial, at least 24–48 hours after exercise when muscle protein synthesis and breakdown remain elevated.

The type of ingested protein influences both acute rates of muscle protein synthesis and degradation as well as chronic resistance training adaptations. Ingestion of high-quality proteins including milk (both slowly digested casein and rapidly metabolised whey) and soy have been reported to stimulate muscle protein synthesis. However, both acute and chronic resistance training responses have been observed to vary depending on the specific protein ingested, most likely because of differences in the amino acid profile and/or rates of protein digestion. Essential amino acids, and specifically the branched-chain amino acid leucine, rather than the non-essential amino acids are required to promote protein synthesis. Approximately 2–3 g of leucine is required to maximally stimulate protein synthesis, an amount easily achieved from the ingestion of a range of whole foods. Foods naturally high in branched-chain amino acids, and specifically leucine, are specified in Table 17.3.

When standardised for essential amino acid consumption, acute post-exercise whey ingestion stimulates muscle protein synthesis to a greater extent than either soy protein or casein (Tang et al., 2009). Replicated over a series of training sessions, whey

Table 17.3 Leucine and branched-chain amino acid content of various foods.[a]

Food	Leucine (%)	Branched-chain amino acids (%)
Whey protein isolate	14	26
Milk protein	10	21
Egg	9	22
Muscle protein	8	18
Soy protein isolate	8	18
Wheat protein	7	15

[a] Values reflect the grams of amino acids per 100 g of protein from the specified foods.

ingestion results in greater skeletal muscle hypertrophy (Hartman et al., 2007). This may be due to its rapid digestion or higher leucine content, the combination of which likely results in higher blood leucine concentrations that approach a critical leucine threshold required to maximally stimulate protein synthesis (Tang et al., 2009). Soy is also rapidly digested but the resultant amino acids appear to be more completely extracted in the splanchnic bed and contribute less to peripheral protein accretion, an effect also observed for other rapidly metabolised proteins. Taken together, the daily distribution and amount of protein ingested at each eating occasion plus the amino acid profile and digestion rate influences both the acute and chronic resistance training response.

Co-ingestion of other nutrients and lean mass gain

Resistance training sessions are partially dependent on glycogenolysis for energy production, resulting in significant reductions in muscle glycogen levels. Given that resistance training typically forms only one component of an athlete's training schedule, recovery strategies proven to enhance restoration of muscle glycogen stores such as post-exercise carbohydrate ingestion should be routinely implemented following resistance training. Carbohydrate ingestion also reduces muscle protein breakdown and thus enhances net protein balance, though to a lesser degree than amino acid ingestion. The combined ingestion of carbohydrate and protein acutely following resistance training results in more favourable restoration of muscle glycogen stores and muscle protein metabolism than the ingestion of either nutrient alone, especially when the intake of either is less than optimal. There is also preliminary evidence suggesting that concurrent fat ingestion enhances amino acid uptake into peripheral tissues. The mechanism by which this occurs remains to be elucidated, although a slowing of protein digestion or associated increase in total energy intake appears plausible.

Energy intake and lean mass gain

While dietary protein is important, total daily energy intake also plays a critical role. At any given protein intake, increasing energy intake creates a more positive nitrogen balance, presumably because the additional energy allows more of the ingested protein to be directed to protein synthesis. A positive energy balance also creates an anabolic hormonal profile, promoting lean body mass gain, even when undertaken independent of resistance exercise. In fact, upwards of half the weight gain may come from lean body mass, although individual responses vary markedly. Despite long-standing awareness of this, little is known about the optimal energy surplus to promote gains in muscle mass. Amongst sedentary individuals, the energy cost of weight gain is about 34 000 kJ/kg gained (Forbes *et al.*, 1986), although this also varies. While interesting, application of these findings to resistance-trained athletes aiming to gain only lean mass is problematic. The optimal energy surplus to maximise gains in muscle mass while minimising the impact on body fat is undetermined as is the nutrient composition of the energy surplus and its distribution throughout the day or training week.

Estimating daily energy needs of athletes is notoriously difficult because of the variability in expenditure associated with training. Creation of a moderate energy surplus (~1000–4000 kJ/day) presuming the athlete is weight stable (and thus in energy balance) and monitoring adaptations closely via regular assessment of body mass and composition is usually effective. This 'monitored titration' of energy intake can result in lean mass gains of 0.25–0.5 kg/week with no appreciable change in body fat. Faster rates of gain are more likely to result in fat deposition. The extent of energy surplus required depends on the individual athlete, the genetic profile, resistance training history and presenting body composition plus time frame available to prioritise muscle hypertrophy. The source of additional energy may depend on practical issues, in particular a requirement to

fuel other training and opportunities to increase food/fluids throughout the day.

For some athletes, increasing energy intake can be a real challenge. Frequent and/or prolonged training sessions can limit opportunities for meals and snacks while intense training can curb appetite (see p. 215). Novel strategies like eating energy-dense snacks and drinks may overcome such obstacles. Failure to recognise the importance of increased energy intake will compromise resistance training adaptations. Regular athlete support and monitoring is required with significant contribution from the sports coach, conditioning specialist and dietitian required.

17.8 Role of physique assessment

Physique assessment enables the effectiveness of diet and training interventions to be evaluated and if necessary modified. Anthropometric, bioelectrical impedance (BIA), radiographic (computed tomography, magnetic resonance imaging, dual energy X-ray absorptiometry or DEXA) and metabolic (creatinine, 3-methylhistidine) techniques are available. Suitable selection requires evaluation of both technical factors (e.g. safety, validity, precision and accuracy) and practical factors (e.g. financial implications, portability, invasiveness, time effectiveness, and available technical expertise). Consideration must be given to assessment methodologies that accommodate measurement of unique physique traits characteristic of some athletes, including particularly tall, broad and muscular individuals or those with extremely low body fat levels. Routine monitoring of physique traits amongst athletes is typically undertaken using one of the following three techniques: DEXA, BIA or surface anthropometry.

Dual energy X-ray absorptiometry

DEXA, originally developed for the diagnosis of osteoporosis, remains the gold standard tool for bone density assessment. In recent years, DEXA has also been widely used as a method to assess soft tissue body composition. In addition to fat mass (FM) and fat-free mass (FFM), DEXA provides information on regional body composition (i.e. arms, legs, trunk, left/right differences), which is particularly appealing to athletes undertaking targeted training programmes or injury rehabilitation. Whole-body scans are rapid, non-invasive and associated with low radiation doses, making the technology safe for longitudinal monitoring.

Of particular relevance to athletic populations is the available scanning area, typically limited to 60–65 × 193–198 cm depending on the manufacturer. Whole-body DEXA scans on particularly tall or broad and muscular athletes are difficult to perform. Taller individuals are either scanned without the head or feet or with knees bent so the body fits within the scanned area. Alternatively, data are summed from two partial scans. To optimise accuracy, special consideration should be given to standardised measurement protocols and, in athletes, measurement in a fasted euhydrated state (Vilaca et al., 2009).

Furthermore, DEXA with only two ('dual') energy beams means it can only determine two different tissue densities at any one measurement point, measured per pixel. Consequently, proportions of FM versus FFM can only be determined in soft tissues, i.e. where there is no bone. Approximately 60% of the pixels in a whole-body scan do not contain bone, so here body composition can be calculated with sophisticated calculations to compute body composition and make assumptions for the remaining bone-containing areas. This is problematic due to differences in fat distribution and for individuals with limited or excessive adipose tissue (Jebb, 1997).

Bioelectrical impedance

BIA is a safe and non-invasive body composition method based on the differing electrical conductivity of FM and FFM (Kyle et al., 2004a,b). FFM contains water and electrolytes and is a good electrical conductor, while anhydrous FM is not. Because of the reliance on body water for conductivity, BIA may not be valid for assessment of subjects with abnormal hydration and this is an issue for athlete assessment. Acute food and fluid intake increases measurement error, and fasting for at least 8 hours with measurement in a euhydrated state is recommended. The practicality and achievement of these conditions in athletes can be challenging.

Although foot to foot (stand-on) BIA analysers are popular, inexpensive and easily purchased, the current is only circulated through the legs and lower trunk with results extrapolated to the whole body, limiting accuracy. 'Athlete' mode is likely most appropriate but unfortunately parameters defining 'athlete'

and details of equations used for calculation of body composition are typically not provided by the manufacturer. Single frequency BIA analysers (usually incorporating four electrodes placed on the wrist, hand, ankle and foot) are also available but more frequently used by health professionals or researchers. While raw impedance data can be extracted and substituted into population-specific equations, overcoming issues with equation specificity, limited equations are available for athlete populations.

Although measurement by BIA appears practical and relatively simple, it has less than optimal accuracy compared with DEXA and hydrodensitometry. Error is often attributed to arm positioning, skin temperature, gastrointestinal tract contents and hydration status plus technical issues like electrode placement. If used, standardised protocols are essential and accuracy limitations should be acknowledged.

Surface anthropometry

Practical, portable and cost-effective, surface anthropometry is often used to assess body composition in athletic populations. The technique evaluates anthropometric traits (body mass, stature, subcutaneous skinfold thicknesses, girths and lengths) at specific anatomical landmarks to describe and monitor physique. Highly skilled technicians are required if reliable data are to be collected. Technicians need to be meticulous with accurate site location and measurement technique, with recognised training through groups like the International Society for the Advancement of Kinanthropometry (ISAK) strongly encouraged. Measurements just 1–2 cm away from a defined site can produce significant differences in results (Hume & Marfell-Jones, 2008). If repeat measurements are to be taken over time, it is important that the same technician collect the data.

Estimates of body density, FM and/or FFM can be derived from raw skinfold data, with more than 100 regression equations to predict body fat from skinfolds available. The value of prediction equations for assessment of change in body fat has not been widely assessed but evidence suggests they lack sensitivity for tracking small but potentially important changes (Silva et al., 2009). As such, conversion of skinfold sum to percent fat is not encouraged. Rather, interpretation of change to raw anthropometric data (i.e. results from individual skinfold sites and sum of sites measured, in millimetres) and subsequent comparison to individual or athlete population norms is likely superior and more sensitive for tracking change and assessing the appropriateness of body composition to competitive success.

Skinfold sum measurement in athletes is robust and not readily influenced by hydration or gastrointestinal tract contents (Norton *et al.*, 1998). However, interpretation of body composition is typically undertaken in conjunction with body mass, which can be acutely influenced by hydration and meal consumption, independent of changes in fat or skeletal muscle mass. Consequently, body mass should be measured at the same time of day (preferably before breakfast or training after voiding bladder and bowel) wearing minimal clothing to minimise variability associated with these factors. The calibration and consistency of scales used, menstrual cycle phase in women, and hydration status also warrant attention.

All physique assessment tools have limitations and are subject to error. An appreciation of this allows practitioners to distinguish between a measured change that could be predominantly error or an actual change in body composition. In general, physique assessments should not be undertaken any more regularly than every 4–8 weeks, depending on the individual athlete and his or her body composition goals. When conducting physique assessments, the physical and emotional well-being of the athlete remains a priority. Sensitivity should be shown to cultural beliefs and tradition. Procedures should be explained to those unfamiliar, with information provided in advance on what testing is to be undertaken, the reason for profiling and any specific requirements such as clothing to be worn. Where appropriate, consideration should be given to gender compatibility between the technician and athlete, with privacy in measurement, data collection and reporting always assured.

17.9 Adjunctive agents for weight/fat loss or lean mass gain

Pharmacological agents to promote weight loss

A number of pharmacological agents are available and demonstrated as effective to promote weight or fat loss. The use of pharmacotherapy to promote weight/fat loss in athletes is inconsistent with the recommended prescription of these medications, which are designed for treatment of obesity in combination with diet, exercise and behaviour modification. Most agents are not permitted by sports drug agencies (reviewed by O'Connor & Caterson, 2010). Their use in athletes is not recommended.

Dietary supplements to promote weight loss

Efficacy of dietary supplements for weight or fat loss, including L-carnitine, chromium picolinate and β-hydroxy-β-methylbutyrate (HMB), are questionable (see Chapter 9). The effectiveness of herbal supplements is reviewed elsewhere (Hasani-Ranjbar *et al.*, 2009). Thermogenic agents including caffeine and green tea extract generally produce a small, not clinically meaningful benefit in the obese, with efficacy yet to be evaluated in athletes. Stimulants such as ephedrine are not permitted by sports drug agencies and use is associated with negative and potentially serious side effects (reviewed by O'Connor & Caterson, 2010). Contamination of weight loss supplements with ephedrine or similar stimulants (e.g. Ma Huang) has been frequently reported (Geyer *et al.*, 2008). In athletes, complementary or over-the-counter weight loss supplements risk inadvertent doping, offer unproven or insignificant clinical benefit and are therefore not recommended.

Dietary supplements to promote weight gain

Individuals attempting to increase muscle mass may be particularly vulnerable to supplement marketing. Weight gain products tend to be popular among athletes competing in strength/power sports and include protein and specific amino acid supplements, buffering agents like sodium bicarbonate and β-alanine, creatine monohydrate, HMB, caffeine and nitric oxide-stimulating supplements (Tipton *et al.*, 2007). Recognising the nutritional value of food sources of protein and essential amino acids, creatine monohydrate appears to be the only supplement which consistently enhances skeletal muscle hypertrophy and functional capacity in response to resistance training (Hespel & Derave, 2007). However, liquid meal supplements rich in carbohydrate and protein may be particularly valuable in the post-exercise period to boost total energy and specific nutrient intake at a time when the appetite is often suppressed. Further details on these supplements, including protocols for ingestion, where appropriate, are provided in Chapter 9. However, it is important to recognise that any benefit of creatine or other supplement ingestion to further enhance skeletal muscle hypertrophy will be very small relative to the adaptations that result from a suitably designed training programme and strategic nutrition support. As with supplements touted to support weight loss, careful consideration should be given to contamination of products that may have both doping and health implications.

References

American College of Sports Medicine. Nutrition and athletic performance. Med Sci Sports Exerc 2009; 41: 709–731.

Bray S, Hagberg MJ, Pérusse L *et al.* The human gene map for perfomance and health-related phenotypes. The 2006–2007 update. Med Sci Sports Exerc 2009; 41: 34–72.

Burd NA, Tang JE *et al.* Exercise training and protein metabolism: influences of contraction, protein inrake and sex-based differences. J Appl Physiol 2009; 106: 1692–1701.

Fogelholm M. Effects of bodyweight reduction on sports performance. Sports Med 1994; 18: 249–267.

Forbes GB, Brown MR *et al.* Deliberate overfeeding in women and men: energy cost and composition of the weight gain. Br J Nutr 1986; 56: 1–9.

Geyer H, Parr MK *et al.* Nutritional supplements cross-contaminated and faked with doping substances. J Mass Spectrom 2008; 43: 892–902.

Hartman JW, Tang JE *et al.* Consumption of fat-free fluid milk after resistance exercise promotes greater lean mass accretion than does consumption of soy or carbohydrate in young, novice, male weightlifters. Am J Clin Nutr 2007; 86: 373–381.

Hasani-Ranjbar S, Nayebi N, Larijani B, Abdollahi M. A systematic review of the efficacy and safety of herbal medicines used in the treatment of obesity. World J Gastroenterol 2009; 15: 3073–3085.

Heaney S, O'Connor H, Naughton J, Gifford J. Towards an understanding of the barriers to good nutrition for elite athletes. Int J Sports Sci Coach 2008; 3: 391–401.

Hespel P, Derave W. Ergogenic effects of creatine in sports and rehabilitation. Subcell Biochem 2007; 46: 245–259.

Hume P, Marfell-Jones M. The importance of accurate site location for skinfold measurement. J Sports Sci 2008; 26: 1333–1340.

Jebb SA. Measurement of soft tissue composition by dual energy X-ray absorptiometry. Br J Nutr 1997; 97: 151–163.

Khosla T, McBroom VC. Age, height and weight of female Olympic finalists. Br J Sports Med 1988; 9: 96–99.

King NA, Burley VJ, Blundell JE. Exercise-induced suppression of appetite: effects on food intake and implications for energy balance. Eur J Clin Nutr 1994; 48: 715–724.

Knechtlet B, Schwanke M, Knechtlet P, Kohler G. Decrease in body fat during an ultra-endurance triathlon is associated with race intensity. Br J Sports Med 2008; 42: 609–613.

Kyle UG, Bosaeus I *et al.* Bioelectrical impedance analysis. Part I: review of principles and methods. Clin Nutr 2004a; 23: 1226–1243.

Kyle UG, Bosaeus I *et al.* Bioelectrical impedance analysis. Part II: utilization in clinical practice. Clin Nutr 2004b; 23: 1430–1453.

McMillan-Price J, Brand-Miller J. Low glycemic index diets and body weight regulation. Int J Obes 2006; 30: S40–S46.

Major GC, Chaput J-P, Ledoux M *et al.* Recent developments in calcium related obesity research. Obes Rev 2008; 9: 428–445.

Manore M, Thompson J. Energy requirments of the athlete: assessment and evidence of energy efficency. In: Clinical Sports Nutrition (Burke L, Deakin V, eds). Sydney: McGraw-Hill, 2010, pp 98–115.

Maughan RJ, Leiper JB. Sodium intake and post-exercise rehydration in man. Eur J Appl Physiol Occup Physiol 1995; 71: 311–319.

Moore DR, Robinson MJ *et al.* Ingested protein dose response of muscle and albumin protein synthesis after resistance exercise in young men. Am J Clin Nutr 2009; 89: 161–168.

Norton K, Olds T. Morphological evolution of athletes over the twentieth century: causes and consequences. Sports Med 2001; 31: 763–783.

Norton K, Hayward S *et al.* The effects of hypohydration and hyperhydration on skinfold measurements. Presented at Sixth Scientific Conference of the International Society for the Advancement of Kinanthropometry, Adelaide. International Society for the Advancement of Kinanthropometry, 1998.

O'Connor H, Caterson I. Weight loss and the athlete. In: Clinical Sports Nutrition (Burke L, Deakin V, eds). Sydney: McGraw-Hill, 2010, pp 116–148.

O'Connor H, Olds T, Maughan RJ. Physique and performance for track and field events. J Sports Sci 2007; 25 (Suppl 1): S49–S60.

Oppliger RA, Case HS *et al.* American College of Sports Medicine position stand. Weight loss in wrestlers. Med Sci Sports Exerc 1996; 28: ix–xii.

Oppliger RA, Landry GL *et al.* Wisconsin minimum weight program reduces weight-cutting practices of high school wrestlers. Clin J Sport Med 1998; 8: 26–31.

O'Rahilly S, Farooqi S, Yeo GSH, Challis B. Human obesity: lessons from monogenic disorders. Endocrinology 2003; 144: 3757–3764.

Saarni SE, Rissaen A, Sarna S *et al.* Weight cycling of athletes and subsequent weight gain in middle age. Int J Obes 2006; 30: 1639–1644.

Sacks FM, Bray GA, Carey VJ *et al.* Comparison of weight loss diets with different compositions of fat, protein and carbohydrates. N Engl J Med 2009; 360: 859–873.

Silva AM, Fields DA *et al.* Are skinfold-based models accurate and suitable for assessing changes in body composition in highly trained athletes? J Strength Cond Res 2009; 23: 1688–1696.

Simpson SJ, Raubenheimer D. Obesity: the protein leverage hypothesis. Obes Rev 2005; 6: 133–142.

Stannard SR, Buckley AJ, Edge JA, Thompson MW. Adaptations to skeletal muscle eith endurance exercise training in the acutely fed versus overnight fasted state. J Sci Med Sport 2010; 13: 465–469.

Steen SR, Brownell KD. Patterns of weight loss and regain in wrestlers: has the tradition changed? Med Sci Sports Exerc 1990; 22: 762–768.

Stepnicka X. Somatotype in relation to physical performance and body posture. In: Kinanthropometry III (Reilly T, Watkins J, Borms J, eds). London: E & F. N. Spon, 1986, pp 39–52.

Stubbs RJ, Johnstone AM, Mazlan N, Mbaiwase E, Ferris S. Effect of altering the variety of sensorially distinct foods, of the same macronutrient content, on food intake and body weight in men. Eur J Clin Nutr 2001; 55: 19–28.

Tang JE, Phillips SM. Maximizing muscle protein anabolism: the role of protein quality. Curr Opin Clin Nutr Metab Care 2009; 12: 66–71.

Tang JE, Moore DR *et al.* Ingestion of whey hydrolysate, casein, or soy protein isolate: effects on mixed muscle protein synthesis at rest and following resistance exercise in young men. J Appl Physiol 2009; 107: 987–992.

Thomas D, Elliott EJ, Baur L. Low glycaemic index or low glycaemic index load diets for overweight and obesity. Cochrane Database Syst Rev 2007; (3): CD005105.

Tipton KD, Jeukendrup AE *et al.* Nutrition for the sprinter. J Sports Sci 2007; 25 (Suppl 1): S5–S15.

Trapp EG, Chisholm DJ, Freund J, Boutcher SH. The effects of high-intensity intermittent exercise training on fat loss and fasting insulin levels of young women. Int J Obes 2008; 32: 684–691.

Tremblay A, Simoneau JA, Bouchard C. Impact of exercise intensity on body fatness and skeletal muscle metabolism. Metabolism 1994; 43: 814–818.

Vilaca KH, Ferriolli E *et al.* Effect of fluid and food intake on the body composition evaluation of elderly persons. J Nutr Health Aging 2009; 13: 183–186.

Wadden TA, Foster GD. Behavioural treatment of obesity. Med Clin North Am 2008; 84: 441–461.

Walberg-Rankin J. Making weight in sports. In: Clinical Sports Nutrition, 4th edn (Burke L, Deakin V, eds). Sydney: McGraw-Hill, 2010, pp 148–170.

Walberg-Rankin J, Ocel JV *et al.* Effect of weight loss and refeeding diet composition on anaerobic performance in wrestlers. Med Sci Sports Exerc 1996; 28: 1292–1299.

Williams L, Williams P. Evaluation of a tool for rating popular diet books. Nutr Diet 2003; 60: 185–197.

Wroble RR, Moxley DP. Acute weight gain and its relationship to success in high school wrestlers. Med Sci Sports Exerc 1998; 30: 949–951.

Further reading

American College of Sports Medicine. American College of Sports Medicine position stand on weight loss in wrestlers. Med Sci Sports 1976; 8: xi–xiii.

Anonymous. Hyperthermia and dehydration-related deaths associated with intentional rapid weight loss in three collegiate wrestlers: North Carolina, Wisconsin, and Michigan, November-December 1997. MMWR 1997; 47: 105–108.

Anonymous. Alert: protein drinks. You don't need the extra protein or the heavy metals our tests found. Consum Rep 2010; 75(7): 24–7.

Børsheim E, Cree MG, Tipton KD, Elliott TA, Aarsland A, Wolfe RR. Effect of carbohydrate intake on net muscle protein synthesis during recovery from resistance exercise. J Appl Physiol. 2004; 96: 674–678.

Bos C, Metges CC, Gaudichon C *et al.* Postprandial kinetics of dietary amino acids are the main determinant of their metabolism after soy or milk protein ingestion in humans. J Nutr 2003; 133: 1308–1315.

Burke LM, Slater G, Broad EM, Haukka J, Modulon S, Hopkins WG. Eating patterns and meal frequency of elite Australian athletes. Int J Sport Nutr Exerc Metab 2009; 13: 521–538.

Calloway DH, Spector H. Nitrogen balance as related to caloric and protein intake in active young men. Am J Clin Nutr 1954; 2: 405–412.

Cisar CJ, Housh TJ, Johnson GO, Thorland WG, Hughes RA. Validity of anthropometric equations for determination of changes in body composition in adult males during training. J Sports Med Phys Fitness 1989; 29: 141–148.

Clarys JP, Martin AD, Marfell-Jones MJ, Janssens V, Caboor D, Drinkwater DT. Human body composition: a review of adult dissection data. Am J Hum Biol 1999; 11: 167–174.

Deglaire A, Fromentin C, Fouillet H *et al.* Hydrolyzed dietary casein as compared with the intact protein reduces postprandial peripheral, but not whole-body, uptake of nitrogen in humans. Am J Clin Nutr 2009; 90: 1011–1022.

Dixon CB, Ramos L, Fitzgerald E, Reppert D, Andreacci JL. The effect of acute fluid consumption on measures of impedance and percent body fat estimated using segmental bioelectrical impedance analysis. Eur J Clin Nutr 2009; 63: 1115–1122.

Elliot TA, Cree MG, Sanford AP, Wolfe RR, Tipton KD. Milk ingestion stimulates net muscle protein synthesis following resistance exercise. Med Sci Sports Exerc 2006; 38: 667–674.

Forbes GB, Brown MR, Welle SL, Underwood LE. Hormonal response to overfeeding. Am J Clin Nutr 1989; 49: 608–611.

Genton L, Hans D, Kyle UG, Pichard C. Dual-energy X-ray absorptiometry and body composition: differences between devices and comparison with reference methods. Nutrition 2002; 18: 66–70.

Going SB, Massett MP, Hall MC *et al.* Detection of small changes in body composition by dual-energy x-ray absorptiometry. Am J Clin Nutr 1993; 57: 845–850.

Gonzalez-Alonso J, Heaps CL, Coyle EF. Rehydration after exercise with common beverages and water. Int J Sports Med 1992; 3: 399–406.

Greiwe JS, Staffey KS, Melrose DR, Narve MD, Knowlton RG. Effects of dehydration on isometric muscular strength and endurance. Med Sci Sports Exerc 1998; 30: 284–288.

Haff GG, Lehmkuhl MJ McCoy LB, Stone MH. Carbohydrate supplementation and resistance training. J Strength Cond Res 2003; 17: 187–196.

Hargreaves M, Hawley JA Jeukendrup A. Pre-exercise carbohydrate and fat ingestion: effects on metabolism and performance. J Sports Sci 2004; 22: 31–38.

Jentjens R, Jeukendrup A. Determinants of post-exercise glycogen synthesis during short-term recovery. Sports Med 2003; 33: 117–144.

Lambrinoudaki I, Georgiou E, Douskas G, Tsekes G, Kyriakidis M, Proukakis C. Body composition assessment by dual-energy X-ray absorptiometry: comparison of prone and supine measurements. Metabolism 1998; 47: 1379–1382.

Lemon PW. Effects of exercise on dietary protein requirements. Int J Sport Nutr 1998; 8: 426–447.

Leveritt M, Abernethy PJ, Barry BK, Logan PA. Concurrent strength and endurance training. A review. Sports Med 1999; 28: 413–427.

Lewiecki EM. Clinical applications of bone density testing for osteoporosis. Minerva Med 2005; 96: 317–330.

Lohman M, Tallroth K, Kettunen JA, Marttinen MT. Reproducibility of dual-energy x-ray absorptiometry total and regional body composition measurements using different scanning positions and definitions of regions. Metabolism 2009; 58: 1663–1668.

Miller SL, Tipton KD, Chinkes DL, Wolf SE, Wolfe RR. Independent and combined effects of amino acids and glucose after resistance exercise. Med Sci Sports Exerc 2003; 35: 449–455.

Mitchell JB, Voss KW. The influence of volume on gastric emptying and fluid balance during prolonged exercise. Med Sci Sports Exerc 1991; 23: 314–319.

Mitchell JB, Grandjean PW, Pizza FX, Starling RD, Holtz RW. The effect of volume ingested on rehydration and gastric emptying following exercise-induced dehydration. Med Sci Sports Exerc 1994; 26: 1135–1143.

Oppliger RA, Harms RD, Herrmann DE, Streich CM, Clark RR. The Wisconsin wrestling minimum weight project: a model for weight control among high school wrestlers. Med Sci Sports Exerc 1995; 27: 1220–1224.

Pasiakos SM, Vislocky LM, Carbone JW et al. Acute energy deprivation affects skeletal muscle protein synthesis and associated intracellular signaling proteins in physically active adults. J Nutr 2010; 140: 745–751.

Phillips SM, Tipton KD, Aarsland A, Wolf SE, Wolfe RR. Mixed muscle protein synthesis and breakdown after resistance exercise in humans. Am J Physiol 1997; 273: E99–E107.

Phillips SM, Tang JE, Moore DR. The role of milk- and soy-based protein in support of muscle protein synthesis and muscle protein accretion in young and elderly persons. J Am Coll Nutr 2009; 28: 343–354.

Rodriguez FA. Physical structure of international lightweight rowers. In: Kinanthropometry III (Reilly T, Watkins J, Borms J, eds). London: E. & F.N. Spon, 1986, pp 255–261.

Rozenek R, Ward P, Long S, Garhammer J. Effects of high-calorie supplements on body composition and muscular strength following resistance training. J Sports Med Phys Fitness 2002; 42: 340–347.

Silva A, Minderico C et al. Calibration models to estimate body composition measurements in taller subjects using DXA. Obes Res 2004; 12: A12.

Steinacker JM. Physiological aspects of training in rowing. Int J Sports Med 1993; 14 (Suppl 1): S3–S10.

Swartz AM, Swartz AM, Jeremy Evans M, King GA, Thompson DL. Evaluation of a foot-to-foot bioelectrical impedance analyser in highly active, moderately active and less active young men. Br J Nutr 2002; 88: 205–210.

Tarnopolsky MA, Atkinson SA, MacDougall JD, Chesley A, Phillips S, Schwarcz HP. Evaluation of protein requirements for trained strength athletes. J Appl Physiol 1992; 73: 1986–1995.

Tarnopolsky MA, Cipriano N, Woodcroft C et al. Effects of rapid weight loss and wrestling on muscle glycogen concentration. Clin J Sport Med 1996; 6: 78–84.

Tipton KD, Gurkin BE, Matin S, Wolfe RR. Nonessential amino acids are not necessary to stimulate net muscle protein synthesis in healthy volunteers. J Nutr Biochem 1999; 10: 89–95.

Tremblay A, Déspres J-P, Bouchard C. The effects of exercise-training on energy balance and adipose tissue morphology and metabolism. Sports Med 1985; 2: 223–233.

van Nieuwenhoven MA, Vriens BE, Brummer RJ, Brouns F. Effect of dehydration on gastrointestinal function at rest and during exercise in humans. Eur J Appl Physiol 2000; 83: 578–584.

18
Eating Disorders and Athletes

Jorunn Sundgot-Borgen and Ina Garthe

Key messages

- Disordered eating (DE) occurs on a continuum that ranges from dieting and restrictive eating, to abnormal eating behaviour and finally to clinical eating disorders (ED) with medical complications.
- Studies show that prevalence of ED is high in those sports in which leanness and/or a specific weight is considered important for performance.
- Since dieting is the primary precursor to the development of DE and EDs, unnecessary dieting should be prevented.
- The medical staff of teams and parents must be able to recognise symptoms indicating risk for EDs. Coaches and leaders must accept that DE can be a problem in the athletic community and that openness regarding this challenge is important.
- If a change in body mass or body composition is wanted by the athlete and recommended by healthcare professionals for health

and/or performance, the weight goal should be based on objective measurements of body composition and prior to weight-loss intervention. There should also be a screening including weight history and weight goal, menstrual history for females, an estimate of body composition and energy/nutritional status, and questions regarding motivation, dietary habits, thoughts and feelings about body image, body weight and food. If there is a history of DE/ED, a more intense and longer period of follow-up is needed.
- Change in body composition should be monitored on a regular basis including a period of at least 2 months after the weight or body fat percentage goal has been reached to detect any continued or unwarranted losses or weight fluctuations.
- Normal-weight athletes under the age of 18 years should be discouraged to lose weight.

18.1 Introduction

Elite athletes often embody the concept of physical perfection. However, not all athletes have, or have a feeling, that their bodies are adapted to the optimal body type of their specific sport. Those athletes often experience pressure to achieve this 'ideal' body type. In addition to the socio-cultural demands placed on male and females to achieve and maintain an ideal body shape, athletes are also under pressure to improve performance and conform to the specific requirements of their sport. They are also evaluated by coaches on an almost daily basis. These factors may lead to dieting, use of disordered eating (DE) behaviours and development of severe eating disorders (EDs). Although dieting is considered one important risk factor, it is not necessarily dieting *per se* that triggers DE or ED, but whether dieting is guided or not. Controlled weight loss intervention in

elite athletes indicates that athletes do not increase the risk for DE or EDs when guided by a professional sports nutritionist. The consequences of DE can be severe in terms of both health and performance, and proper prevention and treatment strategies are therefore necessary. Signs and symptoms of EDs in competitive and elite athletes are often ignored. Thus the aims of this chapter are to present an overview of the following aspects of DE and EDs: (i) the DE continuum, (ii) the prevalence, (iii) risk factors, (iv) health and performance consequences, (v) how to approach athletes with symptoms of DE and those who want to lose weight, and (vi) preventive strategies.

18.2 The disordered eating continuum

There is a continuum model of DE, ranging from energy balance and healthy body image to clinical EDs such as anorexia nervosa (AN), bulimia nervosa

Sport and Exercise Nutrition, First Edition. Edited by Susan A Lanham-New, Samantha J Stear, Susan M Shirreffs and Adam L Collins.
© 2011 The Nutrition Society. Published 2011 by Blackwell Publishing Ltd.

Table 18.1 Diagnostic criteria for anorexia nervosa.

1	Refusal to maintain body weight at or above a minimally normal weight for age and height (e.g. weight loss leading to maintenance of body weight <85% of that expected; or failure to make expected weight gain during period of growth, leading to body weight <85% of that expected)
2	Intense fear of gaining weight or becoming fat, even though underweight
3	Disturbance in the way in which one's body weight or shape is experienced, undue influence of body weight or shape on self-evaluation, or denial of the seriousness of the current low body weight
4	In post-menarcheal females: amenorrhoea, i.e. the absence of at least three consecutive menstrual cycles. (A woman is considered to have amenorrhoea if her periods occur only following hormone, e.g. oestrogen, administration)

Specify type

Restricting type: during the episode of anorexia nervosa, the person has not regularly engaged in binge-eating or purging behaviour (i.e. self-induced vomiting or the misuse of laxatives, diuretics or enemas)

Binge eating/purging type: during the current episode of anorexia nervosa, the person has regularly engaged in binge-eating or purging behaviour (i.e. self-induced vomiting or the misuse of laxatives, diuretics or enemas)

Reproduced from American Psychiatric Association. Diagnostic and Statistical Manual of Mental Disorders, 4th edn. Washington, DC: American Psychiatric Association, 1994.

(BN) and ED not otherwise specified (EDNOS). For the purposes of this chapter, we define relevant terms below.

- *Dieting* may be included on a continuum ranging from energy balance to energy deficiency, including healthy dieting (such as a moderate energy restriction to achieve slow and steady weight loss), harmful dieting, and DE (various abnormal eating behaviours such as restrictive eating, fasting, frequent skipping meals, diet pills, laxatives, diuretics, enemas, overeating, binge-eating and purging).
- *The Female Athlete Triad* refers to the interrelationship between energy availability, menstrual function and bone mineral density (BMD). This triad may have clinical manifestations including EDs, functional hypothalamic amenorrhoea, and osteoporosis. Athletes may induce low energy availability in an attempt to lose weight or body fat by restricting the caloric intake using abnormal eating behaviours without meeting the criteria for an ED.
- *Energy availability* can be defined as dietary energy intake minus exercise energy expenditure and thus the amount of dietary energy remaining for other body functions after training.
- A *negative energy balance* is a result of consuming less energy than needed to meet the energy costs of daily living, plus those expended in exercise. In addition, young athletes must also meet the energy costs of growth. In AN, the athlete believes

he or she is overweight even though being 15% or more below ideal body weight. Amenorrhoea is one of the DSM-IV diagnostic criteria in female individuals with BN, who follow a cycle of food restriction or fasting leading to overeating or binge eating followed by purging. Purging may include vomiting and the use of laxatives, diuretics, enemas and excessive exercise. For athletes, excessive exercise means more exercise than originally planned to achieve the desired performance level. It is therefore easy for coaches and/or team medical staff to detect this indicator of DE. Athletes suffering from BN also usually have a 'normal' body weight. In both AN and BN, there are restricting and binge/purging categories. Athletes who meet the criteria for EDNOS also often have a 'normal' body weight, but they are focused on body image, weight and guilt surrounding eating. The EDNOS category refers to disorders of eating that do not meet the criteria for any specific ED. This category acknowledges the existence and importance of a variety of eating disturbances and EDNOS is more prevalent among athletes than AN and BN. On this continuum athletes are struggling with body image, eating behaviours and performance issues. Athletes constitute a unique population, and special diagnostic considerations should be made when working with this group. Tables 18.1–18.3 summarise the DSM-IV diagnostic criteria for AN, BN and EDNOS.

Table 18.2 Diagnostic criteria for bulimia nervosa.

1	Recurrent episodes of binge-eating. An episode of binge-eating is characterised by both of the following: (i) eating, in a discrete period of time (e.g. within any 2-hour period), an amount of food that is definitely larger than most people would eat during a similar period of time in similar circumstances; and (ii) a sense of lack of control over eating during the episode (e.g. a feeling that one cannot stop eating or control what or how much one is eating)
2	Recurrent inappropriate compensatory behaviour in order to prevent weight gain, such as self-induced vomiting; misuse of laxatives, diuretics or other medications; fasting; or excessive exercise
3	The binge-eating and inappropriate compensatory behaviours both occur, on average, at least twice a week for 3 months
4	Self-evaluation is unduly influenced by body shape and weight
5	The disturbance does not occur exclusively during episodes of anorexia nervosa

Specify type

Purging type: the person regularly engages in self-induced vomiting or the misuse of laxatives, diuretics or enemas

Non-purging type: the person uses other inappropriate compensatory behaviours, such as fasting or excessive exercise, but does not regularly engage in self-induced vomiting or the misuse of laxatives, diuretics or enemas

Reproduced from American Psychiatric Association. Diagnostic and Statistical Manual of Mental Disorders, 4th edn. Washington, DC: American Psychiatric Association, 1994.

Table 18.3 Diagnostic criteria for eating disorders not otherwise specified (EDNOS).

1	For females, all of the criteria for anorexia nervosa are met except that the individual has regular menses
2	All of the criteria for anorexia nervosa are met except that, despite significant weight loss, the individual's current weight is in the normal range
3	All the criteria for bulimia nervosa are met expect that the binge-eating and inappropriate compensatory mechanisms occur at a frequency of less than twice per week or for a duration of less than 3 months
4	The regular use of inappropriate compensatory behaviour by an individual of normal body weight after eating small amounts of food (e.g. self-induced vomiting after the consumption of two cookies)
5	Repeatedly chewing and spitting out, but no swallowing, large amounts of food
6	Binge-eating disorder: recurrent episodes of binge-eating in the absence of the regular use of inappropriate compensatory behaviour characteristics of bulimia nervosa

Reproduced from American Psychiatric Association. Diagnostic and Statistical Manual of Mental Disorders, 4th edn. Washington, DC: American Psychiatric Association, 1994.

18.3 Prevalence of disordered eating and eating disorders in athletes

Up to 70% of elite athletes competing in weight class sports are dieting and have abnormal eating behaviours to reduce weight prior to competition, and a higher frequency of DE in athletes competing in sports that emphasise leanness or a low body weight has also been reported. A controlled study showed that the prevalence of EDs is significantly higher in Norwegian male and female elite athletes (8% and 22%) than in non-athletic male and female controls (0.5% and 10%), and more common among those competing in sports in which leanness, high power-to-weight ratio and/or weight classes are important. In contrast, some studies on high-school athletes report no greater risk for the development of an ED than controls. In a recent study by Rosendahl *et al.* (2009) 59% of the young male elite athletes were dissatisfied with their body, 19% were dieting and 11% had DE. The prevalence of DE was 10%, 17% and 42% for endurance, weight-class and anti-gravitation sports, respectively. In a Norwegian study on adolescent male elite athletes, 13% reported symptoms associated with EDs. The differences in prevalence between different studies can be attributed to different methodological issues, such as different sports, different competitive level, different screening instruments, different investigators (coaches, researchers), different periods (on-off season) and different age groups.

18.4 Risk factors for the development of disordered eating and eating disorders

The cause of EDs is multifactorial and different factors predispose, precipitate and perpetuate the disorder. In sports, predisposing factors (e.g.

individual, family, culture) can be triggered by a precipitating factor (e.g. comment on body weight), and then maintained by perpetuating factors (e.g. initial success, approval by coach). As regards to the DE continuum as a whole, it is not known whether the risk or causative factors are the same as the different included EDs. Athletes restricting caloric intake, whether inadvertent or by intent, could therefore be considered at risk for DE. Risk factors can be divided into two categories: the first involves general factors that place an individual, athlete or non-athlete at risk of developing DE. The second category involves factors specific to athletes, including personality factors, pressure to lose weight leading to restricted eating and/or frequent weight cycling, body dissatisfaction, early start of sport-specific training, injuries, symptoms of over-training and the impact of coaching behaviour. Another risk factor in the athletic environment is the fact that in some sports, a decrease in body fat/weight can enhance performance. Often an initial loss of weight leads to a better performance and this initial success can force the athlete (and other athletes observing this) to continue efforts to lose weight and unknowingly slip into an ED. Thompson and Trattner-Sherman (2009) have suggested that some traits desired by coaches in their athletes (referred to as 'good athlete' traits) are similar to traits found in individuals with EDs, such as excessive exercise, perfectionism and (over-) compliance. Leon (1991) suggested that these athletes may also have evidence of psychological traits such as high achievement orientation and obsessive–compulsive tendencies commonly associated with EDs, but also essential for successful competitions. Therefore, such athletes should be considered as at increased risk for EDs. Such attitudes and behaviours are apt to be rewarded in the sport environment. Thus, rather than identifying an individual who is in need of treatment, sport personnel are, without knowing, apt to increase the frequency of EDs through their reinforcement of attitudes and behaviours. Most sports have appearance and body paradigms. For example, distance runners are 'thin' and female elite rhythmic gymnasts are 'tiny'. Thus, it can be difficult to identify athletes with EDs who fits the paradigm. Most researchers agree that coaches do not cause ED in athletes, although through inappropriate coaching the problem may be triggered or exacerbated in vulnerable individuals. In most cases, the role of coaches in the development of EDs in athletes should be seen as a part of a complex interplay of factors.

18.5 Why are athletes dieting?

For elite athletes, the cause of starting to diet are related to (i) a perception of the 'ideal' body appearance in his or her sport, (ii) perceived performance improvement benefits, and (iii) socio-cultural pressures for thinness or an 'ideal' body composition or shape. In some sports it is desirable to have a high lean body mass and low body fat mass to achieve a high power-to-weight ratio. There are sports that require horizontal (e.g. running and long jump) or vertical (e.g. high jump, gymnastics, ski jumping) movements of the body where excessive fat mass is considered a disadvantage. A high fat mass increases energy demands and could therefore affect performance negatively. Furthermore, in sports where aerodynamics and reduced resistance or drag is important (e.g. cycling, swimming) body composition plays an important role (although not always associated with low body fat). A high lean body to fat mass ratio is also desirable in sports for aesthetic reasons (e.g. figure skating, rhythmic gymnastics, diving, body-building and sports dance). Finally, in sports with weight categories such as wrestling, judo, karate and rowing, athletes wish to get a competitive advantage by obtaining lowest possible body weight with greatest possible strength. Thus they often compete in a weight class below their natural body weight and therefore start dieting due to their experience of the specific body weight/composition demands in their sport. It is also possible that especially female athletes competing in sports such as sprinting, speed skating and cycling experience that their sport-specific muscular body type does not fit the socio-cultural ideal body shape characterised by thinness. Therefore, these athletes try to change their body composition by dieting, despite the fact that they might abandon the paradigm body composition of their sport. Thus, for many athletes who start dieting, weight concerns, dieting and use of abnormal eating behaviours become a focus of their athletic existence and some may be diagnosed with an ED. Because DE and ED often start with dieting, in this chapter we emphasise the importance of guided weight loss for athletes.

Also, some younger athletes may unknowingly slip into an ED because they are unaware of the energy demands of their increased training loads (e.g. going from junior to senior). Longer periods of unintentionally low energy availability, and perhaps enhanced performance for a brief period, probably increases the risk of developing DE. This may also be the case for athletes who gradually reduce intake by reducing what they classify as 'bad' food for different reasons (e.g. meat, fatty food, dairy products). Lack of nutrition knowledge can put the athlete at risk for DE and ED.

18.6 Health and performance consequences of disordered eating and eating disorders

Longer periods with low energy availability, with or without DE, can impair health and physical performance. Medical complications involve the cardiovascular, endocrine, reproductive, gastrointestinal, renal and central nervous systems. In several studies, the negative effects of rapid weight loss (e.g. fasting, dehydration) and longer periods of restricted energy intake on performance, growth, cognitive function and health have been discussed. Dieting athletes may slip into DE, which in turn can lead to a serious ED, disruption of the normal menstrual cycle, and eventually imbalance in bone remodelling leading to osteopenia or osteoporosis. Although any one of these problems can occur in isolation, the emphasis on weight loss in risk individuals can start a cycle in which all three diseases occur in sequence, hence the term the 'Female Athlete Triad'. Also, in male competitive cyclists and long-distance runners with a low percentage body fat, low BMD values have been found and as many as 63% of male cyclists have been diagnosed with osteopenia. In a recent study, 25% and 9% of male cyclists were diagnosed with osteopenia and osteoporosis, respectively (Smathers et al., 2009). Psychological problems associated with EDs include low self-esteem, depression and anxiety disorders. For athletes, the stress of constantly denying hunger, obsessing about food, agonising over body weight and fearing high body weight is mentally exhausting. Moreover, this preoccupation interferes with the athlete's daily activities as well as his or her training and competition. Mortality rates in athletes with EDs are not known, but 5.4% ($n = 5$) of those diagnosed in one study reported suicide attempts.

18.7 How to approach athletes with symptoms of disordered eating and eating disorders

Identifying athletes with ED must go beyond focusing on those who meet diagnoses for EDs to include those who have too low energy availability and/or those who are practising pathogenic weight control behaviours. Since no controlled longitudinal studies, treatment studies or controlled prevention studies on athletes have been published, the recommendations presented in the latest position papers on the Female Athlete Triad and our experience from 20 years of work with elite athletes and EDs have been used in this chapter. If an athlete has been identified as engaged in DE or is believed to be at risk for abnormal eating behaviours or an ED by medical staff, athletic trainer, coaching staff or team-members, the following procedures are based on recommendations by Drinkwater et al. (2005).

The athlete should be referred to a qualified sports nutritionist/dietitian for a nutritional assessment and meal planning. The focus should be educational with the aim of helping the athlete understand the nutritional needs for good health and performance. The nutritionist should ask questions needed to determine whether the athlete has an optimal energy intake or not. If the athlete is not able to improve the intake by guidance, the athlete should be referred to the team physician or general practitioner where appropriate. The physician should take a detailed medical history review and perform a physical examination, obtain blood and biochemical tests and perform dual energy X-ray absorptiometry (DEXA) to determine body fat and bone health. The physician should also determine whether further medical specialist consultations are necessary (e.g. psychiatry, endocrinology and gynaecology). It is not enough to document behaviours; the emotional and psychological state of the athlete must also be examined.

Special attention should be paid to male athletes who exhibit signs and symptoms of DE since men have no diagnostic hallmark such as amenorrhoea for detecting EDs. Athletes diagnosed with DE, but no other underlying medical disorder, who are unable or unwilling to follow the eating recommendations made by the nutritionist and/or physician should be referred to an ED treatment specialist experienced in working with athletes. If the physician and/or ED specialist recommends treatment, the athlete should be considered injured and agree to treatment in order to later be allowed to return to training and competition. For athletes who agree to treatment, eligibility to continue training and competing while symptomatic would be determined on an individual basis by treatment staff. At the minimum, the athlete would have to be cleared medically and psychologically, his or her training/competition should not be used as a means to diet or control his or her weight, and he or she would be required to follow a prescribed set of health maintenance criteria. These criteria are individual and would generally include, but not be limited to:

(1) being in treatment, complying with the treatment plan, and progressing toward therapeutic goals;
(2) maintaining a weight of at least 90% of expected and, in accordance with Behnke's theoretical concept of minimal body mass, a body fat above 5% for male athletes and above 12% for female athletes, or more if prescribed by the treatment team;
(3) eating enough to comply with the treatment plan regarding weight gain or weight maintenance.

In some cases it is important to be able to negotiate with the athlete when it comes to energy intake and return to training and competition. However, it must be clear that the DE/ED treatment team makes the decision and that the athlete's health has priority. For athletes willing to follow the recommended treatment and who include their coach (if the athlete and the coach have a positive relationship) in the treatment, and, if appropriate, also the parents for young athletes, the compliance and prognosis is expected to be good.

To be allowed to train the athlete must be able to maintain a weight of at least 90% of therapeutic goal. The body weight must gradually increase during the training period and any indication of decreased body weight will discontinue the training. The athlete may return to competition when the goal weight or body composition is reached and when the athlete is mentally prepared. As stated above any indication of decreased body weight or return to DE will mean withdrawal of the athlete from competitions as well as training. For athletes who refuse treatment, training and competition should be withheld until they agree to participate in treatment.

Finally, maintaining open lines of communication between the coaches and members of the ED team is important. Coaches are in a prime position to monitor their athletes' behaviours and reactions. It should be noted that coaches may have difficulty discussing sensitive issues related to DE/ED with either treatment team members or athletes. While there are probably still some instances in which a coach directly contributes to an athlete's DE/ED, most coaches are aware of the liabilities involved and are careful not to overstep their boundaries regarding weight and dieting issues. Thus it is important to avoid placing blame. Coaches need to be held accountable for their athletes in a way that is not threatening. The best way to do this is to make DE/ED a health and safety issue and not a coaching issue.

18.8 The athlete and the healthcare team

The various types of DE/ED treatment strategies have been described in detail elsewhere. When it comes to athletes, controlled treatment studies have not been published. Thus, our recommendation is based on results from treatment studies on non-athletes with EDs and our experience from treating elite athletes and an ongoing controlled treatment study on elite athletes. We recommend a multidisciplinary approach combining nutritional guidance, alternative or adjusted training, and cognitive and psychodynamic therapy. The treatment team should consist of a physician who monitors medical status, a dietitian/nutritionist with experience in DE/ED and sports nutrition, trainer/physiologist who supports training and performance, and a psychiatrist or a cognitive therapist with experience in DE/ED to address mental issues. For athletes under 18 years old, parents should be involved.

Athletes with DE/ED seem more likely to accept the idea of going for a single consultation than committing themselves to prolonged treatment. The treatment of athletes with DE/EDs should be undertaken by healthcare professionals. It is our experience that it is easier to establish a trusting relationship when the athlete understands that the healthcare professionals know their sport in addition to being trained in treating DE/ED patients. Healthcare professionals who have good knowledge about DE/EDs and know the various sports will better understand the athlete's training setting, daily demands and relations that are specific to the sport/sport event and competitive level. To build such a relationship includes respecting the athlete's desire to be lean for athletic performance, and to express a willingness to work together to help the DE/ED athlete to become lean and healthy. The treatment team needs to accept the athlete's fears and irrational thoughts about food and weight, and then present a rational approach for achieving self-management of healthy diet, weight and training programme.

18.9 Training, energy expenditure and energy intake during treatment

It is our experience that a total suspension from training during treatment is not a good solution for the following reasons: (i) to minimise the frustration and prevent depression during the rehabilitation period and (ii) to control gains in fat mass during weight gain. Therefore, unless severe medical complications such as electrolyte imbalance or arrhythmia are present, training at a lower volume and at a decreased intensity should be prescribed. Sometimes it is necessary to focus on aspects other than the short-term sport-specific training. High-intensity endurance training may be replaced with strength training and alternative recreational training in order to make the goal set for the individual athlete. In athletes with low BMD, strength training should be involved to maintain or aim at increasing BMD on the site-specific bone. In general, it is recommended that athletes do not compete during treatment in order to avoid a message of sport performance as more important than their health. Nevertheless, competitions during treatment might be considered for individuals with less severe DE/ED. This will depend on the athlete's total medical condition, progression in treatment and type of sport/competitive event.

On our experience, rapid weight gain should be avoided in athletes who have to gain weight for health reasons. It is safer, both psychologically and physically, for the athlete to gradually increase energy intake. A predictable small weight gain corresponding to 0.5–1 kg/week over a longer period (depending on the severity of the initial weight loss) seems to make the process easier for the athlete. Even though the athlete starts out with a suboptimal meal plan with energy intake below what is considered healthy or appropriate

for him or her, it is considered more important that the meal plan increases over time and that the athlete is committed, rather than providing an optimal meal plan that the athlete is not ready to commit to. However, for athletes with reduced BMD it is important to ensure calcium intake (about 1500 mg/day when combining the amount included in the diet and supplements) (Nattiv *et al.*, 2007) and adequate vitamin D in combination with strength training to reduce further loss of bone mass or, in some cases in young athletes, regain bone mass. For athletes who binge and/or purge, it is more difficult to set a goal. Perhaps the athlete is normal weight or has a relatively high fat percentage, but has menstrual disturbances. The goal will not be weight gain, but stabilisation of a healthy body composition with a frequent meal pattern and reduced binge/purge episodes until regular cycles have been achieved. Most DE/ED athletes need to meet with the nutritionist once a week at least for the 6 first weeks; depending on treatment progress, most athletes can meet every other week and keep in contact by phone and/or mail if followed by the (team) physician or psychiatrist/therapist. It is considered important that there is a consensus in the team surrounding the athlete, to avoid unnecessary anxiety and ambivalence in an already vulnerable athlete.

Most DE/ED athletes want to continue their sport. However, the question regarding his or her motivation is important because some want to quit and that should be taken into consideration during the treatment plan. If the athlete wants to compete again, then this should be used as a motivational agent during treatment. It is our experience that few athletes are critically ill and although ambivalent about treatment, most are motivated to get well and to compete again. This may be used as an advantage in this situation, for example it is easier for an athlete to accept a higher-energy meal plan if she or he is allowed to train. However, there are cases in which the athletes actually want to quit sport and it is therefore important to ask questions related to this.

18.10 Prevention of disordered eating and eating disorders

Existing preventive programmes that have been evaluated with athletes as participants are limited. Thus we focus on issues that are expected to help prevent DE and ED in athletes.

Information and guidelines

In order for coaches to adequately perform a supportive function, many need factual information on nutrition, factors determining weight, risks and causes of DE/ED, menstrual (dys)function, and psychological factors that both negatively and positively affect health and athletic performance. Coaches and athletes should learn to know that female athletes with menstrual dysfunction are at increased risk of injuries. Sports governing organisations and federations should give support to the coaches and provide education regarding DE/ED for coaches and athletes. Each federation should have position statements with guidelines, and support to make the difficult decisions with respect to affected athletes as to whether they will be in treatment or be allowed to train and compete.

De-emphasise weight

The best way to de-emphasise weight is to avoid weighing athletes for non-health-related issues, avoid frequent measurements of the athlete's body composition and avoid verbal and non-verbal comments regarding body composition and/or body weight. Dieting and weight issues should never be a theme from the coach, but be presented according to the athlete's wishes. In such cases, the coach should take the athlete's initiative seriously and refer to professional help. The focus should be on performance enhancement via non-dieting strategies: improved nutrition, improved health, mental and psychological approaches (i.e. positive imagery, concentration, anxiety management) and physical aspects (i.e. enhancement of speed, quickness, endurance such as in middle distance running and speed skating).

Weight loss and dieting

Unnecessary dieting (dieting performed where there is no excess fat and unaccompanied by professional guidance) is considered one of the most important risk factors for development of DE/ED and should be prevented. Coaches should avoid putting pressure and/or telling an athlete to lose weight. This is especially important when it comes to athletes representing weight class sports. Most weight-class athletes are fit and lean, but want to reduce weight to compete in a lower weight class. Most weight-class athletes consider this 'part of the game' and do not question methods or consequences. In such case the coach and healthcare team should rather motivate the athlete to improve strength and compete in a higher weight class. Healthcare providers should educate athletes and coaches that weight loss does not necessarily lead to improved athletic performance. Furthermore, since athletes are eager to perform, it is important to inform about the side effects of undereating and abnormal eating behaviour, such as fatigue, anaemia, electrolyte abnormalities and depression. If the coach is concerned about an athlete's eating behaviour, body image and/or weight or body fat level, he or she should be referred to a sports nutritionist for further evaluation and consultation. If a change in body mass or body composition is desired by the athlete and recommended by healthcare professionals for health and/or performance, our recommendations for weight loss are as follows.

- The weight goal should be realistic and based on objective measurements of body composition rather than weight-for-height standards.
- Prior to weight-loss intervention, there should be a thorough screening including weight history and weight goal, menstrual history for females, an estimate of body composition and energy/nutritional status, and questions regarding motivation, dietary habits, thoughts and feelings about body image, body weight and food. If there is a history of DE/ED, a more intense and longer follow-up is needed.
- The weight-loss period should be done off-season to avoid interference with competitions and sports-specific training loads.
- The athlete should commence a 4-day (3 weekdays + 1 weekend day) or a 7-day diet registration (weighed or household measurements) as a base for the diet plan. Objective measurements on body mass, fat mass and BMD should be done (DEXA) as well as blood tests. If a blood test indicates any specific micronutrient needs (e.g. iron, vitamin B_{12}), these vitamins should be provided and biochemical changes monitored during the period. A multivitamin multimineral supplement and ω-3 fatty acids should be provided during the weight-loss period to ensure sufficient micronutrient intake and essential fat intake. Measurements of body composition should be done in private to reduce the stress, anxiety and embarrassment of public assessment and the results should be explained and discussed with the athlete.

- The athlete should consume sufficient energy to avoid menstrual irregularities and aim for a gradual weight loss corresponding to about 0.5 kg/week. To induce a weight loss of 0.5 kg/week an energy deficit similar to 500 kcal/day is needed. This can be achieved by reduced energy intake, increased energy expenditure, or a combination of the two.
- A sports nutritionist who knows the demands of the specific sport should plan individual nutritionally adequate diets. Throughout this process, the role of overall good nutrition practices in optimising performance should be emphasised. The diet should aim to have a protein intake of 1.4–2 g/kg, a carbohydrate intake of 4–6 g/kg, and 20% fat or more. The focus should be on low-energy/high-nutrient density foods that provide satiety as well as food variety and a frequent meal pattern making sure that the athlete is not fatigued during training sessions. Emphasise recovery meals containing carbohydrates and protein within 30 min after training sessions to optimise recovery, and include dairy food sources to meet Recommended Dietary Intakes of calcium.
- It is important that the weight loss does not compromise lean body mass and performance. Thus strength training should be included during the weight-loss period. A moderate energy restriction combined with strength training alleviates the negative consequences on lean body mass and performance.
- Body fat percentage should be no lower than 5 for males and 12 for females after weight loss. However, individual evaluation should be taken. Some athletes are genetically disposed to have a lower fat percentage, whereas others cannot 'tolerate' a low percentage.
- Change in body composition should be monitored on a regular basis, including a period of at least 2 months after the weight or body fat percentage goal has been reached to detect any continued or unwarranted losses or weight fluctuations.
- Weight-class athletes are encouraged to be no more than about 3% over competition weight and to suffer no more than 2% in rapid weight loss (dependent on time from weigh-in to competition and recovery strategies) to avoid large weight fluctuations and impaired performance.
- Normal-weight athletes under the age of 18 should be discouraged to lose weight.

Recognition of disordered eating and increased openness

The main goal in secondary prevention should be to better identify athletes with DE in order to introduce education and treatment. Earlier treatment results in fewer health risks for the athlete and also an earlier return to training and competition. Finally, identification could be facilitated through the de-stigmatisation of receiving an ED diagnosis, as well as through proper and supportive management of the athlete following identification. Regarding DE stigmatisation, coaches have to accept that DE and EDs exists in many sports and not deny it and, furthermore, be able to talk about this and other psychiatric disorders.

18.11 Summary

The prevalence of DE/ED is higher among elite athletes competing in sports focusing on leanness and/or a specific weight, but in studies on younger athletes the prevalence of DE seems to be lower among athletes than controls. There is no hard evidence for sport-specific risk factors for EDs. Thus, longitudinal quantitative and qualitative studies are warranted. The diagnosis of an ED in female athletes can easily be missed unless specifically searched for. DE and EDs may result in amenorrhoea and low BMD because of energy deficit. If untreated, ED can have long-lasting physiological and psychological effects. Treating athletes with EDs should be undertaken only by qualified healthcare professionals. Ideally, these individuals should also be familiar with, and have an appreciation for, the sport environment. Since dieting is the primary precursor to the development of DE and EDs, unnecessary dieting should be prevented. The team staff and parents must be able to recognise the physical symptoms and psychological characteristics that indicate a risk for DE/EDs. The sport environment must focus on increased openness regarding challenges such as EDs among both male and female athletes. If the coach is concerned about an athlete's eating behaviour, body image and/or weight or body fat level, he or she should be referred to a sports nutritionist for further evaluation and consultation. Athletes who do need to change weight or body composition should get professional guidance, and ideally weight reduction should be performed during the off-season.

References

Drinkwater B, Loucks A, Sherman R, Sundgot-Borgen J, Thompon R. International Olympic Committee Medical Commission Working Group Women in Sport. Position stand on the female athlete triad. Available at http://multimedia.olympic.org/pdf/en_report_917.pdf. 2005.

Leon GR. Eating disorders in female athletes. Sports Med 1991; 4: 219–227.

Nattiv A, Loucks AB, Manore MM, Sanborn CF, Sundgot-Borgen J, Warren MP. The female athlete triad. Special communications: position stand. Med Sci Sports Exerc 2007; 39: 1867–1882.

Rosendahl J, Bormann B, Aschenbrenner K, Aschenbrenner F, Strauss B. Dieting and disordered eating in German high school athletes and non-athletes. Scand J Med Sci Sports 2009; 19: 731–739.

Smathers AM, Bemben MG, Bemben DA. Bone density comparisons in male competitive road cyclists and untrained controls. Med Sci Sports Exerc 2009; 41: 290–296.

Thompson RA, Trattner-Sherman R. Eating Disorders in Sports. New York: Routledge, 2009.

Further reading

American College of Sports Medicine. Position stand: weight loss in wrestlers. Med Sci Sports Exerc 1996; 28: ix–xii.

American College of Sports Medicine. Position stand: nutrition and athletic performance. Med Sci Sports Exerc 2009; 41: 709–731.

American Psychiatric Association. Diagnostic and Statistical Manual of Mental Disorders, 4th edn. Washington, DC: American Psychiatric Association, 1994, pp 539–550.

Andersen AE. Diagnosis and treatment of males with eating disorders. In: Males with Eating Disorders (Andersen AE, ed.). New York: Brunner/Mazel, 1990, pp 133–162.

Beals KA. Disordered Eating Among Athletes. A Comprehensive Guide for Health Professionals. Champaign, IL: Human Kinetics, 2004, chapter 11.

Beals KA, Hill AK. The prevalence of disordered eating, menstrual dysfunction, and low bone mineral density among US collegiate athletes. Int J Sport Nutr Exerc Metab 2006: 16: 1–23.

Beals KA, Manore MM. The prevalence and consequences of sub-clinical eating disorders in female athletes. Int J Sport Nutr 1994; 4: 175–195.

Brownell KD, Steen SN, Wilmore JH. Weight regulation practices in athletes: analysis of metabolic and health effects. Med Sci Sports Exerc 1987; 6: 546–560.

Clark N. How to help the athlete with bulimia: practical tips and case study. Int J Sport Nutr 1993; 3: 450–460.

Dummer GM, Rosen LW, Heusner WW. Pathogenic weight-control behaviors of young competitive swimmers. Physician Sportsmed 1987: 5: 75–86.

Fogelholm M. Effects of bodyweight reduction on sports performance. Sports Med 1994: 4: 249–267.

Gadpaille WJ, Sanborn CF, Wagner WW. Athletic amenorrhea, major affective disorders and eating disorders. Am J Psychiatry 1987; 144: 939–942.

Garner DM, Olmsted MP, Polivy J. Manual of Eating Disorder Inventory. Odessa, FL: Psychological Assessment Resources, 1984, pp 1–19.

Garthe I, Raastad T, Refsnes PE, Koivisto A, Sundgot-Borgen J. Is it possible to maintain lean body mass and performance during energy-restriction in elite athletes? [Abstract] Med Sci Sports Exerc 2009; 41 (5 Suppl): 7.

Gresko RB, Rosenvinge JH. The Norwegian School-based prevention model: development and validation. In: The Prevention of Eating Disorders (Vandereycken W, Noordenbos G, eds). London: Athlone Press/New York: New York Univerisity Press, 1998.

Hausenblas HA, Carron AV. Eating disorder indices and athletes: an integration J Sport Exerc Psychol 1999; 21: 230–258.

Hetland ML, Haarbo J, Christiansen C. Low bone mass and high bone turnover in male long distance runners. J Clin Endocrinol Metab 1993; 77: 770–775.

Heyward VH, Wagner DR. Applied Body Composition Assessment, 2nd edn. Champaign, IL: Human Kinetics, 2004.

Koral J, Dosseville F. Combination of gradual and rapid weight loss: effects on physical performance and psychological state of elite judo athletes. J Sports Sci 2009; 27: 115–120.

Manore MM. Dietary recommendations and athletic menstrual dysfunction. Sports Med 2002; 32: 887–901.

Marquart LF, Sobal J. Weight loss beliefs, practices and support systems for high school wrestlers J Adolesc Health 1994; 15: 410–415.

Martinsen M, Eriksson A, Sanda SB, Sundgot-Borgen J. Dieting to win or to be thin? A study of dieting and disordered eating among adolescent elite athletes and non-athlete controls. Br J Sports Med 2010; 44: 70–76.

Nichols JF, Rauh MJ, Lawson MJ, Ji M, Barkai HS. Prevalence of the female athlete triad syndrome among high school athletes. Arch Pediatr Adolesc Med 2006; 160: 137–142.

O'Connor H, Caterson I. Weight loss and the athlete. In: Clinical Sports Nutrition, 4th edn (Burke L, Deakin V, eds). Sydney: McGraw-Hill Australia, 2010.

O'Connor PJ, Lewis RJ, Kirchner EM. Eating disorder symptoms in female college gymnasts. Med Sci Sports Exerc 1995; 27: 550–555.

Rector RS, Rogers R, Ruebel M, Hinton PS. Participation in road cycling vs running is associated with lower bone mineral density in men. Metabolism 2008; 57: 226–232.

Roemmich JN, Sinning WE. Weight loss and wrestling training: effects on growth-related hormones J Appl Physiol 1997; 82: 1760–1764.

Rosen LW, McKeag DB, Hough DO. Pathogenic weight-control behaviors in female athletes. Phys Sportsmed 1986; 14: 79–86.

Rosenvinge JH, Gresko RB. Do we need a prevention model for eating disorders? Eating Disorders 1997; 5: 110–118.

Shisslak CM, Crago M, Estes LS. The spectrum of eating disturbances. Int J Eat Disord 1995; 18: 209–219.

Smathers AM, Bemben MG, Bemben DA. Bone density comparisons in male competitive road cyclists and untrained controls. Med Sci Sports Exerc 2009; 41: 290–296.

Smolak LS, Murnen R, Ruble AE. Female athletes and eating problems: a meta-analysis. Int J Eat Disord 2000; 27: 371–380.

Steen SN, Brownell KD. Pattern of weight loss and regain in wrestlers: has the tradition changed? Med Sci Sports Exerc 1990; 22: 762–768.

Stiegler P, Cunliffe A. The role of diet and exercise for the maintenance of fat-free mass and resting metabolic rate during weight loss. Sports Med 2006; 36: 239–262.

Sundgot-Borgen J. Prevalence of eating disorders in elite female athletes. Int J Sport Nutr 1993; 3: 29–40.

Sundgot-Borgen J. Risk and trigger factors for the development of eating disorders in female elite athletes. Med Sci Sports Exerc 1994; 4: 414–419.

Sundgot-Borgen J. Eating disorders, energy intake, training volume and menstrual function in high-level modern rhythmic gymnastic gymnasts. Int J Sport Nutr 1996; 2: 100–109.

Sundgot-Borgen J, Klungland M. The female athlete triad and the effect of preventive work. Med Sci Sports Exerc 1998; Suppl 5: 181.

Sundgot-Borgen J, Larsen S. Nutrient intake and eating behavior of female elite athletes suffering from anorexia nervosa, anorexia athletica and bulimia nervosa. Int J Sport Nutr 1993; 3: 431–442.

Sundgot-Borgen J, Torstveit MK. Prevalence of eating disorders in elite athletes is higher than in the general population. Clin J Sport Med 2004; 14: 25–32.

Thompson RA, Sherman RT. Helping Athletes with Eating Disorders. Champaign, IL: Human Kinetics, 1993.

Thompson RA, Sherman RT. 'Good athlete' traits and characteristics of anorexia nervosa: are they similar? Eating Disorders 1999; 7: 181–190.

Torstveit MK, Sundgot-Borgen J. The female athlete triad: are elite athletes at increased risk? Med Sci Sports Exerc 2005a: 37: 184–193.

Torstveit MK, Sundgot-Borgen J. The female athlete triad exists in both elite athletes and controls. Med Sci Sports Exerc 2005b: 37: 1449–1459.

Torstveit MK, Rosenvinge J, Sundgot-Borgen J. Prevalence of eating disorders and the predictive power of risk factor models in female elite athletes: a controlled study. Scand J Med Sci Sports 2008; 18: 108–118.

Umeda T, Nakaji S, Shimoyama TA, Yamamoto Y, Sugawara K. Adverse effects of energy restriction on changes in immunoglobulins and complements during weight reduction in judoists. J Sports Med Phys Fitness 2004; 44: 328–334.

Van Hoeken D, Seidell J, Hoek HW. Epidemiology. In: Handbook of Eating Disorders, 2nd edn (Treasure J, Schmidt U, Van Furth E, eds). Chichester: Wiley, 2003, pp 11–34.

Walberg Rankin J. Weight loss and gain in athletes. Curr Sports Med Rep 2002; 4: 208–213.

Wilmore JH. Eating and weight disorders in the female athlete. Int J Sport Nutr 1991; 1: 104–117.

19
Bone Health

Charlotte (Barney) Sanborn, David L Nichols and Nancy M DiMarco

---

Key messages

- Bone tissue has three main functions: (i) to provide structural and mechanical support for soft tissues and to serve as attachment points for skeletal muscle to aid in locomotion; (ii) to maintain calcium homeostasis and act as a storage site for other minerals such as phosphate, magnesium, potassium and bicarbonate; and (iii) as a primary site of blood cell formation.
- The skeleton comprises 80% cortical bone and 20% trabecular bone.
- Trabecular bone is more metabolically active than cortical bone. Trabecular bone is more sensitive to changes in biochemical, hormonal and nutritional status and more susceptible to loss of bone. Hence, the majority of osteoporotic fractures occur in areas with a large proportion of trabecular bone: the spine, proximal hip (femoral neck and greater trochanter), and distal radius and ulna.

- The major nutrients associated with bone health are calcium, protein, vitamin D, vitamin K, potassium, phosphorus, fluoride and vitamin C.
- Vitamin D status should be evaluated regularly as it is frequently deficient/suboptimal and can play a significant role in optimising bone health and other health outcomes such as immune function.
- The three components of disordered eating, amenorrhoea and osteoporosis are called the Female Athlete Triad. Existence of one or more components of the triad, alone or in combination, poses a health risk for the physically active and athletic female.
- Energy availability is calculated as dietary energy intake minus exercise energy expenditure divided by kilogram fat-free mass (FFM). Optimal dietary intake for an athlete is estimated at an energy availability of 45 kcal/kg FFM. Reproductive and skeletal health problems occur at a minimal energy availability calculated at 30 kcal/kg FFM.

19.1 Introduction

The goal of bone health or skeletal integrity is to prevent osteoporotic fractures as an elderly adult. In addition, for an athlete or physically active individual, the objective is to prevent stress fractures. The primary strategies for the prevention of osteoporosis are twofold: (i) maximise peak bone mass during the bone accrual years and (ii) reduce the rate of bone loss as an adult. Overall, a benefit of participating in athletics and exercising, specifically weight-bearing exercise such as running or weight-lifting, is an increased bone density compared with non-athletes and sedentary individuals. However, low bone density for age has been found in female athletes who suffer from amenorrhoea and/or have an eating disorder. These interrelated, cascading events of disordered eating, amenorrhoea and osteoporosis have been

termed the *Female Athlete Triad*. Further, low bone mass has also been associated as a contributing factor for stress fractures among athletes and military recruits, especially among women.

The focus of this chapter is on risk factors specific to the athlete, and primarily the female athlete. The chapter begins with an overview of bone physiology and diagnostic techniques, followed by sections on optimal nutrition for bone health and then sport, exercise and bone health. The final sections cover the Female Athlete Triad and stress fractures. The conclusion and recommendations are based upon a nutritional care process for athletes throughout the life cycle specifically related to bone health. A lifetime approach for the athlete is divided into the following major periods: childhood, adolescence, college and adulthood. The nutritional assessment recommendations for the athlete are based upon the

---

Sport and Exercise Nutrition, First Edition. Edited by Susan A Lanham-New, Samantha J Stear, Susan M Shirreffs and Adam L Collins.
© 2011 The Nutrition Society. Published 2011 by Blackwell Publishing Ltd.

mnemonic ABCDE: *A*nthropometric measurements, *B*iochemical tests, *C*linical examinations, *D*ietary assessments and *E*nvironmental factors.

19.2 Bone physiology

Bone tissue has three main functions. The primary function is to provide structural and mechanical support for soft tissues and to serve as attachment points for skeletal muscle to aid in locomotion. The skeleton also helps maintain calcium homeostasis and is a storage site for other minerals such as phosphate, magnesium, potassium and bicarbonate. Finally, bone is the primary site of blood cell formation.

There are two types of bone tissue, cortical bone and trabecular bone. Cortical bone is found in the shafts of the long bones and comprises approximately 80% of the skeleton. Trabecular bone, also known as cancellous bone, constitutes the remaining 20% of the skeleton. Trabecular bone is found in the flat bones, such as the pelvis and vertebral bodies, and in the ends of the long bones such as the head and neck of the femur. Trabecular bone is arranged in a honeycomb pattern of trabeculae and is more metabolically active than cortical bone, with an annual bone turnover rate of 25% compared with an annual bone turnover rate of 2–3% in cortical bone. Therefore, trabecular bone is more sensitive to changes in biochemical, hormonal and nutritional status and more susceptible to a loss of bone. It is for this reason that a majority of osteoporotic fractures occur in areas with a large proportion of trabecular bone: the spine, proximal hip (femoral neck and greater trochanter), and distal radius and ulna.

Maintenance and growth of the skeleton occurs through the process of bone modelling and remodelling. Both the child and adult skeleton undergo a constant process of bone resorption and bone formation, referred to as bone remodelling. Bone remodelling serves to maintain the architecture and strength of the bone, maintain mineral homeostasis and prevent fatigue damage. Remodelling is also important during periods of growth when the majority of adult bone mass is laid down. During growth, an increase in both length and size of the bone is accomplished by bone modelling in which bone formation occurs without prior bone resorption.

The processes of both bone remodelling and modelling are complex but, in a simplistic sense, bone

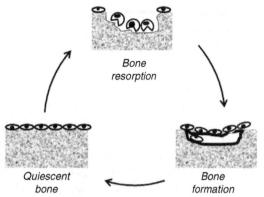

Balanced bone turnover and maintenance of bone mass:
bone formation = bone resorption

Figure 19.1 A simplistic view of bone remodelling. The bone remodelling cycle begins with the bone resorption stage, which creates a cavity as old bone is removed by osteoclasts (☻). During the bone formation stage, new bone is produced by osteoblasts (◉) to fill in the cavity. Maintenance of bone mass occurs when the amount of bone resorbed is equal to the amount of bone formed.

resorption is carried out by bone cells known as osteoclasts, whereas bone cells called osteoblasts form new bone. The complete remodelling cycle takes several months and leaves a new Haversian system in cortical bone and a new 'packet' of bone in trabecular bone. Modelling and remodelling are influenced by both hormonal and nutritional status; remodelling can also be affected by mechanical strain such as exercise (Figure 19.1).

During both childhood and adult life, if increases in mechanical strain are sufficient, the bone remodelling cycle can be altered and increases in bone mass and strength will occur. However, increases in mechanical strain will not affect the bone modelling cycle. On the other hand, if during the growth period severe deficits in mechanical strain occur, such as immobilisation, a loss in bone mass and reduced growth in bone length will occur.

Nutritional deficits have differing effects depending on the stage of life. If caloric intake is insufficient during childhood, when bone modelling is still occurring, the body will sacrifice increases in length of bone to maintain bone strength. Nutritional deficits will cause decreases in bone mass and strength after late adolescence when bone growth has ceased.

For women, oestrogen deficiency for any reason at any stage of life after puberty results in rapid bone loss. However, prior to puberty, the effects of oestrogen on the skeleton are small, with changes in both bone mass and length influenced primarily by growth hormone and insulin-like growth factors. In men, testosterone plays a similar role as oestrogen does in women, although men do not experience a rapid decline in testosterone such as occurs in women at menopause.

In general, bone loss occurs when there is disruption at any point during the remodelling cycle of resorption and formation. During young adulthood these two processes are balanced and bone loss is minimal, with peak bone mass being attained by the end of the second decade. There appears to be some age-related bone loss (approximately 0.5–1.0% per year) experienced by both men and women after approximately age 40 years.

19.3 Diagnostic techniques

Changes in bone tissue are primarily determined by measuring bone mineral density (BMD), often referred to as bone mass. Dual-energy X-ray absorptiometry (DEXA) is the most commonly used technology for measuring BMD. DEXA uses low-dose X-rays to emit photons at two different energy levels. BMD is calculated based on the amount of energy attenuated by the body. DEXA measurements are reported in grams per square centimetre (g/cm^2), so they are not a true density but rather area density measurements. DEXA is capable of differentiating between bone and soft tissue and so can also be used to measure regional and total body composition. The advantages of DEXA are that it is capable of measuring small changes in BMD over time, has a precision of 0.5–2.0%, requires short examination times (5–10 min) and provides low radiation exposure.

Quantitative computed tomography (QCT) can also be used to assess changes in bone mass and has two distinct advantages over DEXA. First, QCT provides a precise three-dimensional anatomic localisation for direct measurement of true bone density. Second, QCT is capable of differentiating between trabecular and cortical bone and is used to examine the anatomy of trabecular regions within the spine. However, QCT is less practical than DEXA for routine screening due to expense and higher radiation exposure.

However, QCT may be a better choice for measuring bone changes in children. Because the bone is also growing in length in children, quantifying increases or decreases in bone mass is problematic especially when obtaining an area measurement of bone density with DEXA. Some have suggested converting area bone density measurements obtained with DEXA to a 'volumetric' density, but this approach has not been determined clinically useful. Because of the expense of QCT, peripheral QCT (pQCT) has gained some support for measuring bone mass in children, but currently there are no reference databases for comparison in children. Additionally, pQCT is limited to measurements of the forearm and tibia, and thus more clinically relevant sites such as the lumbar spine and proximal femur cannot be measured.

BMD is reported not only in g/cm^2 (DEXA) or g/cm^3 (QCT), but also in terms of standard deviations, or T-scores. The likelihood of sustaining a fracture increases 1.5–3 fold for each standard deviation decrease in BMD. The World Health Organisation Consensus Development Conference has developed diagnostic criteria for osteoporosis based on this relationship. Normal BMD is that which is less than 1.0 standard deviations below the mean for young adults. A BMD that is 1.0–2.5 standard deviations below the young adult mean is considered low bone mass or osteopenia. Osteoporosis is defined as BMD more than 2.5 standard deviations below the young adult mean, and is considered 'severe' if accompanied by one or more fragility fractures. These criteria were originally developed for diagnosis of osteoporosis at the proximal femur in post-menopausal women, and recent recommendations from the International Society for Clinical Densitometry (ISCD) suggest that T-scores not be used with all populations. Instead Z-scores and other criteria should be used for children and young adults; Z-scores indicate the number of standard deviations below the age-matched mean.

19.4 Optimal nutrition for bone health

Distribution and function of calcium and phosphorus

The predominant minerals found in bone include calcium and phosphorus, with over 99% of the calcium found in the matrix as hydroxyapatite in bones (and teeth). The other 1% of calcium circulates in the plasma, with 50% in the active ionised form, 40% bound to albumin, and 10% complexed with citrate, phosphate or sulphate. The 0.5% that exists in the active ionised form participates in blood coagulation, neuromuscular contraction, cell adhesion, neuronal transmission, cell membrane stability, signal transduction, enzyme activation, and as a trigger for hormonal secretion. The concentration of intracellular calcium is about 100 nmol/l and is primarily sequestered in the endoplasmic reticulum (ER) and mitochondrial matrix. In response to hormone stimulation, the cytosolic concentration of calcium increases by transport out of the ER and mitochondrial matrix, which then allows calcium to carry out its myriad of functions including action as a second messenger and involvement in smooth and skeletal muscle contraction. Phosphorus and magnesium also make up large percentages of the bone matrix, with over 88% and 60% of those minerals deposited, respectively.

Absorption and excretion of calcium

Calcium is only absorbed in the ionised form (Ca^{2+}) but is present in most foods as insoluble salts. It must therefore be solubilised prior to absorption after exposure to stomach acid. Calcium is absorbed via two processes: a saturable active process involving calbindin and regulated by calcitriol (1,25-dihydroxyvitamin D_3) and a non-saturable passive process that depends on the amount of calcium ingested. The active process occurs in the presence of 1,25-dihydroxyvitamin D_3 when low to moderate amounts of calcium are included in the diet at less than 400 mg. Typically, the non-saturable process takes place in the jejunum and ileum when excess amounts of calcium are consumed. Calcium is one of the threshold nutrients, meaning that any intake above 400–500 mg is simply excreted. Calcium balance studies with premenopausal women have indicated that a calcium intake of 800–1000 mg/day is sufficient to maintain bone health. Children absorb up to 75% of the calcium from the diet in contrast to adults who absorb about 30%.

Calcium is excreted primarily in the urine (100–240 mg/day) and faeces (45–100 mg/day) with some skin losses (60 mg/day). To gain an idea of calcium balance, assume individuals ingest about 1 g calcium each day and only absorb 36%. However, 19% goes back into the lumen, being derived from gut secretions and epithelial losses, so net absorption of calcium in someone in calcium balance is only 17%. This amount is exactly equal to urinary losses.

Current intakes of calcium

According to the United States Continuing Survey of Food Intakes of Individuals (CSFII) national survey of Americans in 1994–1996, among 6–11 year olds, approximately 44% of boys and 58% of girls did not meet the recommendations for calcium intake; among those aged 12–19 years, those not meeting the calcium recommendations comprised 64% of boys and 87% of girls; for those aged 20 years or older, 55% of men and 78% of women did not meet the recommendations for calcium intake. The US 1999–2000 National Health and Nutrition Examination Survey (NHANES) showed that average calcium intakes were 1081 and 793 mg/day for boys and girls aged 12–19 years, respectively; 1025 and 797 mg/day for men and women aged 20–39 years; and 797 and 660 mg/day for men and women aged 60 years or older. Adequate intakes for calcium are shown in Table 19.1.

Dietary sources and supplements

The best food sources of calcium include milk and dairy products; good sources include sardines, clams, oysters, turnip greens, broccoli, legumes and dried fruit, and poor sources include most plants that contain phytate and oxalate that chelate calcium and make it unavailable for absorption from the gut.

Most individuals consume their calcium from dairy sources such as milk but often misconceptions about milk and milk products as high-fat foods cause people to avoid them altogether. Another reason that people do not consume milk is that they are or believe themselves to be lactose intolerant. While a valid reason, most individuals with lactose intolerance are able to consume up to two cups of milk without gastrointestinal distress over a day. Indeed, many products on the market today are lactose-free, or calcium-fortified. Reasons for not consuming enough calcium in the diet are not justified.

The best food sources of calcium (Table 19.2) are typically those from dairy sources because they are not only rich sources of calcium but also provide many other nutrients that are essential for bone health such as vitamin D, magnesium, phosphorus w

Table 19.1 Adequate intakes for calcium.

	USA	UK	Australia
Children			
4–8 years	800 mg[a]	550 mg[b]	700 mg[c]
Males and females			
9–18 years	1300 mg	F, 800 mg	9–11 years, 1000 mg
		M, 1000 mg	12–18 years, 1300 mg
19–50 years	1000 mg	700 mg	19–70 years, 1000 mg
51–70+ years	1200 mg	700 mg	>70 years, 1300 mg
Pregnancy and lactation			
<18 years	1300 mg		
19–50 years	1000 mg	Pregnancy: 700 mg	Pregnancy: 1000 mg
		Lactation: as above for age group, plus another 550 mg	Lactation: 1200 mg
Tolerable Upper Limit, all ages: 2500 mg			

[a] United States, Food and Nutrition Board, National Academy of Sciences Institute of Medicine, 1997.
[b] United Kingdom, Department of Health, Recommended Daily Intakes (children 7–10 years).
[c] Australia. Commonwealth Department of Health, Recommended Dietary Intakes.

protein. It is difficult to obtain enough calcium and bone-building nutrients from food alone, so if dairy products are not consumed regularly supplementation may be necessary.

The two main types of calcium supplements are calcium carbonate and calcium citrate. Calcium carbonate contains 40% of its weight as elemental calcium, making it the supplement that contains the most calcium. It is also one of the cheapest supplements making it attractive to those on budgets. Calcium carbonate is not as easily digested and should be consumed with meals due to the increase in stomach acid production that aids absorption later in the gut. As people age, some individuals produce less stomach acid, and absorption of calcium carbonate may become problematic. Calcium citrate, on the other hand, contains 21% calcium by weight, and an individual would have to consume larger amounts to obtain the same amount of calcium as contained in calcium carbonate. An advantage of using calcium citrate is that because it already is an acid, it does not require the acidic environment necessary for calcium to be absorbed. Therefore, it can be consumed without food. It is recommended that no more than 500 mg of calcium is consumed at one time to ensure optimal absorption and that the calcium supplements are taken three times per day, depending on the type of supplement. Other supplements are salts of calcium including gluconate, lactate, di- and tri- calcium phosphate, and each has very small percentages of calcium by weight. Therefore, much larger doses would be needed to receive the same amount as contained in calcium carbonate or citrate. There is a lack of evidence to suggest that one form of calcium salt is superior to another in terms of absorbability, but there are differences in cost, absorbability, and safety of some supplements sold in health food stores, grocery markets, etc. Naturally occurring calcium carbonate sources, such as bone meal, dolomite and oyster shell, may contain heavy metals, including lead. The Food and Drug Administration (FDA) sets an upper limit for the amount of lead a calcium supplement can contain at 7.5 μg/kg of calcium. Pregnant and lactating women and children should consume as little lead as possible because of the devastating effects on the nervous system and development. It is recommended that the consumer test the supplement for digestibility by dissolving a tablet in 168 g (6 ounces) of white vinegar. A supplement should dissolve within 30 min. Consumers should look for the United States Pharmacopeia (USP) seal or check www.ConsumerLab.com to research a particular supplement and determine whether it has been evaluated for truth in advertising, safety and efficacy.

Table 19.2 Selected food sources of calcium.

Food	Milligrams (mg) per serving	Percent DV[a]
Bread, white, 1 ounce (28 g)	31	3
Bread, whole-wheat, 1 slice	20	2
Broccoli, raw, ½ cup (113 g)	21	2
Cheddar cheese, 1.5 ounces (42.5 g)	306	31
Cheese, cream, regular, 1 tablespoon (14.8 ml)	12	1
Chinese cabbage, raw, 1 cup (227 g)	74	7
Cottage cheese, 1% milk fat, 1 cup unpacked (237 ml)	138	14
Frozen yoghurt, vanilla, soft serve, ½ cup (118 ml)	103	10
Ice cream, vanilla, ½ cup (118 ml)	85	8.5
Instant breakfast drink, powder prepared with water, 8 ounces (237 ml)	105–250	10–25
Kale, cooked, 1 cup (227 g)	94	9
Kale, raw, 1 cup (227 g)	90	9
Milk, buttermilk, 8 ounces (237 ml)	285	29
Milk, lactose-reduced, 8 ounces[b] (237 ml)	285–302	29–30
Milk, non-fat, 8 ounces (237 ml)	302	30
Milk, reduced-fat (2% milk fat), 8 ounces (237 ml)	297	30
Milk, whole (3.25% milk fat), 8 ounces (237 ml)	291	29
Mozzarella, part skim, 1.5 ounces (42.5 g)	275	28
Orange juice, calcium-fortified, 6 ounces (177 ml)	200–260	20–26
Pudding, chocolate, instant, made with 2% milk, ½ cup	153	15
Ready-to-eat cereal, calcium-fortified, 1 cup (227 g)	100–1000	10–100
Salmon, pink, canned, solids with bone, 3 ounces	181	18
Sardines, canned in oil, with bones, 3 ounces (85 g)	324	32
Sour cream, reduced fat, cultured, 2 tablespoons (29 ml)	32	3
Soy beverage, calcium-fortified, 8 ounces (237 ml)	80–500	8–50
Spinach, cooked, ½ cup (113 g)	120	12
Tofu, firm, made with calcium sulphate, ½ cup[c]	204	20
Tofu, soft, made with calcium sulphate, ½ cup[c]	138	14
Tortilla, corn, ready-to-bake/fry, 1 medium	42	4
Tortilla, flour, ready-to-bake/fry, one 6 inch diameter	37	4
Turnip greens, boiled, ½ cup (114 g)	99	10
Yoghurt, fruit, low fat, 8 ounces (237 ml)	245–384	25–38
Yoghurt, plain, low fat, 8 ounces (237 ml)	415	42

[a] DV, Daily Value. The DV for calcium is 1000 mg for adults and children aged 4 and older. Foods providing 20% or more of the DV are considered to be high sources of a nutrient, but foods providing lower percentages of the DV also contribute to a healthful diet. The US Department of Agriculture's Nutrient Database website, www.nal.usda.gov/fnic/foodcomp/search, lists the nutrient content of many foods. It also provides a comprehensive list of foods containing calcium at www.nal.usda.gov/fnic/foodcomp/Data/SR20/nutrlist/sr20a301.pdf.
[b] Calcium content varies slightly by fat content; the more fat, the less calcium the food contains.
[c] Calcium content is for tofu processed with a calcium salt. Tofu processed with other salts does not provide significant amounts of calcium.

Factors that impact calcium absorption

In addition to those discussed above, there are a number of factors that can increase or decrease calcium absorption, and there are some dietary sources that when consumed in excess can increase calcium losses from the body. Factors that improve calcium absorption in the intestine include vitamin D as well as consumption of foods that contain lactose when ingested at the same time as calcium-containing foods. Sugar alcohols such as xylitol and protein can also enhance calcium absorption.

Nutrients or substances that inhibit calcium absorption include fibre and phytates (myoinositol hexaphosphate). Many foods such as cereals, nuts and legumes contain both fibre and phytate that can bind calcium. Oxalates, found in rhubarb, spinach, squash, strawberries, pecans and peanuts, can bind calcium by chelation and increase the excretion of calcium through the faeces. High intakes of dietary sodium, protein or caffeine can increase urinary excretion of calcium by decreasing the reabsorption of renal calcium.

Although the negative effects of caffeine may have been overstated in the past, especially since there are positive effects of flavonoids on bone health from tea, fruit and vegetable consumption, it may be necessary to study anew the role of caffeinated beverages, especially energy drinks such as Red Bull® and Monster®, that contain significant amounts of caffeine. Full Throttle® 16 oz contains 144 mg caffeine, Red Bull® 8.5 oz contains 80 mg caffeine and Monster Energy Assault® 8 oz contains 80 mg caffeine. In comparison, 224 g (8 ounces) of brewed coffee contains 134–240 mg caffeine, tea 48–175 mg caffeine and carbonated beverages 22–46 mg caffeine. Anecdotal information indicates that these energy drinks may be consumed in very large amounts by young people that may put them at risk for decreased BMD as a result of displacement of calcium and other vital bone nutrients from their diets in favour of these beverages. College students are consuming energy drinks to offset lack of sleep, to increase energy, and to consume with alcohol. Additionally, physical symptoms of headaches and heart palpitations have been noted. Small amounts of caffeine (100 mg) consumed by women in the third decade of life does not appear to be detrimental to bone health, and consumption of up to 400 mg/day by healthy adults is not associated with adverse effects. Children should consume no more than 2.5 mg/kg and women of reproductive age should limit their intake to no more than 300 mg/day.

Other nutrients/conditions related to bone metabolism

Alcohol
Both animal and human studies have shown that chronic heavy drinking has serious detrimental effects on bone. Bone density, growth, volume and strength were all significantly reduced when alcohol was provided long term to young growing rats during adolescent growth. In fact, cell proliferation and longitudinal growth at the ends of the long bones ceased.

The US Government defines moderate drinking as no more than one drink per day for women and no more than two drinks per day for men. Standard values/pub measures are 360 ml of beer, 125 ml of wine and 35 ml of spirits. In middle-aged men who abuse alcohol, osteoporosis with decreased amounts of trabecular bone as well as thickness of the bone struts was seen. Decreased osteoblastic activity, and reduced levels of osteocalcin (a biochemical marker of bone formation) are consistent with these observations in adult males. Fewer studies have been performed on adult females who ingest alcohol in large amounts. In contrast to men, women who are heavy drinkers tend to have higher bone mass compared with women who do not drink at all. Post-menopausal women who drink alcohol appear to have even greater bone density as alcohol may increase circulating levels of oestrogen that decreases bone remodelling. No studies have been done on children or adolescents concerning the effect of alcohol on bone formation and growth but extrapolation from animal studies suggests that consuming alcohol during prime bone-building years may predispose individuals to increased fracture risk and increased risk for osteoporosis because of decreased BMD.

Protein
Protein is necessary to build and maintain bone mass and prevent bone loss in adulthood. Protein contributes to the collagen scaffold that serves as the matrix into which minerals are deposited. Because the protein–mineral matrix constantly turns over, it must be continuously supplied with a daily supply of amino acids. However, controversy about protein and its role in maintenance of bone density continues to exist, and protein intake has been shown to have both positive and negative effects. Estimates have suggested an increase of 1 mg urinary calcium excreted for every gram of protein intake but only if the protein comes from purified sources, not food sources. Conversely, other studies have shown that increased BMD and decreased risk of fracture resulted from increased protein intakes and may determine peak bone mass in pre-menopausal women. Among elderly patients who suffered a hip fracture, those who received an additional 20 g/day of an oral protein supplement had shortened hospital stays, improved recoveries, and return to independent living.

A more likely explanation for the effect of protein on bone mass is that the amount of calcium in the diet also plays a role. Although protein intake does cause an increase in urinary calcium, the amount of calcium in the diet will determine whether the individual remains in positive or negative calcium balance. Athletes will more than likely not have problems as they usually consume more protein. They could potentially have problems if they begin to restrict calories, as many who participate in body conscious sports often do.

Vitamin D

Vitamin D status, as measured by plasma concentrations of 25-hydroxyvitamin D, is positively associated with BMD in middle-aged and elderly women. Further, the amount of calcium consumed and absorbed throughout life is also positively associated with the female adult BMD. The absorption of calcium occurs throughout the small intestine but there are two major processes. The first one is dependent on the presence of calcitriol, or 1,25-dihydroxyvitamin D_3, which is stimulated when intakes of less than 400 mg calcium is ingested at one time by the body. If blood calcium levels decrease, parathyroid hormone (PTH) is released from the parathyroid gland which causes calcitriol to be formed in the kidney. Calcitriol regulates calcium absorption in a three-step sequential process that is saturable in the duodenum and jejunum and which comprises transport across the epithelial lining of the small intestine, movement of calcium across the brush border of the enterocyte and, finally, release of calcium on the basolateral portion of the enterocyte. Calcitriol activates the synthesis of calbindin, a calcium-binding protein that facilitates movement of calcium from the brush border into the cytoplasm of the enterocyte, and extrusion from the basolateral portion in an active process. The second process by which calcium is absorbed in the small intestine typically occurs when the amount of calcium ingested is over 400 mg at one time. This process is non-saturable, passive and occurs between the cells (paracellular) in the jejunum and ileum, predominantly.

When the concentration of blood calcium is below 8.5 mg/dl (normal serum calcium concentration is 8.5–10.5 mg/dl), PTH increases the release of calcitriol to stimulate increased renal reabsorption of calcium via a different calbindin protein. Finally,

in bone, PTH will initiate activation of osteoclastic action by binding with its receptor on osteoblasts. Bone degradation is promoted by lysosomal proteases that cause bone demineralisation and release of calcium into the blood to cause blood calcium levels to increase. These three processes, increased calcium absorption in the gut and reabsorption in the kidney, coupled with bone demineralisation, cause blood calcium levels to increase back into the normal range.

If blood calcium levels increase above 10.5 mg/dl, calcitonin is released from the parafollicular cells of the thyroid gland to cause osteoblastic activation, inhibition of osteoclasts and uptake of calcium into the bones for incorporation into the bone matrix. In addition, calcitonin also causes decreased kidney reabsorption, and activation of vitamin D leading to decreased blood calcium levels.

Phosphorus

Second only to calcium in abundance in the body, about 85% of phosphorus is found in the bones as part of the hydroxyapatite complex ($Ca_5(PO_4)_3OH$). The other 15% is associated with muscle (14%) and blood and body fluids (1%) as proteins, nucleic acids, ATP and lipids, functioning in cell membranes, acid–base balance and oxygen availability. Phosphorus is found in nearly every type of food in both organic and inorganic forms, but some of the best sources include eggs, milk and milk products, meat, fish and poultry, nuts, cereals and grains. The Recommended Dietary Allowance (RDA) for phosphorus is 700 mg/day for males and females over age 19 years.

Phosphorus is absorbed in its inorganic form after hydrolysis from organic forms occurs in the lumen of the small intestine, either by a saturable carrier-mediated active process that is promoted by calcitriol, or by a concentration-dependent diffusion process. The absorption of phosphorus can be facilitated by the presence of vitamin D, as is calcium, or inhibited by phytates, found in grains and legumes, and excess intakes of aluminium, calcium or magnesium. Anywhere from 50 to 70% of dietary phosphorus is absorbed depending on the source and increases linearly, with greater amounts being absorbed with larger intakes. Plasma concentration of phosphorus is in the range 2.5–4.5 mg/dl but it is not as tightly controlled as calcium. The same hormones that regulate calcium metabolism also regulate phosphorus metabolism, i.e. PTH, calcitriol and calcitonin. PTH stimulates both bone phosphorus resorption and kidney excretion while calcitonin increases bone mineralisation with phosphorus. Calcitriol increases phosphorus absorption in the gut and, in combination with PTH, promotes bone resorption. Phosphorus is excreted primarily in the urine with up to 30% excreted in the faeces.

Potassium

Potassium is an important nutrient for human health, with most countries recommending almost four times more dietary potassium than calcium to meet daily human needs. The Adequate Intake (AI) of potassium is 4.7 g while that of calcium is 1.2 g. Potassium is the major intracellular cation and serves roles in acid–base balance and nerve transmission. What is not well understood is the relationship of potassium to bone health. A large proportion of the American population does not consume adequate amounts of calcium (30% over age 2), potassium (<3%) and magnesium (55%), according to the latest NHANES report. Bone acts as an alkaline (base) reserve to buffer acids in the blood and other tissues that are generated during metabolic processes. The average Western diet causes more acid production, primarily from excessive protein and cereal grains, less than adequate amounts of calcium, and few potassium and bicarbonate-rich fruits and vegetables, especially after age 50 when people tend to produce more acid. On the other hand, fruits and vegetables cause more alkali (base) to be produced and thus may play a role in helping to decrease the incidence of osteoporosis. Fruits and vegetables contain large amounts of potassium, mostly in the form of potassium salts such as potassium citrate, potassium malate and potassium gluconate. When they are consumed, the body converts them to potassium bicarbonate, which is then used to buffer acids produced during metabolism. If individuals do not consume adequate amounts of fruits and vegetables containing potassium salts, the body will resorb bone to obtain the neutralising alkali found in the bone mineral matrix causing increased mineral losses in urine. Urinary calcium levels are elevated when an individual consumes a diet containing little potassium (few fruits and vegetables) and the reverse is also true. Consumption of fruits and vegetables

may also offset losses occurring when consuming a diet high in sodium chloride. More recent studies have shown that increased incidence of hip fracture is associated with an increased intake of animal protein (acid producing) compared with intake of vegetable protein (base producing). In fact, countries with large amounts of animal protein in their diets, such as Germany and the USA (199.3 hip fractures per 100 000 person-years, 120.3 hip fractures per 100 000 person-years, respectively), have much greater incidences of hip fracture compared with countries such as China and Nigeria (2.9 hip fractures per 100 000 person-years, 0.8 hip fractures per 100 000 person-years, respectively) that consume very little animal protein. The average animal protein versus protein intakes in these countries are Germany 62.4 g/day vs. 35.3 g/day; USA 70.1 g/day vs. 32.9 g/day; China 10.7 g/day vs. 51.2 g/day; Nigeria 8.1 g/day vs. 40.2 g/day.

Vitamin C

Humans are one of the few mammals incapable of synthesising vitamin C and as such must consume adequate amounts of vitamin C on a daily basis. Total body vitamin C is found primarily in adrenal and pituitary glands, brain, eyes and white blood cells, and its amount varies by tissue, but there is less than 2 g found in the adult. The primary function of vitamin C is to act as an antioxidant to scavenge free radicals, but it also functions as a co-factor of enzymes involved in the synthesis of carnitine, collagen, neurotransmitters norepinephrine and serotonin, and regulates absorption, transport and storage of iron. Some of the best food sources include citrus fruits, cantaloupe, green peppers, kale, broccoli, tomatoes, potatoes and strawberries. The RDA is 90 mg for men over age 30 and 75 mg for women over age 30. It is recommended that daily intake of vitamin C not exceed 2000 mg. People who smoke should consume 35 mg additional vitamin C. Individuals regularly exposed to second-hand smoke may need additional vitamin C. Vitamin C is absorbed throughout the small intestine by a sodium-dependent active process. It is transported freely in the plasma in the range 0.4–1.7 mg/dl.

Vitamin C is related to bone health because of its function in collagen formation. In a recent study using participants in the Framingham Osteoporosis Study, bone density of 213 men and 393 women, average age 75, was assessed at the beginning of a 4-year period to determine what effect intake of vitamin C had on bone density. Males who consumed the largest amounts of vitamin C lost the least amount of bone measured at the femoral neck but the same was not true for females.

Fluoride

Fluoride is considered a micromineral as it is present in only trace amounts in the human body. Specifically, fluoride replaces the hydroxyl groups of the hydroxyapatite complex forming fluorohydroxyapatite, a stronger less acid-soluble compound than hydroxyapatite. Tooth enamel seems to be especially capable of taking fluoride into the matrix and strengthening its structure. In addition, fluoride also makes the teeth more resistant to the lactic acid produced by the bacteria in the mouth and decreases the actual amount of acid production. The American Dental Association considers the use of fluoride in water to be completely safe as long as it is not consumed in amounts above 4 mg/l, as set by the Environmental Protection Agency. Approximately 70% of the population of the USA drinks fluoridated water but that is uncharacteristic in comparison to the rest of the world. Europe primarily relies on fluoridated toothpastes for tooth fortification.

When consumed as sodium fluoride at 40–80 mg/day, plus calcium supplements, fluoride stimulates osteoblastic activity, primarily in trabecular bone of the spine. The use of fluoride as a therapeutic option for the treatment of osteoporosis is not without controversy as not all studies have shown benefits. Vertebral fracture rate has been reduced in individuals in some studies while other studies have not shown a positive effect.

Fluoridated water is the best source of fluoride in communities where it is added or occurs naturally in the water supply (1–2 ppm). Food is quite low in fluoride but some grains, cereal products and fish contain small amounts. The adequate intake of fluoride is 4 mg/day for males and 3 mg/day for females. Nearly 100% of fluoride is absorbed if it is consumed as sodium fluorosilicate from fluoridated water or monofluorophosphate from toothpaste. When consumed with food or beverages that contain calcium, the absorption of fluoride is reduced to 50–80%. Calcium forms an insoluble complex with fluoride that reduces its absorption.

Vegetarianism

Individuals who practise vegetarianism, or the exclusion of meat, fish and poultry, and those who practise veganism, or the exclusion of all animal products from the diet, constitute approximately 4% of the US population. Vegetarianism is increasing in popularity for its perceived health or societal benefits. Vegetarian diets are typically higher in fibre, vitamins A, C and E, potassium, magnesium, phytonutrients, and lower in saturated fat, cholesterol, vitamins B_{12} and D, calcium, iron, zinc and ω-3 fatty acids. Individuals who practise these lifestyles tend to be thinner, have lower blood pressure, lower serum cholesterol and other blood lipids, and reduced risk for developing heart disease. Most studies have concluded that those who follow vegetarian/vegan diets have a small but significant reduction in BMD compared with those who follow omnivorous diets. However, there is growing support of the beneficial effects of fruits and vegetables on BMD. Many confounding variables, such as differences in body weight, physical activity levels, and rate of smoking, have made research in this area complicated. At present, the practice of vegetarianism is not a serious issue for risk for osteoporosis but determination of which aspects of the vegetarian diet are most beneficial to bone health remain to be determined.

19.5 Sport, exercise and bone health

The mechanical strain on the skeleton as a result of participation in athletics should increase BMD, especially in the child, high school and college athlete. Positive effects on bone health from sports-specific training have been found in a number of studies, although it appears that impact loading sports such as gymnastics, rugby or volleyball tend to produce a better overall osteogenic response than sports without impact loading such as cycling, rowing or swimming. The intensity of training will also play a role in the response of the bone. Unfortunately, the optimal intensity has not been determined nor is there sufficient data to understand site-specific responses of bone to sports training.

At some point, an athlete may reach his or her genetically determined maximal bone mass, and further increases will not be seen after that, regardless of the intensity or type of training. It is also possible that over-training can result in decreases in bone density, especially if energy deficits or disruptions in hormone secretion occur. An important point for the female athlete is that regardless of the type or intensity of training, the mechanical strain of sports will not be sufficient to overcome the loss of bone that will occur if there is a cessation of menses.

Increases in BMD from typical exercise programmes are generally only 2–6% above non-exercise controls, which is one of the dilemmas regarding the effect of sports participation on bone density. Physically active men and women typically fail to attain the benefits of exercise on bone health that might be expected based on the BMD seen in athletes. The reason for the discrepancy is most likely the differences in the amount and intensity of training as well as the fact that many athletes begin training before puberty when the impact of exercise on BMD may be greater.

19.6 Female Athlete Triad

Since the passage of Title IX in 1972, the number of girls and women engaging in sports has grown exponentially. Regarding athletics, Title IX requires that women have an equal opportunity to play in sports as men, as well as receive proportional athletic scholarships as men. Participation for girls in high school athletics has increased over 900% and for women in collegiate athletic by approximately 450% The overall benefits of being physically active and involvement in athletics are far too numerous and beyond the scope of this chapter. With this backdrop, the concerns in the 1970s revolved around the finding of menstrual dysfunction, specifically amenorrhoea, among long-distance runners and ballet dancers. The following menstrual function terms have been defined for the female athlete.

- Anovulation: menses without ovulation.
- Amenorrhoea: no menses for more than 90 days.
  - Primary amenorrhoea: delay in menarche; no menses after the age of 15 years.
  - Secondary amenorrhoea: menarche has occurred with subsequent absence of menses.
- Eumenorrhoea: ovulation with menses about very 26–32 days.
- Gynaecological age: current age minus age at menarche.

- Luteal suppression: luteal phase <11 days or low levels of progesterone.
- Menarche: age at first menstrual cycle.
- Oligoamenorrhoea: long menstrual cycles ≥36 days.
- Short menstrual cycles: menses <24 days.

In the general population, the median age for menarche is 12.4 years, primary amenorrhoea is very rare at less than 1% and secondary amenorrhoea is also low at 2–5%. Delayed menarche and an elevated prevalence of menstrual irregularities have been found in adolescent athletes. In sports that emphasise leanness, such as gymnastics, cheerleading and diving, primary amenorrhoea has been reported as high as 22%. A higher occurrence of secondary amenorrhoea has also been reported for athletes, ranging from 10% to as high as 45% among long-distance runners and 69% among ballet dancers. Finally, the diagnosis of luteal suppression or anovulation requires further medical screening other than the reporting of menstrual cycle length. Therefore, the occurrence of these subclinical menstrual dysfunctions may go unreported or underestimated. Luteal deficiency or anovulation may be as high as 75% among athletes.

The high frequency of amenorrhoea observed among runners and ballet dancers provided insight into the possible aetiology or mechanism(s). From 1980 to the early 1990s, initial research focused on the common factors between these athletes: low body fat, strenuous training, psychological stress, training at a young age, often before menarche, and late menarche. A common association emerged between disordered eating, amenorrhoea and low bone mass (osteoporosis) which became known as the *Female Athlete Triad*. The first Female Athlete Triad position stand by the American College of Sports Medicine was published in 1997 detailing the research and link between the three components.

In 2007, the American College of Sports Medicine (ACSM) Position Stand for the Female Athlete Triad was revised. The three components of disordered eating, amenorrhoea and osteoporosis are now viewed as a continuum of potential cascading intertwining health issues (Figure 19.2). Each factor has an optimal health level, but also a spectrum where an athlete or physically active woman may move down a path to subclinical health concerns to frank medical health problems. Existence of one or more components of

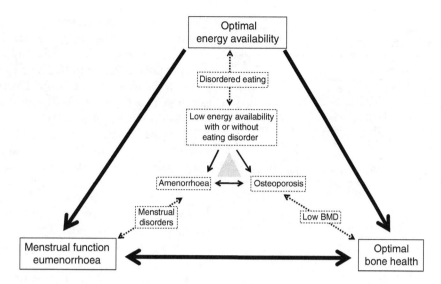

Figure 19.2 The spectrum of the Female Athlete Triad from optimal health to medical health issues. Optimal energy availability is the key component of the Triad where an athlete has increased her dietary intake to offset the increased exercise energy expenditure. Reduced energy availability with or without an eating disorder can lead to menstrual dysfunction and amenorrhoea and subsequently to low bone mineral density (BMD) and osteoporosis. (Reproduced from Nattiv A, Loucks AB, Manore MM, Sanborn CF, Sundgot-Borgen J, Warren MP, American College of Sports Medicine position stand, The female athlete triad, Med Sci Sports Exerc, 2007, 39(10):1867–1882. With permission from Wolters Kluwer Health.)

the triad, alone or in combination, poses a health risk for the physically active and athletic female.

To date, the key component in the Female Athlete Triad appears to be energy availability. Energy availability is calculated as dietary energy intake minus exercise energy expenditure divided by kilograms fat-free mass (FFM). At the optimal energy availability spectrum, the athlete has increased her dietary intake to compensate for the increased energy expenditure due to exercise. The combination of optimal energy balance and normal menstrual cycle function along with bone-loading activities promotes bone health. A potential health issue arises when the female athlete is in energy deficit or reduced energy availability because of consuming fewer calories than her energy expenditure through exercise. As the athlete 'slides' down the spectrum from optimal energy availability to low energy availability with or without frank clinical eating disorders, normal menstruation can follow a similar path from sub-clinical menstrual disorders to amenorrhoea. Finally, bone health can become compromised by low energy availability and menstrual dysfunction, alone or in combination. At the extreme end, amenorrhoea can lead to low BMD and subsequently osteoporosis.

Also, reduced energy availability and frank eating disorders can result in low BMD and osteoporosis.

Energy balance in young healthy women is estimated at energy availability of 45 kcal/kg FFM (Table 19.3). For menstrual cycle function, low energy availability has been proposed to occur below a daily energy availability of 30 kcal/kg FFM (Table 19.4). Increasing dietary intake alone, or in combination with a decrease in exercise, has been found to reverse abnormal hormonal patterns. Subclinical menstrual cycle dysfunction, i.e. suppression of luteinising hormone (LH) pulsatility, can occur after 3 days of training when dietary energy intake is reduced in regularly menstruating women. When dietary intake was increased, hormonal patterns returned to normal. Decreasing training by 1 day per week and increasing dietary caloric intake by approximately 350 kcal/day has also been shown to restore LH pulsatility to normal patterns in athletes with amenorrhoea. For increasing BMD, the athlete may need to gain weight and thus a higher energy availability of 45 kcal/kg FFM may be necessary.

A considerable population of women who combine moderate diet and exercise regimens for fitness and weight control may fall below the energy availability

Table 19.3 Optimal energy availability (kcal) for body weight and body fat is calculated at 45 kcal/kg FFM.

Body weight (kg)	Body fat (%)				
	10	15	20	25	30
45	1823	1721	1620	1519	1418
50	2025	1913	1800	1688	1575
55	2228	2104	1980	1856	1733
60	2430	2295	2160	2025	1890
65	2633	2486	2340	2194	2048

Table 19.4 Minimal energy availability (kcal) for body weight and body fat is calculated at 30 kcal/kg FFM.

Body weight (kg)	Body fat (%)				
	10	15	20	25	30
45	1215	1148	1080	1013	945
50	1350	1275	1200	1125	1050
55	1485	1403	1320	1238	1155
60	1620	1530	1440	1350	1260
65	1755	1658	1560	1463	1365

threshold. Thus, female athletes, dancers, cheerleaders and soldiers would be among those groups most frequently not obtaining an adequate energy balance. A surprise finding has been the low total caloric intakes reported by female athletes regardless of their menstrual status. Overall, athletes with amenorrhoea tend to consume fewer calories per day than do regularly menstruating athletes; however, the differences have not always been significant because of the large variability reported. The average recommended energy intake for light to moderately active women aged 15–24 years is 2200 kcal/day. However, the mean total consumption for female athletes has been reported to be as low as 1272 kcal/day. These athletes would appear to be in a reduced energy availability or caloric deficit.

Female athletes, dancers, cheerleaders and soldiers are often under intense pressure to have low body fat or meet weight standards, which often leads to dieting and, in many cases, disordered eating. No sport involving either males or females should be considered exempt from participants susceptible to an eating disorder. The term 'disordered eating', adopted for the triad, refers to a wide spectrum of abnormal patterns of eating that range in severity from restriction of food intake, using diet pills, diuretics or laxatives, periods of binging and purging to anorexia nervosa and bulimia nervosa at the extreme end of the spectrum. The incidence of eating disorders is much higher among athletes (15–62%) than in the general population (1–3%). Female soldiers also experience the interrelated conditions of the Female Athlete Triad. Military women are very physically active and experience pressure similar to the athlete to meet weight standards as often as every 6 months. A high percentage of females in basic training or on active duty have been reported to chronically or repeatedly engage in pathogenic dieting practices.

The revised ACSM position stand addresses the spectrum of bone health to low bone mass and/or fractures or osteoporosis. In general, eumenorrhoeic athletes in weight-loading sports have a lumbar BMD 5–15% higher compared with sedentary individuals. Athletes in non-weight-bearing activities such as swimming tend to have BMD similar to, if not lower than, non-athletes. The findings hold true also for femoral neck BMD, with gymnasts having some of the highest values reported, reflecting the high impact forces generated in this sport. Again, swimmers may have lower BMD than non-athletes. Further, physically active women also have a BMD 2–5% greater than sedentary women.

The majority of studies examining amenorrhoeic athletes have reported 10–25% lower BMD at the spine compared with eumenorrhoeic control subjects. There are three major concerns regarding the bone loss among amenorrhoeic athletes. First, it appears that amenorrhoeic athletes may not regain former BMD levels, which questions whether peak bone mass may be compromised. Second, without restoration of menstrual function, amenorrhoeic athletes continue to lose BMD. Third, a relationship has been found between low bone density and stress fractures. Thus, amenorrhoeic athletes are at a greater risk for stress fractures. In the revised ACSM position stand, 'low BMD' is defined as a Z-score between −1.0 and −2.0 in combination with the following risk factors: a history of disordered eating, hypo-oestrogenism, stress fractures, and/or other secondary clinical risk factors for fracture. For female athletes, osteoporosis is

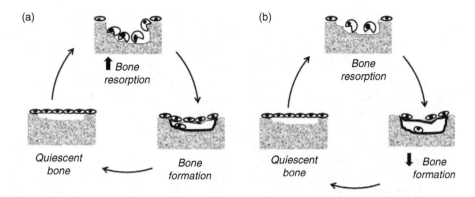

Figure 19.3 A simplistic view of bone loss. Net loss of bone will occur when bone resorption (🖤) exceeds bone formation (🖤), such as occurs with (a) lack of oestrogen (amenorrhoea) or (b) when leptin values are decreased.

defined as a BMD Z-score −2.0 or less with clinical risk factors for fracture.

The mechanism for bone loss in amenorrhoeic athletes may be more than the altered pattern of bone remodelling attributed to oestrogen deficiency (Figure 19.3). In addition, amenorrhoeic athletes have been shown to have a reduced bone turnover, bone formation and bone resorption. A possible explanation for the reduced bone turnover could be energy deficiency as documented by the finding of elevated cortisol, low T3 syndrome, deficiency of insulin-like growth factor (IGF)-1, and low leptin levels. Leptin is a regulator of energy intake and energy expenditure and thought to be an important inhibitor of appetite. Further, leptin may have a direct role in the bone loss because leptin receptors have been found on bone. Amenorrhoeic athletes have been found to have abnormal leptin secretion. Leptin may represent a mechanism other than hypo-oestrogenism that could account for low bone density.

19.7 Stress fractures

Chronic leg pain is an injury that plagues many athletes and military personnel. The two most frequent forms of exercise-induced leg pain are medial tibial stress syndrome ('shin splints') and stress fractures. The diagnosis of medial tibial stress syndrome is based on the criteria of pain located along the posteriomedial border of the tibia that occurs during exercise and can last for several hours or days after exercise. A stress fracture is defined as a partial or complete fracture of bone due to its inability to withstand rhythmic non-violent stress applied repeatedly in a submaximal manner. Stress fractures also present themselves with one common theme: pain. In the early phases of a stress fracture the pain is usually more intense after some kind of physical training. If this injury goes unnoticed, the pain can increase to the point where normal daily activities such as walking can become painful. Training sessions start to suffer as the pain aggravates any and all movements around the stress fracture site. Often, the injury reaches this point before the athlete or recruit actually presents for evaluation. The majority of stress fractures occur in the tibia, with some also occurring in the metatarsals or femur or, in rare cases, the pelvis.

Stress fractures are a common overuse injury attributed to strain damage from repetitive weight-bearing loads such as running, jumping and marching. In female athletes, annual stress fracture rates have been reported to be the highest for track athletes (52%), runners (37%) and gymnasts (27%). Ballet dancers also experience high rates (22–45%). In the US military, the estimated incidence of stress fractures varies from 1 to 21% in women and from 1 to 9% in men. In military studies, a higher occurrence is commonly found in women versus men and in whites compared with non-whites. In contrast to the military, a gender difference has not been observed in the athletic population.

The aetiology of stress fractures is multifactorial and complex. The major risk factors that have been identified for the development of stress fractures include training errors, anthropometric differences, low bone density, bone geometry, menstrual disturbances and dietary insufficiency. Abrupt changes that occur in physical activity are referred to as 'training errors' and may be the most important cause of running injuries. Training errors can include sudden increases in training volume or intensity, changes in footwear or improper footwear for training (e.g. military boots versus running shoes), or hard training surfaces. Stress fractures were first described in the military as 'march fractures' and corresponded to a recruit placed in a short intense period of basic training wearing combat boots. Not surprisingly, the initial fitness level of the recruit has been found to be a strong predictor for the development of stress fractures. When a longer, progressive training period has been implemented in the military, the occurrence of stress fractures has been significantly reduced. The following training changes have also resulted in a reduction in stress fractures: reduction in marching speed, softer running surfaces, interval training versus the traditional middle distance runs, and individualised step lengths versus marching in formation.

Anthropometric characteristics have been theoretically linked both directly and indirectly to stress fractures. Leg-length discrepancy, less leg muscle, smaller calf girths, shorter tibial length, narrower tibial widths and lower cortical bone area in the tibia have been found to be distinguishing factors in athletes and military recruits with stress fractures. The association between muscle mass and stress fractures might be explained by lower bone density or by fatigue damage under repetitive loading. Based on Frost's mechanostat theory, muscle forces cause an osteogenic response; therefore, it is theorised that smaller muscles correspond to less of a stimulus resulting in less bone mass. Muscles may also have a protective role in resisting mechanical stress, where weaker muscles may contribute to fatigue damage, thus leading to stress fractures. This hypothesis is supported by the finding of reduced calf girth in female athletes with stress fractures, and smaller muscle cross-sectional area in female runners with a history of stress fractures.

Low bone mass may be a contributing factor in athletes and military recruits with stress fractures especially among women. Compared with sedentary individuals, physically active women with stress fractures have an average BMD decrease of 6% in the lumbar spine, 4% in the femur and 4% in the tibia/fibula. For the physically active woman with a stress fracture, the finding of low bone mass is often accompanied by amenorrhoea and disordered eating. A relationship between stress fractures and amenorrhoea has been reported in athletes, ballet dancers and female recruits. Amenorrhoeic athletes have a relative risk for stress fracture that is two to four times greater than regularly menstruating athletes. Female recruits with menstrual irregularities may also be predisposed to stress fractures.

19.9 Prevention, screening and treatment recommendations for the Female Athlete Triad and stress fractures

Optimal nutritional status is critical for all athletes to perform at their maximum potential. For the female athlete, adequate energy availability and meeting daily nutrient requirements are the first key steps in prevention of the triad. The athlete, coach and parent need exercise and sports nutrition education, preferably from a registered dietitian who is a board certified specialist in sports nutrition or CSSD. Screening for the triad begins with a thorough assessment at an athletic pre-participation examination and/or annual health screening examination. Signs of any component of the triad should warrant further evaluation and referral to appropriate healthcare professionals. The complex clinical components of the triad require a multidisciplinary treatment approach, including a physician, a registered dietitian and, if needed, psychiatrist for an eating disorder. If appropriate and available, other members of the team should include the coach, parents, athletic trainer and exercise physiologist.

Initial treatment for the triad is to regain optimal energy availability by increasing caloric intake and/or reducing energy expenditure through exercise. Athletes with signs of disordered eating such as low energy availability or restrictive eating habits should be quickly identified and provided with guidance to normal eating patterns. Disordered eating patterns, especially at a young age, can lead to frank eating disorders. Menstrual dysfunction and amenorrhoea should not be assumed to be functional hypothalamic amenorrhoea and need further evaluation to rule out other potential causes of amenorrhoea.

Table 19.5 Nutrition care process for athletes throughout the life cycle.

	Child (prepuberty)	Adolescent (puberty to 18 years)	College (18–24 years)	Adult (>25 years)
Anthropometric	BMI (*% Body fat*)	BMI (*% Body fat*)	BMI (*% Body fat*)	BMI (*% Body fat*)
Biochemical	(*Growth hormone*) (*IGF-1*)	(*Menstrual dysfunction*) (*Eating disorders*)	Vitamin D (*Menstrual dysfunction*) (*Eating disorders*)	Vitamin D (*Menstrual dysfunction*) (*Eating disorders*)
Clinical	Physical exam. Medical history (*DEXA*)	Physical exam. Medical history Menstrual history (*DEXA*) (*Stress fractures*)	Physical exam. Medical history Menstrual history (*Luteal phase length*) (*DEXA*) (*Stress fractures*)	Physical exam. Medical history Menstrual history (*Pregnancies, length of postpartum amenorrhoea*) (*DEXA*) (*Stress fractures*)
Dietary	Dietary record (*Calcium, protein, vitamin D*)	Dietary record Energy availability	Dietary record Energy availability	Dietary record (*Energy availability*)
Environmental	Training log Injury history Nutrition education: parent, basics	Training log Injury history Nutrition education: basics, diets, supplememts	Training log Injury history Nutrition education: cooking, eating out, etc.	Training log Injury history Nutrition education: meal planning

Italic terms in parentheses would be indicated for further assessment if warranted by initial screening.
BMI, body mass index; DEXA, dual-energy X-ray absorptiometry; IGF, insulin-like growth factor.

Low leg pain in combination with or without the other two triad components should be referred to a physician for a comprehensive physical examination to confirm a diagnosis of stress fracture. Typical rehabilitation involves a reduction in training and a gradual return to exercise activity. Assessment of BMD is recommended for an athlete with a history of a stress fracture or a 6-month history of amenorrhoea, oligoamenorrhoea, disordered eating or eating disorder. At this time, the first aim of treatment for low bone density in young girls and pre-menopausal female athletes is to restore normal menstrual function and optimal energy balance and increased body weight. Bisphosphonates, though approved for post-menopausal osteoporosis, should not be used in the young athlete because of unknown efficacy and concerns for potential harm during pregnancy. Weight gain, not hormone replacement therapy and/or oral contraceptive pills, has been shown to be more effective in increasing BMD. For athletes less than 16 years of age, oral contraceptive pills have not been recommended because of concern for early closure of growth plates.

19.10 Nutrition care process for athletes throughout the life cycle

The bone health recommendations are based on a nutrition care process for athletes throughout the life cycle (Table 19.5). A lifetime approach for the athlete is divided into the following major periods: child, adolescent, collegiate and adult. The **ABCDE** nutritional assessment mnemonic corresponds to **A**nthropometric measurements, **B**iochemical tests, **C**linical examinations, **D**ietary assessments and **E**nvironmental factors. The major recommendations for each age and nutritional assessment are specific for skeletal growth and maintenance. These assessments should occur during the pre-participation examination or annual health screening examination. Further assessments may be warranted based on the initial screening or when any signs and symptoms of nutritional deficiencies, hormonal dysfunction and/or stress fractures occur.

Measuring weight and height and calculating body mass index (BMI) is the fundamental anthropometric assessment at all ages. The addition of estimating body fat and FFM is recommended after puberty to calculate optimal energy availability for the athletes. Calculating percentage body fat and FFM for the prepubescent athlete may also be recommended if energy deficiency is a concern.

During prepubescence, bone modelling and remodelling are critical for bone growth. Biochemical assessment of growth hormone and IGF-1 may be indicated when severe energy deficits are occurring. After puberty, the female athlete is vulnerable to low energy availability and disordered eating, which could develop into a frank eating disorder, and subclinical menstrual disorders and amenorrhoea. Biochemical evaluations may be necessary for diagnosis of functional hypothalamic amenorrhoea and for excluding other potential causes. Thyroid function tests, urinalysis and other blood chemistry profiles may be indicated for an athlete with disordered eating or an eating disorder. Vitamin D assessment may also be warranted in this age group because of lack of milk consumption, lack of sunlight exposure and lack of other foods that contain vitamin D.

A thorough physical examination and medical history should be obtained every year. Menstrual histories should include age at menarche and a log of menses and oral contraceptive usage. Since luteal suppression or deficiency is problematic among young female athletes, further clinical screening may be necessary. The duration of postpartum amenorrhoea needs to be monitored to rule out subsequent development of secondary amenorrhoea. BMD should be assessed in female athletes who have a stress fracture or have a 6-month history of hypo-oestrogenism (amenorrhoea, oligoamenorrhoea), disordered eating or an eating disorder. Additional diagnostic imaging such as plain radiography and bone scans may be required to confirm the diagnosis of a stress fracture.

Dietary records are needed to assess dietary patterns, macronutrients and micronutrients and supplementation for all athletes regardless of age. The challenge arises in obtaining accurate detail and compliance from the athlete. For the child, a parent will provide the dietary record, usually for 3 days, including two weekdays and a weekend day, to begin to understand typical eating patterns, food sensitivities, food aversions and food intolerances. As the individual becomes an adolescent, more of the food choices are made by him or her and the parent exerts less control. In the US, particularly, milk

consumption decreases with age at the same time bone is accruing. Particular attention should be paid to the consumption of calcium-rich foods and vitamin D along with adequate protein to ensure optimal bone mass. Three-day diet records, food frequency records or diet histories may be used with older athletes to gain a better picture of their relationship with food. In addition, if disordered eating is noted during the nutritional assessment, energy availability should be determined based on an assessment of energy intake, exercise energy expenditure and body composition based on DEXA ideally. Specific environmental assessments for the athlete include a training log, injury history and nutrition education programmes. Athletes tend to overestimate the time, intensity and duration of their workouts; therefore, a training log is needed for an accurate calculation of their energy expenditure. Exercise and sports nutrition education is vital for not only the athlete but the coach and parent. Topics should include proper nutrition during the competitive season and off-season, as well as before, during and after the athletic event. During adolescence, the pressure to be thin or have low body fat becomes intensified for many female athletes; therefore, dieting and supplements should be discussed. For the first time, collegiate athletes are living away from home and will need strategies for eating in the dorms and eating out at restaurants. How to grocery shop on a limited budget and cooking lessons are additional lessons for collegiate athletes. The adult athlete will be balancing a training schedule and work, and for some a family as well. Nutrition education should include meal planning.

19.11 Summary

The skeleton undergoes a constant process of modelling and remodelling. During childhood, bone growth in length and size is accomplished by bone modelling. Bone remodelling occurs throughout life and serves to maintain the architecture and strength of the bone, maintain mineral homeostasis, and prevent fatigue damage. Overall, eumenorrhoeic athletes who participate in weight-bearing sports have a greater BMD than sedentary individuals. All athletes should have a thorough physical examination, a medical history and a dietary record assessment.

Particular attention should be paid to the consumption of calcium-rich foods and vitamin D along with adequate protein to ensure optimal bone mass. Energy availability should be calculated to determine if the athlete is in optimal energy balance and has increased her dietary intake to compensate for the increased energy expenditure due to exercise. However, reduced energy availability and frank eating disorders can result in low BMD and osteoporosis.

Acknowledgements

The authors wish to thank Ms Jimmie Lyn Harris for her invaluable help with the literature searches and citations.

Further reading

Abraham SF, Beumont PJ, Fraser IS, Llewellyn-Jones D. Body weight, exercise and menstrual status among ballet dancers in training. Br J Obstet Gynaecol 1982; 89: 507–510.

American Psychiatric Association. Treatment of Patients with Eating Disorders, 3rd edn, 2006. Available at www.psychiatryonline.com/pracGuide/pracGuideTopic_12.aspx. Accessed 28 May 2010.

American Psychiatric Association. Treating Eating Disorders: A Quick Reference Guide. Available at www.psychiatryonline.com/content.aspx?aid=146929. Accessed 28 May 2010.

Bachrach LK. Measuring bone mass in children: can we really do it? Horm Res 2006; 65 (Suppl 2): 11–16.

Bailey W, Duchon K, Barker L, Maas W. Populations receiving optimally fluoridated public drinking water: United States, 1992–2006. MMWR 2008; 57: 737–741.

Barr SI, Rideout CA. Nutritional considerations for vegetarian athletes. Nutrition 2004; 20: 696–703.

Bass SL. The prepubertal years: a uniquely opportune stage of growth when the skeleton is most responsive to exercise? Sports Med 2000; 30: 73–78.

Bass SL, Eser P, Daly R. The effect of exercise and nutrition on the mechanostat. J Musculoskelet Neuronal Interact 2005; 5: 239–254.

Beals KA, Manore MM. Disorders of the female athlete triad among collegiate athletes. Int J Sport Nutr Exerc Metab 2002; 12: 281–293.

Bennell KL, Brukner PD. Epidemiology and site specificity of stress fractures. Clin Sports Med 1997; 16: 179–196.

Bennell KL, Malcolm SA, Thomas SA et al. Risk factors for stress fractures in track and field athletes. A twelve- month prospective study. Am J Sports Med 1996; 24: 810–818.

Bennell K, Matheson G, Meeuwisse W, Brukner P. Risk factors for stress fractures. Sports Med 1999; 28: 91–122.

Benson JE, Engelbert-Fenton KA, Eisenman PA. Nutritional aspects of amenorrhoea in the female athlete triad. Int J Sport Nutr 1996; 6: 134–145.

Bianchi ML, Baim S, Bishop NJ et al. Official positions of the International Society for Clinical Densitometry (ISCD) on DXA evaluation in children and adolescents. Pediatr Nephrol 2010; 25: 37–47.

Bonjour JP, Carrie AL, Ferrari S, Clavien H, Slosman D, Theintz G. Calcium-enriched foods and bone mass growth in prepubertal girls: a randomized, double-blind, placebo controlled trial. J Clin Invest 1997; 99: 1287–1294.

Brukner P, Bennell K. Stress fractures in female athletes. Diagnosis, management and rehabilitation. Sports Med 1997; 24: 419–429.

Chan GM, Hoffman K, McMurry M. Effects of dairy products on bone and body composition in pubertal girls. J Pediatr 1995; 126: 551–556.

Chavassieux P, Seeman E, Delmas PD. Insights into material and structural basis of bone fragility from diseases associated with fractures: how determinants of the biomechanical properties of bone are compromised by disease. Endocr Rev 2007; 28: 151–164.

Chumlea WC, Schubert CM, Roche AF et al. Age at menarche and racial comparisons in US girls. Pediatrics 2003; 111: 110–113.

Dawson-Hughes B. Interaction of dietary calcium and protein in bone health in humans. J Nutr 2003; 133: 852S–854S.

Dawson-Hughes B, Harris SS. Calcium intake influences the association of protein intake with rates of bone loss in elderly men and women. Am J Clin Nutr 2002; 75: 773–779.

Dawson-Hughes B, Tosteson AN, Melton LJ III et al. Implications of absolute fracture risk assessment for osteoporosis practice guidelines in the USA. Osteoporos Int 2008; 19: 449–458.

Dawson-Hughes B, Harris SS, Palermo N, Casteneda Sceppa C, Rasmussen HM, Dallal G. Treatment with potassium bicarbonate lowers calcium excretion and bone resorption in older men and women. J Clin Endocrinol Metab 2009; 94: 96–102.

De Souza MJ, Miller BE, Loucks AB et al. High frequency of luteal phase deficiency and anovulation in recreational women runners: blunted elevation in follicle-stimulating hormone observed during luteal-follicular transition. J Clin Endocrinol Metab 1998; 83: 4220–4232.

Dew TP, Day AJ, Morgan MR. Bone mineral density, polyphenols and caffeine: a reassessment. Nutr Res Rev 2007; 20: 89–105.

Downey PA, Siegel MI. Bone biology and the clinical implications for osteoporosis. Phys Ther 2006; 86: 77–91.

Dueck CA, Matt KS, Manore MM, Skinner JS. Treatment of athletic amenorrhoea with a diet and training intervention program. Int J Sport Nutr 1996; 6: 24–40.

Edwards PH Jr, Wright ML, Hartman JF. A practical approach for the differential diagnosis of chronic leg pain in the athlete. Am J Sports Med 2005; 33: 1241–1249.

Ervin RB, Wang C-Y, Wright JD, Kennedy-Stephenson, J. Dietary intake of selected minerals for the United States population: 1999–2000. Adv Data 2004; 341: 1–5.

Frassetto L, Morris RC Jr, Sebastian A. Worldwide incidence of hip fracture in elderly women: relation to consumption of animal and vegetable foods. J Gerontol 2000; 90: 831–834.

Frost HM, Ferretti JL, Jee WS. Perspectives: some roles of mechanical usage, muscle strength, and the mechanostat in skeletal physiology, disease, and research. Calcif Tissue Int 1998; 62: 1–7.

Gibson R. Principles of Nutritional Assessment, 2nd edn. New York: Oxford University Press, 2005.

Hannan MT, Tucker KL, Dawson-Hughes B, Cupples LA, Felson DT, Kiel DP. Effect of dietary protein on bone loss in elderly men and women: the Framingham Osteoporosis Study. J Bone Miner Res 2000; 15: 2504–2512.

Heaney R. Bone as the calcium nutrient reserve. In: Calcium in Human Health (Weaver CM, Heaney RP, eds). Totowa, NJ: Humana Press, 2006, pp 7–12.

Heaney R. Nutrition and risk for osteoporosis. In: Osteoporosis, 3rd edn, Vol 1 (Marcus R, Feldman D, Nelson DA, Rosen CJ, eds). Amsterdam: Elsevier, 2008, pp 799–836.

Heaney RP, Layman DK. Amount and type of protein influences bone health. Am J Clin Nutr 2008; 87: 1567S–1570S.

Hogan HA, Sampson HW, Cashier E, Dedoux N. Alcohol consumption by young actively growing rats: a study of cortical bone histomorphometry and mechanical properties. Alcohol Clin Exp Res 1997; 21: 809–816.

Johnston CC, Miller JZ, Slemenda CW et al. Calcium supplementation and increases in bone mineral density in children. N Engl J Med 1992; 327: 82–87.

Klopp SA, Heiss CJ, Smith HS. Self-reported vegetarianism may be a marker for college women at risk for disordered eating. J Am Diet Assoc 2003; 103: 745–747.

Konig D, Muser K, Dickhuth HH, Berg A, Deibert P. Effect of a supplement rich in alkaline minerals ion acid–base balance in humans. Nutr J 2009; 8: 23–30.

Lanham-New SA. The balance of bone health: tipping the scales in favour of potassium-rich bicarbonate-rich foods. J Nutr 2008; 138: 172S–177S.

Lanham-New SA. Is 'vegetarianism' a serious risk factor for osteoporotic fracture? Am J Clin Nutr 2009; 90: 910–911.

Lauder TD, Dixit S, Pezzin LE, Williams MV, Campbell CS, Davis GD. The relation between stress fractures and bone mineral density: evidence from active-duty Army women. Arch Phys Med Rehabil 2000; 81: 73–79.

Lewiecki EM, Gordon CM, Baim S et al. Special report on the 2007 adult and pediatric Position Development Conferences of the International Society for Clinical Densitometry. Osteoporos Int 2008; 19: 1369–1378.

Loucks AB, Thuma JR. Luteinizing hormone pulsatility is disrupted at a threshold of energy availability in regularly menstruating women. J Clin Endocrinol Metab 2003; 88: 297–311.

Loucks AB, Verdun M, Heath EM. Low energy availability, not stress of exercise, alters LH pulsatility in exercising women. J Appl Physiol 1998; 84: 37–46.

Malinauskas BM, Aeby VG, Overton RF, Carpenter-Aeby T, Barber-Heidal K. A survey of energy drink consumption patterns among college students. Nutr J 2007; 6: 35.

Marcus R, Cann C, Madvig P et al. Menstrual function and bone mass in elite women distance runners. Endocrine and metabolic features. Ann Intern Med 1985; 102: 158–163.

Massey LK, Whiting SJ. Caffeine, urinary calcium, calcium metabolism and bone. J Nutr 1993; 123: 1611–1614.

Mawrot P, Jordan S, Eastwood J, Rothstein J, Hugenholtz A, Feeley M. Effects of caffeine on human health. Food Addit Contam 2003: 1–30.

Myburgh KH, Hutchins J, Fataar AB, Hough SF, Noakes TD. Low bone density is an etiologic factor for stress fractures in athletes. Ann Intern Med 1990; 113: 754–759.

Nattiv A, Loucks AB, Manore MM, Sanborn CF, Sundgot-Borgen J, Warren MP. American College of Sports Medicine position stand. The female athlete triad. Med Sci Sports Exerc 2007; 39: 1867–1882.

New SA. Do vegetarians have a normal bone mass? Osteoporos Int 2004; 15: 679–688.

Nichols DL, Sanborn CF, Essery EV. Bone density and young athletic women. An update. Sports Med 2007; 37: 1001–1014.

Otis CL, Drinkwater B, Johnson M, Loucks A, Wilmore J. American College of Sports Medicine position stand. The Female Athlete Triad. Med Sci Sports Exerc 1997; 29(5): i–ix.

Otten JJ, Hellwig JP, Meyers LD (eds). Calcium. In: Dietary Reference Intakes: The Essential Guide to Nutrient Requirements. Washington, DC: National Academies Press, 2006, pp 286–295.

Otten JJ, Hellwig JP, Meyers LD (eds). Phosphorus. In: Dietary Reference Intakes: The Essential Guide to Nutrient Requirements. Washington, DC: National Academies Press, 2006, pp 362–369.

Otten JJ, Hellwig JP, Meyers LD (eds). Vitamin C. In: Dietary Reference Intakes: The Essential Guide to Nutrient Requirements. Washington, DC: National Academies Press, 2006, pp 202–210.

Otten JJ, Hellwig JP, Meyers LD (eds). Vitamin D. In: Dietary Reference Intakes: The Essential Guide to Nutrient Requirements. Washington, DC: National Academies Press, 2006, pp 224–233.

Pak CY, Sakhaee K, Rubin CD, Zerwekh JE. Sustained-release sodium fluoride in the management of established postmenopausal osteoporosis. Am J Med Sci 1997; 313: 23–32.

Petit MA, Beck TJ, Kontulainen SA. Examining the developing bone: what do we measure and how do we do it? J Musculoskelet Neuronal Interact 2005; 5: 213–224.

Phipps K. Fluoride and bone health. J Public Health Dent 1995; 55: 53–56.

Popp KL, Hughes JM, Smock AJ et al. Bone geometry, strength, and muscle size in runners with a history of stress fracture. Med Sci Sports Exerc 2009; 41: 2145–2150.

Riggs BL, Hodgson SF, O'Fallon WM et al. Effect of fluoride treatment on the fracture rate in postmenopausal women with osteoporosis. N Engl J Med 1990; 322: 802–809.

Sahni S, Hannan MT, Gagnon D et al. High vitamin C intake is associated with lower 4-year bone loss in elderly men. J Nutr 2008; 138: 1931–1938.

Sampson HW, Chaffin C, Lange J, DeFee B. Alcohol consumption by young actively growing rats: a histomorphometric study of cancellous bone. Alcochol Clin Exp Res 1997; 21: 352–359.

Sanborn CF, Martin BJ, Wagner WW. Is athletic amenorrhoea specific to runners? Am J Obstet Gynecol 1982; 143: 859–861.

Sanborn CF, Horea M, Siemers BJ, Dieringer KI. Disordered eating and the female athlete triad. Clin Sports Med 2000; 19: 199–213.

Schurch MA, Rizzoli R, Slosman D, Vadas L, Vergnaud P, Bonjour JP. Protein supplements increase serum insulin-like growth factor-I levels and attenuate proximal femur bone loss in patients with recent hip fracture. A randomized, double-blind, placebo-controlled trial. Ann Intern Med 1998; 128: 801–809.

Suarez FL, Adshead J, Furne JK, Levitt MD. Lactose maldigestion is not an impediment to the intake of 1500 mg calcium daily as dairy products. Am J Clin Nutr 1998; 68: 1118–1122.

Szulc P, Seeman E. Thinking inside and outside the envelopes of bone: dedicated to PDD. Osteoporos Int 2009; 20: 1281–1288.

Teucher B, Dainty JR, Spinks CA et al. Sodium and bone health: impact of moderately high and low salt intakes on calcium metabolism in postmenopausal women. J Bone Miner Res 2008; 23: 1477–1485.

Turner RT. Skeletal response to alcohol. Alcochol Clin Exp Res 2000; 24: 1693–1701.

Turner RT, Sibonga JD. Effects of alcohol use and oestrogen on bone. Alcohol Res Health 2001; 25: 276–281.

US Department of Agriculture. Results from the United States Department of Agriculture's 1994–1996 Continuing Survey of Food Intakes by Individuals/Diet and Health Knowledge Survey. 1994–1996.

US Department of Health and Human Services and US Department of Agriculture. Dietary Guidelines for Americans, 2005.

Warren MP, Brooks-Gunn J, Hamilton LH, Warren LF, Hamilton WG. Scoliosis and fractures in young ballet dancers. Relation to delayed menarche and secondary amenorrhoea. N Engl J Med 1986: 314: 1348–1353.

Weaver CM. Should dairy be recommended as part of a healthy vegetarian diet? Point. Am J Clin Nutr 2009; 89: 1634S–1637S.

Williams NI, Caston-Balderrama AL, Helmreich DL, Parfitt DB, Nosbisch C, Cameron JL. Longitudinal changes in reproductive hormones and menstrual cyclicity in cynomolgus monkeys during strenuous exercise training: abrupt transition to exercise-induced amenorrhoea. Endocrinology 2001; 142: 2381–2389.

Yates B, White S. The incidence and risk factors in the development of medial tibial stress syndrome among naval recruits. Am J Sports Med 2004; 32: 772–780.

Zanker CL, Swaine IL. Relation between bone turnover, oestradiol, and energy balance in women distance runners. Br J Sports Med 1998; 32: 167–171.

20
Nutrition and the Gastrointestinal Tract for Athletes

Jeni Pearce and John O Hunter

Key messages

- Athletes are advised to trial all food and drinks during training, or in practice sessions, prior to competition.
- Lower gastrointestinal (GI) tract symptoms appear more common than upper tract symptoms and can appear before, during and after exercise.
- Responses vary widely among athletes and advice should be individualised.

- A number of substances can alter GI comfort and cause distress, including caffeine, buffers, glycerol, alcohol, sorbitol, non steroidal anti-inflammatory drugs, meal timing and carbohydrate concentration of beverages.
- Athletes should have a good working knowledge of the function and limitations of the GI tract.

20.1 Introduction: gastrointestinal symptoms and exercise

Gastrointestinal (GI) discomfort and a range of symptoms are well recognised and reported to medical and nutritional support teams by up to 50% of athletes, especially from those involved in high-intensity exercise. These symptoms and discomfort may be exacerbated by exercise or existing conditions. This either results in the athlete withdrawing from training and competition, or competing with discomfort which consequently hinders performance outcomes. The benefit of physical activity in reducing the risk of colon cancer is well recognised. Inactivity is linked to a 1.2–3.6 fold increase in the risk of developing colon cancer, potentially through less contact time between possible carcinogen and the mucosa and factors involved in the immune function and protection of the GI tract.

The frequency of GI distress or symptoms may be twice as high in endurance athletes such as runners compared with cyclists or swimmers and 1.5–3 times higher in elite athletes than recreational athletes. The function and role of the GI tract is dependent on the composition of the food and fluid digested and is influenced by the timing of ingestion before, during and after exercise. Stress may also impact the function of the GI tract, as does undesirable contaminants (bacterial, viral and food-related compounds). Causes of GI distress appear to range from reduced blood flow, altered motility, central nervous system (CNS) influences, hormonal and mechanical effects (pounding with running and compression with bending). Failure to manage and treat GI disturbances could lead to withdrawal from training and competition, in addition to adverse health outcomes. Fortunately, with the exception of GI bleeding, the symptoms are generally transitory. This area requires further research due to conflicting and equivocal data, differing incidence with varying modes of exercise, intensity, duration, training status, gender, dietary intake and age. Advances in techniques to monitor and examine the GI tract make research more feasible. Just as athletes must train the muscle and the mind, so they must also train the GI tract to meet the demands of exercise.

Sport and Exercise Nutrition, First Edition. Edited by Susan A Lanham-New, Samantha J Stear, Susan M Shirreffs and Adam L Collins.
© 2011 The Nutrition Society. Published 2011 by Blackwell Publishing Ltd.

20.2 Gastrointestinal tract

The structure and function of the GI tract has been explained in detail in recent excellent reviews (see Further reading) and the following is therefore a brief overview of key information.

The GI tract is a complex, much coiled tube which passes through the body from mouth to anus. However, it must be understood that the contents of the GI tract are at all times 'outside the body' itself, that is to say, there is a barrier between substances passing along the GI tract and the body's internal environment, which is quite separate. The GI tract has been described as a barrier, both protective and functional.

Food, together with various environmental chemicals, drugs and medications are taken into the mouth where they are mixed with saliva. Saliva is secreted by three pairs of salivary glands which lie beside and below the lower jaw and secrete a watery fluid; this not only allows the food to be broken down by chewing into a soft paste that is easier to swallow, but it also contains an enzyme, amylase, which starts the process of starch digestion. Recent research suggests that the presence of carbohydrate in the mouth may improve performance, without influencing muscle metabolism. These mouth-rinsing studies suggest that ingesting carbohydrate, and possibly taste, may exert a beneficial influence on the brain and CNS (central effect). This is supported by athletes covering increased distances (self-paced) and reporting lower rates of perceived exertion and 'feeling better' with carbohydrate consumption during prolonged running and cycling. A dry mouth (xerostomia) may also increase the risk of infection, bacterial or viral, due to ease of access to the body and reduction in natural defences provided by saliva and its components.

Swallowing is a voluntary act but once food has passed from the mouth through the pharynx and into the oesophagus, its subsequent progress is assured by the contraction of smooth muscle in the wall of the GI tract, over which we have no conscious control. Food passes along the oesophagus, propelled by peristalsis. Gravity is not involved and it has been shown that it is quite possible to swallow food or drink and for it to pass along the GI tract while standing on one's head. At the bottom of the oesophagus lies a small valve, the lower oesophageal sphincter, which serves to provide a degree of protection for the oesophagus from reflux of stomach contents.

The stomach is basically a bag where food can be stored while further digestion occurs. This is mainly done by the secretion of hydrochloric acid, which is strong enough, under certain circumstances, to cause ulcers by burning the lining of the stomach. There is a protective layer of slime, known as mucus, coating the internal stomach wall and this is mixed with bicarbonate which neutralises the acid. It also contains compounds known as prostaglandins, which are very important in protecting not only the stomach but also the intestine from damage.

Food slowly passes out of the stomach into the duodenum. The rate at which this happens depends very much on the food that has been eaten and is partly controlled by hormones secreted by the duodenum, as well as neural mechanisms. Complete gastric emptying may take 30–120 min. Nutrients absorbed directly through the stomach lining include alcohol, caffeine, water and some medications. Glucose and other single molecular carbohydrates may leave the stomach in a relatively short time (sports drinks, depending on volume, can empty within 30 min) while a more complex composition, such as a high-fat meal, could take several hours.

In the duodenum the food is mixed with bile. Bile is produced in the liver and passes along the bile ducts to be stored in the gallbladder, which after a fatty meal contracts as a result of hormone (cholecystokinin) release, expelling the bile into the duodenum. The bile contains compounds called bile salts, which have the property of being water soluble at one end (hydrophilic) and fat soluble at the other (hydrophobic). They form micelles with the fat-soluble ends in the middle. This allows fat to enter so that it can be acted upon by digestive enzymes.

The opening through which the bile passes into the duodenum is also shared by the duct from the pancreas. The pancreas produces further digestive enzymes (trypsin, lipase and amylase) and these break down proteins, fats and starches. It also contains bicarbonate so that at this stage, the acid mixture secreted from the stomach becomes mildly alkaline (pH 7–8).

The partially digested food is further broken down as it passes along the small intestine. To increase the speed of absorption, the lining of the intestine is thrown into finger-like processes called villi, which greatly increase the surface area available for this purpose. Proteins are converted into their component amino acids, which are absorbed for their use in the synthesis of further proteins. Not all amino acids are equally valuable in nutrition, for example those derived from meat and egg can all be used to synthesise the body's proteins and have a high biological value, but only 50% of those from wheat are of value in human metabolism and the remainder must be broken down and excreted in the urine. Fat is broken down into fatty acids and glycerol which, after absorption by the intestinal cell, are combined – three fatty acids to one molecule of glycerol – to form a triglyceride for transportation via the lymphatic system. Starches are broken down into smaller compounds and eventually to monosaccharides such as glucose and galactose, which can easily be absorbed by the intestinal cells. Several enzymes (lactase) are present in these villi and these may be damaged as the result of infection or disease (e.g. coeliac disease), reducing the ability to digest nutrients, leading to fermentation in the lower bowel.

Blood from the intestine, containing the nutrients which have been absorbed, flows through the portal vein to the liver. In the liver, blood is filtered by special cells known as Kuppfer cells and these remove any bacteria that have managed to pass through the intestinal wall, as well as other impurities such as ammonia. The nutrients are removed by the liver cells and used in various metabolic processes, such as the production of glycogen. Fats, however, pass into the blood by a different route. Smaller fatty acids (medium-chain triglycerides or MCT) with a chain length of only 6 or 12 carbon atoms may be absorbed directly from the GI tract into the portal blood (see Chapters 6 and 9 for further information on the role of MCT in sports performance). More complex fatty acids are secreted into ducts running along the intestine called lacteals. These drain into the thoracic duct, thereby entering the general systemic circulation in the great veins (close to the heart). Bile salts, which have been used in the digestion of fat, are reabsorbed at the terminal ileum. They pass back to the liver and are resecreted in the bile.

The small intestine presents a hostile environment for the growth of bacteria and fungi. Most of these are destroyed by the actions of the intestinal enzymes so that in health the small intestine is sterile. In contrast, the large intestine contains many trillions of bacteria, fungi and protozoa. The ileo-caecal valve, between the terminal ileum and the caecum (the first part of the large bowel), is not very strong and it seems likely that in many individuals the lower end of the small bowel may become contaminated by bacteria from the large intestine.

At birth, the large intestine contains no bacteria, but the development of a healthy bacterial flora is crucial to the successful development of the immune system. The baby swallows some of its mother's bacteria as it passes down the birth canal and breast-feeding subsequently (colostrum) promotes the growth of a healthy flora containing lactobacilli and bifidobacteria (see Chapter 9 for more information on colostrum and the athlete). Some researchers suggest that lactobacilli may be secreted in the mother's milk. When the baby is weaned, other bacteria appear and the bowel flora becomes much more complex. However, there is very little oxygen in the large bowel and this means that the great majority of bacteria are anaerobes. A small number of aerobic bacteria also form part of the flora, but in health their numbers are very much fewer than the anaerobes. There may be only 10^5 aerobes compared with 10^{12} anaerobes in every gram of faeces. Considering the fact that there may be 500 different species and strains of bacteria in a normal intestine and that the number of bacterial cells in the bowel is greater than the number of human cells in the whole body, the importance of these bacteria to good health is clear. Undigested food residues passing from the small bowel into the large bowel are fermented by the bacteria. They break down harmful chemicals (such as carcinogens) and synthesise valuable nutrients, including short-chain fatty acids, which are used to nourish the cells lining the large bowel, and a number of vitamins including B_{12}, folic acid and vitamin K. The other major role of the large intestine is to preserve water. A large volume of fluid passes from the small intestine into the large, but most of this is reabsorbed, with the average weight of faeces being only 100–200 g/day.

There is considerable individual variation in the normal excretion of faecal matter on a daily basis. It is still within normal limits to have up to three stools daily, provided that these are formed and not urgent, although some people only pass one stool every 3 days. If this is not associated with abdominal pain, it is within the limits of normality. Consequently, it is difficult to provide an accurate definition of constipation and this may not only include infrequent bowel actions but other problems such as struggling and straining to pass small hard stools.

20.3 The effects of exercise on the gastrointestinal tract

The impact of physical exercise on the GI tract falls into two groups: moderate exercise is clearly beneficial, while severe exercise may cause problems.

Several studies have shown that regular moderate physical activity can accelerate the passage of food, gas and faecal residues along the GI tract. Apart from the well-known effects of moderate exercise on heart and blood pressure, obesity and diabetes, it may also reduce the risk of other GI diseases such as gallstones and diverticular disease. Some studies suggest that it may help constipation and there is good evidence to suggest that it reduces the risk of bowel cancer. Moderate exercise is well tolerated and can benefit patients suffering from inflammatory bowel disease (IBD).

On the other hand, vigorous exercise may lead to GI problems, particularly when it is undertaken in the heat without adequate training and proper attention to hydration. Risks to health and damage to the GI tract (including bowel obstruction and removal of intestinal adhesions) can be linked to dehydration when prolonged intense exercise is undertaken in the heat. During vigorous exercise, blood flow in less active organs and tissues is reduced, placing the GI tract at risk and leading to episodes of bloody stools, diarrhoea, cramping, nausea, vomiting, abdominal pain and other transient GI problems.

Selected specific effects of exercise on the GI tract

Appetite and hunger
There appears to be no evidence that acute exercise triggers adaptation resulting in elevated hunger or increased energy intake. Before exercise, particularly when it is competitive, impulses from the brain lead to stimulation of the sympathetic nervous system and the release of a number of hormones. Some of these (PYY, GLP-1 and PP) slow transit along the small intestine and reduce appetite. Sympathetic stimulation leads to a dry mouth and reduces feelings of hunger, especially after high- to moderate-intensity

exercise. Such 'exercise-induced anorexia' diminishes an hour after exercise, but overall exercise produces a significant decrease in energy intake when the energy expended during exercise has been accounted for. Athletes may delay eating after exercise and should be encouraged to consume small amounts of liquid or semi-solid foods frequently to support future training and performance.

Reduced blood supply to the GI tract
The increased sympathetic nervous activity during exercise allows the heart to increase the amount of blood it pumps to the body. Most of this increased cardiac output flows to the muscles and the skin to provide the nutrients to sustain muscular effort and to help prevent any excessive increase in body temperature. As blood supplies to the heart, brain and kidneys must be maintained at all times to prevent damage to these vital organs, it follows that the amount of blood available to the GI tract may be greatly reduced. It has been shown that the reduction in the blood supply to the stomach and intestine during maximum exercise falls by as much as 80% at 70% Vo_{2max}. This reduction in blood supply makes the lining of the GI tract susceptible to injury and reduces its protective power so that it becomes leakier and substances which would not normally pass through are able to enter the body. The passage of bacteria through the GI tract wall also may be increased under these conditions and they may produce dangerous endotoxins. This can lead to inflammation of the GI mucosa. Reductions in hepatic blood flow of 12–14% have been reported at 30–35% Vo_{2max} and of 30–45% at 35–60% Vo_{2max}. Portal blood flow in cyclists decreased by 57% in 20 min at 70% Vo_{2max} and by 80% after 1 hour.

The increased blood supply to the skin, especially in hot conditions, causes loss of water by sweating. This can be a factor promoting dehydration, which may be made worse because the excitement of competitive exercise causes the release of sympathetic hormones that suppress thirst. High-intensity exercise also slows gastric emptying, further reducing fluid available for absorption in the small intestine. Dehydration is therefore a major problem of vigorous exercise.

Gastric emptying and transit time
Studies on gastric emptying involving vigorous exercise showed that hypertonic drinks caused reflux and GI symptoms that were severe in half of those athletes

reporting symptoms, whereas isotonic drinks lead to symptoms in only one in ten. Athletes susceptible to exercise-related transient abdominal pain reported more GI disturbances (especially bloating) when using fruit juice (>10% solution of carbohydrate) before and during exercise compared with other drinks, including water, 6% carbohydrate sports drinks or where no fluid was provided at all.

Whether exercise affects speed of transit along the small and large bowel is still uncertain. Some studies have suggested that running delays transit through the small bowel, but accelerates it through the large. However, others have found that exercise does not alter transit time in either the small or large bowel and transit time does not appear to be influenced by short bouts of high-intensity exercise and is also independent of the mechanical pounding of abdominal contents. Transit time in sedentary individuals who take up exercise has been reported to be decreased from 35 to 24 hours. This may place weekend or 'fun run' athletes at an increased incidence due to a possible 'unconditioned' (untrained) GI tract.

Mechanical factors

There may be further mechanical effects of exercise on the GI tract. Runners are more likely to suffer GI upsets than cyclists or swimmers and it has been suggested that this may be because running leads to more vibration of the abdominal wall and pounding of the GI tract organs. This effect is less likely to be seen in sports which involve gliding motions such as cycling and swimming. Mechanical compression of the colon and when the abdomen is flexed may also delay emptying and create discomfort for some athletes (cyclists, rowers, canoeists, weight-lifters and wheelchair athletes).

Distance runners are particularly likely to suffer problems arising from the large intestine, including diarrhoea and pain. It seems likely that the cause of this is a combination of all the above factors including dehydration, reduction in blood supply to the GI tract, increased permeability of the GI tract wall, pounding and possible changes in the motility of the large intestine.

What are common symptoms during exercise?

Gastrointestinal problems frequently accompany vigorous exercise. It has been suggested that 20–50%

Table 20.1 Gastrointestinal symptoms reported by athletes.

Upper abdominal problems
Reflux/heartburn
Belching and air swallowing
Bloating
Stomach pain/cramps
Vomiting
Nausea

Lower abdominal problems
Intestinal/lower abdominal cramps
Side ache/stitch
Flatulence
Urge to defecate
Diarrhoea
Intestinal bleeding

of endurance athletes are hampered by GI tract symptoms, which may discourage them from taking part in training and competitive events. However, these acute symptoms are transient and rarely damage health in the long term. The main symptoms suffered are listed in Table 20.1.

Upper abdominal problems
Reflux and heartburn

Although the stomach is lined with mucus to protect it from damage by gastric acid, the oesophagus is not. The lower oesophageal sphincter is a weak valve and a number of factors may allow acid to regurgitate into the oesophagus producing burning and, in severe cases, inflammation of the lining of the lower oesophagus, which may even be sufficiently severe to cause ulceration and bleeding. It has been suggested that 60% of athletes experience reflux of gastric contents, with greater frequency during exercise than at rest and episodes of reflux tending to increase in parallel with exercise intensity.

Gastro-oesophageal reflux normally occurs when the pressure inside the stomach is higher than that of the lower oesophagus. As the stomach lies within the abdominal cavity, raised intragastric pressure is often a reflection of raised intra-abdominal pressure. The commonest reason for oesophageal reflux is obesity, with excess fat laid down in the abdominal cavity increasing intra-abdominal pressure. However, this is rarely relevant to athletes. Increased intra-abdominal pressure (through lifting and bending) may arise during certain sports such as American football, weight-lifting, football and cycling. There may be an increase in gastric contents when gastric emptying is delayed by vigorous exercise, and certain foods that also delay gastric emptying are known to aggravate the condition. These include foods with a relatively high fat content (e.g. crisps, fried foods and oils), coffee and other caffeine-containing drinks, red wine, orange juice and other citrus drinks (including grapefruit, fresh pineapple and some fruit smoothies), spicy foods (curry and chilli based) and possibly peppermint, cinnamon and vinegar. Iron supplementation may also induce reflux in some athletes. The effects and reactions are highly individual, with some athletes having no reaction to eating these foods. Athletes are encouraged to identify any foods inducing their symptoms.

In one recent study, symptoms of heartburn and chest pain persisted in volunteers who were given omeprazole, a drug that blocks gastric acid secretion, thereby suggesting other factors in athletes rather than reflux of gastric acid. Because these symptoms could not be due to gastric acid reflux, the reflux of alkaline bile might possibly have produced pain. Exercise reduces the frequency, duration and amplitude of oesophageal contractions. Thus, any fluid refluxed may have remained in the oesophagus longer than normally expected and would have contributed to symptoms.

A further factor that affects reflux both in athletes and sedentary persons is the swallowing of air (aerophagia). This is discussed in more detail in the section on belching. Smoking is another factor which promotes gastric acid reflux and should of course be studiously avoided by athletes. Smoking directly relaxes the muscle of the lower oesophageal sphincter, thus making reflux more likely.

It is important to remember that heartburn, a pain in the centre of the chest, may be easily confused with angina, the pain that arises when the blood supply to the heart muscle is reduced because of narrowing of the coronary arteries. In middle-aged patients, the development of heartburn on exercise must always be investigated fully in order to exclude this possibility. Angina may occur even in younger athletes, as was shown by the recent tragic death of a Spanish footballer aged 26 years.

Those suffering gastro-oesophageal reflux may control their symptoms by lifestyle modification. Athletes frequently eat shortly before bedtime after late-night training or evening competitions such as rowing, day/night games of cricket, swimming and athletics. This is not a habit to be encouraged, as lying flat removes the normal effect of gravity in reducing reflux and, furthermore, the presence of a full stomach makes reflux more likely. Ideally, it is sensible to aim to eat at least 4 hours before bedtime, avoiding both exercise after the meal and eating those foods that relax the lower oesophageal sphincter (mentioned above). They should avoid eating large meals and excess alcohol. Sleeping on at least two pillows to promote oesophageal clearance by gravity is recommended. Drugs that reduce gastric acid secretion, such as omeprazole and ranitidine, may be very valuable and, if overweight, reducing body mass may assist in alleviating symptoms.

Belching

Belching is a common symptom which of itself is rarely serious. It is often a feature of disease of the gallbladder, when it is associated with characteristic dyspeptic pain. By far the most common cause of belching, however, is air swallowing.

Excess air swallowing may arise for a number of reasons, including heartburn and a blocked nose, but perhaps the most common cause is anxiety. Anxious persons often develop an abnormal form of rapid yet shallow breathing known as over-breathing, hyperventilation or 'breathing pattern disorder'. Abnormal breathing involves the muscles of the upper chest and is rapid and shallow. Because the breathing is rapid, it is more likely to be through the mouth than the nose. The airways resistance when taking a breath through the nose is very much greater than that when taking a breath through the mouth and, for this reason, people who breathe rapidly tend also to be mouth breathers. Breathing through the mouth increases the amount of air going down the oesophagus into the stomach. This may produce belching but also bloating, abdominal rumblings and pain. In severe cases of air swallowing, the amount of air in the stomach may be sufficient to raise the pressure in the stomach enough to cause gastro-oesophageal reflux and sometimes even vomiting. Prolonged exercise may cause an oxygen debt which leads to mouth breathing. This involves less effort but may cause air swallowing. Athletes may swallow air by gulping meals and fluids. It is also possible to swallow air with fluid from bottles and cups during training and competitions. Further research is needed into the

Table 20.2 Foods which cause flatulence.

Drinks

Drinks containing air (carbonated drinks) such as soft drinks, mineral water, sparkling wine, beer, ginger beers and ciders

Foods

Foods that may not be completely digested and absorbed in the bowel. Bacterial enzymes cause these by-products to be fermented and produce the wind (or flatus). Baked beans and legumes are a common cause of wind from this effect. A full list is shown below.

Kidney beans, onions, split peas, navy beans, black eye peas, baked beans, lima beans, green peppers, broccoli, pimentos, brussels sprouts, radishes, cabbage, sauerkraut, cauliflower, scallions, corn, shallots, cucumbers, soyabeans, leeks, turnips, lentils, raw apples, apple juice, avocados, cantalope, honeydew melon, watermelon, rock melon, gums (used as bulking agents, psyllium)

area of air intake with fluid delivery; changing to a wider bottle dispensing greater volume may assist.

Perhaps the most important message is that if athletes belch when they are at rest, this is probably a sign of anxiety. Consequently, it is sensible to seek instruction on the development of proper diaphragmatic breathing and to continue with that training until it becomes second nature.

Bloating

Bloating or distension of the abdominal wall is extremely common in the general population. It may of course be a consequence of air swallowing as described above. If gas is not belched back up, it may pass through the stomach and along the small bowel causing distension, bloating, rumblings and pain as it passes through, followed eventually by excess rectal flatulence.

Another important cause of bloating is excessive fermentation in the large bowel, producing increased amounts of hydrogen, methane and carbon dioxide. This sort of bloating differs from that of air swallowing in that it is rarely associated with belching.

Athletes may anecdotally report that some foods appear to cause gas formation and bloating more frequently than others, with the response being highly individualised. The normal intestine processes 7–10 l of gas (nitrogen, oxygen, carbon dioxide, hydrogen and methane) each day with most of it being reabsorbed into the blood. Two indigestible carbohydrates, raffinose and stachyose, are largely responsible for the discomfort. Too much or excessive wind is a common complaint and the correct term for this is 'flatulence'. Excessive intakes of wholegrain and bran produces gas in the initial 2–3 weeks, but this usually settles (introduce bran and wholegrain foods gradually and slowly). The response to these foods varies widely and

Table 20.3 Strategies to avoid excess flatulence.

Eat slowly, chewing with the mouth closed, and avoid drinking through straws
Eat slowly and in a relaxed environment, to avoid swallowing air
Chew food thoroughly
Limit or avoid drinks containing gas (fizzy drinks, beer)
Avoid chewing gum
Take care with foods that may be fermented in the bowel and avoid large or overly frequent intakes
Use water and drink bottles with good free flow of fluid
Smoking and stress may also increase bloating and flatulence
Avoid excess intakes of simple sugars especially fructose, sorbitol
Any increase in fibre or complex carbohydrate should be gradual

excessive gas may also be the result of swallowing air whilst eating or drinking (as above) (see Tables 20.2 and 20.3 for food and nutrition strategies).

Nausea and vomiting

During the swim phase of triathlons, it is not uncommon for athletes to vomit into the ocean, river or lake water (this may be due to a combination of gels, sports foods, sports drinks, pre-race meal content and sea water), especially for those who report eating within 30 min of the race start. Nausea and vomiting also occur quite frequently after high-intensity and prolonged exercise. These symptoms are usually attributed largely to delayed gastric emptying, although air swallowing may also be important. The emptying of liquids and solids from the stomach is delayed by high-intensity exercise, although gastric acid secretion in response to meal ingestion is not. Alterations in small bowel activity may also be involved in these symptoms, because exercise affects the motility of the duodenum or jejunum, without affecting the oral–caecal transit time. After strenuous exercise, the activity of the duodenum is significantly reduced and this effect is more likely to occur during running than cycling. The interruption of this motility pattern occurs sooner after fluid supplementation with a carbohydrate sports drink than with tap water. However, no connection between glucose levels in the blood and the activity of the duodenum has been observed. It is clearly important not to undertake heavy exercise until sufficient time has elapsed from the previous meal.

Despite the rapid and scientific advances in sports nutrition, athletes continue to eat foods in the pre-event phase which are unfamiliar and new. This may be in response to poor catering recommendations, or failure of sports and team management to consult, or engage, sports dietitians and nutritionists in the menu planning for foreign competitions. Athletes may be accommodated in hotels where a full cooked breakfast is included in the room bookings. A number of factors, such as the food available (fried cooked breakfast, buffet), hunger, fatigue, finances or a lack of experience, may lead to athletes selecting food combinations that are less than ideal and not in keeping with pre-competition planning and recommendations. Another behaviour response of athletes is attempting to eat 'healthily' or 'do the right thing' in the pre-competition meal. This may include eating high-fibre cereals and breads, higher than usual intakes of fruit and over-eating, where the athlete's GI tract is unaccustomed to these foods, causing GI distress, discomfort, gastro-oesophageal reflux, urgency to defecate, increased bowel frequency, bloating and distension.

Stomach pain and cramps

These appear to be rather non-specific symptoms, which may occur in association with any of those previously discussed. They are likely to be related to a reduced blood supply to the GI tract, exacerbated by other factors such as dehydration and reduced gastric emptying and duodenal motility. This may also be related to incorrect mixing of sports drinks, which increases the osmolality of the beverage, due to the fact that many athletes fail to use correct measurements in powder to water ratios. There is a tendency for sports science support practitioners to mix hydration beverages incorrectly in both bulk and individual servings. When mixed correctly, the drink will be isotonic and provoke fewer symptoms. Susceptible athletes may find that carbohydrate content at or above 8% may precipitate GI disturbances.

Upper GI distress in marathon and ultra-marathon events (67–160 km) does appear to be linked to less training and shorter distances covered. It can be severe. There is a tendency for more highly trained athletes to report a lower incidence of GI problems. There appears to be a connection between the tolerance by marathon and ultra-distance athletes of solid foods, fibre intake and use of more concentrated beverages, longer training times and at lower intensity.

Lower abdominal problems
Intestinal/lower abdominal cramp

It is believed that these are due to altered function of the large intestine. Although the small intestine might also be affected, it has been found that the reduction in small bowel activity that accompanies vigorous exercise has no clear effect on the transit time, with the large bowel the most likely source of these problems.

The effect of exercise on transit in the large bowel is still poorly understood. One study showed accelerated times while in another there was no change. Yet another more modern study showed that acute graded exercise decreased the activity of the large bowel. It has been suggested that exercise may reduce the activity of circular muscles, which would reduce resistance to colonic flow. This might lead to a faster passage of stool along the bowel.

Flatulence

This may be a consequence of either air swallowing or of abnormal colonic fermentation; both are discussed in the section on irritable bowel syndrome (IBS).

Diarrhoea

Prevalence in the athlete population is largely unknown and athletes may withhold information about this from coaches and selectors. Acute exercise-induced diarrhoea is often referred to as 'runner trots' and current understanding suggests physiological causes other than dehydration or electrolyte imbalance. As discussed above, although changes in colonic transit may be a factor in producing diarrhoea, it seems likely that the reduction in blood supply to the GI tract is another major contributor. Diarrhoea appears to depend very much on the state of fitness of the runner concerned. It often occurs during exercise and may affect recreational runners as well as elite athletes, although it is more frequent in the latter. Improvement in the state of physical training may reduce the likelihood of diarrhoea in recreational runners and as one of the major effects of training is to increase cardiac output and hence blood supply to the body, it seems distinctly possible that the blood supply to the GI tract is the key to the problem. Although mechanical pounding of abdominal organs has been suggested as also important, a study in which mouth to caecum transit times were performed in runners showed no significant change, suggesting that this particular factor was unlikely to be the cause of this problem. Endotoxaemia (and the leakage of these compounds into the blood, via GI tract, in the later stages of endurance events) may lead to vomiting, nausea and diarrhoea and may increase GI distress with exercise duration. The use of prebiotics and probiotics, food poisoning and travellers' diarrhoea are covered elsewhere (see Chapter 22).

Intestinal bleeding

Bleeding in athletes may take two forms. In some, it is overt with runners passing bloody diarrhoea. In others, it is less easily detected, with small amounts of blood lost into the GI tract that are not sufficient to be visible to the naked eye. However, persistent losses over weeks and months may lead to iron deficiency anaemia.

Reduction in blood supply to the gut has been suggested as the causal mechanism of gastrointestinal bleeding during, and after, exercise. Although blood loss itself may be transient, analysis of stools has revealed the presence of α_1-antitrypsin and lysozyme in raised concentrations, indicating local damage to the bowel lining with an inflammatory response. Examination of the bowel by endoscopy after exercise has shown small ulcers in some athletes; when biopsies are taken and examined under the microscope, the picture seen is that of damage caused by a reduction in blood supply. The effects of this reduction may become critical under extreme exercise conditions, when they may be associated with an increase in body temperature, dehydration, a fall in blood glucose and a relative lack of oxygen. It has also been suggested that, under these circumstances, the blood may become more viscous and the red cells less flexible, which could further compromise local blood flow. The cells lining the bowel become deprived of nutrients, leading to their death and mucosal bleeding. Such changes may, in theory, produce malabsorption of nutrients from the bowel and an increase in intesti-

nal secretion, together with the permeability of the bowel, allowing the passage of bacteria and the development of increased amounts of endotoxins in the blood. However, an increase in intestinal permeability and mild leaking of endotoxins into the portal blood has only been found at very high intensity of exercise.

Colonic fermentation

To date, an effect of exercise on colonic fermentation has not been clearly shown. In patients and athletes with IBS, increased fermentation may be demonstrated by measuring breath hydrogen release after administering a non-digestible sugar such as lactulose. This passes unchanged through the small intestine and is fermented by colonic bacteria. Hydrogen release after lactulose is typically increased in IBS, but when the same procedure was performed in well-trained individuals, no difference was seen in hydrogen release after exercise or at rest.

There is interest in the possible role of healthy bacteria or probiotics. These may modulate the intestinal microbial flora and thus have the potential to reduce disturbances in immune function which occur after severe exercise. For the athlete, the possibility of minimising the duration and severity of diarrhoea and accelerating the return to training or competitions with the use of specific strains or combinations of probiotics and prebiotics is of particular interest. However, much further research is needed before specific recommendations can be made (see Chapter 22 for discussion on probiotics).

Who is likely to experience GI problems?

The prevalence of GI problems varies greatly between different individuals. Generally, women are more likely to experience GI symptoms than are men. This is especially true during menstruation, when women frequently suffer GI problems, even when they are not athletes. Younger athletes appear to be more susceptible to GI tract symptoms than older ones, mainly because they lack experience in both training programmes and choice of suitable nutritional strategies. Training status is certainly negatively correlated with the frequency of GI symptoms. These are very much more common in subjects who are unfit. The frequency of GI disturbances is twice as high in running compared with other endurance sports (such as cycling and swimming) and 1.5–3.0 times higher in elite than recreational athletes. Distance runners appear more susceptible to lower GI problems such as diarrhoea and IBS.

Apart from these risk factors however, there are a number of other matters that change the individual sensitivity of athletes. Many runners only get GI tract symptoms during exercise or shortly afterwards. Others may have them even when they are not exercising at all and it is perhaps not surprising that the latter group are more likely to run into difficulties during exercise. The following factors should be considered.

The menstrual cycle

Many women suffer gastrointestinal complaints that may be related to the stage of their menstrual cycle. Changes in hormone levels during the cycle may produce a variety of symptoms that vary from woman to woman. Many women are symptom-free between the end of menses and the time of ovulation, when the hormone oestrogen has the strongest influence. After ovulation, however, oestrogen levels fall and the picture changes. Whether or not conception has occurred, progesterone levels rise (to protect a possible embryo) and at this stage the woman is more likely to suffer symptoms. GI tract symptoms are very common and many women report that they have diarrhoea or constipation, in addition to temporary weight gain and bloating, just before their menses starts. All these symptoms rapidly clear once menstruation begins.

Many women gain weight in the week before their period due to fluid retention and this may be associated with feelings of bloatedness. The fluid retention may be so marked as to make rings and clothes tight and to cause the ankles to swell. Breast symptoms can be particularly severe, with tenderness, enlargement, heaviness and pain. If such symptoms in the second half of the menstrual cycle become severe enough to require medical attention, they may be referred to as pre-menstrual syndrome (PMS). Many female athletes find that they develop problems in the days leading up to and during menstruation. These changes may be sufficiently severe as to impair their performance.

The cause of these hormonal changes is not yet completely understood. Many consider that the problem is largely psychological and certainly the condition is difficult to study because symptoms vary widely from woman to woman; various theories have been put forward concerning the balance between oestrogen and progesterone, or excessive production of other hormones such as prolactin. None of these have been confirmed. One of the few indisputable facts is that PMS disappears if the ovaries are removed.

The usual ovarian hormonal cycle can be blocked by putting women on the oral contraceptive, which prevents the release of eggs from the ovary and the development of the corpus luteum which produces progesterone. This will often relieve peri-menstrual symptoms satisfactorily. However, not every woman wishes to use oral contraceptives. Some find that pyridoxine (vitamin B_6) is helpful. It is customary to recommend 100 mg daily, but doubts have been raised about the safety of this and nowadays 50 mg daily is more usual. Fluid retention and weight gain may be reduced by taking diuretics to increase the flow of urine. The use of any diuretics by an athlete requires medical support and clearance due to the potential risks linked to a positive doping result.

In recent years, there has been increasing interest in the possible nutritional management of symptoms related to the menstrual cycle. There is now evidence that the bowel bacteria may be more metabolically active under the influence of progesterone and thus it may be possible to reduce their activity by changing the diet. Some women find that low-residue enteral formulations, such as Ensure, satisfactorily control these symptoms so as not to interfere with their capacity for exercise. Others may benefit from following an exclusion diet, as described in the section on IBS.

Travel

Many people find that they develop changes in bowel function and GI symptoms when travelling. In one study performed in the US, 108 consecutive patients attending a travel clinic who were reassessed on their return had developed the following during their trip: diarrhoea (63%), constipation (9%), bloating (45%), dyspepsia (16%) and symptoms suggestive of IBS (24%). Many of these patients found that their symptoms persisted after their return home. Travel to tropical and subtropical climates may carry an increased risk of food poisoning and diarrhoea. It has been shown that the risk of developing IBS increased 12-fold in subjects who had already experienced a bout of proven bacterial gastroenteritis.

However, many other people have symptoms which are much less obviously infective in cause, such as constipation and dyspepsia. Many of these symptoms may be because travel often brings with it changes in customary lifestyle. It may be difficult to maintain normal dietary patterns away from home and this applies to drinks as well as food. People who consume less alcohol are more likely to become dehydrated if their consumption increases (e.g. on holiday, post-match events). Added to this are the inevitable anxieties associated with travel, flight connections and settling in unfamiliar environments. All these factors may increase the likelihood of GI symptoms in athletes who are travelling to compete away from home.

Food intolerances/food allergy

Nowadays, food intolerances are greatly in vogue. They are widely discussed in newspapers and magazines and widely misunderstood. This is because there are several different mechanisms by which food may produce unpleasant symptoms.

The oldest and best understood of these is when foods combine with circulating IgE antibodies to produce an immune complex, which can rapidly trigger an allergic response. This may come on very quickly after a small amount of the food concerned has been digested. Peanuts are a typical example. Susceptible people may develop swelling of the lips and throat, breathlessness and shock (anaphylactic shock) and if not promptly treated this can be fatal. This form may be diagnosed by detecting the relevant IgE antibodies by blood test (RAST) or by skin-prick testing. Other food causing similar responses include seafood, especially shellfish.

Food intolerance is far more common than genuine food allergy. Here, there are no circulating antibodies in the blood and anaphylaxis does not occur. Foods may produce symptoms because of a lack of enzymes to digest them, for example alactasia in lactose intolerance, pharmacological effects of substances contained in foods such as caffeine, monosodium glutamate or ethanol (alcohol), and also by malfermentation of undigested food residues that pass into the lower bowel. The latter is a common cause of IBS (see below). Usually, much larger amounts of the food must be eaten to provoke a food intolerance reaction, compared with that which provokes a genuine allergy.

The diagnosis of food intolerance may be difficult. At present, no simple test exists. Blood tests, hair tests, and techniques such as kinesiology and Vega machines have been shown to be highly unreliable. It is also unsatisfactory merely to remove a food group from the diet. This frequently leads to progressive dietary restrictions that are not only unsuccessful but may also be dangerous, potentially leading to malnutrition and in extreme cases death. The only reliable way is to seek advice from a specialist dietitian, who can provide advice on a suitable exclusion diet, to resolve symptoms and allow reliable prospective food testing.

Common food intolerances

Dairy products The milk sugar lactose is widely blamed for unfortunate reactions to this group. The enzyme lactase which breaks down the milk sugar lactose is present in the small intestine in childhood but disappears around puberty in most races, except for white people in northern Europe. People who genuinely lack the enzyme may get wind, pain and diarrhoea after consuming dairy products (mainly milk). Athletes with lactose intolerance can tolerate small amounts of milk without adverse effects and management of the condition is to avoid foods containing lactose (e.g. milk, soft cheese, ice cream, yoghurt, custards, smoothies and cream soups). For the athlete, special significance is the use of sports bars and shakes containing milk and milk powders. Athletes are advised to read ingredient labels for milk sugars (lactose) and milk products. Non-carbohydrate-containing protein powders are available and soy-based powders are suitable. Temporary or transitory lactose deficiency can occur due to damage to the intestinal mucosa (following gastroenteritis, inflammation and coeliac disease). Calcium and possibly vitamin B_2 are nutrients which may be at risk if dairy products are vigorously excluded. However, dairy products may also upset people who have normal levels of lactose in the GI tract and these are usually caused by dairy fats.

Gluten Many people have problems eating gluten, which is found in foods made from wheat, barley and rye. Classical IgE allergy to gluten is infrequent, but malfermentation by the GI tract bacteria of cereal residues containing gluten is very common and may cause a range of symptoms that affect not only the GI tract but which also lead to migraine, fluid retention and general malaise.

A special form of gluten intolerance is seen in coeliac disease where a different form of immune reaction (from IgE allergy) takes place, leading to damage to the lining of the upper small intestine, with loss of villi. Absorption of nutrients is compromised and this may lead to diarrhoea and weight loss, together with complications such as loss of bone density, and iron and vitamin B_{12} deficiency anaemias. A simple blood test (tissue transglutaminase) will indicate the possibility of coeliac disease, but the final diagnosis is confirmed by an endoscopic biopsy of the small bowel, which reveals the characteristic changes. Athletes are recommended to consult a Clinical Dietitian or specialist and join local coeliac societies for advice and support. Composition of sports foods requires care, especially bars, shakes and gels, and the ingredient list must be carefully checked (see Further reading).

Fructose There has recently been interest in the possibility that fructose, a sugar found in fruit, may be important in provoking GI tract symptoms. Some people have a much reduced capacity to absorb fructose and it is suggested that these individuals may be better on a diet that avoids fructose and related compounds. However, diets low in these are usually also low in foods containing gluten and it is probable that the benefits ascribed to them are due to reducing the intake of gluten rather than fructose. Early research on using fructose as a significant source of carbohydrate during events reported GI distress in athletes. This is not to be confused with the recent studies highlighting the use of combinations of carbohydrates, including fructose, to improve the delivery of carbohydrate through use of different transporters (GLUT5), leaving less in the GI tract and therefore reducing the risk of adverse symptoms.

Irritable bowel syndrome

IBS is the most common GI complaint seen in the developed world. It is said to occur in as many 15% of the population and is more common in women than men. It is characterised by abdominal pain, associated with a change in bowel habit, either to diarrhoea or constipation. This may be accompanied by excess wind and bloating, together with symptoms outside the GI tract, such as difficulty in concentrating and fatigue. Although these symptoms may prove very distressing, there has been no pathological abnormality discovered, despite intensive investigation with endoscopy and radiography or analysis of blood and stool. IBS is a diagnosis of exclusion, which can only be accepted when more serious gastrointestinal diseases such as cancer and IBD have been ruled out. In order to achieve some consistency, the Rome II Criteria for IBS were drawn up in 1999 and have been upgraded twice since first proposed.

The Rome II Criteria 1999

At least 12 weeks or more (not necessarily consecutive), in the preceding 12 months, of abdominal discomfort or pain having two of the following three features:

(1) relieved by defecation and/or
(2) onset associated with a change in the frequency of stool and/or
(3) onset associated with a change in the form/appearance of stool.

Other features that were part of the more complex Rome I criteria are no longer required, but are often present, including:

(1) abnormal stool frequency
(2) abnormal stool form
(3) abnormal passage of stool (straining, urgency or feeling of incomplete evacuation)
(4) passage of mucus
(5) bloating or feeling of abdominal distension.

Many physicians take a negative view of IBS. They believe it is largely psychological and that it is caused by day-to-day stresses in the lives of patients/athletes. However, careful psychological analysis has suggested that this is unlikely. Patients who had recently developed symptoms of IBS showed no sign of psychological features or problems such as anxiety and depression. However, those where the condition had persisted for more than 5 years frequently showed such psychological abnormalities, suggesting that if there is a psychological factor, it is a consequence of poor treatment of IBS rather than its cause.

It has been suggested that there are several different forms of IBS which respond to different treatments.

Colonic malfermentation

The balance of the bowel bacteria has been shown to be abnormal. There is a slight reduction in the numbers of lactic acid bacteria (lactobacilli and bifidobacteria) and considerable increase in facultative aerobic bacteria. This produces changes in the fermentation processes in the large bowel, with the production of greatly increased amounts of hydrogen. This can be reduced by antibiotics which kill off many of the bacteria concerned. Unfortunately, when the antibiotics are stopped, the bacteria return to the previous levels and therefore this does not represent a long term-strategy. Exclusion diets have been shown to reduce hydrogen production and to relieve symptoms very effectively. Foods most likely to produce problems are grains, dairy products, caffeinated drinks, citrus fruit, yeast and certain starchy vegetables such as potatoes, onions and sweetcorn. This form of IBS may follow bacterial gastroenteritis, which increases the risk of developing IBS 12-fold, or a treatment course of antibiotics, which increases the risk fourfold. This form of IBS may be helped by the use of probiotics.

Overload and overflow

This form of IBS produces intermittent bouts of diarrhoea every 7–10 days and leads patients to take anti-diarrhoeal drugs when, in fact, these make the problem worse. On specific enquiry, patients have a history of constipation between bouts of diarrhoea. They have strained to produce small, hard, bitty stools and on examination the colon is easily palpable, being full of faeces. In fact, these patients have a form of constipation and if the bowel is emptied by a suitable purge and bowel transit speeded up by a non-fermentable bulking agent such as cracked linseed or sterculia, their symptoms are well controlled.

Air swallowing and anxiety

This accounts for 20% of IBS cases. These patients develop breathing pattern disorder. This may be caused by anxiety or it may follow an abdominal operation, where a surgical scar has led to considerable discomfort on moving the diaphragm. It is also often seen in asthmatics who have to breathe more forcefully to overcome obstruction of the airways. Women may develop it in pregnancy. Essentially, a bad habit develops whereby breathing is with the upper chest rather than with the diaphragm. The respiratory rate increases and, particularly if there is also a tendency to mouth breathe (as with nasal obstruction or during high-impact exercise), the amount of air swallowed increases dramatically. This leads to wind, bloating and pain, which in turn may increase anxiety, setting up a vicious cycle whereby the problem is prolonged and exacerbated. Some athletes are trained to hold in the abdominal muscles to support the lower back when exercising and this may be a contributory factor. Physiotherapy is necessary to retrain using diaphragmatic breathing. If anxiety is a factor, this should be dealt with and nasal obstruction may be corrected by decongestant or, if necessary, surgery.

Constipation

Constipation is a vitally important cause of IBS. A normal bowel habit, as mentioned previously, may be quite variable and the most important symptom is that the faeces are hard and difficult to pass. Faulty technique when going to the toilet is a common cause of constipation, especially in women who are multi-tasking and begrudge time spent in the toilet. A combination of haste and poor position can lead to real problems with opening the bowel. The muscles of the pelvic floor may also be damaged during childbirth. Treatment for constipation depends on the underlying cause (see section Overload and overflow). In general, it helps to increase fluid and fibre intake. Sometimes laxatives are necessary and advice should be sought from a colorectal nurse and a sports nutritionist. Different types of fibre have different roles to soften and assist motility. Soluble fibre is found in gums, pectin (fruit), dried beans (kidney beans, baked beans, lentils and lima beans), oats, barley, some vegetables (carrots) and seeds such as psyllium (used in many bulking agent laxatives). Insoluble fibre (cellulose, hemicellulose and lignin) are found in wholegrains, most vegetables and wheat bran. Insoluble fibre may help prevent diverticulitis and haemorrhoids.

Menstrual-related IBS

As mentioned above, IBS symptoms are common at the time of menstruation and may respond to an oral contraceptive, or to temporary changes in diet such as low-residue liquid feeds. For the majority, the changes are mild but can be severe for some.

Musculoskeletal problems

Many patients are told they have IBS when there is nothing wrong with their GI system at all. Abdominal pain may arise from damage to the muscles of the abdominal wall and the nerves and bones that supply and support it. This may easily occur if athletes undertake unusual exercises for which they are not prepared. As this pain does not arise from the GI tract, it is not associated with other disturbances of GI tract function, such as diarrhoea. The pains tend to be persistent rather than cyclical and get worse towards the evening. They may be provoked by movements such as lifting, bending or even just rolling over in bed. The pain may radiate to the back or leg. In this instance, physiotherapy is essential. Pain may be relieved by local ultrasound, mobilisation and manipulation of the torso and exercises to strengthen the muscles concerned.

People and athletes with IBS frequently find that their symptoms are worse when they are exercising, but also occur at rest. Clearly, it is necessary to master IBS in order to prevent problems during training or competition. The condition is discussed in detail in the book *Irritable Bowel Solutions* (see Further reading). For further information on IBD (including Crohn's disease and ulcerative colitis), please see Further reading. Involvement of a medical specialist and dietitian are required for care, diagnosis and management of IBS.

Reactive hypoglycaemia

Factors maintaining a normal blood glucose are discussed elsewhere. Normally, these are highly effective. In some individuals, however, there appears to be increased sensitivity to the effects of insulin so that after eating sugar the blood glucose level may fall so low as to provoke symptoms of fatigue, hunger, dizziness, palpitations and sweating. Eating sugary foods will rapidly relieve these symptoms but will provoke further excessive insulin release, so that the symptoms quickly return. It is better to take foods which are broken down slowly to release glucose as these may maintain a stable blood level without excessive insulin release. Such foods include protein snacks, for example chicken, ham, cheese or complex carbohydrates, oats, muesli bars. A low blood glucose level may provoke bouts of hyperventilation and air swallowing (see above).

20.4 Low-residue diets and sports performance

Depending on the sex and the body size of the athlete, additional support can be provided through the use of a low-residue diet for weight-making classifications and goals in sport. Currently, there is no research in athletes supporting the benefit of these regimens, which have been adapted from preparations for GI surgical and investigative procedures. Low-residue diets were developed to assist surgeons performing procedures by clearing the residue from the large and small intestine. The amount of weight lost will be dependent on the athlete's size, usual diet and length of the GI tract. Athletes need to receive advice on the change and often absence of bowel motions, which is not to be confused with constipation, when using low-residue diets.

These diets are unusual and are designed to reduce the volume of the faecal contents of the bowel. Foods with a moderate and high fibre content, milk products and meat with connective tissue are all excluded. As this diet is nutritionally inadequate, it can only be used for short periods of time, may require supplementation with a multivitamin and multimineral and can lead to malnutrition if used for an extended time. Low-residue diets must be tested during training and refined to suit the individual athlete and the specifics of the sport. The diet is generally used for 3 days leading up to an event where the athlete is required to weigh in and meet the restrictions or requirements of a weight class. It is also valuable where there is a performance advantage in an athlete reducing body mass to assist with momentum (over a bar, for jumping sports) and possibly sports where the body weight is carried (running and cycling). Weight loss will be in the range 300–800 g only, depending on the size of the athlete's GI tract. Low-residue diets are not to be confused with liquid diets, or clear fluids. Carefully designed by a clinical or sports dietitian, sufficient total energy, adequate carbohydrate and protein are easily provided. Sources of carbohydrate include sports drinks, strained fruit juices and for protein, a selection of lean chicken and fish.

General guidelines for low-residue diet

- Remove all wholegrain, grainy and wholemeal breads, cereals and bran. This includes food and products made with these foods.

- Remove food containing seeds, nuts, popcorn, legumes (dried beans and lentils), potatoes and coconut. Remove skins and foods with pips.
- Use only fruit juices and vegetables juices rather than whole fruits and vegetables.
- Avoid meat and shellfish with tough connective tissue (often referred to as gristle) such as mussels and those found in meats.
- Limit the use of milk, milk products and foods containing milk (yoghurt, smoothies, ice cream) to two cups or less per day. This includes protein powders, ready to drink shakes, flavoured milk and smoothies.
- Restrict the use of prebiotics and probiotics to assist in reducing faecal residue.
- To maintain bowel function drink 250 ml (1 cup) of strained prune juice daily.
- Laxative use is discouraged as this causes dehydration and disruptions to the sense of well-being. Fluid and electrolyte balance adversely affect performance and their use is banned in some sports (e.g. boxing).
- Ensure adequate energy balance (provide regular intake of fruit juices, jelly, sports drinks, meringue, eggs, fish, sports gels, low residue formulas, boiled sweets and candy, puréed fruit, chicken, beef and vegetable stocks, white bread, white crackers, rice crackers, tea and coffee) and nutrient intake.

20.5 Substances potentially altering GI comfort (Table 20.4)

It is well known that *caffeine* increases motility and has a laxative effect on the GI tract when used as a supplement. Use of caffeine has also been linked to reflux, by promoting an increase in gastric acid or decreasing the lower oesophageal sphincter pressure. Other foods which may have a similar effect include fat, oils, fried food, chocolate, alcohol and peppermint. Athlete responses to the elimination of caffeine to relieve symptoms are very individual.

Carbonated beverages (sparkling waters, sodas, energy drinks and some varieties of sports drinks) are consumed by athletes to provide both fluid and carbohydrate. Anecdotally, athletes report upper GI distress and bloating with the use of carbonated beverages, and de-gassing beverages prior to use is a common practice. Studies have reported no effects of carbonation on gastric emptying or subjective effects

Table 20.4 Substances potentially causing GI distress.

High-fibre diets and sudden increase in fibre intake
Consuming fibre and fat before and during events
Unaccustomed high carbohydrate intakes
Milk and lactose intolerance
NSAID use
High doses of caffeine
Buffers: sodium bicarbonate, sodium citrate
High doses of mineral supplements (iron)
Unfamiliar changes in dietary intake and timing
Incorrectly mixed sports drinks and hypertonic beverages including fruit juice
High intake of foods containing sorbitol
High intake of alcohol

of GI comfort with exercise. An influence of carbohydrate content has been reported and as the carbohydrate content of many carbonated beverages is above 8% (commonly 10–12%), this may contribute to the expression of adverse GI symptoms.

Buffers such as sodium bicarbonate and sodium citrate used in high-intensity short-duration events of 1–3 min are reported to cause severe GI discomfort and distress (vomiting and diarrhoea). This can be avoided by tailoring the delivery and the dose to suit the athlete and trialling in a series of practice sessions. Trials should be held under different conditions and intensities, starting with a moderate dose and progressing as the athlete's GI tract becomes more accustomed. Suggestions include splitting the dose into several intakes over 1 hour, using capsules, ensuring the purity of the product and using well-tolerated clinical medications (used for renal and urinary tract infections) or developing bespoke formulations (see Chapter 9 for discussion on the role and use of buffers).

Glycerol (a rapidly absorbed three-carbon alcohol), used by athletes to obtain a possible performance advantage through hyperhydration (increased fluid retention) and reduced negative effects of fluid loss on thermoregulation and the cardiovascular system during exercise, has been reported to cause symptoms of GI distress (possibly due to the high osmolality of drinks influencing fluid absorption). Athletes are advised that results vary, responses are individual, and that they should practise the use of glycerol and the relevant dose during training; they are also reminded that this substance is currently banned under the World Anti-Doping Agency (WADA) code (see Chapter 9 for further information).

Alcohol is a well-recognised laxative, with the action thought to be via changes in motility and effects on the hormonal system. Its effects on the kidney may lead to dehydration, further reducing blood flow to the gut. As alcohol also lowers sphincter pressure in the oesophagus and increases gastric acid secretion, the risk of reflux is increased.

Sorbitol is a sugar substitute (sugar alcohol) that is well known for a laxative effect on the lower GI tract, its ability to aggravate IBS, and as a cause of abdominal pain, gas and possibly diarrhoea if sufficient amounts are consumed. Found most commonly in chewing gum, sports bars and cereal bars, it is added to provide moisture (humectants) and to reduce the total carbohydrate content. The discomfort is caused by fermentation of any unabsorbed sugar alcohol by bacteria in the large intestine. Other commonly used sugar alcohols include mannitol and xylitol. Athletes should be aware of supplements containing sorbitol, especially if consumed frequently.

Non-steroidal anti-inflammatory drugs (NSAIDs) are commonly used by athletes for pain relief. Examples are aspirin and ibuprofen. These are also known to cause ulceration and possible perforation of the GI tract (increase and aggravate mucosal damage) with bleeding, nausea and vomiting. Frequent usage and high doses may cause GI distress, especially GI bleeding. Athletes should be aware of the risks for GI distress and the potential to cause mucosal damage. Paracetamol is usually better tolerated.

Iron supplementation may induce GI discomfort including constipation, increased stool frequency, black stools, abdominal discomfort such as cramping, and in some cases diarrhoea, nausea and vomiting. If iron supplements are taken with food, the symptoms usually subside.

20.6 Sports food, practices and GI distress

The use of sports foods, drinks and gels in sport requires practice and there are wide individual responses to their use. Unaccustomed intake in both volume and timing may lead to increases in GI symptoms or distress. In a recent study in runners, the use of gels (providing 90 g/hour carbohydrate for 16 km) was well tolerated by the majority of the athletes, although some had severe GI discomfort. This rein-

forces the message that athletes must practise and trial their fuel and fluid intakes prior to competing in high-intensity training and competition, as tolerance varies widely between individual athletes.

When undertaking carbohydrate loading, it is important to ensure that the food selected does not lead to excess fibre intake, especially in athletes who are susceptible to GI disturbances. As total carbohydrate intake increases, fibre intakes and faecal residue can increase above previously tolerated levels, resulting in a greater urge to defecate and more frequent and bulky stools prior to, and during, the race or competition. Unless tolerated, high-fibre intakes prior to endurance, ultra-endurance and high-intensity training and competitions are not recommended.

20.7 Summary

> ### Dietary strategies to minimise exercise-related GI symptoms or distress
>
> (1) Use foods and practices which are familiar and well rehearsed.
> (2) Limit or avoid solid food in the 3 hours prior to exercise.
> (3) Mix sports drinks correctly.
> (4) Practise drinking suitable fluids during training and have an individual fluid/hydration plan for competition.
> (5) Liquid meals, foods and fluids are suitable before training and competition, and during training and events, when well tested and practised.
> (6) Where the provision of fuel and carbohydrate are equally important, isotonic beverages are encouraged and must be trialled and practised in a range of training sessions.
> (7) A liquid lower residue meal or formula may assist athletes with frequent diarrhoea or persistent urge to defecate during training or competitions.
> (8) Athletes may need to learn to evacuate bowels prior to competition, in order to reduce the urge to defecate during competitions.
> (9) Foods which enhance GI tract motility should be restricted or avoided prior to exercise or competition. These include caffeine, high-fibre foods, alcohol and unaccustomed spicy foods.

Lower GI symptoms do not always appear during exercise and can occur as frequently after competition. GI discomfort is more common during hard exercise than easy and is affected by both pace and intensity. The following factors must be taken into consideration by all athletes experiencing GI distress and discomfort, especially if severe and recurring: training, lifestyle, meal composition and timing, choice and composition of sports drinks, foods and gels, hydration status and strategies, food allergy, food intolerance, stress levels, the use of medications and clinical investigations. These are all areas of consideration for athletes experiencing GI distress, especially if severe and recurrent. If symptoms are persistent, these should be clinically investigated to rule out any underlying pathology.

Further reading

De Oliveria EP, Burini RC. Impact of physical exercise on the gastrointestinal tract. Curr Opin Clin Nutr Metab Care 2009; 12: 533–538.

Fallon K. Athletes with gastrointestinal disorders. In: Clinical Sports Nutrition, 3rd edn (Burke L, Deakin V, eds). Sydney: McGraw-Hill, 2006, pp 721–738.

Gassull M, Cabre E. The gastrointestinal tract. In: Clinical Nutrition (Gibney MJ, Elia M, Ljunggvist O, Dowsett J, eds). Oxford: Blackwell Science, 2005.

Glace B, Murphy C, McHugh M. Food and fluid intake and disturbances in gastrointestinal and mental function during an ultramarathon. Int J Sport Nutr Exerc Metab 2002; 12: 414–427.

Hunter J. Irritable Bowel Solutions. London: Vermillon Press, 2007.

Hunter J. Inflammatory Bowel Disease. London: Vermillon Press, 2010.

Maddison KJ, Shepherd KL, Hillman DR, Eastwood PR. Function of lower esophageal sphincter during and after high-intensity exercise. Med Sci Sport Exerc 2005; 37: 1728–1733.

Manas M, de Victoria E, Gil, Yago M, Mathers J. The gastrointestinal tract. In: Nutrition and Metabolism (Gibney MJ, Roche HM, MacDonald IA, eds). Oxford: Blackwell Science, 2003.

Martins C, Morgan LM, Bloom SR, Robertson MD. Effects of exercise on gut peptides, energy intake and appetite. J Endoccrinol 2007; 193: 251–258.

Morton DR, Aragon-Vargas LF, Callister R. Effect of ingested fluid composition on exercise-related transient abdominal pain. Int J Sport Nutr Exerc Metab 2004; 14: 197–208.

Murray B, Stofan J, Sallis B. Return to competition following ischemic colitis caused by severe dehydration. J Sport Rehabil 2007; 16: 271–276.

Peters HP, Van Schelven FW, Verstappen PA, De Boer RW, Bol E, De Vries WR. Gastrointestinal problems as a function of carbohydrate supplements and mode of exercise. Med Sci Sport Exerc 1993; 25: 1211–1224.

Peters HP, De Vries WR, Vanberge-Henegouwen GP, Akkermans LM. Potential benefits and hazards of physical activity and exercise on the gastrointestinal tract. Gut 2001; 48: 435–439.

Pfeiffer B, Cotterill A, Grathwohl D, Stellingwerff T, Jeukendruo A. The effect of carbohydrate gels on gastrointestinal tolerance during a 16-km run. Int J Sport Nutr Exerc Metab 2009; 19: 485–503.

Rehrer N, Van Kemenade M, Messter W, Brouns F, Saria W. Gastrointestinal complaints in relation to dietary intake in triathletes. Int J Sport Nutr Exerc Metab 1992; 2: 48–59.

Riddoch C, Trinick T. Gastrointestinal disturbances in marathon runners. Br J Sports Med 1988; 22: 71–74.

Shi X, Hron MK, Osterberg KL et al. Gastrointestinal discomfort during intermittent high intensity exercise: effect of carbohydrate-electrolyte beverage. Int J Sport Nutr Exerc Metab 2004; 14: 673–683.

Simren M. Physical activity and the gastrointestinal tract. Eur J Gastroenterol Hepatol 2002; 14: 1053–1056.

Zachwieja JL, Costill DL, Beard GC, Robergs RA, Pascoe DD, Anderson DE. The effects of carbonated drink on gastric emptying, gastrointestinal distress, and exercise performance. Int J Sport Nutr Exerc Metab 1992; 2: 239–250.

21
Immunity

Glen Davison and Richard J Simpson

Key messages

- Athletes appear to be at increased risk of infection (especially of the upper respiratory tract) during periods of heavy training and competition. The cause of this is not completely understood but could be due to environmental factors, increased exposure to pathogens, viral reactivations, psychological stress and poor nutritional practices.
- The immune system comprises a complex network of molecules, cells and tissues that protect the host from infection. Most components of the immune system can be altered in response to acute (and sometime chronic) exercise, but it is unknown if these immune changes (which are usually transient) are mechanistically involved in the infection-like symptoms commonly reported by athletes.
- Many of the immune changes that occur in response to high-intensity exercise are often perceived as being detrimental and immunodepressive. There are certain nutritional interventions that can influence the immune response to exercise and potentially impact on exercise-induced immunodepression; these can be considered to have either direct or indirect effects on immunity.

- Maintaining a healthy and balanced diet that is sufficient in total energy and macronutrient and micronutrient intake during periods of heavy training is important to help prevent the occurrence of detrimental immune disturbances with exercise. Of particular importance to endurance athletes is the maintenance of adequate carbohydrate intake, as low muscle glycogen stores are known to elicit a number of negative effects on immunity in response to exercise.
- Certain supplements might benefit athletes with a known nutritional deficiency; however, there is little scientific evidence supporting the use of many so-called immune-enhancing supplements at preventing exercise-induced immunodepression. More research is required to investigate the impact of certain supplements at attenuating the immunodepressive effects of acute exercise to assist with the provision of appropriate recommendations to coaches and athletes.

21.1 Introduction: exercise and immunity

Immunity is defined as the resistance of an organism to disease and infection. Interest in the immune response to exercise stemmed from a series of anecdotal reports of athletes incurring a high frequency of infections during periods of heavy training and competition. These anecdotes triggered a large number of epidemiological studies during the late 1980s and early 1990s that attempted to link the volume and type of exercise training undertaken with symptoms of infection in both athletes and non-athletes.

These studies, which are mostly survey-based and rely on memory recall and self-reported symptoms, revealed that athletes appear to be more susceptible to upper respiratory tract infections (URTIs) – or the associated symptoms so this is sometimes referred to as upper respiratory illness – especially when training for and competing in long-distance endurance events. It also became evident that the risk of contracting a URTI is greater in elite athletes compared with their non-elite exercising counterparts, and appears to be related to training volume and intensity. Such observations led to the development of the pioneering J-shaped model by David Nieman in

Sport and Exercise Nutrition, First Edition. Edited by Susan A Lanham-New, Samantha J Stear, Susan M Shirreffs and Adam L Collins.
© 2011 The Nutrition Society. Published 2011 by Blackwell Publishing Ltd.

(a)

(b)

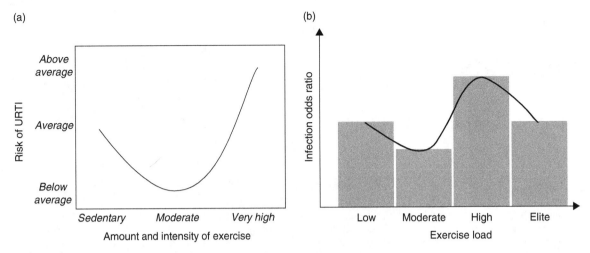

Figure 21.1 Exercise and infection models showing the relationship between exercise load and infection risk. (a) J-shaped model. (Reprinted from Nieman 1994, with permission from Wolters Kluwer Health.) (b) S-curve model. (Reprinted with kind permission from Malm 2006. Copyright © with permission from Wiley-Blackwell.)

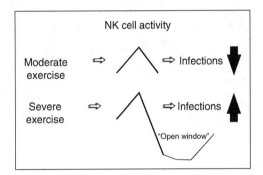

Figure 21.2 The open window hypothesis: strenuous (and/or prolonged) exercise may lower the immune system presenting a temporary 'open window' during which opportunistic infections may take hold. (Reproduced from Pedersen & Ullum 1994, with kind permission from Wolters Kluwer Health.)

1994, which depicts an apparent paradoxical relationship between activity level and risk of contracting an infection (Figure 21.1). Other exercise and infection models that have been developed include the S-curve model and 'open-window' hypothesis (Figures 21.1 and 21.2), each with their own scientific merit and theoretical framework.

The precise mechanisms that underpin this apparent increased infection risk in athletes are not completely understood at present but are likely to be multifactorial, with environmental factors (i.e. pollution, air temperature, altitude), increased exposure to pathogens, psychological stress and poor nutritional practices all purported to play a role. If an athlete should contract an infection then this will undoubt-

edly have an impact on performance, by inhibiting optimal performance, preventing an athlete from competing and/or interfering with their training, and increasing infection risk in other athletes (i.e. team mates) who are in close proximity to the infected athlete, particularly if the infection is contagious. Hence, it is important to understand the relationship between exercise and the immune system and potential interventions to maintain immunity and reduce infection risk in athletes.

21.2 Immune system and immune functions

The immune system is made up of a collection of cells, tissues and molecules that function to protect the host from pathogens, i.e. microorganisms that cause infectious disease. Although scattered throughout the body, the cells of the immune system are highly connected, interactive and interdependent. The orchestrated response of the cells and molecules of the immune system to infectious microbes or organisms (e.g. viruses, bacteria, fungi and parasites) is known as an immune response. The immune system also interacts with other tissues and organs in the body such as the brain and the liver.

Two major divisions of the immune system are recognised: innate (natural or non-specific) and adaptive (acquired or specific) immunity. Despite this stratification, these are two very interactive systems that work synergistically, and most immune responses involve different elements of both innate and adaptive immunity. For example, a macrophage is an immune cell that participates in both the innate system (i.e. during phagocytosis) and adaptive system (i.e. as an antigen-presenting cell or APC). In brief, the innate response is immediate but lacks antigen specificity (i.e. it will elicit the same response regardless of the type of challenge it incurs) and immunological 'memory', while the adaptive response has both antigen specificity (i.e. to a particular pathogen) and 'memory' properties, but takes much longer to develop on initial exposure to an infectious agent. While the innate immune system provides an immediate defence against invading pathogens, its response does not alter on repeated exposure to an infectious agent or other immunogen. The adaptive response, however, increases in tempo and magnitude with successive encounters with the immunogen and the 'memory' component associated with this response can confer lifelong immunity.

Innate immune response

An innate immune response will occur due to tissue damage or any pathogen that attempts to enter and infect the body. In terms of evolution, the innate immune response is much older and less sophisticated than the adaptive response, but because of its immediate response is highly effective at preventing the initial spread of an infectious agent. Innate immunity comprises a variety of cellular, anatomical (mechanical), chemical and other obstacles, providing a system of non-specific antimicrobial functions.

Anatomical/chemical barriers

Skin and mucous membranes, and epithelial cell surfaces comprising mucous membranes, form barriers that microbes and other pathogens have difficulty penetrating. Epithelial cells secrete mucus, which traps microbes, dust and other substances and which can be actively expelled via ciliary action ('immune exclusion'). The chemical properties of the innate immune system also contribute to microbial resistance. For example, sebum (secreted by sebaceous glands) forms a protective layer over the skin. Sweat contains the enzyme lysozyme, which can degrade the cell walls of some bacteria, and the low pH of gastric juice (pH 1.2–3.0), together with its enzymatic activity, destroys many bacteria. If the anatomical

barriers are breached and pathogens do gain entry, then soluble factors (i.e. in body fluids) and innate cellular defences are the next line of defence.

Soluble factors
Complement system
Complements are a group of proteins normally present in the blood (in an inactive form). They function in the innate system as they are activated by pathogens such as bacteria. Essentially, this stimulates the breakdown/cleavage of complement into 'fragments' and it is these cleaved fragments which possess biologically active properties, including the stimulation of phagocytosis, phagocytic 'killing' functions as well as some direct antimicrobial effects. For example, a number of complement proteins, when activated, form a functional unit, the membrane attack complex. This can insert into the cell membrane of target cells such as bacteria, causing water to flow into the cell until it lyses and dies.

Antimicrobial factors in fluids/secretions
Antimicrobial factors like the antimicrobial proteins and peptides (AMPs) such as lysozyme, lactoferrin and defensins, can contribute to the barrier and exclusion functions discussed above to protect the body surfaces, internal surfaces and mucosal surfaces. They also have a key role in mucosal immunity, as discussed below. However, many antimicrobial substances also function in the body fluids (e.g. blood) where they act as innate defences and/or modulate some cellular components of the immune system. There are hundreds of AMPs and many have been shown to work synergistically with each other and other areas of the immune system. In general, AMPs have broad-spectrum antimicrobial and antiviral properties and have been shown to be effective against many pathogens. Hence, they perform important effector functions as part of innate immunity. Indeed, many AMPs have been shown to be important for both the prevention and clearance of infection.

Cellular defences
In terms of cellular components, innate immunity is mediated by neutrophils, monocytes/macrophages and natural killer (NK) cells. The innate system is different from the adaptive immune system (discussed below) in that it does not recognise specific pathogens, but rather generic markers/molecules common to

certain groups of pathogens (e.g. bacteria) or non-self material (e.g. pathogen-associated molecular patterns or PAMPs), which explains the non-specific response. Some elements of the human innate immune response are highly conserved. For example, a type of receptor important in recognition of microorganisms (Toll-like receptors or TLRs) are found on human cells but are also responsible for fungal immunity in the fruit fly *Drosophila*. TLR activation causes secretion of inflammatory cytokines (hormone-like signalling molecules of the immune system) and upregulation of co-stimulatory molecules that are required for antigen presentation and activation of cells of the adaptive immune system.

There are two major innate cellular functions, phagocytosis (the ingestion of a microorganism for destruction) and extracellular killing. Phagocytic cells include neutrophils, macrophages and dendritic cells. Neutrophils are the major phagocytes (they constitute 50–60% of total white blood cells in the circulation). Macrophages (these exist as monocytes in the blood and mature into macrophages when they migrate into tissue) are also phagocytes and may kill engulfed microorganisms. They also possess tumour cytotoxic capacities. However, they also act as APCs and produce cytokines that stimulate some types of lymphocyte, showing the relationship with adaptive immunity. Dendritic cells are capable of phagocytosis but their primary role is presenting antigen, for activation of the adaptive immune system. NK cells are a type of lymphocyte capable of inducing the death of other cells (i.e. those infected by a virus) as part of the innate immune response. They cause apoptosis (programmed cell death) via insertion of perforin and release of various other substances into target cells, leading to death. Perforin inserts into the membrane of target cells, allowing the entry of other substances that induce apoptosis and cell death. The eosinophils are also capable of extracellular killing (but this is usually against large parasites).

Bacterial lipids directly activate monocytes and neutrophils and trigger the release of hormone-like cell-signalling molecules known as cytokines and chemokines, which are capable of activating other immune cells (i.e. T-cells) and tissues (i.e. the liver). Some cytokines are considered proinflammatory, such as tumour necrosis factor (TNF), interleukin (IL)-1β, IL-12 and IL-15, while others are anti-inflammatory, such as IL-4 and IL-10. The ratio of proinflammatory to anti-inflammatory cytokine release loosely dictate the type of immune response that will occur. TNF is the principal mediator of the immune response to infection with Gram-negative bacteria. Along with IL-1 and IL-6, it impacts directly on the liver to activate the acute-phase response. This response augments innate immunity and is characterised by the release of acute-phase proteins such as C-reactive protein (CRP), fibrinogen and hapto-globin from activated hepatocytes into the plasma. CRP is a bacterial opsonin, which binds bacteria and activates complement, increasing bacterial phagocytosis by macrophages.

Viruses can also be recognised by cells of the innate immune system. During adaptive immune responses, T-cells are highly efficient at recognising viral peptides presented to them by APCs (i.e. macrophages or dendritic cells) via major histocompatibility (MHC) molecules; however, some viruses are capable of turning off MHC synthesis in cells allowing the virus to evade certain aspects of the immune system. Absence of the MHC molecule in virally infected cells can be recognised by NK cells and destroyed via a process called antibody-dependent cell cytotoxicity (ADCC).

Adaptive immune response

The adaptive immune response is a more complex process, has a high level of specificity and is capable of eliciting immunological 'memory'. T-cells (matured in the thymus) and B-cells (matured in the bone marrow) carry antigen-specific receptors allowing them to mediate specific adaptive immune responses following pathogen incursion. A component of this adaptive immune response is long-term immunological memory. This means that the response to a virus or bacterium is 'remembered' for many years by cells of the adaptive immune system, allowing a more rapid and effective response on re-exposure to the same antigen.

The lymphatic system plays a major role in adaptive immunity as it transports T-cells and APCs to the lymph nodes where antigen presentation takes place before eliciting the appropriate adaptive immune response. Adaptive immunity is a complex process as T-cells are incapable of binding free antigen in soluble form and must have it presented to them

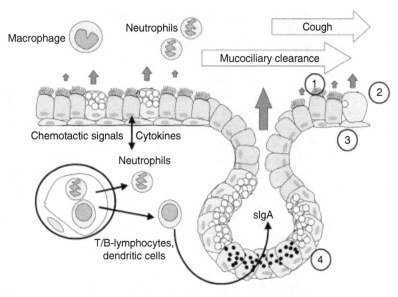

Figure 21.3 Defence mechanisms of the respiratory epithelium. 1, Ciliated cell; 2, goblet cell; 3, basal cell; 4, mucous and serous gland cell. Secretory IgA (sIgA) is transported across the epithelial membrane by the polymeric immunoglobulin receptor (pIgR). Innate and adaptive mechanisms provide protection of the epithelial surfaces. Immune exclusion occurs via ciliary action. Phagocytic cells and antimicrobial factors (i.e. AMPs) provide innate protection. It has also been demonstrated that the innate system is involved in the induction of secretory IgA (sIgA) secretion into the mucosa (i.e. into saliva). Furthermore, immunoglubulins may work synergistically with innate defences (i.e. AMPs) showing the intricate interrelationship between the innate and adaptive systems. (Reproduced from Bals 2000, with permission from BioMed Central.)

by MHC molecules on the membranes of APCs. This allows the T-cell to recognise portions of protein antigens (peptides) bound to the MHC molecules. Two classifications of MHC molecules are recognised: MHC class I, which displays peptides to CD8$^+$ T-cells (cytotoxic cells); and MHC class II, which displays peptides to CD4$^+$ T-cells (helper cells). Antigenic stimulation causes T-cells to proliferate (undergo clonal expansion via cell division) and differentiate into effector T-cells that perform specialised functions, such as cytokine secretion, the recognition and killing of target cells, and the activation of macrophages and antibody-producing B-cells. This proliferation, which results in an expansion of antigen-specific clones, generally occurs within 1–2 days after activation. T-cells in the periphery may generally be considered as naive, memory or effector cells. Naive cells have not encountered antigen since leaving the thymus. When stimulated, some T-cells become effector cells whilst others form long-lived memory cells. Memory cells have previously encountered antigen but returned to a resting state (long-lived). Effector cells derive from naive or memory cells several days after antigenic stimulation and perform specialised functions (i.e.

cytokine secretion, destroy target cells). Many of these are short-lived cells in a highly activated state and further stimulation is required before their effector functions are performed. Following infection resolution, many of the effector cells undergo apoptosis, while others form part of the memory T-cell pool in case of a further encounter with the same antigen.

Mucosal immunity

The mucosal immune system encompasses innate and adaptive components and is primarily composed of networks of tissues that protect the gut and respiratory systems. Together, these aspects of mucosal immunity make up the common mucosal immune system, incorporating the structures and systems responsible for protecting the body's 'inner' surfaces, such as the gut, urinary tract, respiratory tract (incorporating the salivary and nasal glands) and all other mucous membranes throughout the body. Mucosal immunity provides protection against infection by exclusion methods and functions as discussed above (see Figure 21.3). A common example of this, and one particularly relevant in a sport and exercise context, is the continual flow of saliva providing mechanical 'washing' of mucosal surfaces in the mouth and throat. In addition to this mechanical effect, many soluble factors of the innate immune system (such as AMPs) can be detected in mucosal secretions such as saliva, which also contribute to host protection. However, specific (and non-specific) immunity is also provided by secretory immunoglobulins (e.g. sIgA, sIgM). The innate antimicrobial substances may be secreted locally (i.e. by the salivary glands or local epithelial cells, or by innate immune cells such as neutrophils) and/or may move passively into the mucosa from the systemic circulation. Immunoglobulins, on the other hand, are secreted locally by B-cells which are predominantly located in mucosa-associated lymphoid tissue (MALT). After polymeric immunoglubulins are secreted by B-cells, they are transported across the epithelial membrane by the polymeric immunoglobulin receptor (note that the predominant secretory immunoglobulin is IgA).

Assessing immune function

Immune function and biomarkers of the immune system are assessed in a number of ways. The following provides a brief description of the more common assays that have been used in sport and exercise immunology research.

Identification and counting of leucocytes

Cells can be identified and counted in bodily fluids (usually peripheral blood, i.e. venous blood samples). This can be done simply by manual counting, with histological staining and microscopic examination, or by using automated equipment such as a haematology analyser or a flow cytometer. This technique allows the determination of both a total and a differential (i.e. leucocyte subtypes) blood leucocyte count, which might be important for monitoring immune changes in athletes during training and competition (discussed later in this chapter).

Surface expression of CD antigens

Cells of the immune system are typically identified via receptors expressed on their cell surface known as cluster of differentiation/designation (CD) antigens. For example, T-cells are identified by their expression of CD3 (said to be CD3$^+$) and subtypes can be identified by the expression of other CDs. For instance, CD8$^+$ T-cells (CD3$^+$ CD8$^+$) are cytotoxic T-cells while

CD3$^+$ CD4$^+$ are helper T-cells. At present, there are 350 known CD antigens in humans, many of which have distinctive functional characteristics. For instance, CD69 is the earliest observable surface antigen expressed on T-cells when they become activated and has been used as a marker of cell responsiveness. Flow cytometers are typically used to detect the expression of cell surface molecules and most commercially available flow cytometers allow up to four markers to be assessed simultaneously on a single cell. This allows researchers to identify specific immune cell populations of interest and, in some cases, their functional status (i.e. state of activation, markers of dysfunction, intracellular expression of cytokines, cell surface homing receptors). This technique is useful for assessing the frequency of specific immune cell populations in the blood compartment in response to exercise and nutritional interventions.

Natural killer cell activity

Tumour cells are known to be specific targets for NK cells. The K562 tumour cell line is commonly used as an NK-cell target for *in vitro* assays. The target cells are usually labelled with a radioactive substance and, when destroyed by the NK cell, the substance is released into the cell culture medium, which can be measured and quantified using a gamma counter. To account for exercise-induced changes in NK-cell number after exercise, the amount of K562 cell killing (lytic activity) is typically divided by the number of NK cells in the sample. This mathematical correction of the NK-cell response to exercise has received a great deal of criticism but is still used in exercise immunology research today.

Cytotoxic T-cell activity

The killing capacity of cytotoxic T-cells (mostly of the CD8$^+$ subset) is assessed in a similar manner to NK-cell function, but with virally infected target cells (e.g. P815 cell line).

Lymphocyte activation and proliferation

These assays measure cell activation and division, and the consequential increased number of cells in response to a stimulus. For proliferation, this is typically measured as the incorporation of radioactive labelled thymidine into the DNA of the dividing cells. To activate the cells and induce proliferation *in vitro*, mitogens are used to activate T-cells in a process known as mitogen-induced stimulation/proliferation. Antibodies against specific cell surface receptors such as CD3 and CD28 have also been used to trigger activation and proliferation.

Cell migration

The movement of cells towards particular stimuli is known as chemotaxis. The ability of specific immune cell populations to move towards certain stimuli can be measured *in vitro* using supernatants of virally infected cells (for T-cell migration) or specific chemoattractants such as leukotriene B_4 and IL-8.

Phagocytosis

Bacteria, sheep red blood cells, yeast particles or latex beads are typically used in neutrophil and monocyte phagocytosis assays. Flow cytometry allows the measurement of both the number of cells actively performing phagocytosis and the phyagocytic activity per cell. This can be measured alongside bacterial killing and measures of oxidative burst.

Neutrophil oxidative burst activity and degranulation

Oxidative burst activity (OBA) involving superoxide generation by phagocytic cells of the immune system (i.e. neutrophils and monocytes) can be measured in response to bacteria and bacterial peptides. Stimulatory agents are used to activate the phagocytic cells in the presence of a non-fluorescent compound that is oxidised by superoxide (and other reactive oxygen species generated during the oxidative burst). The amount of oxidation of the compound (the fluorescent probe) can be measured by flow cytometry, allowing the quantification of OBA following activation of the phagocytic cells. Similar methods can be performed in single tubes or on multiwell microplates with luminescent probes (i.e. compounds which produce luminescence when exposed to reactive oxygen species, named chemiluminescence) or other compounds that can be detected with simple absorbance readers. The release of granular contents (e.g. elastase, myeloperoxidase) in response to stimulation can be determined with similar methods. The cells are typically stimulated (e.g. with bacterial lipopolysaccharide) and incubated for a short time. The substance of interest (e.g. elastase) can be measured in plasma from stimulated and unstimulated samples using ELISA assays (see below) to work out the stimulated release (or degranulation capacity) relative to the number of neutrophils in the sample. Such assays can be performed on whole blood or isolated cells.

Viral reactivation

When certain viruses are reactivated, viral DNA can be detected in saliva or plasma using polymerase chain reaction (PCR). The number of copies of viral DNA detected is indicative of the viral load.

Enzyme-linked immunosorbant assays (ELISA)

This is one of the most commonly used techniques in sport and exercise immunology research to detect the presence of proteins in blood plasma (and other bodily fluids) that are known to influence the immune system. Plasma samples from humans (or supernatants from cell culture assays) are usually loaded on to a 96-well plate that contains specific detection antibodies against a protein of interest. The amount of protein bound to the antibody is subsequently measured and quantified on a plate reader. The ELISA technique is typically used to measure antimicrobial proteins in saliva, plasma cytokines, specific enzymes (e.g. elastase) and immunoglobulins, and also to determine whether an individual has antibodies against certain viruses.

Assessing mucosal immune function

Mucosal immunity is commonly assessed, in a sport and exercise context, by measuring the concentration and secretion of substances in saliva (e.g. s-IgA, AMPs). The major advantage is that saliva is relatively easy and non-invasive to obtain and may be particularly relevant in relation to protection against URTIs. However, it is important to be mindful of the fact that there are numerous ways in which salivary analytes can be expressed. For example, it may be appropriate to look at the rate of secretion of the analyte, IgA for example, into saliva (secretion rate can be obtained by the product of saliva flow rate and analyte concentration), which may give a better indication of acute exercise-induced alterations in mucosal immunity. Also, exercise can cause variations in hydration status and/or mucosal 'drying', resulting in a short-term pseudo-concentrating effect. Hence, it is often desirable to normalise analyte concentration relative to a 'stable' salivary substance. Some early investigations normalised relative to salivary total protein (e.g. s-IgA/protein) but this may not be appropriate as exercise can induce marked changes in many salivary proteins (i.e. total protein is too variable). Specific proteins such as albumin have been suggested to be more appropriate (e.g. s-IgA/albumin), as has salivary osmolality (s-IgA/osmolality). There is no general consensus as to which is the 'best' method and it is common practice for researchers to present results for salivary parameters using more than one method.

21.3 Impact of exercise (and other stressors)

In humans there is not much research that has established direct links between exercise-induced changes in immunity and infection. This is not to say that the link does not exist, just that research in this area is logistically difficult. Direct links between changes in immunity and infection risk have been difficult to establish/confirm in a sport and exercise context. One of the difficulties is due to the known redundancy in the immune system. This means that there are compensatory mechanisms and numerous components that can provide similar overall protective/defence functions, so that a deficiency in any one component does not necessarily mean that 'overall' defence is compromised. A good example of this is observed in patients with low salivary IgA, whereby high salivary IgM can compensate for the IgA deficiency and as such URTI incidence is normal. However, those who are also deficient in IgM suffer a higher than 'normal' rate of URTIs. So changes in a single area may not necessarily result in an increased infection risk. However, exercise has been shown to affect most areas of the immune system in some way and it is reasonably well accepted that athletes participating in regular intensive training, especially endurance athletes, may be more susceptible to URTI as discussed above. It should be noted, however, that most of this evidence is based on epidemiological surveys and self-reported symptoms. Such studies are open to selection bias and have many limitations that could potentially confound the interpretation of these results. Also, it has become apparent that not all self-reports of illness in athletes may actually be caused by an infection. For example, some athletes may present with upper respiratory tract symptoms (such as a sore throat) but this might

not necessarily be a true infection, but rather an effect of some localised inflammation in the upper airways. Another problem with the use of self-reported symptoms is that athletes are more likely to notice or report minor symptoms that others would simply dismiss as being insignificant. However, strenuous exercise may also be associated with acute inflammation in the upper airways (caused by factors such as increased ventilation, especially of cold dry air during training and/or the switch from the nose to mouth breathing that occurs during intense exercise), which may cause typical symptoms of URTI without an actual infection being present. It is often difficult to distinguish between true infection and other causes of URTI-type symptoms without clinical investigation and many researchers have taken to using the terminology 'upper respiratory illness symptoms' in order to acknowledge this fact. Despite these challenges, recent studies have confirmed (with the use of clinical examination of athletes and laboratory confirmation of infection, i.e. from nasal and throat swabs) that athletes do pick up infections more often, just that the actual incidence may not be as high as the original models proposed (see Figure 21.1). However, clinical investigations also have limitations in that it is not always possible to test for every single infection-causing pathogen. Indeed, an infection may exist causing URTI-like symptoms by a pathogen not screened for or detected. Moreover, there appears to be an assumption that an exercise-induced URTI will be caused by exposure to some external pathogen, although a reactivating latent virus (i.e. shedding of Epstein–Barr virus) could also be responsible. Although true infections may be much more serious that non-infective symptoms, whether these are due to an underlying infection can be rendered irrelevant if the symptoms persist and there is the potential to debilitate the training and performance of the athlete. Therefore, any intervention than can minimise symptoms (whether caused by a true infection or not) may be beneficial.

Although it is clear that the effects of exercise on infection incidence are not fully understood, physical exercise is known to cause profound changes in immune system function that might have some influence on the susceptibility to infection in athletes. For this reason, the response of the immune system to both acute and chronic exercise has been extensively researched and reported in the exercise immunology literature. However, it is difficult to completely confirm such theories in humans since, even when immune defences are lowered, the individual will not contract an infection unless exposed to a pathogen (hence lowered immunity is sometimes referred to as an infection risk factor). Exposure to infection/pathogens is very difficult to control in human experimental studies. However, animal models have provided us with some strong evidence and support for the exercise–infection risk models discussed above. For example, studies in rodents inoculated with pathogens (e.g. influenza, herpes simplex virus) have shown that, compared with control/inactive animals, moderate exercise (shortly before or after inoculation) may reduce infection symptoms and mortality whereas prolonged or strenuous exercise may increase infection and mortality.

Acute and chronic effects

The acute changes in the immune system following prolonged/strenuous exercise have been well reported in the exercise immunology literature and are often described as being similar, in many respects, to the responses induced by infection. As an example, these changes may include the following.

- Increases in the plasma concentrations of various substances that are known to influence leucocyte functions, including:
  - some cytokines, such as TNF-α, IL-1, IL-6, IL-10 and IL-1 receptor antagonist (IL-1ra);
  - several hormones known to have immunomodulatory effects, including catecholamines and cortisol (stress hormones).
- A transient increase in the number of circulating leucocytes, primarily neutrophils (there is also an initial increase in circulating lymphocytes followed by a significant decrease below resting values).
- The function of many immune cells is also affected:
  - neutrophil functions are often seen to be decreased;
  - NK cell cytotoxic activity may increase immediately after exercise but soon decreases below resting values for up to 6 hours;
  - a number of monocyte/macrophage functions may be decreased following prolonged exercise, including TLR expression and function and antigen-presenting functions.

  - a number of lymphocyte functions may be diminished, including mitogen-stimulated lymphocyte proliferation and cytokine production and B-lymphocyte production of immunoglobulins.
- The concentration and secretion of mucosal secretory immunoglobulin (sIgA and sIgM) may also be decreased.

It is these transient perturbations in immunity that are believed to underpin the 'open window' hypothesis, which represents a time-frame when opportunistic infections have an increased likelihood to invade the host and evade the immune system. This 'open-window' may last for a number of hours; however, many of the immune changes that occur usually return to normal within 24 hours after cessation of exercise, suggesting that a single bout of acute strenuous exercise is incapable of eliciting any chronic effects on the immune system. Any chronic effects that are observed in some athletes are most likely due to the effects of an acumulation of repeated bouts of acute strenuous exercise, coupled with inadequate recovery. The magnitude of the acute effects are determined by the nature of the exercise/stress (duration, intensity) and the chronic/cumulative effects are also influenced by the frequency, duration and recovery between exercise. Hence, when prolonged and/or strenuous exercise is repeated with insufficient recovery, the acute effects may cumulate in a state of chronically lowered immune function (i.e. even at rest), presenting a more prolonged 'open window'. With this in mind, it is clear that the nature (i.e. magnitude, direction) of the acute effects of exercise are of key importance and intricately related to the chronic effects. Hence, a lot of attention in the exercise immunology literature has been devoted to determination of the acute effects.

The chronic effects of exercise seem to be most evident in the mucosal immune system in athletes. For example, chronic decreases in mucosal immunity (i.e. IgA and/or AMP levels) have been observed over the course of a competitive season in a variety of sports (i.e. football, rugby, swimming, rowing). In some studies comparison with a control group have ensured that these changes are likely a result of the activity/sport and not just down to seasonal variation (see Figure 21.4). Some researchers have been able to observe significant relationships between changes in mucosal immunity (IgA levels) over the course of a competitive season and incidence of URTI, supporting the idea that low IgA may be associated with decreased protection against opportunistic infection, should the individual be exposed to a pathogen. Indeed, sIgA levels are one of the best established immunological 'risk factors' for URTI occurrence in athletes. Given the important role of IgA in protecting the mucosal surfaces, such as the respiratory tract, the chronic effects of exercise that may exist in some athletes certainly goes some way to explaining the higher than 'normal' URTI incidence often observed in high-level athletes.

Psychological stress

Psychological stress may also cause or add to the effects of exercise on the immune system. Psychological stress is known to induce stress responses (i.e. increase stress hormones) which could have both direct and indirect effects on immunity. Also, athletes are known to be exposed to additional stressors related to serious training or competition (e.g. competitive stress and anxiety, and pressures associated with selection, performance expectations, media, personal life) that can be experienced concomitantly with the physical and physiological stress of their sport. It is possible therefore that the immunodepressive effects of exercise would be exacerbated under these conditions of additional/psychological stress.

Exercise, acute stress and viral reactivation

In addition to the many external pathogens that could cause infection in athletic populations, there are also lifelong infections that individuals carry. Reactivations of latent viruses during periods of heavy exercise or competition could pose a threat to athlete immune health. This is a particular problem for athletes working in training camps, as healthy athletes might live in close proximity to athletes carrying a latent virus that has been reactivated. Herpesviruses are known to infect humans and establish lifelong latency. After primary infection, which for most herpesviruses occurs during childhood and adolescence, the infection remains dormant in various cells of the body. Each of these viruses has the potential to be reactivated as a result of lowered immunity (i.e. resulting from psychological stress associated with competition, heavy exercise,

poor nutritional practices, sleep disturbances or many of these effects combined). While reactivating viruses can cause illness directly, evidence of viral shedding also indicates that the immune system might be weakened leaving the athlete susceptible to other infections. For instance, continued control of latent viruses requires vigilant immune surveillance. When immunity has been compromised, latent viruses have the chance to reactivate. There are currently eight known herpesviruses that infect humans, of which the best known are herpes simplex virus (HSV-1 and HSV-2), varicella zoster virus (VZV), Epstein–Barr virus (EBV) and cytomegalovirus (CMV). While HSV reactivation can cause blisters, such as cold sores, to develop on mucous membranes, VZV causes chickenpox on primary infection and manifests as shingles when subsequently reactivated. EBV causes infectious mononucleosis (glandular fever) and is also linked with B-cell malignancy (Burkitt's lymphoma) as well as Hodgkin's lymphoma, and nasopharyngeal carcinoma. CMV is often regarded as a 'harmless' infection as it is clinically asymptomatic in immunocompetent hosts; however, it can cause problems for the severely immunocompromised athlete and is also known to accelerate biological ageing of the immune system, increasing infection risk in later life. Not everyone is infected (seropositive) with all latent virses (e.g. in people aged 18–35 years in Western society, about 50–60% are infected with CMV and 70–80% with EBV) but the frequency appears to be similar in elite-level athletes.

It is therefore some what surprising that very few studies have been undertaken to assess the impact of heavy training and competition on latent viral reactivations in athletes. In a group of elite female swimmers, EBV viral DNA was detected in 64% of the EBV-seropositive athletes during a 30-day period of intensive training. Almost all the EBV-seropositive swimmers who had detectable viral DNA in their saliva reported symptoms of URTI, while no URTI symptoms were reported in the EBV-seronegative swimmers. Interestingly, EBV viral DNA had the tendency to appear before the onset of URTI symptoms, indicating that EBV could have a mechanistic role to play in the aetiology of URTI in athletes. At the very least, this would suggest that viral shedding might serve as an immune monitoring tool to highlight compromised immunity and URTI susceptibility in

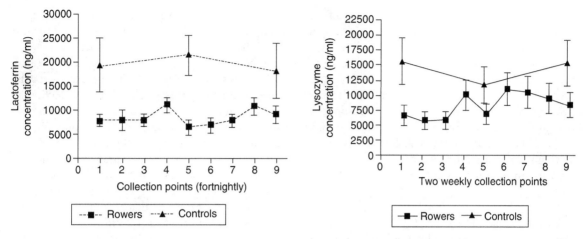

Figure 21.4 Chronic effects of heavy training on innate salivary defences (AMPs). This study monitored salivary AMPs (lactoferrin and lysozyme) over a 5-month training period in well-trained rowers and made comparisons with a control group. The AMPs tended to be lower in the athletes, suggesting a chronic lowering associated with heavy training. (Reprinted from West *et al*. 2010. Copyright © with permission from BMJ Publishing Group Ltd.)

athletes. Detecting viral shedding in athletes during periods of heavy training might also allow an early intervention countermeasure to be put in place and mitigate the risk of subsequent clinical infections. Maintaining good nutritional practices might reduce the frequency of latent viral reactivation and thus help to keep athletes healthy during periods of heavy training and competition. It is known that certain reactivating viruses, such as HSV-1, have been linked with vitamin A deficiency; however, no studies have been conducted to assess the impact of nutritional interventions on exercise-induced latent viral reactivation. This should be a major focus of sport and exercise immunology research over the years to come.

Mechanisms of exercise-induced immunodepression

Exercise is known to elicit many changes in a host of immune system biomarkers and functions. While the clinical relevance of these, for the most part, is relatively unknown, it is generally perceived that declines in certain functional aspects of immunity (T-cell proliferation, neutrophil degranulation, NK-cell cytotoxicity, salivary IgA secretion, etc.) with exercise are indicative of immune system depression. The term 'exercise-induced immunodepression' has been used to describe the impact of exercise (either acute or chronic effects) on immune system functional changes that can be perceived as being negative responses.

Many of the depressive effects of exercise on immune functions are thought to be largely mediated, either directly or indirectly, by increased levels of hypothalamic–pituitary–adrenal (HPA) axis stress hormones (particularly glucocorticoids and catecholamines) and some cytokines; metabolic factors and substrate availability; leucocyte redistribution; and possibly oxidative stress.

Stress hormones

It has been suggested that glucocortocoids, particularly cortisol, may have a direct inhibitory effect on some immune cells. Also, catecholamines and glucorticoids may act indirectly. For example, cortisol may induce/contribute to leucocyte redistribution. Also, IL-6 (released from active skeletal muscle) may contribute to exercise-induced cell trafficking, by directly stimulating the mobilisation of neutrophils into the circulation or indirectly by inducing an increase in plasma cortisol concentration.

Saliva flow/secretion is under neural control so the stress response (i.e. sympathetic activation, release of catecholamines, etc.) may cause vasoconstriction to the vessels supplying the salivary glands, reducing saliva flow and/or affecting the secretion of proteins. Also, repeated activation during acute heavy exercise may chronically deplete the body's stores, possibly explaining the chronically lowered levels of 'effector' proteins of mucosal immunity (Figure 21.4).

Exercise-induced alterations in immune cell functions may also be caused by alterations in intracellular signalling and/or activation pathways. This could be mediated by direct effects (i.e. from stress hormones) or by an altered subpopulation of immune cells induced by leucocyte redistribution, as discussed below. Also, exercise may cause activation of some cells of the immune system (possibly in response to tissue damage and/or other 'non-infective' stimuli), leaving them in a refractory state and affecting their capacity to respond to other stimuli, such as a pathogen.

Substrate availability

Decreased substrate availability (i.e. muscle glycogen depletion, decreased blood glucose concentration) may act indirectly by exacerbating the stress responses discussed above. Also, many cells of the immune system have a high metabolism and energy demand and reduced substrate availability, such as glucose, can limit their capacity to function properly.

Exercise-induced leucocyte redistribution

Exercise causes a number of leucocyte redistribution effects, which may influence overall immune function. Strenuous exercise causes an initial increase in the number of circulating leucocytes (leucocytosis), depending on the exercise intensity and duration. This leucocytosis is predominantly influenced by increases in the neutrophil (neutrophilia) and lymphocyte (lymphocytosis) counts. For intense short-duration exercise the response is biphasic: leucocytosis during and immediately after the exercise bout, followed by a return to baseline during the recovery phase of exercise. The recovery phase is characterised by a further (delayed) leucocytosis at 1–3 hours after exercise. However, this is dominated by the granulocytes (i.e. neutrophilia) as the lymphocyte count typically decreases, and may even decrease below baseline levels (lymphocytopenia). For prolonged exercise lasting more than 90 min the leucocytosis is not biphasic as the two components tend to be superimposed on one another. Neutrophil numbers may increase up to fourfold or more following prolonged exercise (and some subpopulations, such as immature cells, may have compromised functional capacity). Numbers normally return to baseline by 1–6 hours after exercise. There may be slight lymphocytosis after prolonged exercise, but there is a rapid efflux of lymphocytes from the blood compartment that results in a lymphocytopenia, usually within 30–120 min after cessation of exercise. Lymphocyte numbers during the recovery phase of exercise can be as much as 50% lower than the pre-exercise counts and are often reported to fall below 1.0×10^9/L (particularly after very prolonged exercise, over 2 hours), which is considered to be the clinically lower limit for blood lymphocyte counts. Although the actual clinical significance of this exercise-induced lymphocytopenia is unknown (blood lymphocyte counts are usually restored after 24 hours of recovery), many scientists have proposed that this presents an 'open window' for opportunistic infections.

Exercise-induced oxidative stress

It has been proposed that exercise-induced oxidative stress can, in certain situations, lead to damage or modification to immune cells and tissues that results in impaired function. Oxidative stress is known to occur when the generation of free radicals, which can be either nitrogen centred (reactive nitrogen species) or oxygen centred (reactive oxygen species), outweighs the antioxidant defence system, negatively disturbing the redox balance. Strenuous or prolonged (>2 hours) exercise can cause disturbances to cellular redox balance, leading to oxidative stress and lipid peroxidation. The human body has natural defence mechanisms to counteract the potentially detrimental effects of free radical production in the form of antioxidant enzymes and compounds but they may be overwhelmed during prolonged exercise bouts and/or when the stressor is unfamiliar. This is not uncommon in athletes who may progressively increase training volume and intensity (i.e. to satisfy the training principles of overload and progression). Hence, dietary antioxidants (e.g. vitamins A, C, E) intake may be particularly important in helping to maintain optimal antioxidant defences in athletes (as discussed later).

21.4 Effects of nutrition

Nutrition and dietary intake

It is well known that diet can influence the immune system, for example a poor diet or dietary deficiency (especially of carbohydrate, total energy, protein and some micronutrients) has been shown to have negative effects on most aspects of immunity. There is little doubt that malnutrition (including both under-nutrition and over-nutrition) can have a negative effect on the immune system. Indeed malnutrition, in particular nutritional deficiency, is believed to be one of the major causes of secondary immunodeficiency. It is quite uncommon for such severe malnutrition to be evident in healthy athletes but this certainly highlights the important role of diet in maintaining optimal immune function. Nutrient availability can have either a direct or an indirect effect on immunity. A nutrient is said to have a direct effect when addition or depletion of the nutrient will impact solely on the particular immune system component with little or no influence from other immune system regulators (e.g. glucose being used by T-cells as a fuel source for biosynthesis). An indirect effect is when addition or depletion of the nutrient elicits changes in other organs, cells and/or their components that act as immune system regulators or influence immunity in some way (e.g. blunting of the stress hormone response).

The combination of poor diet and exercise can result in even greater negative effects on the immune system. Nutritional deficiencies may further exacerbate exercise-induced immune impairment and/or hinder the recovery of normal immune function following exercise. Indeed, suboptimal nutrition can cause immunodepression in response to exercise that would not normally depress (or would even enhance) immune function. In addition to the negative effects of chronic (or relatively long-term) malnutrition, acute nutritional intake has also been shown to significantly influence the immune responses to exercise. For example, when considering the potential mechanisms of exercise-induced immunodepression mentioned above (direct and indirect) it becomes apparent that some of these could be counteracted by acute nutritional interventions. For example, direct substrate availability effects (e.g. glucose) can be minimised by the ingestion of carbohydrate (CHO), which also acts indirectly by attenuating stress hormone and leucocyte trafficking responses (Figure 21.5).

Total energy intake

A deficiency of total energy intake (negative energy balance) may have direct and indirect effects on immune responses to exercise. Direct effects may include the effects mediated directly by energy avail-

ability to immune cells. Negative energy balance may also have indirect effects by exacerbating stress responses (i.e. increased secretion of stress hormones), which may worsen exercise-induced immunodepression. Also, a total energy deficiency means that at least one of the macronutrients must be deficient in the diet, which can have other direct and indirect effects on immunity, as discussed below. Furthermore, such deficiencies are also likely to result in a suboptimal intake of micronutrients, some of which may be important for optimal immune function, as discussed below.

Carbohydrate

Of all the macronutrients, CHO availability appears to have the greatest impact on exercise-induced immune changes. It has become apparent that athletes who consume less than the recommended amount of CHO will be at a greater risk of immune disruption during exercise. This is likely to be due to a combination of both direct and indirect effects of CHO availability on immunity. Conversely, extreme (very high) intakes of CHO may result in a dietary imbalance which could mean insufficient intake of protein, leading to negative effects on immunity as discussed in the protein section below.

It has been demonstrated that exercising in a glycogen-depleted state, or after only a few days on a low-carbohydrate diet, causes greater immune disturbance (increased stress responses, greater leucocyte redistribution, and depressed immune function) compared with exercise on a normal or high-CHO diet (or when not glycogen depleted). Exercise in a glycogen-depleted state has been shown to negatively affect many aspects of immune function (such as T-cell, neutrophil and NK-cell functions) compared with the same exercise in a non-glycogen-depleted state. This may be related to direct effects, such as glucose availability, although a number of indirect mechanisms may also be involved. In fact, the indirect mechanisms may be the major contributing factors for most aspects of adaptive immunity affected by exercise.

Exercise with low CHO intake, or depleted CHO stores, is associated with greater stress responses, including greater HPA axis activation (i.e. cortisol secretion), catecholamine release, and muscle IL-6 production and release (see Figure 21.5). This may be associated with inhibitory effects on some aspects of immunity and other indirect effects via mobilisation

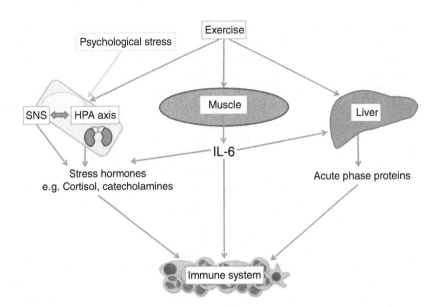

Figure 21.5 Stress responses during exercise can influence the immune system. Exercise (and psychological stress) can stimulate the sympathetic nervous system (SNS) and the hypothalamic–pituitary–adrenal (HPA) axis resulting in a 'stress response' and the release of stress hormones and catecholamines (e.g. cortisol, adrenaline, noradrenaline). The main biological effects are geared towards maintaining plasma glucose concentration and substrate availability (i.e. promotion of gluconeogenesis and hepatic glucose output; lipolysis and increased free fatty acid availability; increased free amino acid availability). Glycogen depletion during prolonged exercise also causes release of IL-6 from the active skeletal muscle. The main effects are also geared towards maintaining substrate availability (directly, by inducing hepatic glucose output, and indirectly by inducing cortisol secretion) but IL-6 also induces an acute-phase response. In particular, these stress responses (if excessive/prolonged, i.e. during prolonged exercise) may have a number of direct and indirect, potentially depressive, effects on the immune system. The above responses are substantially blunted if glucose availability is maintained (prevented from decreasing) during exercise (i.e. by the ingestion of CHO at a rate of 30–60 g/hour).

of (immature) leucocytes. This has been demonstrated for a variety of types of exercise but is most evident with prolonged/endurance exercise. It has also been shown that for some types of exercise there is a significant depression of immunity under glycogen-reduced conditions that do not normally exist under conditions of normal CHO status. For example, there is considerable research on the effects of single bouts of intermittent exercise, simulating the physiological demands of football, on immune parameters. A number of studies have demonstrated that there are minimal acute immune disturbances following such exercise when athletes have consumed a normal mixed diet in the days prior. However, when muscle glycogen stores have been depleted in the preceding days, without optimal restoration, such exercise causes notable immunodepression (Figure 21.6).

Acute carbohydrate intake

The importance of CHO availability on immune function is further demonstrated by the fact that

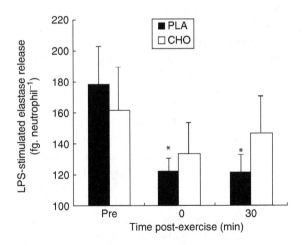

Figure 21.6 Effects of CHO intake on neutrophil function following intermittent exercise. A 90-min intermittent exercise protocol (simulating the physiological demands of a football match) was performed the morning after muscle glycogen lowering exercise. There was a significant decrease in neutrophil function (assessed by stimulated degranulation) after exercise but the decrease was blunted if CHO was consumed during the exercise. (Reprinted, with permission, from Bishop *et al.* 2002.)

acute CHO ingestion significantly blunts or prevents many aspects of exercise-induced immunodepression (also evident in Figure 21.6). CHO ingestion affects exercise-induced immunodepression via a number of mechanisms, for example by counteracting or preventing many of the immunodepressive responses highlighted in Figure 21.5. For example, CHO ingestion prevents the fall in plasma glucose, insulin, HPA axis activation, and associated stress responses, providing avenues by which CHO consumption has direct and indirect effects on immune responses to exercise. Most measures of immunity (certainly cellular) that are shown to be decreased following exercise are positively affected by acute CHO ingestion before and during exercise. This includes blunting of exercise-induced increases in leucocytosis (i.e. neutrophilia), post-exercise lymphocytopenia and the decrease in most leucocyte functions that typically occurs after prolonged and/or strenuous exercise.

The amount of CHO ingested in studies showing beneficial effects is typically in the region of 30–60 g/hour. This is usually delivered by the consumption of a CHO beverage at regular intervals before and during exercise. Typically these drinks contain about 6% w/v CHO (equivalent to most commercially available sports drinks), indicating that around 150–300 ml is consumed before and at 15–20 min intervals during exercise in most studies (the precise amount is usually prescribed based on body mass, i.e. 2–3 ml/kg every 15–20 min). This has been shown to be beneficial on many aspects of innate immunity (as seen for neutrophil function in Figure 21.6) as well as many aspects of adaptive immunity. CHO consumption during exercise has also been shown to lower the impairment of T-cell functions associated with prolonged exercise. There are beneficial effects on functions such as T-cell proliferative capacity (in response to mitogens, influenza and tetanus toxoid for example), and the ability of T-cells to migrate towards infected tissue in culture.

Protein

Protein has an important role in many aspects of the immune system. For example, activated immune cells may need to divide/replicate (proliferation) or produce substances and proteins involved in immune regulation (i.e. cytokines) or functions, namely substances involved in intracellular (phagocytes) or extracellular (NK cells) killing such as granular enzymes and AMPs. Also, many aspects of innate immunity (e.g. many of the soluble factors) derive largely from protein (and often rely on other protein-containing substances to activate them). Other key immune tissues (e.g. lymphoid tissues) also rely on protein to maintain their normal/healthy state. Hence, prolonged protein malnutrition will have numerous adverse effects on the immune system. Conversely, an excessive intake of protein may also be detrimental to immune functions. Likewise, the consumption of individual amino acids, in excessive amounts, may affect the balance of amino acids in the free pool (either increasing the relative proportion of the ingested amino acids or depleting the relative proportion of others), which may have some negative effects on immune function.

While protein deficiency is known to impair immunity and increase susceptibility to infection, it is generally accepted that athletes who maintain a reasonably well-balanced diet will receive adequate amounts of protein to keep them healthy. However, there are certain athletes, particularly in endurance sports, who may be more likely to fall short of their individual specific requirements (e.g. some vegetarians, or those adhering to periods of food restriction). This, combined with the fact that protein turnover is known to increase during periods of heavy training, could put the athlete at an unnecessary risk of infection and poor athletic performance.

Glutamine

Some of the earliest studies in the area of exercise immunology hypothesised that availability of the amino acid glutamine could be implicated in exercise-induced immunodepression (the glutamine hypothesis). Glutamine can be used as an energy substrate by many immune cells (especially mononuclear cells such as lymphocytes and monocytes) and its depletion, as observed after severe trauma or injury, is associated with immunodepression. Glutamine is a non-essential amino acid but leucocytes are incapable of synthesising their own glutamine and are therefore dependent on synthesis by other tissues (mostly skeletal muscle). The proliferative response of T-cells to mitogens *in vitro* is influenced by glutamine in a dose-dependent manner. The ideal concentration of glutamine for optimal T-cell proliferation is reported to be 600 µmol/l (equivalent to 'normal' concentrations observed in resting individuals), which led to the hypothesis that a fall in plasma glutamine below this level will debilitate adaptive immune system responses, the basis of the glutamine hypothesis. Plasma glutamine concentration is decreased after prolonged or strenuous exercise (by 20% or more) but this usually recovers within 24 hours. However, chronic decreases may manifest during heavy training as it has been reported that plasma glutamine levels are lower (at rest) in overtrained compared with healthy athletes. However, the glutamine hypothesis has lost scientific support over recent years. This is mainly due to the inability of orally ingested glutamine supplements to prevent declines in immune system function after exercise despite being able to increase and maintain plasma glutamine concentrations. It has been suggested that exercise does not deplete body glutamine enough to cause immunodepression and that glucose is a more important fuel source for leucocytes anyway. Although supplementing athletes with glutamine can prevent exercise-induced falls in plasma levels, this does not appear to prevent the declines in T-cell proliferation, NK-cell killing capacity, salivary IgA concentration or neutrophil degranulation that have been observed after prolonged exercise. Although some studies have documented benefits of glutamine supplementation on self-reported symptoms of URTI in the days and weeks following a major endurance competition, it has been suggested that this may be mediated by other mechanisms and not glutamine *per se* (i.e. indirectly, simply by the provision of additional protein, or by antioxidant mechanisms as glutamine is important for maintaining levels of the endogenous antioxidant glutathione). Furthermore, it is important to note that orally ingested glutamine supplements do prevent exercise-induced declines in plasma glutamine and there does not appear to be any adverse effects, meaning that athletes can take this supplement relatively safely (as long as this does not lead to excessive total protein intake).

Fat

Fat, as a nutrient, is often undervalued by athletes and/or perceived as being unhealthy. While excessive intake of dietary fat can have negative health effects, it should not be overlooked that fat, in the correct proportions, is an essential part of a healthy and balanced diet. The intake of fat, in a healthy diet, helps to ensure athletes obtain adequate energy (i.e. 20–30% of total energy intake) to maintain energy balance. Therefore, a deficiency of fat may contribute to a deficiency of total energy, which may negatively affect immune function as discussed above. Deficiency of essential fatty acids may also result in deficiencies of lipid-soluble micronutrients (including antioxidant vitamins, see below), which can also have a negative effect on immunity. For example, dietary antioxidant restriction has been shown to reduce antioxidant protection and increase oxidative stress responses to exercise, and excessive oxidative stress in response to exercise has been implicated as a possible mechanism for exercise-induced immunodepression. Lipids are also important components of cell membranes and can also act as an energy substrate (though a less important fuel than glucose) for cells of the immune system, and as such are important for immune cells.

The effect of dietary fat on immunity is a difficult, and often confusing, area. For example, supplemental fatty acids have been shown to have positive and negative effects on immunity, depending on energy and lipid balance, the type of fat studied, and factors such as quantity and amount of supplemental fatty acids relative to normal dietary intake. However, some generally agreed notions are that fat is an important component of a normal balanced diet and that both excessively low and high intakes negatively affect immune function, which may be more evident in athletes. The general dietary recommendations for athletes (i.e. obtain 20–30% of total energy intake from fat) can also be considered appropriate for maintaining optimal immune function in athletes or exercisers.

Micronutrients

Athletes with high energy requirements may have an increased need for many micronutrients. This increased requirement is usually achieved with an appropriate increase in energy intake to maintain energy balance and deficiencies are unlikely if the diet is well balanced and varied. However, under certain circumstances, athletes (or certain groups) may be at an increased risk of dietary deficiency (e.g. those adopting an imbalanced diet or excluding certain foods, and those experiencing increased losses or gastrointestinal and malabsorption problems). A deficiency of certain micronutrients can have negative effects on immune function. This has led some to believe that additional

(a)

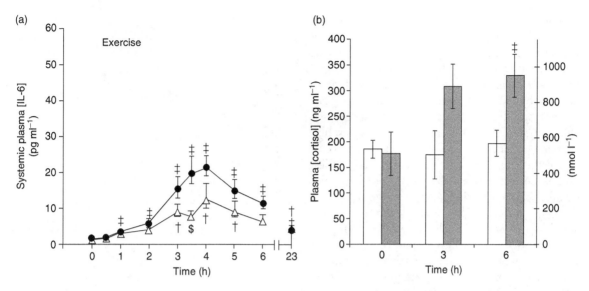

(b)

Figure 21.7 Effects of antioxidant vitamins (C and E) on IL-6 and cortisol responses to prolonged exercise. In this study subjects either consumed high dosages of antioxidants daily for 28 days (including 500 mg vitamin C and 400 IU vitamin E per day) or a placebo before performing 3 hours of exercise. The antioxidant supplementation completely blunted cortisol and attenuated IL-6 systemic responses that were evident in the placebo group. The study also demonstrated (not shown here) that IL-6 synthesis within the active muscles was not affected by the antioxidants but rather the release from muscle (i.e. into the blood) was attenuated. This study also provides evidence for the role of exercise-induced IL-6 release in the cortisol response to prolonged exercise. The non-shaded data represent the antioxidant group and the shaded data represent the placebo group. (Reproduced with kind permission from Fischer *et al.* 2004, with permission from Wiley InterScience.)

intakes of these substances (i.e. vitamins and minerals) will boost the immune system. However, if a deficiency is corrected immune function is usually restored to normal but additional intake above the normal (individual-specific) requirement, for most micronutrients, does not provide any additional benefits. There is some evidence in support of the idea that additional intake of some micronutrients (i.e. many fold greater than the RDA) has beneficial effects on the immune system and infection susceptibility in athletes (see below), although this could simply reflect a higher than normal requirement in these individuals.

Antioxidants

Deficiencies can have negative effects on immunity in athletes (e.g. vitamin A deficiency is associated with the reactivation of certain latent viruses, as discussed above; antioxidant deficiencies may decrease protection against oxidative stress, which may negatively affect some immune functions). Although, as a general rule for micronutrients, intakes in excess of normal requirements appears to offer little additional protection and in some cases might actually be detrimental, beneficial effects have been observed for some antioxidants (such

as vitamins C and E). For example, megadoses (i.e. in the region of 10 times RDA) have been shown to reduce infection incidence in ultra-endurance athletes. This was originally thought to be mediated indirectly by the effects of antioxidants on minimising stress hormone and cytokine responses but this has more recently been called into question. It is quite clear that supplementing with high doses of antioxidants (typically 2–8 weeks of daily supplementation with vitamin C, vitamin E and/or other dietary antioxidants; see Figure 21.7 for example) is capable of blunting the cortisol and IL-6 responses to exercise. However, recent research has demonstrated that in well-nourished healthy individuals this has little effect on most aspects of immunity and URTI incidence. A few studies have demonstrated some beneficial effects of antioxidants on neutrophil functions following prolonged exercise, but these effects may be more related to increased antioxidant protection of these cells. One theory is that athletes (endurance athletes in particular) have particularly high requirements for antioxidants due to the production of free radicals and reactive oxygen species during heavy training. It has been suggested that this can deplete endogenous antioxidant pools, which may have negative effects on some immune functions. Natural endogenous antioxidant defences (i.e. antioxidant enzymes such as superoxide dismutase) are naturally upregulated in response to training but athletes may have a substantially higher than normal requirement, which may need to be obtained by additional dietary antioxidants.

Another antioxidant that has received a considerable amount of attention in the sport and exercise immunology field is the bioflavonoid quercetin. Quercetin is found naturally in many foods including onions, some fruits and berries (especially apples, cranberries and cherries), green leafy vegetables and teas. Typical dietary intake is less than 50 mg/day but supplemental dosages in the region of 1000 mg/day have been used in nutritional intervention studies. Laboratory research has suggested that quercetin also has anti-inflammatory and 'immune-stimulating' properties *in vitro*; however, supplementation in exercising subjects, compared with a placebo, tends not to elicit any changes in a wide array of immune function markers, including NK-cell activity, neutrophil OBA, mitogen-induced T-cell proliferation and salivary IgA output. However, one study did report that quercetin supplementation reduced the occurrence of self-reported URTI symptoms during the 2 weeks after a 3-hour laboratory-based cycling protocol despite inducing no change in a number of immune system functional markers. Quercetin is known to have direct antimicrobial and antiviral properties *in vitro*. Therefore, some researchers have theorised that supplementation provides protection against infection (as observed in the study just mentioned) by increasing the antimicrobial and antiviral properties of bodily fluids, making it more difficult for opportunistic infections to gain a foothold, although this requires further investigation.

A practical consideration for antioxidants

Whether antioxidant supplementation is beneficial for athletes (from an immune perspective) during periods of heavy training is an ongoing debate. For example, there is an emerging body of evidence showing that exercise-induced free radicals and reactive oxygen species serve as important intracellular signalling molecules with integral roles in many physiological processes and responses. Indeed, there is some evidence that the mechanisms by which antioxidant supplementation modulates the systemic cortisol and cytokine responses to exercise is by inter-

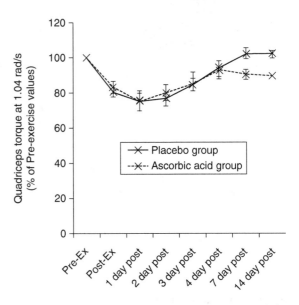

Figure 21.8 Effects of high-dose vitamin C supplementation on the recovery of muscle function after damaging exercise. In this study subjects performed downhill running (i.e. eccentrically biased action of the quadriceps, compared to level running) to induce acute muscle damage and delayed-onset muscle soreness (DOMS). Subjects either consumed a high dose (1000 mg) of vitamin C or placebo before and every day after the exercise for a 2-week period. The study showed that the exercise caused peak torque (a measure of strength) to decrease for at least a few days whilst perceived soreness (DOMS, not shown here) was increased. However, the placebo group recovered their maximal strength more quickly, suggesting that very high levels of vitamin C may interfere with recovery, remodelling and adaptation processes. (Data from Close *et al.* 2006, with permission from Cambridge University Press.)

fering with redox sensitive intracellular signalling pathways involved in gene expression and transcription. Interfering with these processes may have deleterious effects on normal regulatory and adaptation responses to stressors such as exercise. Furthermore, the release of cortisol during exercise may be considered part of the normal physiological response. It has been demonstrated, for example, that high-dose vitamin C supplementation slows the recovery of muscle function after eccentric exercise (inducing muscle damage and soreness; Figure 21.8). This is likely mediated by antioxidant interference with cellular signalling processes involved in the normal physiological responses and subsequent adaptation. It may also interfere with aspects of innate immunity (i.e. phagocytes are involved in early inflammatory processes and may be important for clearing debris and damaged tissue/cells and initiating the remodelling process). Indeed, some recent evidence has suggested that excessive antioxidant consumption reduces the rate of performance improvement in response to an endurance training programme (i.e. blunts the training response), which is obviously not desirable for athletes.

Minerals

Iron deficiency may compromise some components of immunity (cellular), as may excessive intake. Furthermore, if prolonged deficiency occurs and results in anaemia, this could have indirect effects by affecting the ability to endure and tolerate heavy training and the subsequent stress responses. Zinc has an important role in the development and functioning of many immune cells. Hence, zinc deficiency is associated with compromised function of NK cells and phagocytes. Likewise, excessively large intakes may also be associated with negative effects on the function of phagocytes (especially in athletes or in response to exercise). The effects of zinc deficiency on adaptive immune function include impaired T-cell proliferation to mitogens, and lower synthesis of the cytokine IL-2 (important for eliciting adaptive immune responses such as T-cell proliferation). However, there is a distinct lack of studies that have explored the effects of many dietary minerals on exercise-induced immune changes in athletes. Many studies in this area have obtained mixed results, so it is not completely clear whether supplementation, especially with single nutrients, is beneficial or detrimental to exercise-induced immune perturbations. One difficulty is that there are some beneficial and detrimental effects associated with these nutrients. For example, although iron deficiency is associated with compromised immunity, an increase in free iron may increase the risk of bacterial infection as bacteria need free iron to thrive. Indeed, the antimicrobial protein lactoferrin works partly by binding free iron to prevent bacterial growth/replication. So iron deficiency may actually reduce susceptibility to bacterial infections (although there would obviously be many other negative health, performance and immune effects from deficiency). With this in mind, and the known negative health/toxicity effects and the potential to interfere with the absorption of other nutrients that can occur with excessive intakes of some minerals such as iron and zinc, a prudent recommendation for athletes is to obtain these nutrients from a healthy and balanced diet (and certainly avoid the intake of single nutrient supplements).

Fluids

The majority of studies on the effects of CHO on exercise-induced immune responses have delivered the CHO in the form of a beverage. This led some researchers to question whether the beneficial effects observed in such studies were solely a result of the CHO or whether there were any effects from the fluid. Subsequent studies have confirmed that most of the effects on the immune system are due to the CHO. However, it has been determined that the provision of fluid alone provides some benefits for acute prolonged exercise, including maintaining saliva flow (important as an innate 'washing' defence, as discussed above) and reducing some stress hormones. Furthermore, prolonged fluid restriction (i.e. over a number of days) has been shown to augment the reduction of salivary IgA secretion caused by sustained (2 days) physical exertion in military recruits. Taken together, these results highlight the importance of hydration and suggest that optimal fluid intake can also contribute to minimising the negative effects of exercise on immunity.

Caffeine

A few recent studies have demonstrated beneficial effects of acute caffeine ingestion on T-cell responsiveness, neutrophil and NK-cell functions following fixed intensity and duration exercise (which induces immunodepression). As caffeine is an ergogenic aid (and may reduce perceptions of effort and exertion) these effects could be related to a reduction of some aspects of psychological stress (i.e. exercise is perceived as easier, less stressful and more tolerable). However, a direct mechanism may also exist. For example, caffeine is known to exert some of its stimulant effects via the antagonism of adenosine receptors in the brain/CNS. However, some immune cells are known to have a relatively high density of adenosine receptors. For example, the activation (agonism) of A_{2a} adenosine receptors on neutrophils is known to diminish some neutrophil functions (such as OBA). Hence, it is possible that the (blocking) antagonism of these receptors may help to maintain neutrophil OBA capacity. This is proposed as a likely mechanism to explain attenuated neutrophil immunodepression after prolonged submaximal exercise with caffeine (compared with placebo) ingestion. However, the overall effects of caffeine depend on the nature of the exercise. Caffeine is also known to enhance the secretion of catecholamines, which may have immunodepressive effects and amplify the stress response to exercise (see Figure 21.5). For example, typical ergogenic caffeine doses of 6 mg/kg (usually ingested 1 hour before exercise) have been shown to elevate plasma adrenaline concentrations both before and after exercise. This in turn has been shown to exacerbate the lymphopenia of both CD4+ and CD8+ T-cells during the recovery phase of exercise, as well as increasing the activation status of T-cell subsets as measured by CD69 expression. While the increased immune cell activation and egress of specific immune cells from the blood compartment during the recovery phase of exercise could be considered as a negative immune perturbation, the clinical impact of caffeine ingestion, as it pertains to exercise and immunity, remains to be established. The effects of caffeine on the immune responses to exercise will depend on the balance between potentially beneficial effects (i.e. adenosine receptor antagonism) and the potentially negative effects (i.e. catecholamines). For example, with submaximal fixed intensity and duration exercise the effects may be mainly beneficial but when performance is not fixed in terms of intensity/duration (i.e. time-trial and competition, where maximal effort is exerted) caffeine may allow more work/intense exercise to be performed and/or exacerbate catecholamine and stress responses. Under these circumstances (which are believed to be more representative of real sporting situations), the beneficial effects of caffeine seem to be lost. From another perspective, performance is generally enhanced and immunodepression is no different to placebo conditions, which may be viewed as a beneficial effect (i.e. more work/better performance is achieved for the same amount of immunodepression).

Nutritional 'immune-enhancing' supplements

As is the case with any kind of supplement, athletes should always be aware of the potential risk of contamination with banned substances and exercise caution. There are a number of products that are claimed to enhance the immune system and provide protection for athletes. However, evidence for the vast majority of these 'immune-enhancing' supplements is often limited. That said, there are a few apparent immune-enhancing substances for which there is growing evidence for beneficial effects, including echinacea, bovine colostrum and probiotics.

Echinacea

Echinacea is a genus of plant species (coneflower) indigenous to North America. There are a number of variations within the genus but the most commonly used (in immune intervention studies) is *Echinacea purpurea* (purple coneflower). A number of derivatives have been isolated for human consumption (such as pressed juice, plant extracts). Early (non-exercise) studies have suggested that supplementation with echinacea can have some beneficial effects on the incidence (or duration) of symptoms of URTI, although there is still some disagreement in the literature. However, a recent meta-analysis did show that echinacea can reduce the incidence of common cold by over 50% and can significantly reduce the duration of infection, in those that did become infected. This has led to some interest in the exercise immunology literature, investigating whether this supplement is effective at reducing exercise-induced immunodepression and/or incidence of URTI although there are relatively few conclusive studies. Echinacea has been shown to have 'stimulatory' effects on some aspects of immunity (i.e. phagocytic cells, NK cells, IgA output). One study found that a commercial echinacea product taken daily for 28 days (compared with a placebo) reduced the decrease of sIgA concentration and secretion caused by an acute bout of strenuous exercise, i.e. three repeated Wingate anaerobic (30-s maximal sprint) tests. This did not reduce the incidence of self-reported URTI episodes, although the average duration that symptoms persisted was shorter in the group receiving echinacea (~3 days) compared with the group receiving placebo (~9 days). However, the mechanisms for any beneficial effects are unclear at present but may be related to bioactive compounds of the plant, such as caffeic acids and derivatives (e.g. phenolic compounds), flavonoids and alkamines.

Bovine colostrum

Bovine colostrum ('early milk') is the initial milk from cows after birthing (usually obtained within the first 48 hours). Like normal milk, it is a rich source of

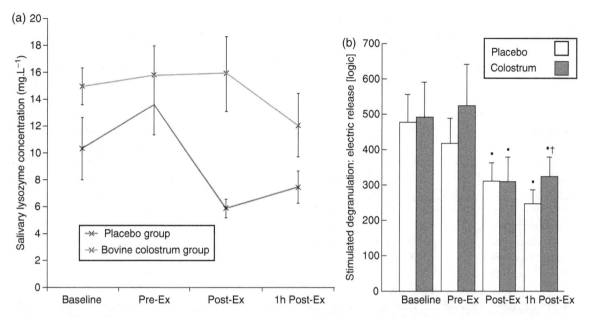

Figure 21.9 Effects of bovine colostrum supplementation on innate immune markers before and after prolonged exercise. In this study subjects either consumed bovine colostrum (20 g/day) or a placebo for 28 days before undertaking a prolonged (2 hours) exercise bout. The exercise-induced decrease in salivary lysozyme concentration (a) was blunted in the bovine colostrum group (a similar pattern was evident for lysozyme secretion rate, not shown here). Exercise caused a similar decrease in neutrophil function (b) in both groups but it appeared to recover more quickly in the bovine colostrum group. There were no other differences between placebo and colostrum groups in measured stress responses that are known to affect the immune system, suggesting that the beneficial effects observed with bovine colostrum were due to direct effects on the immune system. (Data from Davison & Diment 2010, with permission from Cambridge University Press.)

nutrition, in terms of both macronutrients and micronutrients but is also abundant in bioactive components with significant roles within the immune system (such as immunoglobulins and antimicrobial proteins). It is of obvious importance for protection against infection for newborn calves and there is growing interest in this dairy product as a potential dietary supplement to counteract immunodepression in athletes. It has been shown to reduce the incidence of self-reported URTI symptoms in athletes, which may be related to the enhancing effects that have been observed, for a variety of immune functions, at rest and/or in response to exercise. For example, bovine colostrum has been shown to enhance the humoral immune response to vaccination and modulate cell-mediated immunity. It has also been shown to increase salivary IgA concentration. Also, a few very recent studies (Figure 21.9) have observed that bovine colostrum intake can enhance aspects of innate and/or mucosal immunity at rest and in response to prolonged exercise or intensified training. The underlying mechanisms responsible for such immune-enhancing effects of colostrum are not

completely clear at present, although preliminary evidence suggests that some of the bioactive compounds directly stimulate and prime key aspects of immunity. Bovine colostrum has also been consistently shown, in a number of well-controlled studies, to prevent increases in gut permeability induced by drugs and stress (including exercise and/or heat stress), which may assist in innate protection by direct effects on the gut and gut epithelia.

Probiotics

Supplementation with probiotics is able to modulate the intestinal microbial flora and may enhance gut immune function (including effects on gut barrier functions). As the gut microbial flora is able to interact with intestinal epithelial cells and a number of specific immune cells, this can exert beneficial effects on the skin and upper respiratory tract, which could have important implications for athletes in heavy training. Unfortunately, there are not many studies on the effects of probiotic supplementation on aspects of immunity in athletes at present. Theoretically, beneficial effects on the gut may be beneficial to host immune defences. Although probiotic supplementation is considered to be a promising practical strategy for enhancing and maintaining intestinal immunity in athletes, further research is required to explore its usefulness in a sport and exercise context.

21.5 Potential immune monitoring in athletes

At present, there are no known immune biomarkers that can conclusively predict infection risk or underperformance in athletes. Although many guidelines have been offered to help preserve immunity in athletes during training and competition, many are based on anecdotes and speculation. Nevertheless, there are many immune system variables that are known to change as a result of high-volume training and which have been linked with compromised immunity and URTI in athletes. These could serve as immune system biomarkers to monitor immune risk in athletes, which could allow an early intervention countermeasure to be put in place and potentially mitigate the risk of subsequent clinical infections. For instance, detecting evidence of latent viral shedding (e.g. EBV, VZV or CMV) in blood or saliva might indicate a weakened immune system and increased susceptibility to infection. Increases in the plasma levels of CRP could indicate that the athlete has a bacterial infection, although CRP can also be elevated as a result of inflammation associated with exercise-induced muscle damage. In terms of cellular markers, elevated neutrophil counts and/or low lymphocyte counts might highlight inadequate recovery from a previous training session or a current immune response to an infection. An inverted T-cell CD4$^+$/CD8$^+$ ratio is also indicative of impaired immunity and elevated infection risk, while the presence of activation markers on the surface of T-cells (i.e. CD69) might indicate that there is an active viral infection. Elevated monocyte counts might be indicative of a chronic infection or low-level inflammation, while increased numbers of eosinophils suggest an allergic reaction such as asthma or hay fever. In addition, blood sampling is a useful technique for identifying deficiencies in certain micronutrients that could compromise immunity and inhibit athletic performance.

While blood samples are useful for obtaining the more sophisticated measures of the immune system, it is not always practical to take frequent blood samples, as these techniques are invasive and inconvenient for athletes. More and more researchers are investigating the use of saliva to monitor changes in the immune system in athletes. For instance, immunoglobulins and a number of antimicrobial proteins can be detected in saliva, as can viral shedding, all of which may be useful markers as discussed above. However, immune biomarkers are costly and often require a degree of expertise and specialised equipment, which is not always practical. It is also important to create a profile of the individual athlete using as many of the available techniques as possible. Identifying a 'normal' profile for an individual athlete, in conjunction with available normative values, will be useful for future monitoring. In addition to biomarkers, training diaries, mood states, sleep patterns, diet logs, exercising (and resting) heart rate and performance will all help to identify if an athlete does not match up to their normal profile and might be at risk of subsequent infection.

21.6 Summary and future directions

It is generally accepted that the prevalence of infections (especially of the upper respiratory tract) is higher in athletes and individuals involved in heavy training programmes and/or prolonged bouts of exercise. This is likely related, at least in part, to exercise-induced changes in immune system functions presenting 'open windows' for opportunistic infection (or viral reactivation). It is known that nutrition has a significant role in maintaining optimal immune functions and that certain nutritional interventions can influence the immune response to exercise, potentially impacting exercise-induced immunodepression. In general, it can be said that athletes are able to minimise their risk of immune disruption and potentially infection if they consume a healthy and balanced diet that is sufficient in total energy and macronutrient and micronutrient intake. However, it is important to remember that there is, at present, no known immune biomarkers that can conclusively predict infection risk in athletes. So whilst a great deal of sport and exercise immunology research has demonstrated the role of various nutritional practices and strategies in modulating exercise-induced immune changes, the clinical relevance of this to athlete infection risk remains to be fully determined. Hence, key future directions in this area should identify which interventions are best able to offer protection against exercise (and other stressor)-induced alterations in 'clinically' relevant outcomes, such as infections caused by external pathogens but also latent reactivating infections. In summary, although it is difficult to provide any clear recommendations at this time due to the lack of scientific evidence, it appears that, at the very least, athletes should aim to eat a well-balanced diet during periods of heavy training and competition. It is particularly important that athletes, especially those partaking in endurance-based training, maintain adequate amounts of CHO in the diet. The immunodepressive effects of exercise are more pronounced during periods of glycogen depletion, indicating that athletes lacking in appropriate CHO stores will be at increased risk of immune impairment. The use of certain supplements might benefit athletes with a known nutritional deficiency; however, there is little scientific evidence supporting the use of many so-called immune-enhancing supplements at preventing exercise-induced immunodepression. More research is urgently required to investigate the impact of certain supplements at attenuating the immunodepressive effects of acute exercise before further recommendations can be given to coaches and athletes.

Further reading

Albers R, Antoine JM, Bourdet-Sicard R et al. Markers to measure immunomodulation in human nutrition intervention studies. Br J Nutr 2005; 94: 452–481.

Bals R. Epithelial antimicrobial peptides in host defence against infection. Respir Res 2000; 1: 141–150.

Bishop NC, Blannin AK, Walsh NP, Robson PJ, Gleeson M. Nutritional aspects of immunosuppression in athletes. Sports Med 1999; 28: 151–176.

Bishop NC, Gleeson M, Nicholas CW, Ali A. Influence of carbohydrate supplementation on plasma cytokine and neutrophil degranulation responses to high intensity intermittent exercise. Int J Sport Nutr Exerc Metab 2002; 12: 145–156.

Close GL, Ashton T, Cable T et al. Ascorbic acid supplementation does not attenuate post-exercise muscle soreness following muscle-damaging exercise but may delay the recovery process. Br J Nutr 2006; 95: 976–981.

Davison G, Diment BC. Bovine colostrum supplementation attenuates the decrease of salivary lysozyme and enhances the recovery of neutrophil function after prolonged exercise. Br J Nutr 2010; 103: 1425–1432.

Fischer CP, Hiscock NJ, Penkowa M et al. Supplementation with vitamins C and E inhibits the release of interleukin-6 from contracting human skeletal muscle. J Physiol 2004; 558: 633–645.

Gleeson M (ed.). Immune Function in Sport and Exercise. London: Elsevier, 2006.

Gleeson M. Immune function in sport and exercise. J Appl Physiol 2007; 103: 693–699.

Gleeson M, Pyne DB. Special feature for the Olympics: effects of exercise on the immune system: exercise effects on mucosal immunity. Immunol Cell Biol 2000; 78: 536–544.

Gleeson M, Pyne DB, Austin JP et al. Epstein–Barr virus reactivation and upper-respiratory illness in elite swimmers. Med Sci Sports Exerc 2002; 34: 411–417.

Gleeson M, Nieman DC, Pedersen BK. Exercise, nutrition and immune function. J Sports Sci 2004; 22: 115–125.

Malm C. Susceptibility to infections in elite athletes: the S-curve. Scand J Med Sci Sports 2006; 16: 4–6.

Maughan RJ. Contamination of dietary supplements and positive drug tests in sport. J Sports Sci 2005; 23: 883–889.

Nieman DC. Exercise, upper respiratory tract infection, and the immune system. Med Sci Sports Exerc 1994; 26: 128–139.

Nieman DC, Bishop NC. Nutritional strategies to counter stress to the immune system in athletes, with special reference to football. Sports Sci 2006; 24: 763–772.

Nieman DC, Henson DA, Gross SJ et al. Quercetin reduces illness but not immune perturbations after intensive exercise. Med Sci Sports Exerc 2007; 39: 1561–1569.

Niess AM, Dickhuth HH, Northoff H, Fehrenbach E. Free radicals and oxidative stress in exercise: immunological aspects. Exerc Immunol Rev 1999; 5: 22–56.

Pedersen BK, Hoffman-Goetz L. Exercise and the immune system: regulation, integration, and adaptation. Physiol Rev 2000; 80: 1055–1081.

Pedersen BK, Ullum H. NK cell response to physical activity: possible mechanisms of action. Med Sci Sports Exerc 1994; 26: 140–146.

Peters EM, Goetzsche JM, Grobbelaar B, Noakes TD. Vitamin C supplementation reduces the incidence of post-race symptoms of upper respiratory tract infection in ultramarathon runners. Am J Clin Nutr 1993; 57: 170–174.

West NP, Pyne DB, Renshaw G, Cripps AW. Antimicrobial peptides and proteins, exercise and innate mucosal immunity. FEMS Immunol Med Microbiol 2006; 48: 293–304.

West NP, Pyne DB, Kyd JM, Renshaw GM, Fricker PA, Cripps AW. The effect of exercise on innate mucosal immunity. Br J Sports Med 2010; 44: 227–231.

22
Travel

Bronwen Lundy and Elizabeth Broad

Key messages

- Planning is the key to success when it comes to travel. Troubleshooting on arrival is important but most problem areas require safeguarding before departure.
- Use key people within the support team to help manage nutrition issues if you will not be travelling with the team.
- There are many distractions during travel and it often occurs at key times such as competition or important training periods. The team nutritionist can act as a reminder to athletes to keep them focused on the areas that could most impact on performance e.g. hydration, food safety.

- Long-haul flights and jet lag can interfere with hydration, digestion and appetite. Be aware which types of trips are most likely to cause problems and plan for this prior to departure.
- Travellers' diarrhoea is common during travel to certain destinations. Whilst not completely protective it would seem wise to warn athletes about high-risk foods and drinks to avoid and to discuss the possibility of using a probiotic or combined prebiotic/probiotic preparation in the lead up to and during travel to high-risk countries.

22.1 Introduction

Travel is inevitable at some time in any athlete's career, and can be a regular, even weekly, occurrence for some. Any form of travel which removes athletes from their home environment can result in discomfort and fatigue, and influence their ability to train and perform to their optimum if not managed well. This chapter outlines key issues athletes face when travelling to either train or compete, and ways to manage this more effectively.

The support of a sports nutrition professional in an athlete's travel management requires research and preparation. The sports nutrition professional needs to understand the needs of the athlete, including factors such as age, gender, type of sport, whether travelling for competition and/or training, experience with travelling, and any specific nutritional needs (e.g. food allergies/intolerances, vegetarian). This information must then be matched with an understanding of where athletes are travelling to,

what the method of travel is, and how they will access food when away.

22.2 Travel planning

Any travel undertaken by athletes requires research in advance. Athletes can be guided in the process or it may be the responsibility of the sports nutrition professional to undertake this on their behalf (such as in a team environment). It is likely this will require communication with the team manager (or similar) in order to determine logistics such as timing, travel mode(s) and accommodation. Recommendations can then be prepared in writing and presented to team staff and/or athletes. Examples of the planning which may be required include the following.

- Eating logistics. Are the athletes to be self-catering, catered for in one location all the time (such as a hotel), given an allowance and allowed to choose for themselves, or will they eat at a range of venues?

Sport and Exercise Nutrition, First Edition. Edited by Susan A Lanham-New, Samantha J Stear, Susan M Shirreffs and Adam L Collins.
© 2011 The Nutrition Society. Published 2011 by Blackwell Publishing Ltd.

- Are there volunteers or food service professionals catering for the athletes? Guidelines for feeding athletes should always be offered, especially where there are specific needs, likes/dislikes or allergies/intolerances which need to be catered for. Many hotels will treat athletes like any guest, and hence the food served can be higher in fat, lower in carbohydrate (CHO), and smaller in serve sizes than is preferred.
- Climate. Hotter and more humid climates, and increases in altitude, will require additional fluids to ensure athletes maintain hydration. Making athletes familiar with the impact of climate changes on their sweat losses and daily fluid needs prior to departure is important (see Chapter 7).
- Location and type of supermarkets or food outlets should be investigated. This is particularly important where athletes are self-catering, or require 'top-up' snacks to be purchased. In many countries, the variety of foods and/or the opening hours of supermarkets are not the same as in the UK.
- If the athlete is travelling outside the UK, what are the food customs of the destination country? Many countries have their main meal at lunch and a late supper. It can create difficulty for an athlete to eat out at restaurants if they do not open until after 8 pm, or to find a suitable lunch if the whole area shuts for a 2-hour siesta at lunch time.
- What is the food culture in the destination? The traditional food preferences may not suit the athletes. For example, many countries eat minimal cereal at breakfast, and do not have a large variety of cereals available, making it useful for athletes to carry breakfast cereals individually. Similarly, traditional foods may appear spicy, bland, repetitive or simply inedible by athletes who have not travelled previously.
- Where athletes are competing at large events, the catering at the hotel and/or the venue may be for all teams and modifications may not be possible. In these instances, the athlete and staff should be provided with as much information as possible and a range of strategies they can employ to ensure nutritional requirements continue to be met. This may include taking some of their own food.
- What are the customs regulations of the country the athletes are travelling to? This is important if athletes are relying on certain food items brought from home.

Short-duration travel (bus, car, train, short plane trips)

Travelling over short distances may not appear as complex as long-haul travel, but can still result in inappropriate food choices. Planning remains important to ensure adequate amounts of suitable fluids are available (such as water) to maintain adequate hydration throughout the trip. Useful foods to pack include sandwiches, fresh fruit, yoghurts and cereal bars so that athletes are less likely to opt for inappropriate foods such as chocolate, confectionary and potato crisps en route.

Long-haul flights

Watches should be set to local time at destination as soon as possible after boarding a long-haul flight so that sleep and eating times can be adjusted to the new destination. Athletes are advised to plan sleep or naps to coincide with night time at the new destination, and to keep themselves awake at other times. Taking a range of activities that can aid wakefulness, such as reading material, board or card games or music, is recommended as there can be times when the in-flight entertainment is restricted or not working. Ear plugs, eye masks and loose-fitting clothing are useful for supporting effective sleep during long-haul flights.

Meals are generally served around 1 hour after take-off and 2 hours before landing on long-haul flights, with snacks generally being made available between meal services. Athletes can choose to pre-order a special meal for flights (e.g. vegetarian, low fat) which are generally served first. Alternatively, athletes are encouraged to choose the healthier option. Athletes should also take their own snacks on flights, including fresh fruit, dried fruit and nut mixes and muesli bars, since meal serve sizes tend to be small and are padded out with energy-dense 'extras'. It is important for athletes to plan regular fluid intake to counteract the dryer air, choosing water as the primary source (working on 250 ml of fluid per hour of flight) and avoiding alcohol. Passengers are restricted in taking fluids through security for international flights, although most boarding lounges have drinking water dispensers so athletes are encouraged to take empty water bottles with them which they can fill in the boarding gate to take on board. Empty bottles can then be refilled once on board to ensure adequate fluid intake and prevention of dehydration during the flight.

Avoidance of deep-vein thrombosis (DVT) is critical during long-haul flights. The risk of DVT is increased with duration of periods of inactivity, and subsequent pooling of blood in the legs. It is recommended that athletes and support staff move around the plane periodically during the journey, and undertake light stretching every 2 hours or so. Compression socks are also recommended for this purpose. Maintaining hydration levels during the flight will also encourage the need to move around in order to go to the bathroom. It is recommended athletes choose aisle or exit-row seats to enable greater freedom of movement.

Jet lag

Jet lag refers to the feelings of disorientation, reduced alertness, poor psychomotor coordination, light-headedness, impatience, lack of energy, loss of appetite, difficulty sleeping at night yet tired during the day, altered bowel function, reduced motivation and general discomfort that follow travelling across time zones and can persist for several days. This does not include fatigue or stiffness from travel northwards or southwards within the same time zone, but rather travel eastwards or westwards. Eastward travel tends to cause difficulty in falling asleep, while westward travel usually interferes with sleep maintenance. Whilst arousal and alertness can adapt more rapidly, it takes about 1 day for each time zone crossed for body temperature, upon which many performance and physical factors are based, to adapt completely. It is during this period of desynchronisation between body temperature and arousal that physical performance may be below normal. The impact is equally problematic in support personnel as it is in athletes. The readjustment period can be influenced by the direction of travel, being faster with westward travel than with eastward travel, unless a full 12-hour time difference is achieved. Melatonin, a natural hormone released by the body, is a key influence on the biological clock. Numerous studies have investigated the use of exogenous melatonin supplementation on speeding adaptation to a new time zone. In general, melatonin works opposite to light exposure: melatonin in the evening can advance circadian rhythms to earlier, which is useful for eastward flight adjustments.

Factors which can speed adaptation to training/competing in a new time zone include the following.

- Adjustment of daily patterns (such as sleeping, eating and exercising) to the new environment as soon as possible (even prior to departure, or at least on the trip).
- Avoid napping, especially at times which correlate with normal sleep times at home/place of origin, since this acts to anchor circadian rhythms to their former phase.
- Exposing athletes to daylight as this inhibits melatonin and is the key signal that helps readjust the body clock to the new environment. Exposure to light in the morning can advance circadian rhythms to earlier, which aids the shift across time zones going eastward. Exposure to light later in the day delays circadian rhythms to later, which aids the shift in time zones going west. Tables of appropriate times for sunlight exposure have been developed (Table 22.1).
- The use of melatonin supplementation should be discussed with a sports physician prior to departure. If used, ensure it is taken at the most appropriate time: in the evening for eastward flight, in the morning for westward flight.
- Retiring to bed earlier than normal in the first few days after westward flight to help speed the phase delay in circadian rhythm.
- Exercising more in the evening than the morning after eastward flight.
- If travelling across multiple time zones (more than 10-hour time difference), some athletes prefer an overnight stopover during the journey to help with the shift.
- Choosing flights with a later rather than earlier arrival time at the destination where possible so that athletes have the opportunity to take a full sleep at night in the new time zone sooner after arrival.
- Developing a personal strategy for coping with jet lag.
- If travelling for competition, start training at the time of day that the upcoming competition will occur as soon as practical.

Circadian rhythm has been shown to influence performance. Performance in many sprint and strength-related competitive events is generally greater in the late afternoon/early evening than in the

Table 22.1 Recommendations for the use of bright light to adjust body clock after time-zone transitions.

	Bad local times for exposure to light	Good local times for exposure to light
Time zones to the west		
3	0200–0800[a]	1800–0000[b]
4	0100–0700[a]	1700–2300[b]
5	0000–0600[a]	1600–2200[b]
6	2300–0500[a]	1500–2100[b]
7	2200–0400[a]	1400–2000[b]
8	2100–0300[a]	1300–1900[b]
9	2000–0200[a]	1200–1800[b]
10	1900–0100[a]	1100–1700[b]
11	1800–0000[a]	1000–1600[b]
12	1700–2300[a]	0900–1500[b]
13	1600–2200[a]	0800–1400[b]
14	1500–2100[a]	0700–1300[b]
Time zones to the east		
3	0000–0600[b]	0800–1400[a]
4	0100–0700[b]	0900–1500[a]
5	0200–0800[b]	1000–1600[a]
6	0300–0900[b]	1100–1700[a]
7	0400–1000[b]	1200–1800[a]
8	0500–1100[b]	1300–1900[a]
9	0600–1200[b]	1400–2000[a]
10	Can be treated as 14 hours to the west[c]	
11	Can be treated as 13 hours to the west[c]	
12	Can be treated as 12 hours to the west[c]	

[a] Promotion of a phase advance of the body clock.
[b] Promotion of a phase delay of the body clock.
[c] Body clock adjusts to large delays more easily than to large advances.
This table is based on a T_{min} of 0400; other values for T_{min} would need the times to be adjusted accordingly. For example, an individual with a T_{min} at 0600 should, after a journey across three time zones to the west (see row 1), avoid light at 0400–1000 and seek it at 2000–0200.
Reprinted from Waterhouse *et al.* 2007, copyright © 2007 with permission from Elsevier.

morning, generally coinciding with the peak in body temperature. Hence, when travelling across time zones to compete, it is important to assess what time of day the competition is to be staged when deciding how many days to leave prior to competition, as well as the impact of the travel duration and mode itself.

Caffeine can be considered for use in order to provide temporary relief of fatigue, but should be avoided in the late afternoon/evening where onset of sleep early in the evening is important. Some research has been undertaken regarding the manipulation of macronutrient content of meals (e.g. CHO, protein) to improve sleep onset and maintenance, although this has not been undertaken with specific reference to jet lag. There is some evidence to suggest that the CHO content of a meal can impact on the onset of

sleep since the presence of insulin allows the amino acid tryptophan a competitive advantage in crossing the blood–brain barrier for its conversion to serotonin. In essence, it is useful to encourage athletes to consume an evening meal containing CHO in order to aid sleep onset as well as ensure adequate glycogen stores.

22.3 Meal service options when travelling

Many athletes find it challenging to adapt to a different supply of food from their home environment. There are many ways athletes, teams and staff can manage food access when travelling, all of which have benefits and problems associated with them. Team staff should always consider the range of options available and what is likely to suit the athletes the most when deciding on meal options for travel. The sports nutritionist's role becomes very important in educating athletes and staff, and potentially the food service providers, as to appropriate meal service for athletes and issues around food safety. If the sports nutritionist cannot be present on the trip, then it is also important that this individual trains another staff member to understand how to manage any issues which arise.

Restaurant/buffet/large dining hall

Hotels usually cater for people on holiday or business, rather than for athletes. There are several methods the sports nutrition professional can utilise when working with hotels/restaurants. Whichever one is used, it is important to make requests early to enable time for chefs to understand your needs, to negotiate suitable menus, and to order in specific food items. It is also important to recognise the food budget of the group, and ensure that the methods of food provision, the scope of the menu and the types of foods provided are aligned with this budget. It can also be useful to ask that the athletes are seated in a separate area, away from other guests. The sports nutrition professional may even supply specific recipes to support the request.

(1) Send the restaurant/dining hall guidelines on catering for athletes, including examples of suitable foods they could serve, serving sizes and methods of serving. Then request the chefs to put together a menu based around these guidelines, which can then be checked to ensure suitability and altered if necessary. If this is the case, it is important to recognise the cultural differences between countries and adapt the recommendations.

(2) Request a standard menu from the restaurant/hotel and set a menu for the team/athletes from this. It may be possible to add some different items or request adjustments to the menu (e.g. to reduce the fat content or increase the CHO content).

(3) Send the restaurant/hotel/dining hall a specific menu for them to follow. This can be suitable when athletes travel within their own home country and the foods will be very recognisable. This may be particularly important for the

pre-competition meals, where familiarity is very important.

(4) If athletes are eating as a large group where plated meals are the preferred serving option over a buffet, it can be useful to arrange a way of pre-ordering the meal so that the food is ready to serve as soon as the group arrives. Offering an abbreviated menu (three or four options) can be useful, and make sure a record is kept of the order to prevent confusion when the meals are served. Bread, salad and water can be placed on the table in bulk. This prevents delays in ordering and cooking, especially in a busy restaurant, and ensures that the meal service is prompt and efficient.

Common traps

- There are times when restaurants/hotels fail to respond to any requests. In this situation, it is important to have a member of staff travelling with the team who understands how to manage complications that may arise and who will be able to implement an alternative plan in case the messages have not been understood.
- Hotels/restaurants may interpret guidelines differently so that, for example, a meal may be served which tastes and looks different than intended (such as a 'stir fry'). This can be the case in different languages and cultures. If the sports nutrition professional is not travelling with the team, a staff member should be trained in ways to manage these situations if they occur, recognising that the meals may still fall within the guidelines provided and may therefore be suitable.
- For larger teams, it may be necessary to also request snack items to be available in a 'team room' for mid-meal snacks, especially when the athletes' energy requirements are high. Examples of foods which could be included are fresh fruit, yoghurts, toast and spreads, and low-fat muffins/cakes. It is important that the foods chosen will create minimal mess and to ensure that athletes are aware of their personal responsibility for keeping this food area clean and tidy.

Self-catering

When athletes are travelling for extended periods of time and/or in smaller groups, it can be useful to consider self-catering as a means of obtaining meals. This can be a more economical means of travelling. Many countries offer self-contained units or apartments that can be very suitable, and it is often a preferred catering choice. The sports nutrition professional can assist athletes and support staff by ensuring that all athletes are capable of cooking at least a few simple recipes using ingredients that are easy to find in the location they will be travelling to, by researching accessibility to food stores and by investigating the actual cooking facilities available. This may not be a suitable option for younger athletes unless there is sufficient willing staff to supervise meal preparation.

Common traps

- Cooking and food storage facilities in some small hotel/motel units can be quite limited. They may have no oven, only one or two cookers, a very small refrigerator and a limited range of cooking utensils. In these situations, practical cooking sessions may need to be organised well in advance, and a range of suitable recipes should be provided which allow for such limitations yet still enable variety in choices.
- If athletes are only staying for short periods in one location, consider recipes that ensure minimal wastage, for example incorporating condiments and dry ingredients. A short menu cycle could be developed for athletes which reuses ingredients, or arrange sharing of ingredients between athletes in larger groups.
- It is important to ensure that food stores are within walking distance of accommodation, otherwise private or public transport will be necessary and the cost of this factored in.

Larger-scale dining halls

At large competitions (e.g. Olympic or Commonwealth Games, and some world championships), athletes access the majority of their meals from large-scale dining halls. It is unlikely that single nations will have any mechanism of input into the menu plans for such events since they are catered for by large-scale catering companies. However, there is usually information that can be made available, as in most instances there has been input to the menu through the International Olympic Committee or contracted by the catering company. The sports nutrition professional can then provide advice to their athletes via a newssheet or other means as to how the meal service will operate.

Meal allowances

Some athletes and teams will operate on a meal allowance rather than any pre-organised meal provisions when travelling. This leaves the meal choice up to the individual athlete, and usually means they are reliant on cafés, take-aways, restaurants and/or supermarkets/markets for their daily food needs. In this situation, it is important to educate athletes in advance regarding suitable food choices in restaurants and take-aways, food and fluid safety, and the importance of their meal plans and goals so that they do not compromise their diet in order to save money. It may also be worthwhile suggesting the group organise some team functions/meals, especially the night prior to any competition which can then be organised in advance to suit pre-competition nutrition goals.

Examples of foods, food alternatives and utensils which may be useful to send/take with the athletes include:

- cereal bars;
- breakfast cereal;
- powdered milk;
- dried fruit and nuts;
- quick cook rice/noodles;
- liquid meal supplement powders (such as Complan);
- sports drink powder;
- canned beans, tuna and/or soup if baggage weight is not of concern;
- sports bars and gels;
- special products for allergies (such as gluten-free pasta and/or flour);
- bowls/spoons;
- kettle.

22.4 Typical nutrition issues during travel

- Lack of variety in meals and food types at home makes it more difficult when athletes travel as they find it more difficult to choose a meal they will enjoy. It is important for athletes to familiarise themselves with different food styles prior to travelling.

- Reduced access to fresh fruit and vegetables. Where possible, find a local supermarket or market place to replenish fresh fruit supplies as mid-meal snacks. Reinforce the need for lightly cooked vegetables (without butter/oil) and salads (dressing on the side) to be served with meals in restaurants/buffets.
- Being fed three meals a day in a hotel generally means mid-meal snacks are not readily available. Individual athletes and teams should have a plan for ensuring availability of mid-meal snacks.
- Availability of sports foods. Many countries do not have a wide range of sports drinks/foods available. These may need to be sourced from the home environment and taken with the team/individual. As baggage allowances become tighter and customs checks more stringent at borders, it becomes more expensive and difficult to send products internationally to cover extended travel. Hence, sourcing of products in the local country may be required in advance or suitable food-based alternatives found.
- Food allergies/intolerances can be more difficult to cater for in foreign countries. An interpreter may be required in order to ensure suitable foods are available.
- Eating at 'all you can eat' buffets and athlete dining halls can create many issues, ranging from under-eating (e.g. athletes overwhelmed by choice and/or not willing to try new foods) to over-eating (e.g. taking a taste of everything and hence over-filling the plate, eating hot meals at lunch and dinner rather than once a day, losing focus on individual nutrition goals and being influenced by what other athletes might be eating). Athletes and staff should be educated in advance on ways to avoid these problems.
- Boredom eating. Generally athletes have fewer distractions, such as work, study, friends and family, when they travel. It is important to consider ways of constructively filling this time (DVDs, internet, study) so that athletes are less likely to eat more than they need to fill their time.

22.5 Travel-associated illness

Travel exposes individuals to a range of new pathogens at the same time as defences may be weakened by factors such as lack of sleep, dry air and contact with large numbers of people in confined spaces such as on trains, buses and aeroplanes. Illnesses may range from the minor (e.g. upper respiratory tract infections) to the inconvenient and unpleasant (e.g. travellers' diarrhoea) to the serious (e.g. hepatitis C or malaria). All serious risks should be discussed with the team doctor or a travel clinic in order that appropriate precautions can be arranged. Travellers' diarrhoea (TD) is often associated with diet so will be discussed in greater detail here.

Travellers' diarrhoea

While not usually a severe illness, TD can be very problematic to athletes, causing disruption to training and competition. It is defined as three or more unformed bowel movements occurring within 24 hours and accompanied by other symptoms, most often cramps, nausea, blood in stools and vomiting. The illness is usually self-limited and responds well to antibiotics. The pathogens responsible are wide-ranging and may be multiple, but the most common are *Campylobacter*, *Salmonella*, *Escherichia coli* and *Shigella* species. Food is the major carrier of these infective agents in TD and much of the advice surrounding prevention focus on avoiding high-risk items. TD is most common when travelling to developing countries and may affect more than 60% of visitors. The highest risk, defined as 20–90% incidence of TD per 2-week stay, exists when travelling to Africa, South America and Asia while there is moderate risk in southern Europe and a relatively low risk in northern Europe. While it mostly resolves within 4 days, some individuals may have problems for weeks and there is some evidence that some may go on to develop irritable bowel syndrome. One day of incapacitation is typical and even this could be critical to an athlete's performance. Staying in expensive accommodation does not seem to be protective, with studies showing that five-star hotels have a higher rate of infection than three- or four-star hotels, possibly due to the greater handling of the food. Young adults also appear to have a higher incidence of infection than older adults.

It does appear possible to develop immunity to the infective agents as studies have shown that longer stays in particular regions lower the incidence of infection. Greater risks appear to be associated with lack of avoidance of high-risk foods and with eating in cafeterias or from street vendors.

Table 22.2 Foods and beverages in tropical and semi-tropical areas with expected travellers' diarrhoea risk.

Generally safe
Foods and beverages served steaming hot (>59°C)
Bottles of carbonated drinks including soft drinks and beer
Bottled water with intact seal apparent on opening
Syrups, jellies, jams, honey
Fruits that are peeled
Dry items such as bread and rolls
Any foods carefully prepared in one's own apartment or hotel

Often safe
Tortillas and breads or toast containing butter or sauces
Fruit juices which may have been augmented with tap water
Use of tap water to rinse mouth and toothbrush without swallowing it
Foods served on aeroplanes in developing regions
Few ice cubes

Often unsafe
Fruits and vegetables with intact skins: berries, tomatoes
Hot sauces on tabletop, unpasteurised milk
Moist foods served at room temperature including vegetables and meats
Any food served buffet-style that is maintained at room temperature
Tap water even in hotels claiming filtration systems
Large quantities of ice
Hamburgers not served hot or at fast food restaurants with rapid turnover of prepared hamburgers (hamburger toppings are a major concern in these areas)

From Dupont 2008. Republished with kind permission from Wiley-Blackwell.

Possible preventive measures
Prophylactic antibiotics
These may provide up to 60% protection from TD but present other problems, such as adverse side effects, development of antibiotic-resistant strains, frequency of use required if athletes often travel to high-risk countries, and limitations on what can be taken based on the anti-doping code.

'Boil it, cook it, peel it or forget it'
Several studies have shown that traditional advice regarding food choices does not appear to lower the rate of TD and it may be more related to wider factors such as hygiene when preparing food or appropriate food storage; in addition, pathogens may be so widespread that this advice becomes ineffective. However, it does appear to be common sense to continue to avoid foods known to be high risk and these are described in Table 22.2.

Probiotics
Probiotics have recently received much research attention for their role in minimising infective

diarrhoea. Probiotics have been defined as microbial cell preparations, or components of microbial cells that have a beneficial effect on the health and well-being of the host. The hypothesis behind their protective role in TD is that stress, jet lag and unfamiliar food and water can alter the body's normal bacterial flora and leave it more open to infection. Probiotics could potentially supplement the protective bacteria (bifido-bacteria and lactobacilli) and reduce the risk of infection by competing with disease-causing bacteria for colonisation.

A meta-analysis of the use of probiotics for the prevention of TD found 12 studies undertaken between 1977 and 2005, the analysis showing that probiotics significantly prevented TD (RR 0.85, 95% CI 0.79–0.91; $P < 0.001$). The most effective strains were identified as *Saccharomyces boulardii*, *Lactobacillus acidophilus* and *Bifidobacterium bifidum*. No serious adverse effects were noted, and a very small number reported abdominal cramping. It is worth considering the limitation of this analysis, namely that the study pooled results of different probiotic strains and infection type, which may understate the benefit of some strains and overstate the benefit of others. In addition to preventing TD, probiotics appear to reduce the severity of infection. The main finding of the Cochrane review into probiotics and acute diarrhoea was that the duration of diarrhoea was reduced when a probiotic preparation was taken.

Recent research shows promising signs that probiotics could reduce the incidence and severity of other illnesses such as upper respiratory tract infections in athletes and, while more research is needed, this is an area of interest for the future given the frequency of these in the athletic population and the impact that it can have on training and competition performance.

Prebiotics
Prebiotics are defined as non-digestible food ingredients that beneficially affect the host by selectively stimulating the growth and/or activity of one or more bacterial species in the colon, thereby improving host health. Inulin and oligofructose (also called fructo-oligosaccharide) are the best studied of the prebiotics and support the growth of bifido-bacteria and lactobacilli which have been linked with resistance to infection. The use of prebiotics for the prevention of TD has been less studied but may theoretically be more effective. Prebiotics act as fuel for the beneficial bacteria already in the colon, which

eliminates the issue of strain specificity required with probiotic supplementation. However, this does rely on the right mix of beneficial bacteria being present in the colon in the first place. Of the limited research available the signs are promising, with reductions in the presence of diarrhoea, symptom severity and duration but further investigation is required.

Personal hygiene

Naturally, one of the most important factors in preventing the spread of illness throughout a team is personal hygiene. All athletes should be encouraged to wash their hands with soap or an antiseptic hand wash prior to eating food, and the sharing of utensils (e.g. spoons, water bottles) should be actively avoided.

Dietary management

If athletes do suffer from a bout of diarrhoea or vomiting, in addition to seeing a doctor, they will need to make some adjustments to their diet until their symptoms have settled.

- Keep sipping fluids. Oral rehydration solutions (e.g. Dioralyte) help prevent dehydration due to their high sodium content. Other drink options include water, diluted juice or sports drinks.
- Eating small amounts of plain food frequently, or as tolerated. Plain low-fibre foods such as crackers, plain sweet biscuits, white bread, pasta, white rice, mashed potato or tinned fruit are usually the best tolerated.
- Once symptoms have settled and the athlete is eating a bit more, add some salty foods to help ensure that hydration status returns to normal as quickly as possible. Examples include soup and salty fillings on sandwiches or crackers such as Marmite, ham or cheese.
- While athletes are unwell, they should avoid excessive amounts of fruit juice as the fructose (fruit sugar) may worsen the diarrhoea. Similarly, caffeine can worsen symptoms during the acute phase of illness so tea, coffee and cola drinks are not the best option.
- While athletes are unwell and for a short period afterwards, they may need to avoid milk and other foods containing lactose (the natural sugar found in dairy products, such as yoghurt and milk-based products) as it may worsen diarrhoea and gut discomfort. Athletes should be able to return to eating

these foods within a week or two after the illness by gradually increasing their intake according to tolerance.

Athletes or staff who are unwell should be advised not to handle foods or prepare foods for others while sick as many infections can be passed on.

22.6 Acclimatisation

The process of travel often involves a change in climate and/or altitude, and in fact this is a frequently sought-after outcome for athletes and coaches. This change of environment requires a period of acclimatisation, in addition to managing the impact of jet lag. Hydration is one area of adaptation that may require special attention. Assessment of hydration status via body mass and urine specific gravity or urine colour assessment is recommended for at least the first few days after arrival at a new location in order to reinforce the need for athletes to assess the effectiveness of their acclimation strategies. Readers are referred to Chapter 25 for further advice regarding acclimatisation to different environmental conditions.

22.7 Key tips for travelling athletes

(1) Plan ahead. Know where you are going, how long the travel will take, what sort of food and fluid will be available and how you will access it.
(2) Research your destination. Find out, or ask someone, about food availability, source and hygiene and whether you have a choice.
(3) Organise which foods/fluids/snacks you will need to take with you from home, both for day-to-day use and also training/competition.
(4) For individuals with limited food variety trialling foods typical of the destination before departure may help reduce anxiety about food selection abroad, e.g. finding recipes or restaurants serving those foods.
(5) Have an individualised eating plan and stay focused on your nutrition goals. It is not a holiday!
(6) Treat large-scale buffets like you would at home: serve up *one* meal, rather than tasting a bit of everything.

Practice tips

- Keep records of travel venues for future reference.
- Use frequent travellers who are familiar with the destination to help delineate the right issues for the destination, e.g. team manager, senior athletes/team captain, head coach.
- There are many distractions during travel and it often occurs at key times such as competition or important training periods. The team nutritionist can act as a reminder to athletes to keep them focused on the areas that could most impact on performance, e.g. hydration, food safety.

Example of team travel nutrition guidelines to send to the team hotel

This example could be for a rugby team travelling for an away game within their own country. This might be sent off initially, followed up with a phone call and request for a copy of the planned menus for review. For athletes travelling on a lower budget, the guidelines could be shorter and less prescriptive.

General guidelines for the team

- Low-fat meals: low-fat cooking methods (minimal oil used in cooking, no deep frying), trimming visible fat off meat, removing skin from chicken (chicken breast is preferred), avoiding fatty/processed meats such as salami and sausages, avoiding crumbed or battered foods, avoiding cream or cheese-based sauces; use tomato-based sauces instead and always use low-fat dairy products where possible.
- Carbohydrate-based meals: always include a mixture of rice, pasta, cous cous, noodles or bread.
- Ready access to fluid: provision of jugs of water, juice and squash (regular and no added sugar, labelled) are required on tables at all meals.
- On the day before and the day of competition the players have some special needs. These are listed towards the end of this document.
- All meals to be provided as buffet style.

Breakfast (continental breakfast plus two hot options)

- An array of healthy breakfast cereals, e.g. [insert brand examples for country of visit] plus skimmed and semi-skimmed milks.
- A wide variety of sliced breads, English muffins (fork split) and crumpets plus spreads such as honey, jam (fruit spread), peanut butter. *No* pastries or croissants please.

- Fruit, including pre-sliced fresh fruit, tinned fruit, fruit compote, etc.
- Low-fat flavoured yoghurts, with plenty of variety in flavours.
- Fruit juice, water, tea and coffee.
- One egg item (e.g. poached eggs, scrambled eggs, omelette; each with minimal oil in cooking) or one hot carbohydrate option (e.g. baked beans or spaghetti, pancakes or French toast with maple syrup) to be rotated daily.
- One hot vegetable (e.g. grilled mushrooms, grilled tomatoes, stewed tomato and onion, spinach, creamed corn) to be rotated daily.

Please do *not* provide the following at any breakfast:

- bacon;
- sausages;
- pastries, muffins, croissants;
- hash browns.

Lunch (create your own roll bar plus one or two hot options)
Build your own salad bar

- A variety of fresh breads, bread rolls, individual foccacias, Turkish breads, etc.
- Pre-sliced salad vegetables including lettuce, cucumber, tomato, beetroot, carrot, onion, mushroom, avocado, asparagus, etc.
- Cold cuts of lean meats (low-fat options only). Examples might include ham off the bone, pastrami, corned beef, seasoned skinless chicken/turkey breast fillets, tuna (mixed with low-fat mayonnaise and/or other options like gherkins, etc.) or salmon. No processed or sausage meats please.
- Low-fat cheese slices (<15 g fat per 100 g cheese). For example [insert branded examples here for country of visit]. A few grated cheeses are also available with <15 g fat and are encouraged for use in pizzas, etc.
- Array of spreads, e.g. mustard, chutney, relish, low-fat mayonnaise (<10% fat).
- Sandwich presses for toasting rolls/sandwiches.

Alternate with one to two hot, quick items each day

- Skinless chicken breast and corn risotto with accompanying side of freshly stir fried Asian vegetables.
- Lean beef and vegetable skewers and plain rice.

- Thai fish cakes (baked, not fried) with baked potato wedges.
- Chilli beef and vegetable noodle stir-fry (minimal oil in cooking).
- Build your own burgers using skinless chicken breasts plus the pre-sliced salad vegetables as available above.
- Pizzas made with only small amounts of reduced fat cheese (<15 g/100 g), lean meat and vegetables.
- Low-fat chicken or beef lasagne (using 'diet' chicken mince, extra sheets of lasagne and low-fat cheese) and side salad (fat-free dressings on the side).
- Spiced chicken tenderloin wraps (e.g. chicken, onion, capsicum dish with flat breads, tomato salsa and shredded lettuce).
- Shaved lean roast meat rolls (must be fat trimmed) with low-fat gravy.
- Fish fingers (baked), baked potato wedges and side salads.

Please also provide:

- array of pre-sliced fresh fruit;
- fruit juice and water, squash (regular and no added sugar, labelled), tea and coffee.

Dinner

- Pasta dish, e.g.
  - Bolognaise (with extra lean 'diet' mince only)
  - Napolitana
  - chicken and mushroom on low-fat white sauce
  - lasagne (diet mince and low-fat cheese only)
  - pasta bake, etc.
- Wet dish (lean meat and veggies) with rice, noodles or couscous to accompany, e.g.
  - sweet and sour pork fillets
  - beef and black bean, etc.
  - chicken and mushroom risotto
  - warmed roast pumpkin couscous
  - chilli basil chicken and veggies in noodles.
- Lean roast meat (fat trimmed), seafood or other plain meat option, e.g. cooked to order lean steaks, calamari, grilled tuna steaks, Cajun chicken breasts, leg ham, turkey breast and cranberry sauce.
- Soup (not cream based) and warmed dinner rolls.
- Potato dish, e.g. baked wedges, dry baked potatoes, potato mash (no margarine).
- Cooked vegetables, either separately (e.g. broccoli, cauliflower, peas, honey carrot) or as a stir fry.

- One to two pre-made salads, e.g. garden salad with dressing on the side, pork and mango salad, apple and walnut salad.
- Array of breads, rolls, including herbed breads (avoiding garlic breads and the like that are flavoured with butter).
- One dessert option, e.g.
  - rice pudding made with low-fat milk
  - low-fat custard and jelly
  - low-fat ice cream and fruit salad
  - spiced fruit compote with low-fat custard
  - self-saucing pudding
  - bread and butter pudding made with low-fat milk
  - mousse.
- Pre-sliced fresh fruit either separate or as a fruit salad.
- Juice, water, tea and coffee.

Snacks

Snacks to be available in communal room, e.g. physio room (to be dictated by team management) throughout the day:

- fruit (e.g. bananas, apples)
- cereal bars
- supply of sports drink and water (either in sealed bottles or in large drink coolers where players can fill up their own bottle).

Pre-training snacks

- Low-fat muffins, fruit scrolls/fruit buns.
- Fruit platter.
- Jugs of low-fat smoothies.
- Jugs of juice or water.
- Supply of sports drink and water (either in sealed bottles or in large drink coolers where players can fill up their own bottle).

Competition plan
Day before competition

As usual but:

- no seafood, spicy or chilli dishes
- lunch must contain a pasta dish
- dinner must contain lasagne *plus* one other pasta dish.

Game day

As usual but:

- no seafood, spicy or chilli dishes;
- pre-game meal and lunch should be the same so players can choose when they would like to eat more;

- pre-game meal/lunch (not to be changed)
  - no seafood or chilli
  - choice between spaghetti bolognaise made on extra lean mince (needs to be very low in fat but full of flavour); other pasta with low-fat sauce; lean meat and vegetable wet dish with accompanying rice or noodles, small pieces of meat only.
  - warmed dinner rolls
  - fresh pancake station (plain, banana and berry with accompanying maple syrup plus lemon and sugar)
  - low-fat muffins, including chocolate flavour
  - build your own salad bar (as above)
  - fresh fruit platter and bunch of bananas
  - tea, coffee, water.

Post-game meal
As usual; acceptable to include seafood or spicy dishes.

If you have any questions or comments please feel free to contact me.

[Insert your name and contact details]

Further reading

Afaghi A, O'Connor H, Chow CM. High-glycemic-index carbohydrate meals shorten sleep onset. Am J Clin Nutr 2007; 85: 426–430.

Allen SJ, Okoko B, Martinez EG, Gregorio GV, Dans LF. Probiotics for treating infectious diarrhoea. Cochrane Database Syst Rev 2003; (4): CD003048.

Callister R. Effect of *Lactobacillus acidophilus* probiotic treatment in fatigued athletes with an interferon defect. Med Sci Sports Exerc 2006; 38: S704.

Clancy RL, Pang G. Probiotics: industry myth or a practical reality. J Am Coll Nutr 2007; 26: 691S–694S.

Drakoularou A, Tzortzis G, Rastall RA, Gibson GR. A double-blind, placebo-controlled, randomized human study assessing the capacity of a novel galacto-oligosaccharide mixture in reducing travellers' diarrhoea. Eur J Clin Nutr 2010; 64: 146–152.

Dupont HL. Systematic review: prevention of travellers' diarrhoea. Aliment Pharmacol Ther 2008; 27: 741–751.

Hodge CW, Shlim DR, Echeverria P, Rajah R, Herrman JE, Cross JH. Epidemiology of diarrhea among expatriate residents living in a highly endemic environment. JAMA 1996; 275: 533–538.

McFarland LV. Meta-analysis of probiotics for the prevention of traveler's diarrhea. Travel Med Infect Dis 2007; 5: 97–105.

Oksanen PJ, Salminen S, Saxelin M et al. Prevention of traveler's diarrhea by *Lactobacillus* GG. Ann Med 1990; 22: 53–56.

Reilly T. The body clock and athletic performance. Biol Rhythm Res 2009; 40: 37–44.

Reilly T, Edwards B. Altered sleep–wake cycles and physical performance in athletes. Physiol Behav 2007; 90: 274–284.

Reilly T, Atkinson G, Edwards B et al. Coping with jet-lag: a position statement for the European College of Sport Science. Eur J Sport Sci 2007; 7: 1–7.

Salminen S, Bouley C, Boutron-Ruault MC et al. Functional food science and gastrointestinal physiology and function. Br J Nutr 1998; 80: S147–S171.

Shlim DR. Looking for evidence that personal hygiene precautions prevent traveler's diarrhea. Clin Infect Dis 2005; 41: S531–S535.

Steffan R. Epidemiology of traveler's diarrhea. Clin Infect Dis 2005; 41: S536–S540.

Waterhouse J, Reilly T, Atkinson G, Edwards B. Jet lag: trends and coping strategies. Lancet 2007; 369: 1117–1129.

23
Population Groups: I

Fiona Pelly, Nanna L Meyer and Penny J Hunking

Understanding the nutritional requirements and dietary needs for populations groups involved in physical activity is crucial, particularly given the different physiological stresses at the varying time-points in the life cycle. This chapter focuses attention on children, the female athlete and masters. Key influences with respect to the growing musculoskeletal system, the aged skeleton and the interplay between nutrition (macronutrient and micronutrient intakes) and physical activity at the recreational and competitive sport levels are discussed. The nutritional demands on females engaged in exercise are explored, including the potential detrimental effects of high-intensity training and the link to the Female Athlete Triad. Each sub-chapter has its own core key messages and summary statements.

CHILDREN

Fiona Pelly

Key messages

- Active children require adequate energy intake for growth and maturation, as well as physical activity. Growth should be regularly monitored and energy intake adjusted to meet individual needs.
- Children who consume inadequate energy may end up with delayed maturation, attenuated growth and poor sports performance. Young athletes who are at risk of low energy intakes include those in aesthetic, weight category or endurance sports. Catch-up growth may occur if training intensity is reduced and energy intake increased.
- Suboptimal intake of protein, calcium, iron and zinc may be prevalent in young athletes, particularly during growth spurts, or in those who have restricted energy intakes or undertake intense and/or prolonged training.
- There is evidence that substrate utilisation during exercise differs between children and adults, with children relying more on fat than endogenous carbohydrate (CHO) oxidation. However, there are currently no specific guidelines on quantity and timing of CHO for active children.
- Children and adolescents should practise strategies to ensure adequate hydration before, during and after exercise. Flavoured drinks can assist with increasing fluid consumption.
- The use of performance-enhancing substances in children under 18 years old is not recommended due to their unknown efficacy and potential harmful effects.
- Children and adolescents should be encouraged to be responsible for their own food choices and be educated on how to choose suitable food. A multidisciplinary approach is essential when counselling and educating young athletes.

23A.1 Introduction

A balanced dietary intake is crucial to maintain health and ensure optimal growth and development in children and adolescents. Childhood is vital for providing the foundation for healthy eating practices that can continue throughout life, and assist with reducing long-term chronic disease risk. Regular physical activity in a healthy well-nourished child is crucial for normal skeletal and muscle growth, as well

Sport and Exercise Nutrition, First Edition. Edited by Susan A Lanham-New, Samantha J Stear, Susan M Shirreffs and Adam L Collins.
© 2011 The Nutrition Society. Published 2011 by Blackwell Publishing Ltd.

as the development of cardiovascular fitness, neuro-muscular coordination and cognitive function. In addition to growth, the active child must aim to fuel activity, minimise injury and optimise competition performance. However, there is little research relating to the specific dietary needs of child and adolescent athletes. For the majority of young athletes, nutrient standards specific to age and gender can be used (Dietary Reference Values for the UK, Nutrient Reference Values for Australia and New Zealand and Dietary Reference Intakes for USA/Canada).

23A.2 Factors affecting nutritional intake

There are a number of factors that influence the nutritional needs of children (5–12 years) and adolescents (13–18 years). These include increases in body size (growth) and maturation (progression towards a mature biological state), and changes in physical activity levels. Throughout childhood there is an increase in both bone area (length and width) and bone mass that accelerates at puberty ('growth spurt'), with approximately 80–90% of peak bone mass accrued during this time. Children grow, develop and mature at different rates, and thus skeletal development is considered a better indicator of physiological maturity than chronological age. In the pre-pubertal period, the proportion of fat and muscle in boy and girls is similar. During puberty, boys gain proportionally more muscle than fat and experience greater velocity in growth, which results in more lean body mass per unit of height. Girls tend to start their growth spurt and attain their peak height approximately 2 years earlier than boys (11 years vs. 13 years respectively).

Growth in the young athlete should be regularly assessed using anthropometric measures (height and weight, skinfolds and circumferences). Most active children will typically be between the 25th and 75th percentile of weight for height, although some young athletes may fall outside this range due to a relatively higher muscle mass. There is a risk of false diagnosis of overweight during puberty when increases in height and weight velocity do not coincide. In adolescent girls, peak weight occurs before peak height and therefore pubertal development may make it difficult to attain the ideal physique required by certain sports. Measures of fat mass and fat-free mass (FFM) may be

more appropriate, although care must be taken with the approach due to self-consciousness about their physique. Concerns about body image have been shown to translate into poor dietary habits and disordered eating.

23A.3 Energy requirements

Active children require adequate energy intake for normal growth and maturation, as well as providing for the additional needs of physical activity. Because of the large variability within and between individuals, reference values for energy based on age, height, weight and physical activity level should only be used as an estimate of actual requirements. There is evidence that children are less economical than adults and expend more energy (up to 30%) relative to their body weight for the same activity. Therefore, tables of adult-estimated energy expenditures for specific sports are likely to underestimate the needs of children. More research is needed to determine the energy requirements of children and adolescents undertaking various sports.

A few studies have attempted to measure self-reported energy intakes of young athletes and have shown large variability that is age-, sport- and gender-specific. Despite the limitations with dietary surveys, it is evident that some young athletes are eating well below estimated energy requirements. Chronic negative energy balance during childhood has been shown to result in attenuated growth, delayed maturation, menstrual irregularities, low bone mineral density, increased incidence of injuries, and a greater risk of developing eating disorders. Furthermore, there is evidence that intense training can also have a negative impact on maturation, particularly for those involved in aesthetic sports or where there is an emphasis on leanness (e.g. elite gymnasts). Catch-up growth may occur if training intensity is reduced and energy intake increased. However, this may be compromised if the delay in maturation is severe. Young athletes most at risk of inadequate energy intake are those involved in sports that place importance on a lean physique (distance running), weight category sports (martial arts, rowing) or aesthetic sports (gymnastics, diving). A focus on body image can begin at a young age, particularly in weight-centred sports such as gymnastics and dancing, with girls as young as 5–7 years reporting concern over their weight. Female adolescent athletes are also at risk as they pursue a lighter and leaner physique to offset pubertal changes. In contrast, chronic positive energy balance may lead to obesity and associated negative health consequences.

23A.4 Protein

Protein requirements of children and adolescents are higher than those of adults to support growth and maturation. Protein recommendations for the adult athlete are slightly higher (1.2–1.7 g/kg/day) than nutrient reference values (0.8–1.0 g/kg/day), particularly for those undertaking endurance- and strength-oriented sports. Thus athletic children, especially those engaged in strength/power or endurance sports, may require more protein in comparison to inactive children. Yet few studies have examined the protein requirements of young athletes. Increase in protein requirements may be particularly relevant during growth spurts in those undertaking regular high-volume and high-intensity training. Adequate energy is also critical for growth. Insufficient energy will result in the use of protein as an energy source rather than building lean tissue. In most developed countries, the protein intakes of children and adolescents typically exceed protein requirements, even for those on lower energy intakes. Nevertheless, children or adolescents following a strict vegetarian regimen, experiencing a growth spurt or undergoing high volumes of training may be at risk of inadequate intake.

23A.5 Carbohydrate

The relationship of high-carbohydrate (CHO) diets and performance in the adult athlete are well recognised. However, it is unclear whether young athletes need similar CHO intakes to adults. Substrate utilisation during exercise differs between children and adults, with children relying more on fat than endogenous CHO oxidation during moderate-intensity exercise. Children have been shown to have higher plasma glucose levels than adults after glucose ingestion at the beginning of moderate-intensity exercise, possibly due to decreased insulin sensitivity. There is also evidence for higher rates of exogenous CHO oxidation (CHO consumed during exercise) in children compared with adolescents and adults. This suggests

that children may benefit from CHO consumption during prolonged activity. Furthermore, there are potential gender-related differences in energy substrate utilisation during childhood, with hormonal influences at puberty altering substrate utilisation patterns during exercise. Serum oestradiol levels in girls have been shown to positively correlate with endogenous but not exogenous CHO oxidation, whereas exogenous CHO oxidation rates have been shown to be inversely related to testosterone levels in boys. The development of an adult-like metabolic profile with fully developed glycolytic capacity occurs between mid and late puberty.

Muscle glycogen stores also appear relatively lower in children than adults. Low muscle glycogen content is possibly associated with low activity of glycolytic enzymes and high oxidative capacity. Adult endurance athletes are recommended to consume approximately 7–10 g/kg/day to replenish muscle glycogen. There is currently no evidence for or against this level of intake in children. However, the practice of CHO loading is currently not recommended in children due to potential negative effects. Current guidelines recommend that young athletes consume at least 50% of their total daily energy intake as CHO. Further research is needed to determine the specific CHO needs of child and adolescent athletes.

23A.6 Fat

Children have been shown to have an increased ability to utilise fat as an energy source during exercise, as evidenced by increased fatty acid uptake and lower respiratory exchange ratios. While this may suggest the need for increased fat intake in child athletes, additional dietary fat will not enhance fat oxidation. The average Western diet provides adequate amounts of fat, and current public health guidelines recommend that total fat contributes no more than 30% of total daily energy, with no more than 10% from saturated fat. Furthermore, higher fat consumption often accompanies lower CHO intakes. Therefore, it is prudent to stick to population guidelines for total fat intake, and minimise saturated and *trans* fat consumption in active children. Alternatively, young athletes aiming to reduce body mass or body fat may overly restrict dietary fat intake, resulting in insufficient intake of essential fatty acids and fat-soluble vitamins D and E.

Table 23.1 Reference Nutrient Intakes (RNI) of selected micronutrients for children and adolescents.

Age (years)	Gender	Calcium (mg/day)	Iron (mg/day)	Zinc (mg/day)
4–6	Boys	450	6.1	6.5
	Girls	450	6.1	6.5
7–10	Boys	550	8.7	7.0
	Girls	550	8.7	7.0
11–14	Boys	1000	11.3	9.0
	Girls	800	14.8	9.0
15–18	Boys	1000	11.3	9.5
	Girls	800	14.8	7.0

Adapted from Department of Health 1991. Dietary Reference Values for Food, Energy and Nutrients for the United Kingdom. London: HMSO. Crown Copyright 1991. Crown copyright material is reproduced with the permission of the Controller of HMSO and the Queen's Printer for Scotland.

23A.7 Micronutrients

In a healthy adult population, most micronutrient requirements will be met with a balanced dietary intake that provides adequate energy. Any additional needs of athletes are usually met by an increased consumption of food to meet increased energy expenditure. Research on dietary intakes in young athletes suggests that the intake of most micronutrients is adequate, with the exception of predominantly calcium, iron, and zinc, and vitamins D and E in certain individuals. The Reference Nutrient Intakes (RNI) for calcium, iron and zinc are shown in Table 23.1. Inadequate intake of the B vitamins and vitamin C is less commonly reported, although suboptimal intakes of folate and B$_6$ have been recorded in young athletes on low energy regimens. In adult athletes with restricted energy intakes it is common to see a range of micronutrients below the recommended reference value. Similarly, young athletes who restrict their energy intake (e.g. dancers, gymnasts, wrestlers) may be at risk of suboptimal intakes.

Calcium

Adequate dietary calcium intakes (at least 1000 mg/day) and regular weight-bearing exercise are necessary to optimise bone health during childhood and adolescence. Poor bone quality has been shown to be associated with stress fracture in both boys and girls, particularly those on low calcium intakes (<400 mg/day). While exercise does not increase the need for dietary calcium, low oestrogen levels experienced by some adolescent female athletes can result in decreases in bone mineral density. Under these circumstances, calcium intakes of 1500 mg/day may be necessary. There is recent evidence from an Australian population survey that the majority of girls aged 12–16 years do not meet the recommended intake for calcium, particularly those who restrict their intake of dairy products.

Iron

Iron deficiency may be the result of inadequate intake and/or increased loss, and can result in decreased physical and mental performance. Adolescent athletes, particularly females and vegetarians, are at increased risk of iron deficiency due to higher iron requirements and turnover, menstrual losses and suboptimal intakes. Young athletes undertaking intense or prolonged endurance training also risk iron depletion due to loss via haemolysis and gastrointestinal blood loss. There is evidence that up to 50% of adolescent female athletes have low iron stores (functional iron deficiency) based on serum ferritin levels. However, diagnosis of functional iron deficiency using serum ferritin may be difficult due to growth spurts and expanded plasma volume in response to increases in training, and therefore repeated measures are recommended. Serum transferrin receptor may be a better diagnostic tool for functional deficiency, although current laboratory cut-offs are relevant to non-athletic populations. Overt iron deficiency anaemia in active children is less commonly reported. Treatment is similar to recommendations for the adult athlete.

Zinc

Zinc intakes have been reported to be suboptimal in young female athletes. As animal products are the best source of bioavailable zinc, vegetarian athletes are most at risk. Zinc deficiency can result in reduced growth velocity and delayed sexual development.

Use of dietary supplements

There is evidence that a large proportion of young athletes use some type of vitamin and mineral supplement, with the most commonly reported being multivitamins, vitamin C, iron, calcium, zinc, B vitamins and vitamin A. The common reasons cited for use of supplements include short-term health benefits, prevention or treatment of illness, improved immunity, an energy boost, better sports performance and to rectify a poor diet. While there is no evidence to support the use of supplements in young athletes, a broad range multivitamin and multimineral supplements specifically designed for children may be useful for those with poor dietary habits or restricted energy intakes or if following a special dietary regimen (e.g. vegetarians, gluten free). Children diagnosed with a specific deficiency (e.g. iron deficiency anaemia) may require larger doses of the deficient nutrient. However, medical or dietetic advice should be sought prior to commencing supplementation.

23A.8 Use of performance-enhancing substances

The ergogenic and potentially adverse effects of performance-enhancing substances have not been investigated in subjects younger than 18 years. Young people are vulnerable to peer pressure and product endorsement by sporting heroes, and are likely to be unaware of any potential risks associated with their use. There is evidence that young males, in particular, frequently use muscle-building substances such as protein powders, creatine monohydrate and β-hydroxy-β-methylbutyrate (HMB).

Some supplements may also contain banned ingredients, through inadvertent or advertent contamination, and may result in a positive drug test. Furthermore, the effects of these substances on growth and maturation or long-term health of the young athlete are not known. Young athletes should be made aware that supplements will not instantly improve their performance or change their physique, and may be potentially dangerous. The American Academy of Pediatrics currently condemns the use of any performance-enhancing substance by children and adolescents.

There is increasing concern over the use of energy drinks and caffeinated beverages in children and adolescents. One study of 400 school children showed that a number of boys deliberately used significant amounts of energy drinks prior to sport to enhance their performance. Although there are currently no recommendations on safe levels of consumption, high intakes of caffeine in children may result in headaches and sleep disturbances.

23A.9 Fluids

Children have less developed and less efficient thermoregulatory mechanisms than adults and therefore have traditionally been thought to be at greater risk of heat-related injuries. Children have a larger body surface area to body mass ratio than adults. As a result, they generate more heat per kilogram of body mass. Furthermore, children have immature sweat mechanisms resulting in a lower sweat rate (approximately 2.5 times less) and higher sweating threshold (the core temperature when sweating starts) than adults. Despite these differences, recent evidence suggests that this does not translate into a greater accumulation of body heat or increased risk of heat stress. Similar to the adult athlete, children and adolescents can improve their heat tolerance with improved aerobic fitness and acclimatisation.

Adequate hydration before, during and after exercise is crucial for the prevention of heat injuries. Optimal fluid intake will depend on age, individual sweat rate, exercise intensity, environmental conditions, clothing worn, and degree of acclimatisation. Therefore, it is not possible to recommend a single volume that suits all ages and situations. As with adults, measurement of body mass before and after exercise can indicate fluid loss and help to determine sweat rate. Existing guidelines for fluid consumption in active children and adolescents are outlined in Table 23.2.

Like adults, children and adolescents progressively dehydrate when left to drink *ad libitum*. During exercise, there is evidence that both junior endurance athletes and team players may not take in adequate fluid during and after exercise. In some circumstances, a CHO/electrolyte drink (sports drinks) may help young athletes rehydrate more effectively than water alone. Studies on voluntary drinking habits after exercise in children have shown that they consume more fluid and rehydrate more effectively when flavoured (grape and orange) drinks are offered instead of water. CHO and sodium may also help with fluid absorption and retention. However, further research is needed to determine the ideal concentration of CHO and electrolytes of sports drinks designed for young athletes. In the interim, similar concentrations to sports drinks designed for adults (4–8% CHO) are recommended before, during and after exercise, particularly in hot conditions.

Table 23.2 Summary of existing guidelines for fluid consumption in children and adolescents.

Age	General fluid consumption	Before exercise	During exercise
Up to 10 years	Drink periodically until not thirsty any more then have an extra half glass (100–125 ml) if under 10[a]	150–200 ml 45 min before exercise[b]	150 ml of fluid for children around 40 kg every 20 min[c]
Approximately 15 years	Drink periodically until not thirsty any more then have one glass (200–250 ml) beyond thirst if 10 years or older[a]	300–400 ml 45 min before exercise[b]	250 ml for adolescents around 60 kg every 20 min[c]

[a] Bar-Or & Wilk (1996).
[b] Sports Medicine Australia (1997).
[c] Bar-Or (2001).

23A.10 Dental caries

Parents are commonly concerned about the regular consumption of sports drinks and other sweetened beverages and the risk of dental caries. Sugars found in soft drinks, sports drinks and confectionery, and the acids found in some fruits and drinks, can provide the substrate for enhancing acid production and bacterial growth that can lead to dental caries. Measures to help prevent this occurring include regularly brushing teeth, drinking water after eating, drinking sweetened drinks through a straw or squeeze bottle and consuming plenty of casein-containing foods (e.g. milk and cheese).

23A.11 Eating behaviours

In counselling young athletes, it is important to understand the various influences on their eating habits. Younger, less experienced athletes may follow the dietary advice provided by their coach, trainer or peers and modify their food intake accordingly. Taste and convenience are major influences on adolescent food choice. Body image can become an important issue, particularly in adolescent girls, and lead to dieting and disordered eating. Parents and carers can strongly influence food intake and can assist by modelling healthy eating practices and attitudes towards eating in the home. Nevertheless, children and adolescents should be encouraged to be responsible for their own food choices and be educated on how to choose suitable food. A multidisciplinary approach that includes parents, dietitian, coach and other health professionals is essential when counselling and educating young athletes about their diet. Practical nutrition strategies for the young athlete are summarised in Table 23.3.

23A.12 Summary

Appropriate nutrition for the active child is vital to ensure optimal growth and maturation, as well as better performance and recovery from training and competition. In contrast, young athletes who are not eating well or eating too little may end up with delayed maturation, attenuated growth and poor performance. Young athletes need to eat frequently, and often in large amounts, particularly during a growth spurt, and should be encouraged to consume nutritious snacks that will assist with meeting additional energy and nutrient requirements.

Few studies have examined the specific macronutrient or micronutrient needs of child and adolescent athletes. An increased energy intake with an emphasis on CHO is recommended for young athletes undertaking regular high-intensity and/or high-volume training, although specific guidelines on amounts and timing of CHO is lacking. The limited available research suggests that protein and micronutrient intake is adequate to meet the needs of most young athletes. However, protein, calcium, iron and zinc intake may be suboptimal during growth spurts or in young athletes undertaking intense and/or prolonged training (e.g. swimmers) or on restricted energy intakes (e.g. gymnasts and dancers). The use of

Table 23.3 Practical nutrition strategies for the young athlete.

- Monitor growth and maturation to ensure that individual energy intake is matching energy expenditure. Young athletes need three nutritious meals with snacks in between. Young athletes who are at risk of low energy intakes include those in aesthetic, weight category or endurance sports
- Consume nutritious snacks for additional energy, e.g. baked beans, sandwiches with meat or cheese filling, sports and cereal bars, canned or stewed fruit with yoghurt, scones with jam, pancakes with honey, noodles, dried fruit and nuts, liquid meal supplements, or English muffins with peanut butter
- Include calcium-rich foods for optimal bone development, e.g. smoothies, milk drinks, cheese, yoghurt and dairy desserts
- Encourage intake of iron-rich foods such as lean red meat. If vegetarian, encourage intake of iron fortified cereal, legumes, bread, baked beans and green leafy vegetables
- Discourage the use of any performance-enhancing supplements and the indiscriminate use of vitamin and mineral supplements. Medical or dietetic advice should be sought to determine whether a specific micronutrient supplement is required to correct a deficiency
- Encourage children to drink until they are not thirsty any more, then have a few more gulps. Water is an excellent choice before, during and after exercise. Sports drinks may be of benefit in hot conditions when sweat rates are high. Weighing before and after exercise can help to determine the amount of fluid lost during various activities. Flavoured drinks encourage fluid consumption, while the use of caffeinated beverages should be discouraged
- Encourage children and adolescents to be responsible for their own food choices through education and modelling appropriate eating behaviours. A multidisciplinary approach may be needed to counsel and educate the young athlete

performance-enhancing substances in children under 18 years is not recommended due to their unknown efficacy and potential harmful effects. Children and adolescents should practise strategies to ensure adequate hydration before, during and after exercise. Finally, a multidisciplinary approach that focuses on sports performance is recommended when counselling and educating the young athlete.

FEMALE ATHLETES

Nanna L Meyer

Key messages

- This section discusses the specific nutritional needs of female athletes.
- It describes gender differences in metabolism and performance.
- It discusses energy, macronutrient and micronutrient needs.

- The Female Athlete Triad is described.
- Particular challenges to meet nutritional requirements of female athletes are also highlighted.

23B.1 Introduction

Female athletes have unique nutritional needs that are based on biological differences between men and women. Interestingly, however, female athletes are also surprisingly similar in how they respond to physiological demands and how they manage nutrition as it applies to their training. The most important nutritional issue for female athletes is the Female Athlete Triad, an interrelated syndrome comprising energy availability, menstrual function and bone mineral density. In addition, female athletes are at risk for low energy and nutrient intakes, especially if training is intense and their diets are restrictive. This sub-chapter briefly reviews current knowledge on female athletes' nutritional needs and provides practical recommendations for those who work with the female athlete population.

23B.2 Gender differences in metabolism and performance

With the slow acceptance of female athletes in Olympic competitions and the disproportionate number of scientific studies using male subjects, it is understandable that the evidence showing physiological and performance differences between men and women is still scarce. What has been established is that women show a consistently lower respiratory exchange ratio than men at submaximal exercise intensities, and before and after endurance training. This indicates that women oxidise more fat than their male counterparts at the same absolute and relative intensity. Studies have also shown a consistently higher intramuscular lipid content in women compared with men, and women exhibit a greater whole-body lipolytic response during endurance exercise than men. Contributing factors of these gender differences appear to include muscle fibre type differences and the predominance of female sex steroid hormones. Perhaps these and other physiological differences between men and women would suggest that women are well suited for endurance, and particularly ultra-endurance events, where it has been suggested that women may someday outperform men.

With the aforementioned differences in fat metabolism, do female athletes also differ in the way they store and use carbohydrate (CHO)? Women appear to have similar capacities as men to store muscle glycogen, as long as their energy and CHO intake is high enough. However, women use less muscle glycogen than men at the same relative and absolute exercise intensity. Interestingly, women do not seem to differ greatly from men with respect to their metabolic response (i.e. CHO oxidation) to prolonged exercise when ingesting CHO (e.g. sport drinks). These findings indicate that women can apply similar recommendations for CHO supplementation during exercise with the purpose of improving performance and slowing the onset of fatigue. For CHO loading, female athletes must make an extra effort to consume enough calories and CHO in order to super-compensate their muscle glycogen stores.

Whether there are different requirements for protein in exercising men and women depends on how much protein is oxidised during exercise, whether protein feeding after exercise affects recovery and subsequent performance, and how much overall protein is required to maintain daily nitrogen balance. As is well known, protein oxidation is relatively limited during exercise and it appears that women oxidise even less than men. Regarding the second issue, it is interesting to note that recent research shows that post-exercise protein feeding has little influence on subsequent cycling performance in trained women cyclists as opposed to men. Finally, nitrogen balance data suggest that women require approximately 15–25% less protein than men to maintain net nitrogen balance.

Despite the fact that the scientific data discussed above provides some knowledge of gender differences in substrate metabolism, some of these discoveries have yet to be examined in terms of how they might alter nutritional recommendations for exercising women (e.g. differences in CHO, protein and fat metabolism). Thus, gender-specific nutritional guidelines may integrate some but not all of these concepts along with the unique nutritional issues of exercising women.

23B.3 Energy

Diets of female athletes are often low in energy, and consequentially low in CHO, low in fat and possibly low in protein if the athlete restricts energy intake or limits protein choices. The diets of female athletes are also often low in bone-building nutrients (e.g. calcium, vitamin D, magnesium), low in oxygen transport nutrients (e.g. iron, folate, vitamin B_{12}) and they can be low in certain B vitamins (e.g. riboflavin, vitamin B_6). The following section focuses on the aforementioned nutrients.

Female athletes often fail to meet energy requirements. This has been shown by multiple studies using the doubly-labelled water (DLW) technique. Comparing energy intake from dietary records with total daily energy expenditure (TDEE) measured by DLW, it becomes apparent that energy intake frequently does not match TDEE (Table 23.4).

Interestingly, it is quite common that weight is maintained in these studies despite a large gap between measured TDEE and reported energy intake. This discrepancy may be due to under-eating with or without energy efficiency and/or under-reporting

Table 23.4 Energy expenditure measured by doubly labelled water and energy intake in selected studies on female athletes.

Sport	Total daily energy expenditure (kcal/day)	Energy intake (kcal/day)
Runners[a]	3492	2318
Runners[b]	2990	2039
Lightweight rowers[c]	3957	2214
Cross-country skiers[d]	4373	4350

[a] Haggarty et al. (1988).
[b] Edwards et al. (1993).
[c] Hill & Davies (2002).
[d] Sjödin et al. (1994).

Table 23.5 Macronutrient recommendations for female athletes.

Nutrient	Quantity (g/kg/day)
CHO	
Low intensity or skill-based activities	3–5[a]
Moderate exercise (i.e. 1 hour/day)	5–7[a]
High intensity exercise (i.e. >4–5 hours/ day)	6–10[a]
CHO loading	>8–12[ab]
Protein	
Female athletes at ~25% lower than men	1.2–1.3[b]
Fat	
Acceptable Macronutrient Distribution Range (DRI)	20–35%[c]

[a] Burke et al. in press.
[b] Tarnopolsky (2008).
[c] Dietary Reference Intakes (DRI) (2002).

energy intake and should be taken into consideration when interpreting dietary records of female athletes. However, it is wrong to assume that all female athletes under-report and/or under-eat. In fact, in a study on cross-country skiers, energy turnover (intake and expenditure) was 80 kcal/kg/day. In other words, some female athletes eat adequate quantities of food during high-intensity training and do not experience weight gain or loss.

Nevertheless, more common is that female athletes are struggling to adjust energy intake to changes in exercise volume/intensity. Indeed, in another study on cross-country skiers, it was shown that only male athletes adjusted their energy intake to changes in leisure (exercise) energy expenditure (EEE). Other data have shown similar trends in that female athletes appear to eat the same amount of calories regardless of how intense or prolonged their training or competitions may be. This raises a concern because adequate energy and macronutrients, especially CHO, are needed to fuel intense repetitive training.

23B.4 Carbohydrates

As expected, female athletes consume lower quantities of CHO than male athletes even when adjusted for body mass. Average CHO intake for female endurance athletes is around 5.5 g/kg/day (vs. 7.5 g/kg/day for males), while CHO intakes are below 4 g/kg/day for non-endurance athletes. These CHO intakes are likely too low to maintain a high training intensity and are probably too low to help replete glyco-

gen stores or attempt to super-compensate muscle glycogen. Low CHO intakes may lead to reduced training capacity, mental and physical fatigue, increased risk for injury and illness, and muscle protein breakdown. Female athletes training repetitively for several hours per day should ingest at least 7 g/kg/day (see Table 23.5 for recommendations).

23B.5 Protein

Female athletes who restrict energy intake compromise their protein intake. In particular, if athletes are trying to lose body mass and fat using a low-calorie diet, protein intake should be increased to preserve muscle mass and power. In addition, protein serves many functions beyond muscle protein synthesis and repair, and reduced protein intakes can result in amino acid deficiencies with clinical consequences. Adequate dietary protein is also important in the treatment of female athletes with eating disorders due to the fact that protein is satiating and preserves muscle mass, and that amino acids affect growth, maintenance, immunity and reproduction. Meeting protein needs in female athletes should not be difficult even if women restrict some sources of protein such as red meat or use a vegetarian diet, as long as their energy intake is adequate (see Table 23.5 for recommendations).

23B.6 Fat

Many female athletes try to limit dietary fat in order to lose body mass and body fat or because of misconceptions about fat. If fat intake falls below 10–15% energy intake, the absorption of fat-soluble vitamins and the capacity to meet essential fatty acid recommendations may be impaired, which can lead to nutrient deficiencies. Currently, there are no athlete- or female-specific recommendations for dietary fat intake. Table 23.5 shows current macronutrient recommendations adapted to the female athlete. Note that most macronutrient recommendations are expressed relative to body mass (in kilograms), which can make it quite difficult for some female athletes with caloric restriction to meet daily needs.

23B.7 Micronutrients

Micronutrients of particular concern in female athletes are calcium, iron, magnesium, zinc, B vitamins and vitamin D, especially if energy intake is restricted. Low micronutrient intake can lead to vitamin and mineral deficiencies and impact both health and performance.

Micronutrients vital for bone health include several vitamins and minerals (e.g. vitamin K and magnesium), but most importantly calcium and vitamin D. Average calcium intake in female athletes is typically lower than recommended. If athletes limit dairy products, it is more difficult to meet the recommended levels for calcium. In addition, due to the important role vitamin D plays in calcium absorption and the high prevalence of vitamin D deficiency in the general population and in athletes, bone health may not be optimised at an age when the potential for bone formation is greatest. Further, female athletes with menstrual dysfunction, as part of the Female Athlete Triad, may compromise their ability to optimise bone mass because they lack oestrogen's protective effect on bone, potentially leading to irreversible bone loss. Thus, female athletes should try to meet daily recommendations for calcium and vitamin D, among other bone-building nutrients, and maintain or resume a regular menstrual cycle. Calcium recommendations are 1300 mg/day and 1000 mg/day for females aged 14–18 years and 19–50 yeaars, respectively. For female athletes with the Female Athlete

Triad, the International Olympic Committee Medical Commission recommends 1500 mg/day.

While most calcium intake is provided by the diet, vitamin D sources from food are relatively scarce. The best source comes from the synthesis of vitamin D in the skin as a result of sun exposure. Female athletes, especially if using sunscreen or training indoors, should get their vitamin D status tested throughout the season in order to prevent vitamin D deficiency.

Despite the recent attention on vitamin D deficiency, the most common nutrient deficiency in female athletes continues to be iron deficiency. In particular, stage I iron depletion, indicated by low serum ferritin, is prevalent in about 15–60% of female athletes. At risk for compromised iron status are adolescent female athletes, females competing in endurance or aesthetic sports, and females training and/or sleeping at altitude. There is no evidence suggesting that low serum ferritin, consistent with stage I iron depletion, interferes with performance. However, this marker, along with serum transferrin receptor, is widely used to identify athletes at risk for iron deficiency with anaemia (stage III) and without anaemia (stage II). Among other functions, iron is important for haemoglobin and myoglobin synthesis, and stage III iron deficiency with anaemia reduces the athlete's oxygen-carrying capacity, potentially impairing performance, recovery and training adaptations. Female athletes need to consume at least 18 mg of iron daily and, most importantly, some of this iron should be in the haem form from animal sources due to better bioavailability. Supplementation with iron should only be attempted based on compromised iron status measured periodically in those at high risk for iron deficiency. Self-medication is not advised.

In addition to low iron intake and status in female athletes, several B vitamins such as those participating in haemoglobin synthesis (i.e. vitamin B_{12} and folate), among others important for energy metabolism (e.g. riboflavin, vitamin B_6), and zinc and magnesium can be of concern in active women. In fact, research shows that if energy intake is restricted these micronutrients are not consumed in adequate amounts. Female athletes should ingest 2.4–3.0 mg/day of riboflavin, 1.5–3 mg/day of vitamin B_6, 400 μg/day of folate, 2.4 mg/day of vitamin B_{12}, 350–400 mg/day of magnesium and 8 mg/day of zinc. These recommendations are based on several review articles by experts in the field and some values are higher than recommended for the general, non-athletic female population.

Finally, an important factor to consider is whether female athletes limit their food choices or adhere to fixed dietary rules. Excluding dairy products or meat, practising a vegan lifestyle, or adhering to a highly processed diet can provide a good guiding principle regarding marginal intakes of micronutrients and the potential concern of nutrient deficiencies. A dietary assessment, including usual intake, in combination with food frequency inquiries, can provide insight into both the quantity and quality of the diet. In this situation, female athletes may do best to consume a multivitamin/multimineral supplement that provides close to the recommended amounts for most micronutrients. Attention should be given to athletes, including females, who supplement with chronically high doses of certain vitamins (e.g. vitamin C, vitamin E) and minerals (e.g. zinc, iron).

23B.8 The menstrual cycle of female athletes

The menstrual cycle in female athletes is often different from that of non-athletes. In fact, athletes have a higher prevalence of menstrual dysfunction than non-athletes. Age at menarche may be delayed in female athletes: non-athletic females begin their menstrual cycle at an average age of 12.6 years, while athletic females, especially if their training begins prior to puberty, may present with delayed menarche and/or primary amenorrhoea. If menarche does not occur by 15 years, despite the development of secondary sex characteristics, it is referred to as primary amenorrhoea. Once the menstrual cycle starts, menstrual dysfunction such as oligoamenorrhoea (i.e. cycle length >35 days or four to nine cycles per year), secondary amenorrhoea (complete cessation of menstruation for at least three consecutive months after menarche or less than one to three cycles per year) and subclinical forms such as shortened luteal phase and anovulation are common in female athletes. Menstrual dysfunction in athletes is most likely due to a mismatch between energy intake and TDEE, especially if exercise training is intense or voluminous, which leaves fewer calories to cover basic physiological functions, including reproduction. If female athletes experience menstrual dysfunction they

should consult a physician to rule out other causes such as a pituitary tumour or hyperandrogenism. The relationship between energy derived from the diet and reproductive health in women athletes is part of the Female Athlete Triad and is discussed below.

23B.9 The Female Athlete Triad

Female athletes are at significant risk for the Female Athlete Triad, an interrelated syndrome first identified in 1993. The 2007 American College of Sports Medicine Position Stand illustrates the Female Athlete Triad with each of its components (i.e. energy availability, menstrual function, bone mineral density) on a spectrum, ranging from a healthy athlete to one who is ill. The healthy female matches her energy intake with the amount of energy she expends during exercise and throughout the day. She also has a normal menstrual cycle and optimal bone health, providing all necessary nutrients and the optimal hormonal milieu for reaching a high peak bone mass. A less optimal scenario represents a female athlete who under-consumes calories and does not meet the necessary energy requirement to cover EEE and fulfil all other bodily functions. She thereby begins to compromise her reproductive function and bone mineral density. This female athlete may have disordered eating patterns or may simply be unaware of the additional energy needed for her sport, and therefore is thought to inadvertently under-consume calories, leading to low energy availability (EA). EA represents the amount of dietary energy remaining for other body functions after exercise training. Thus, EA is defined as energy intake minus EEE (expressed per kilogram of FFM per day) and can occur by decreased energy intake, increased EEE or a combination of the two. At the extreme end of the spectrum, the female athlete may present with disordered eating or an eating disorder, attempting to fuel her performance but struggling to achieve or maintain a low body mass or lean physique. Her dieting efforts lead to low EA at a level that has been shown to disrupt normal menstrual function (i.e. <30 kcal/kg FFM/day). This scenario may also coincide with amenorrhoea and requires immediate attention to reduce the risk of osteoporosis and stress fractures, and the focus should be on reversing abnormal eating and providing the necessary nutritional support to maintain bone health, which should include the normalisation of EA and resumption of menstrual function. It is important to note that even at this extreme end of the spectrum, the athlete does not have to present with disordered eating or an eating disorder but may inadvertently under-consume calories due to other factors (e.g. loss of appetite, stress and unfamiliarity of travel, use of medication). The Female Athlete Triad, as depicted on a spectrum from healthy to ill, offers the opportunity for early screening and identification, thereby preventing its most clinical manifestation.

Female athletes with low EA probably interfere with their performance potential, even though initial weight loss may lead to a temporary performance boost. Low EA likely leads to low CHO intake and glycogen depletion. Low EA may also result in low micronutrient intakes necessary for metabolism to function effectively, for bone to strengthen, and for muscle to build. Low EA may also result in reduced protein and essential fatty acid intake and nutrients important for antioxidant protection and immune function.

Treatment of athletes with one or more components of the Female Athlete Triad must primarily include meeting energy requirements, ensuring adequate EA to cover all physiological functions beyond that which is necessary for exercise. It is recommended that EA be at least 30 kcal/kg FFM/day and ideally approach and exceed 45 kcal/kg FFM/day in order to promote growth, training adaptation and success in competition, while maintaining a normal menstrual cycle. It is expected that female athletes struggle the most with these recommendations to optimise EA if an eating disorder prevails, if training intensity or volume are high, or if other stressful events occur (e.g. travelling in areas with unfamiliar food, infections treated with antibiotics, loss of coach, injury) that may interfere with appetite.

If eating disorders have underlying psychopathologies, they must be treated by a psychologist/ psychiatrist experienced with eating disorders in athletes. Triad treatment should also include a sports medicine physician, a sports dietitian, and possibly a physical therapist/athletic trainer and exercise physiologist all experienced in managing athletes with the condition.

The prevalence of the Female Athlete Triad varies by sport, with the greatest occurrence in sports that emphasise leanness such as aesthetic and endurance sports. However, individual components of the Female Athlete Triad should be expected in any sport, and thus screening for risk of the condition should be an integral part of any female athlete sport nutrition programme. Prevention is always more effective than treatment. Thus increasing awareness and providing education to athletes, coaches and parents, and using covert prevention programmes with interactive experiential learning opportunities probably prove most effective, secondary to early screening.

23B.10 Summary

Female athletes differ from their male counterparts and have unique nutritional requirements that must be met to support both success in sport and health promotion. Screening and assessment provide for early identification of potential nutritional issues, including the Female Athlete Triad, and should be an integral aspect of female athlete sport nutrition programming.

MASTERS

Penny J Hunking

Key messages

- Masters athletes compete in an extremely wide variety of sports and participants range from the physically elite to the physically dependent.
- Recommendations for nutrition in Masters athletes should focus on the nutritional requirements of the ageing process and the nutrient needs for exercising.

- The ageing process is associated with age-related changes that may make the older athlete susceptible to hydration problems.
- There is a lack of studies to evaluate the effect of diet and exercise in Masters athletes, especially in the habitually trained. There are no specific recommendations for nutrient intakes for ageing athletes participating in athletic training.

23C.1 Introduction

There are various definitions of the 'Master' athlete but for the purposes of this sub-chapter it is defined as active individuals aged 50 years or older. Ageing brings about a progressive decline in the functioning of all organs and systems. Nutrient recommendations and interventions for Master athletes are based on the physiological changes associated with ageing and their impact on nutrient requirements combined with the additional nutrient requirements as a result of the demands of training and competition.

Participation in sport and exercise by individuals over 50 years appears to be on the increase, possibly because of greater awareness of the health benefits of physical activity regardless of age, stage of life, gender or socio-economic status. In addition, the fact that life expectancy has been steadily increasing for some time means there are simply more people in society over the age of 50 years.

23C.2 Energy

Masters athletes need to consume adequate dietary energy to offset energy expenditure, maintain health, body weight and body composition, and maximise the training effects.

For the most part, young adults have been used in determining the energy costs of specific activities reported in the literature and few data are based on Masters. Masters may well have an energy expenditure not much different from that of young adults when walking at the same rate, but older people tend to walk slower, play sport at less intensity, run less

vigorously and therefore adjustments need to be made accordingly. Ageing is associated with changes in body composition and hence resting energy expenditure. Age-associated loss of fat-free mass (FFM) and a decline in non-training physical activity may contribute to a reduced energy requirement. However, older athletes who practise regular strength training may maintain or increase muscle size, which could in turn have an important impact on energy balance because of an increased metabolic rate and an increase in energy expenditure.

The Dietary Reference Values (DRVs) for energy (Table 23.6) can be used as a guide for establishing energy requirements. However, competitive Masters athletes with heavy training loads could require many more calories to fuel their training and activity.

23C.3 Macronutrients

The energy needs of the Masters athlete are met by the ingestion of carbohydrate (CHO), fat and protein. A high-CHO diet following the usual recommendations for training and competition is still key to support the Masters athlete since CHO absorption and utilisation, in the absence of disease, is unaffected by ageing.

Protein recommendations for Masters athletes have not been established and further research is needed to set definitive guidelines. Ageing athletes may not require as much dietary protein as younger athletes for reasons including age-associated losses of FFM and decreased volume and intensity of training. Studies on the effects of high-protein diets as a means of stimulating protein synthesis and preventing losses of FFM that occur with ageing have not shown

Table 23.6 Estimated average requirements (EAR) for energy.

Age (years)	MJ/day	kcal/day
Men		
19–50	10.60	2550
51–59	10.60	2550
60–64	9.93	2380
65–74	9.71	2330
75+	8.77	2100
Women		
19–50	8.10	1940
51–59	8.00	1900
60–64	7.99	1900
65–74	7.96	1900
75+	7.61	1810

Data from Department of Health, Dietary Reference Values for Food Energy and Nutrients for the United Kingdom. Report of the Panel on Dietary Reference Intakes of the Committee on Medical Aspects of Food Policy. Crown Copyright 1991, Crown copyright material is reproduced with the permission of the Controller of HMSO and the Queen's Printer for Scotland.

Table 23.7 Reference Nutrient Intakes (RNI) for vitamins and minerals for adults (50+ years).

Nutrient	RNI
Calcium (mg/day)	700
Phosphorus (mg/day)	550
Magnesium (mg/day)	270 women, 300 men
Sodium (mg/day)	1600
Potassium (mg/day)	3500
Chloride (mg/day)	2500
Iron (mg/day)	8.7
Zinc (mg/day)	7.0 women, 9.5 men
Copper (mg/day)	1.2
Selenium (µg/day)	60 women, 75 men
Iodine (µg/day)	140
Thiamin (mg/day)	0.8 women, 0.9 men
Riboflavin (mg/day)	1.1 women, 1.3 men
Niacin (mg/day)	12 women, 16 men
Vitamin B_6 (mg/day)	1.2 women, 1.4 men
Folate (µg/day)	200
Vitamin C (mg/day)	40
Vitamin A (µg/day)	600 women, 700 men
Vitamin D (µg/day)	10 after age of 65 years

Data from Department of Health, Dietary Reference Values for Food Energy and Nutrients for the United Kingdom. Report of the Panel on Dietary Reference Intakes of the Committee on Medical Aspects of Food Policy. Crown Copyright 1991, Crown copyright material is reproduced with the permission of the Controller of HMSO and the Queen's Printer for Scotland.

them to be of benefit. In practice, providing enough food is consumed to meet both energy and CHO requirements, then achieving an adequate amount of protein is fairly easy.

No recommendation for dietary fat is available for Masters athletes. Fat is an important nutrient and the diet of the Masters athlete should contain adequate amounts of fat. The American Dietetic Association and the American College of Sports Medicine do not recommend that athletes restrict fat intake below 20% of energy or consume high-fat diets because these practices will not enhance exercise performance.

23C.4 Micronutrients

Usually when energy intakes are met, micronutrients are satisfactory although a small number of dietary intake studies on ageing athletes suggest that some micronutrients (vitamins B_6, B_{12}, D and E, folate, calcium, iron and zinc) may be suboptimal in some groups. Micronutrient deficiencies are most likely to occur in those Masters athletes who restrict energy intake, practise severe methods of weight loss, do not base their diet on nutrient-dense foods or restrict their choice of foods and/or eliminate whole food groups from their diet. Table 23.7 lists the reference nutrient intakes for vitamins and minerals for adults aged over 50 years.

Increased energy demands of training and competition require a higher overall energy intake. Assuming the Masters athlete consumes adequate dietary intake and variety and quality of food choices to meet the increased needs, then he or she is usually likely to meet any increased vitamin or mineral requirements. For those Masters athletes who are habitually consuming low micronutrient intakes, it is recommended they improve their intake through dietary means.

23C.5 Fluid

Hydration is crucial for all athletes but Masters athletes have to pay special attention to fluid intake as there is a reduced sensation of thirst as one ages. In addition, sweat rates, renal adaptation to altered fluid and electrolyte status, and blood flow responses can impair thermoregulation in older athletes. There are no specific recommendations for fluid intake but since older adults have age-related decreased thirst sensitivity when they are dehydrated and tend to be slow to voluntarily establish a normal state of hydration, fluid replacement guidelines should be applied more aggressively in those practising prolonged physical activity (e.g. marathons or triathlons) in the heat. Older athletes have age-related slower renal responses to water and sodium loads and may be at greater risk for hyponatraemia. Generally, in events lasting less than 4 hours symptomatic hyponatraemia is from overdrinking before, during and sometimes after the event. Some of the sodium losses should be replaced over this time, and beverages containing 6–8% CHO and electrolytes, such as isotonic sports drinks, are recommended for exercise events lasting longer than 1 hour.

23C.6 Medications

It is estimated that over 30% of all prescription drugs are taken by older (>65 years) adults and older adults are also the highest users of over-the-counter drugs. Drug–nutrient interactions should therefore always be considered when dealing with Masters athletes. Masters athletes taking medications should always be referred to an appropriate health professional such as a registered sports dietitian.

23C.7 Summary of key dietary recommendations

There are no specific recommendations for nutrient intakes for Masters athletes. Many dietary recommendations do not differ between younger and older adults, and in the UK micronutrient requirements are the same for 51 year olds as for 71 year olds with the exception of vitamin D. The British Nutrition Foundation Task Force Report (2009) aims to identify steps that can be taken from a nutritional perspective to help older adults of tomorrow lead healthier lives and these should be considered when offering dietary advice to Masters athletes (Table 23.8).

Practical strategies: key guidelines

- Take a detailed medical history to determine whether dietary advice is to be influenced by medical concerns.
- Ensure adequate energy intake to sustain training and competition from a variety of foods and drinks.

- Emphasise the inclusion of plenty of whole grains, cereals and legumes.
- Aim for at least five portions of fruit and vegetables every day.
- Ensure sufficient protein intake.
- Maintain calcium and vitamin D intake. Good food sources of calcium include milk and dairy products (e.g. cheese, yoghurt, milk), fish containing soft bones (e.g. tinned salmon, sardines), fortified white flour products (e.g. bread, cereals), dark green leafy vegetables, pulses and seeds. Vitamin D status is mainly determined by the action of sunlight on skin but since vitamin D production tends to reduce as people age, then the Masters athlete may be required to take a supplement. Food sources of vitamin D include oil-rich fish (e.g. salmon, sardines, mackerel, herrings, pilchards), fortified margarines and breakfast cereals.
- Ensure adequate hydration. The Masters athlete must be made aware that dehydration will severely affect training and performance. The athlete should not rely on feeling thirsty as an indicator of fluid needs and should:
  ○ start every training session fully hydrated;
  ○ limit fluid losses to less than 1–2% of body weight;
  ○ avoid drinking too much so they actually gain body weight during exercise;
  ○ drink around 1.5 l of fluid for each kilogram of body weight lost if needing rapid and complete recovery from excessive dehydration after training or competition;
  ○ consume beverages with sodium to help speed up rapid and complete recovery by stimulating thirst and fluid retention.
- Investigate whether the Masters athlete is taking any supplements, assess the value of the product(s) and inform them of current thinking.
- An older athlete may well be living alone so offer practical guidance on shopping and cooking for one.
- Taste and smell diminish with age so suggest the inclusion of foods, herbs, spices and flavourings that make food tasty. Onions, garlic, ginger, chillies, mustards and various seasonings can add an extra 'kick' to meals and snacks.
- Physical challenges such as suffering from arthritis may make food preparation more difficult. Offer guidance to cope with preparation of simple and

Table 23.8 Diet and lifestyle messages emerging from the British Nutrition Foundation Task Force and associated benefits.

	Diet and lifestyle message	Associated benefits include
Fat quality	Decreased SFA and *trans* fatty acids	Decreased risk of CHD and stroke
		Improved insulin sensitivity
	Increased *cis* MUFA and PUFA	
EPA and DHA	Increased EPA and DHA	Decreased risk of CHD and possibly stroke
		Reduced symptoms of rheumatoid arthritis
		May have an effect on eye health and help prevent cognitive decline
		Improved immune function
		Very limited data suggesting improved bone mineral accrual (DHA)
Starchy CHOs	Increased intake	See dietary fibres
Dietary fibres	Increased intake	Improved gut health and cardiovascular health
		Satiety effects with some fibre types, e.g. viscous fibres such as guar gum, pectin, psyllium, β-glucan
Sugars	Moderation	Dental health benefits with moderation of frequency of sugar consumption but regular use of fluoridated toothpaste is the most important message
Alcohol	Moderation	Decreased risk of CHD but high intakes increases risk of stroke, osteoporosis, sarcopenia and some cancers and carries effects associated with dehydration
Protein	Adequate dietary supply	Preserves skeletal muscle mass
		Decreased risk of falls (hence decreased fracture risk)
Vitamin K	Ensure adequate supply	Increased bone mineral density
		Decreased osteoporotic fractures
Salt/sodium	Moderation	Positively associated with blood pressure (raised blood pressure is a major risk factor for stroke and heart disease)
Calcium	Ensure adequate supply	Improves bone health (increased bone mineral density; decreased post-menopausal bone loss)
		Some evidence for decreased colon cancer risk (milk and supplemental calcium)
Vitamin D status	Ensure adequate status	Essential for bone mineralisation
		Decreased sarcopenia risk
		Limited evidence that it may decrease (colon) cancer risk, delay cognitive decline, improve low mood
Vitamin A	Avoid excess	Excess (>1500 mg retinol equivalents/day) associated with low bone mineral density in post-menopausal women
Antioxidant vitamins		Dietary supply (via food and drink) essential for good health
Fruit and vegetables	Increased intake	High intake associated with decreased risk of CHD and of stroke (especially fruit)
		Probably protects against some cancers, limited evidence for a benefit for dementia and bone health
Nuts	In moderation	Positive association with heart health
Whole-grain cereals	Increased intake	Positive association with heart health and gut health (via fibre content)
Soya		Positive association with heart health (via LDL-cholesterol)
Fish (especially oil-rich fish)		Positive association with heart health and cancer risk
		Possible beneficial effect with dementia
Meat		Modest increased risk of colon cancer with processed meat in particular, also some evidence of an increase with red meat particularly in association with low fibre intake (i.e. effect attenuated by high fibre intake)
Low-fat dairy products	In moderation	Calcium content important for bone health
		Decreased blood pressure (as part of the DASH diet)
		Possible decreased risk of colon cancer
Fluid intake		Important for general health and well-being
		Associated with decreased risk of constipation
		Possibly associated with better skin health

CHD, coronary heart disease; DHA, docosahexaenoic acid; EPA, eicosapentaenoic acid; LDL, low-density lipoprotein; MUFA, monounsaturated fatty acid; PUFA, polyunsaturated fatty acid; SFA, saturated fatty acid.
Adapted from Stanner *et al.* 2009.

nutritious meals that require little or no preparation, food labelling education to enable them to choose suitable nutritious ready meals when shopping. and how to choose healthy suitable items from take-away menus.

23C.8 Conclusions

There is a lack of studies to evaluate the effect of diet and exercise in Masters athletes, especially in the habitually trained. In addition, very little is known about the nutrient intakes, nutritional status or nutritional needs of Masters athletes and there are no specific recommendations for nutrient intakes for ageing athletes participating in athletic training. However, when dealing with Masters athletes nutritional recommendations should be based on the following considerations:

- age-related changes in physiology;
- dietary changes that occur with exercise;
- the type of exercise (e.g. strength, power, endurance);
- frequency, intensity and length of training and competition;
- the presence of chronic illness or disease;
- nutrient–medication interactions.

Given the great variety of fitness levels, personal goals and nutrition knowledge, each Masters athlete should be treated as an individual. When dealing with Masters athletes evidence-based guidelines currently available for active adults and competitive athletes need to be adjusted to accommodate their unique concerns regarding health, sports, nutrient needs, food preferences and body weight and body composition goals.

Further reading

Children

American Academy of Pediatrics. Climatic heat stress and the exercising child and adolescent. Pediatrics 2000; 106: 158–159.

American Academy of Pediatrics. Use of performance-enhancing substances. Pediatrics 2005; 115: 1103–1106.

American Academy of Pediatrics. Promotion of healthy weight-control practices in young athletes. Pediatrics 2005; 116: 1557–1564.

American College of Sports Medicine. Roundtable on the physiological and health effects of oral creatine supplementation. Med Sci Sports Exerc 2000; 32: 706–717.

Armstrong LE, Maresh CM. Exercise-heat tolerance of children and adolescents. Pediatr Exerc Sci 1995; 7: 239–252.

Aucouturier J, Baker JS, Duche P. Fat and CHO metabolism during submaximal exercise in children. Sports Med 2008; 38: 213–238.

Bailey DA, McKay HA, Mirwald RL, Crocker PR, Faulkner, RA. A six-year longitudinal study of the relationship of physical activity to bone mineral accrual in growing children: the university of Saskatchewan bone mineral accrual study. J Bone Miner Res 1999; 14: 1672–1679.

Bar-Or O. Temperature regulation during exercise in children and adolescents. In: Perspectives in Exercise Science and Sports Medicine: Youth, Exercise and Sport (Gisolfi C, Lamb D, eds). Indianapolis: Benchmark Press, 1989, pp 335–367.

Bar-Or O. Nutritional considerations for the child athlete. Can J Appl Physiol 2001; 26 (Suppl): S186–S191.

Bar-Or O, Wilk B. Water and electrolyte replenishment in the exercising child. Int J Sport Nutr 1996; 6: 93–99.

Bass S, Inge K. Nutrition for special populations: children and young athletes. In: Clinical Sports Nutrition, 4th edn (Burke L, Deakin V, eds). Sydney: McGraw-Hill, 2010, pp 508–546.

Benardot D, Schwarz M, Heller DW. Nutrient intake in young, highly competitive gymnasts. J Am Diet Assoc 1989; 89: 401–403.

Boisseau N, Delamarche P. Metabolic and hormonal responses to exercise in children and adolescents. Sports Med 2000; 30: 405–422.

Boisseau N, Vermorel M, Rance M et al. Protein requirements in male adolescent soccer players. Eur J Appl Physiol 2007; 100: 27–33.

Bolster D, Pikosky MA, McCarthy LM, Rodriguez NR. Exercise affects protein utilization in healthy children. J Nutr 2001; 131: 2659–2663.

Butte NF. Fat intake of children in relation to energy requirements. Am J Clin Nutr 2000; 72: 1236S–1252S.

Calfee R, Fadale P. Popular ergogenic drugs and supplements in young athletes. Pediatrics 2006; 117: e577–e589.

Cotunga N, Vickery CE, McBee S. Sports nutrition for young athletes. J Sch Nurs 2005; 21: 323–328.

D'Alessandro C, Morelli E, Evangelisti I et al. Profiling the diet and body composition of subelite adolescent rhythmic gymnasts. Pediatr Exer Sci 2007; 19: 215–227.

Delamarche P, Bittel J, Lacour JR, Flandrois R. Thermoregulation at rest and during exercise in prepubertal boys. Eur J Appl Physiol Occup Physiol 1990; 60: 436–440.

Delamarche P, Monnier M, Gratas-Delamarche A, Koubi HE, Mayet MH, Favier R. Glucose and free fatty acid utilization during prolonged exercise in prepubertal boys in relation to catecholamine responses. Eur J Appl Physiol Occup Physiol 1992; 65: 66–72.

Department of Health. Dietary Reference Values of Food Energy and Nutrients for the United Kingdom (Report of the Panel on Dietary Reference Values of the Committee on Medical Aspects of Food Policy). London: HMSO, 1991.

Di Santolo M, Stel G, Banfi G et al. Anaemia and iron status in young fertile nonprofessional female athletes. Eur J Appl Physiol 2008; 102: 703–709.

Dougherty KA, Baker LB, Chow M, Kenney WL. Two percent dehydration impairs and six percent CHO drink improves boys basketball skills. Med Sci Sports Exer 2006; 38: 1650–1658.

Falk B. Effects of thermal stress during rest and exercise in the paediatric population. Sports Med 1998; 25: 221–240.

Falk B, Bar-Or O, MacDougall JD. Thermoregulatory responses of pre-, mid-, and late-pubertal boys to exercise in dry heat. Med Sci Sports Exerc 1992; 23: 688–694.

Gidding SS, Dennison BA, Birch LL *et al.* Dietary recommendations for children and adolescents: a guide for practitioners: consensus statement from the American Heart Association. Circulation 2005; 112: 2061–2075.

Goulding A. Risk factors for fractures in normally active children and adolescents. Med Sport Sci 2007; 51: 102–120.

Inbar O, Morris N, Epstein Y, Gass G. Comparison of thermoregulatory responses to exercise in dry heat among pre-pubertal boys, young adults and older males. Exp Physiol 2004; 89: 691–700.

Inoue Y, Kuwahara T, Araki T. Maturation- and aging-related changes in heat loss effector function. J Physiol Anthropol Appl Human 2004; 23: 289–294.

Iuliano S, Naughton G, Collier G, Carlson J. Examination of the self-selected fluid intake practices by junior athletes during a simulated duathlon event. Int J Sport Nutr 1998; 8: 10–23.

Kaczor JJ, Ziolkowski W, Popinigis J, Tarnopolsky MA. Anaerobic and aerobic enzyme activities in human skeletal muscle from children and adults. Pediatr Res 2005; 57: 331–335.

Lanou AJ, Berkow SE, Barnard ND. Calcium, dairy products, and bone health in children and young adults: a re-evaluation of the evidence. Pediatrics 2005; 115: 736–743.

Loosli AR, Benson J. Nutritional intake in adolescent athletes. Pediatr Clin North Am 1990; 37: 1143–1152.

Lytle L. Nutritional issues for adolescents. J Am Diet Assoc 2002; 102: S8–S12.

MacKelvie KJ, Khan KM, McKay HA. Is there a critical period for bone response to weight-bearing exercise in children and adolescents? A systematic review. Br J Sports Med 2002; 36: 250–257.

Malina RM. Physical activity and training: effects on stature and the adolescent growth spurt. Med Sci Sports Exerc 1994; 26: 759–766.

Massad S, Shier N, Koceja D, Ellis N. High school athletes and nutritional supplements: a study of knowledge and use. Int J Sports Nutr 1995; 5: 232–235.

Meyer F, Bar-Or O. Fluid and electrolyte loss during exercise. The paediatric angle. Sports Med 1994; 18: 4–9.

Meyer F, O'Connor H, Shirreffs SM. Nutrition for the young athlete. J Sports Sci 2007; 25 (Suppl 1): S73–S82.

Montfort- Steiger V, Williams CA. CHO intake considerations for young athletes. J Sports Sci Med 2007; 6: 343–352.

National Health and Medical Research Council (NHMRC). Nutrient Reference Values for Australia and New Zealand. Canberra: Australian Government, 2005.

Naughton GA, Carlson JS. Reducing the risk of heat-related decrements to physical activity in young people. J Sci Med Sport 2008; 11: 58–65.

Nemet D, Eliakim A. Pediatric sports nutrition: an update. Curr Opin Clin Nutr Metab Care 2009; 12: 304–309.

Neumark-Sztainer D, Story M, Perry C, Casey M. Factors influencing food choices of adolescents: findings from focus-group discussions with adolescents. J Am Diet Assoc 1999; 99: 929–937.

Nieper A. Nutritional supplement practices in UK junior national track and field athletes. Br J Sports Med 2005; 39: 645–649.

O'Dea JA. Consumption of nutritional supplements among adolescents: usage and perceived benefits. Health Educ Res 2003; 18: 98–107.

Petrie HJ, Stover EA, Horswill CA. Nutritional concerns for the child and adolescent competitor. Nutrition 2004; 20: 620–631.

Pikosky M, Faigenbaum A, Westcott W, Rodriguez N. Effects of resistance training on protein utilization in healthy children. Med Sci Sports Exerc 2002; 34: 820–827.

Rankinen T, Fogelholm M, Kujala U, Rauramaa R, Uusitupa M. Dietary intake and nutritional status of athletic and nonathletic children in early puberty. Int J Sport Nutr 1995; 5: 136–150.

Rowland T. Thermoregulation during exercise in the heat in children: old concepts revisited. J Appl Physiol 2008; 105: 718–723.

Rowland TW, Black SA, Kelleher JF. Iron deficiency in adolescent endurance athletes. J Adolesc Health Care 1987; 8: 322–326.

Rowland T, Garrison A, Pober D. Determinants of endurance exercise capacity in the heat in prepubertal boys. Int J Sports Med 2007; 28: 26–32.

Sank, L. Dental nutrition. Nutrition Issues Abstracts 1999; 19: 1–2.

Schenkel TC, Stockman NK, Brown JN, Duncan AM. Evaluation of energy, nutrient and dietary fiber intakes of adolescent males. J Am Coll Nutr 2007; 26: 264–271.

Spear B. Adolescent growth and development. J Am Diet Assoc 2002; 102: S23–S29.

Specker B, Vukovich M. Evidence for an interaction between exercise and nutrition for improved bone health during growth. Med Sport Sci 2007; 51: 50–63.

Sports Medicine Australia. Safety Guidelines for Children in Sport and Recreation. Canberra: Sports Medicine Australia 1997.

Stang J. Nutrition in adolescence. In: Krause's Food and Nutrition Therapy, 12th edn (Mahan LK, Escott-Stump S, eds). St Louis, MO: Saunders Elsevier, 2008, pp 236–268.

Stephens BR, Cole AS, Mahon AD. The influence of biological maturation on fat and CHO metabolism during exercise in males. Int J Sport Nutr Exer Metab 2006; 16: 166–179.

Story M, Neumark-Sztainer D, French S. Individual and environmental influences on adolescent eating behaviours. J Am Diet Assoc 2002; 102: S40–S51.

Theintz G. Endocrine adaptations to intensive physical training during growth. Clin Endocrinol 1994; 41: 267.

Thompson JL. Energy balance in young athletes. Int J Sport Nutr 1998; 8: 160–174.

Timmons BW, Bar-Or O, Riddell MC. Oxidation rate of exogenous CHO during exercise is higher in boys than in men. J Appl Physiol 2003; 94: 278–284.

Timmons BW, Bar-Or O, Riddell MC. Influence of age and pubertal status on substrate utilization during exercise with and without CHO intake in healthy boys. Appl Physiol Nutr Metab 2007; 32: 416–425.

Timmons BW, Bar-Or, O, Riddell MC. Energy substrate utilization during prolonged exercise with and without CHO intake in pre-adolescent and adolescent girls. J Appl Physiol 2007; 103: 995–1000.

Unnithan VB, Goulopoulou S. Nutrition for the pediatric athlete. Curr Sports Med Rep 2004; 3: 206–211.

Volpe SL. Micronutrient requirements for athletes. Clin Sports Med 2007; 26: 119–130.

Warren MP, Chua AT. Exercise-induced amenorrhea and bone health in the adolescent athlete. Ann NY Acad Sci 2008; 1135: 234–252.

Winston AP, Hardwick E, Jaberi N. Neuropsychiatric effects of caffeine. Adv Psychiatr Treat 2005; 11: 432–439.

Female athletes

Beals KA, Meyer NL. Female athlete triad update. Clin Sports Med 2007; 26: 69–89.

Burke LM, Cox GR, Cummings NK, Desbrow B. Guidelines for daily CHO intake: do athletes achieve them? Sports Med 2001; 31: 267–299.

Burke LM, Kiens B, Ivy JL. CHOs and fat for training and recovery. J Sports Sci 2004; 22: 15–30.

Burke LM, Loucks AB, Broad N. Energy and CHO for training and recovery. J Sports Sci 2006; 23: 675–685.

Bonci CM, Bonci LJ, Granger LR *et al.* National athletic trainers' association position statement: preventing, detecting, and managing disordered eating in athletes. J Athl Train 2008; 43: 80–108.

Edwards JE, Lindeman AK, Mikesky AE, Stager JM. Energy balance in highly trained female endurance runners. Med Sci Sports Exerc 1993; 25: 1398–1404.

Haggarty A, McGraw BA, Maughan R, Fenn C. Energy expenditure of elite female athletes measured by the doubly-labeled water method. Proc Nutr Soc 1988; 47: 35A.

Hill RJ, Davies PS. Energy intake and energy expenditure in elite lightweight female rowers. Med Sci Sports Exerc 2002; 34: 1823–1829.

International Olympic Committee Medical Commission. Position Stand on the Female Athlete Triad. Available from http://multimedia.olympic.org/pdf/en_report_917.pdf. Accessed 19 May 2010.

Manore MM, Kam LC, Loucks AB. The female athlete triad: components, nutrition issues, and health consequences. J Sports Sci 2007; 25 (Suppl 1): S61–S71.

Manore MM, Meyer NL, Thompson J. Sport Nutrition for Health and Performance. Champaign, IL: Human Kinetics, 2009.

Nattiv A, Loucks AB, Manore MM, Sanborn CF, Sundgot-Borgen J, Warren MP. American College of Sports Medicine Position Stand. The female athlete triad. Med Sci Sports Exerc 2007; 39: 1867–1882.

Sjödin AM, Andersson AB, Hogberg JM, Westerterp KR. Energy balance in cross-country skiers: a study using doubly labeled water. Med Sci Sports Exerc 1994; 26: 720–724.

Stice E, Shaw H. Eating disorder prevention programs: a meta-analytic review. Psychol Bull 2004; 130: 206–227.

Tarnopolsky MA. Sex differences in exercise metabolism and the role of beta-estradiol. Med Sci Sports Exerc 2008; 40: 648–654.

Masters

American Dietetic Association. Position of the American Dietetic Association, Dietitians of Canada, and the American College of Sports Medicine: Nutrition and Athletic Performance. J Am Diet Assoc 2000; 100: 1543–1556.

Burke LM, Deakin V (eds). Clinical Sports Nutrition, 4th edn. Sydney: McGraw-Hill Australia, 2010.

Campbell WW, Geik RA. Nutritional considerations for the older athlete. Nutrition 2004; 20: 603–608.

Department of Health. Dietary Reference Values for Food Energy and Nutrients for the United Kingdom. Report of the Panel on Dietary Reference Intakes of the Committee on Medical Aspects of Food Policy. London: HMSO, 1991.

Evans W, Cyr-Campbell D. Nutrition, exercise and healthy aging. J Am Diet Assoc 1997; 97: 632–638.

Kenney WL. Are there special hydration requirements for older individuals engaged in exercise? Aust J Nutr Diet 1996; 53: S43–S44.

Maughan RJ (ed.). Nutrition in Sport. Oxford: Blackwell Science, 2000.

Maughan RJ, Burke LM, Coyle EF (eds). Nutrition for Athletes. London: Routledge, 2004.

Rosenbloom CA, Dunaway A. Nutrition recommendations for masters athletes. Clin Sports Med 2007; 26: 91–100.

Sawka MN, Burke LM, Eichner ER, Maughan RJ, Montain SJ, Stachenfield NS. Exercise and fluid replacement. Med Sci Sports Exerc 2007; 39: 377–390.

Stanner S, Thompson R, Butriss JL (eds). Healthy Aging. The Role of Nutrition and Lifestyle. The Report of the British Nutrition Foundation Task Force. Oxford: Wiley-Blackwell, 2009.

Stear SJ. Fuelling Fitness for Sports Performance. London: The Sugar Bureau, 2004.

24
Population Groups: II

Weileen Png, Wendy Martinson, Nicola Maffulli and Filippo Spiezia

It is absolutely critical that due consideration is given to how ethnicity, culture and religious beliefs affect dietary patterns. The multicultural society that we live in requires sports nutritionists and dietitians to have a full appreciation of the differences between cultures and be able, multiculturally, to provide the right nutritional guidance, both at the recreational level of physical activity and at the level of competitive sport. It is also key that population groups who follow a particular diet (such as vegetarianism/veganism) are fully investigated and clear guidance provided as to all the benefits/risks associated by following a particular dietary regimen. Of equal importance is the assessment of nutritional requirements to the injured athlete. All these aspects are covered within this chapter, with key messages and summaries provided for each of the different sub-chapters.

ETHNIC GROUPS

Weileen Png

Key messages

- Ethnicity, culture and religion can shape an individual's perception of eating, food choices and habit.
- In order to work with athletes from different ethnic groups, nutrition practitioners are required to be multiculturally competent in delivering appropriate nutrition interventions and programmes.
- To succeed in working with athletes of different ethnicities and cultural backgrounds, nutritionists need to acknowledge similarities and differences among cultures and be prepared to communicate and work in situations that are not typical of their culture.

24A.1 Introduction

Today's athlete is a globetrotter. International training and competition have made it necessary for competitive athletes to jet around the world. With the world development towards globalisation, coupled with the rapid growth of the sports industry, there is an increased trend in athletes migrating from one country to another to gain sporting exposure and international success, thus forming the diverse population within the country. This demographic trend towards globalisation means athletes face the challenge of living in an environment of diverse ethnic and multicultural backgrounds, which can create challenges to an athlete's usual food choices and dietary patterns.

Eating habits are acquired over a lifetime and dietary change requires a conscious effort while practice and commitment are needed to maintain this change. Besides taste and health and nutritional beliefs, ethnicity, culture, religion, social and economic

Sport and Exercise Nutrition, First Edition. Edited by Susan A Lanham-New, Samantha J Stear, Susan M Shirreffs and Adam L Collins.
© 2011 The Nutrition Society. Published 2011 by Blackwell Publishing Ltd.

Table 24.1 Major classification of ethnic groups in Southeast Asia.

	Chinese		
Regions			
Religions	Buddhism	Taoism	Confucianism
Food group Staple	Rice, wheat (noodles, breads) *Others* Mung bean, noodles, etc.	Rice, wheat (noodles, breads) *Others* Mung bean, noodles, etc.	Rice, wheat (noodles, breads) *Others* Mung bean, noodles, etc.
Meat dishes	Strict Buddhism: avoid all meat or animal-derived products although some allow white meat. Generally allows meat alternatives, e.g. tofu, mock meat	Variety of meat, except beef	Variety of meat
Vegetables	Variety of vegetables, except those with strong odours, e.g. garlic, chives, leek, or root vegetables, e.g. potatoes	Variety of vegetables	Variety of vegetables
Fat/oil	Only vegetable-based cooking oils allowed, e.g. sunflower, sesame oil	Variety of animal or vegetable based oils	Variety of animal or vegetable based oils
Others			
Cooking methods	Stir-frying, steaming, frying, stewing		
Dining manner/ etiquette	*Dining etiquette* Communal dinning Main eating utensil: chopsticks *Lifestyle* Reserved Group-oriented Home-oriented Respectful and obedient Prideful Practise traditional Chinese medicine		
Dietary practices	*Buddhism* Most Buddhists practise vegetarian lifestyles (lacto-ovo vegetarians). Some avoid meat and dairy products, while others only avoid beef (affected by cultural, geographical and dietary influences)	*Taoism* Believe that consumption of certain foods might interfere with the body's harmony (e.g. Ying and Yang). Ying refers to 'cold food' believed to reduce body temperature and impart strength and cheerfulness. Yang refers to 'hot food', believed to increase body temperature/spiciness of a food, which affects the body's balance and state of health	*Confucianism* Adjust diet to harmonise with Ying and Yang, e.g. foods are never cooked too fine or minced too well (e.g. meat). Believe art in cooking lies in taste
Nutritional implication(s)	Increased risk of nutrient deficiencies, e.g. iron deficiency for strict vegetarians High fat intake as most of the mock meat used is prepared by frying Higher intake of sodium (soy sauce or condiments) and oil to give flavour as onions and garlic are not allowed in cooking	Increased risk of nutrient deficiencies due to possible food avoidance or improper food choices	

Indian				Malay
North	**South**	**East**	**West**	
Hinduism, Muslim				*Muslim*
Roti (wheat based bread)	Rice	Rice, breads	*Coastal region* (e.g. Goa) Rice *Hilly region* (e.g. Marathi) Wheat, rice, millet, sorghum	Rice, wheat (noodles, breads)
Primarily chicken, goat and lamb	Primarily seafood, variety of meat	Primarily fish and shellfish	*Coastal region* Fish, shellfish *Hilly region* Variety of meat/vegetarian	Variety of meat except pork and animals killed not in accordance with Islamic law
Variety of lentils and vegetables	Variety of lentils and vegetables	Variety of lentils and vegetables	Variety of lentils and vegetables	Variety of vegetables
Ghee (clarified butter), mustard oil	Ghee, coconut milk/oils	Mustard oil	*Coastal region* Coconut milk/oil, vegetable fat *Hilly region* Groundnut oil	Variety of vegetable oil, e.g. coconut oil/milk
Wide use of dairy products	Spices: Sambar, rasam (Chaaru/saaru), tamarind		Wide use of sugar in dishes and desserts	Wide use of spices and coconut milk (*Santan*) in cooking
Simmering, frying, steaming, grilling				Stir-frying, stewing, steaming, frying, baking, grilling

Dining etiquette
Eat sitting on the floor
Family-style serving
Essential to wash hands and mouth prior to eating
No eating utensils, right hand is used to serve food
Eat using right hand (left hand is used for taking foods and drinks)
Food served on plantain or banana leaf
Involves spices in cooking, e.g. Garam masala, cloves, saffron

Lifestyle
Traditional and conservative

Hinduism, Muslim
Avoid foods that cause pain to animals when processing
Consume dairy products, e.g. milk, yoghurt, ghee
Seafood is restricted
Alcohol, onions, garlic and beef are avoided (cow is considered sacred (Krishna's favourite animal))
Prohibited foods: beef (Hindu) and pork (Muslim) are sometimes restricted or avoided
Fasting depends on the person's cast/social standing and occasion

Buddhism
Similar to Chinese Buddhism

Jainism
Devout are complete vegetarians
Jainism ideology: certain foods are *abhaksyas* (not to be eaten)
Restricted/avoided foods: alcohol, honey, meat, vegetables and fruits with many seeds (e.g. eggplant) plus root crops (because believed to destroy infinite souls) such as onions, potatoes and garlic; plus blood-coloured food (because believed to cause death of insects) such as tomatoes and some red-coloured root vegetables

Vegetarian
India (largest vegetarian population in the world)
Mostly lacto-ovo-vegetarians (~90%)
~20% strictly vegetarians
Increased risk of nutrient deficiencies if improper food choices are made particularly if following strict vegetarian diets
May increase risk of iron deficiency due to avoidance of red meat, e.g. beef (Hindus)

Dining etiquette
Eat with right hand
Spoons used to serve food from main dish to individual plate/bowl

Lifestyle
Deeply embedded beliefs
Rural lifestyle

Islam
Avoid Haram foods (prohibited foods), such as pork, alcohol, products with emulsifier made from animal fats, bread products fermented by yeast (may have traces of alcohol)
Require fasting for a month during Ramadan

High fat intake as most of the dishes are prepared by frying, and the use of coconut milk or oil
Increased risk of nutrient deficiencies and dehydration during Ramadan month

influences can shape the athlete's perceptions of eating, food choices and habits. For example, in the case of religions, only kosher foods are permitted by Judaism believers, and halal foods by Islamic believers. In addition, the dietary choices of different countries or regions have different characteristics. For example, athletes accustomed to Western diets may encounter difficulties when training in Asian countries where staple foods are rice and noodles instead of breads and cereals. Foods are often served and shared among a group of people (i.e. communal eating in Southeast Asia) whereas in the Western countries individual set meals are served instead.

The ability to work effectively with athletes from different cultures and in settings where several cultures coexist is of paramount importance for sport nutritionists planning to work in the elite sport industry. Nutrition practitioners working with these athletes are facing greater emphasis on providing culturally appropriate nutrition programmes that can influence athletes' behaviour changes as evidence of effectiveness. Nutrition practitioners are required to be multiculturally competent in delivering appropriate nutrition interventions and programmes; this includes designing menus and recipes that meet the nutrient needs of athlete groups and satisfy a wide variety of individual tastes, expectations and cultural preferences. This would help to minimise any culture shocks that could jeopardise an athlete's usual eating habits and nutrient needs when training and competing in a foreign country.

This sub-chapter focuses on the cultural influences on athletes' food choices and the processes involved in working with athletes of different ethnic and cultural backgrounds.

24A.2 Major classification of ethnic groups in Southeast Asia

It is beyond the scope of this section to describe and provide details of all the ethnic groups in the world. Therefore, we have attempted to simplify the major ethnic groups in Southeast Asia by summarising the major ethnic groups into three broad categories: Chinese, Malay and Indian. The summary provides information on the geographic origin, cultural norms and customs, religious beliefs, dietary practices and its nutritional implications (Tables 24.1 and 24.2).

24A.3 Cultural considerations

Nutrition and food sources

Learning about the common food and cuisines available at the destination will be helpful in planning athletes' meals. It can be beneficial to investigate the main sources of the key macronutrients, carbohydrate (CHO) and protein, fruit and vegetables, and sports foods such as sports drinks and energy bars, available at the destination that can be used as substitutes for the familiar foods often used at home to meet athletes' nutritional needs. Athletes can benefit from familiarising themselves with food choices and dietary customs of the destination by eating in relevant ethnic restaurants offering similar cuisine before leaving home.

Food taboos

Some food and drinks are considered taboo due to religious beliefs, cultural practices or for hygienic reasons. For example, consumption of pork is forbidden among religious followers such as the Muslims, Jews, Seventh-day Adventists, and certain Christian Denominations although it is the most widely eaten meat in most parts of the world.

In some cultures, food taboos include some meats that are generally not accepted as the common range of foodstuff. For example dog meat is widely eaten in China, Korea and Vietnam, although it is considered unacceptable in the USA and Europe. Similarly, horse meat is a common dish in Japan and France but is rarely eaten in the USA, Europe, New Zealand and Australia.

It is therefore important for athletes to be aware of the food available at the destination and plan in advance. It is also important to learn to read the menu and clarify any dishes with the waiters when in doubt, in order to avoid any surprises that are deemed not acceptable or offend the athletes.

Typical meal patterns

In some countries, especially in Asia, the evening meal will be the most substantial meal of the day as it is cultural practice that the family will come together

Table 24.2 Muslim culture backgrounds and dietary habits.

Geographic origin	Practices/festivals	Dietary practices	Culture/customs	Nutrition implications
Islam began in the northwest part of Arabia in the seventh century and spread into Syria, Palestine, Iraq, Iran, Central Asia, Egypt, Libya, Tunisia, Algeria, Morocco, Spain, Portugal and eventually Southeast Asia	• Belief in Islam • Prayer: five times daily • Friday is the holy day in Islamic religion, and a special day of prayer and worship in the mosque, or Islamic temple • Celebrate two major festivals: 1. *Hari Raya Puasa (Aid-il-fitri)* At the end of Ramadan (fasting month) *Ramadan month* - Fasting (abstain from food, drink and smoking from dawn to dusk) to express compassion for the hungry and needy - Mandatory fasting for both males and females - Only consume two meals daily a. Early morning meal (*Sahur*) consumed before dawn, e.g. dates, water, refreshing juices and soups b. Meal consumed after sunset (*Iftar*), e.g. traditional meat dishes, side dishes, salads, flat breads and a variety of sweets 2. *Hari Raya Haji (Aidil Adha/* Pilgrimage festival/Festival of Sacrifice) The end of the Muslim's pilgrimage to Mecca; those who can afford it include the sacrifice of animals (e.g. lamb, cow, goat) and sharing the meat with friends and poor (only one-third consumed by family members)	All food can be used generally as guided by Halal Certified Food (Arabic term for lawful food) - No *Haram* food (Arabic term for unlawful food) - Use only 'clean' (uncontaminated with any *Haram* food) utensils for cooking and eating *Examples of Haram (unlawful) foods* - Animals/birds that died naturally - Animals/birds killed not in accordance with the Islamic law - Shellfish/fish without fins and scales - Blood - Alcohol - Products or food manufactured using gelatins, animal fats or emulsifiers from animals *Typical food taken* • Staple: rice, coconut flavored rice, turmeric rice, noodles, mung bean noodles, bread, etc. • Meat/poultry: beef, mutton, chicken, etc. • Vegetables: all types of vegetables • Egg/legumes: tofu, fermented beans, nuts and variety of beans • Fat/oil: blended vegetable oil, coconut milk (*Santan*)	*Dinning etiquette/manner* - Pray before and after each meal - Eat with right hand - Use spoons to serve food from main dish to individual plate/bowl - Host will expect to start eating first and be the last to finish - Always eat with a washed and wet hand - Wait for everyone to finish before leaving the table or floor cloth *Lifestyle* - Deeply embedded beliefs - Rural lifestyle (simple)	• Food avoidance due to unknown food sources (*Haram*) may leads to inadequate nutrient intake • High consumption of saturated fat due to high intake of coconut milk in dishes and desserts *During Ramadan month* • Increased risk of energy and nutrient deficiencies if inadequate food or inappropriate food choices are made • Increased risk of dehydration

to have dinner after a day's work, whereas in some Western cultures a large midday meal is often taken followed by a light snack in the evening. Therefore, it is an important consideration when organising catering for athletes to have an understanding of the typical meal patterns of the destination in order to make arrangement for meals that meets the athletes training or competition schedule.

Meal-time behaviours

Understanding the typical meal time and operating hours of restaurants and eateries is helpful in arranging catering for athletes. In some countries such as India, dinner is served much later in the evening (7–9 pm) and therefore athletes who have completed training in the evening (5 pm) and want to refuel and return to rest may have problems accessing meals immediately. As such, prior arrangements should be made for meal times with restaurants; alternatively extra food may need to be purchased in advance.

Meal etiquette

In some cultures, communal eating is adopted, where a variety of dishes are expected to be shared among a group. In China, dining tables are round or square rather than long rectangles or oval so that diners are seated equal distances from the dishes. It is also a cultural norm that the host will serve the guests first with food that they consider the best delicacies. In this situation, what the host considers as good food (usually fatty cuts of meat or exotic meats) could differ significantly from the athlete's dietary requirements.

In some religions or customs, a prayer or 'blessing' may be practised at the table before eating. Most prayers are made by the host before the meal is eaten. If invited as dinner guests, athletes may join in or be respectfully silent.

In most Western countries, soups are drunk using a spoon, but in Asian countries like Japan and Korea soups are drunk directly from the bowl. If unsure, observe the host or the locals.

Utensils

Hands, chopsticks, fork and spoon, or knife and fork are all possible utensils used depending on the travel destination. It pays to practice eating with the expected utensils before leaving home. In most Asian countries, when eating a shared meal, it is poor etiquette to use your eating utensils to transfer food to your own plate: always use serving utensils. Remember when eating with your hands to use only one hand, normally the right (watch the locals to determine the correct one).

Dress codes

In most cultures it is highly regarded to be conservatively dressed (no sleeveless shirt, shorts, slippers) for group dining. Athletes in sports gear (i.e. shorts and sleeveless T-shirts) should change out of the sports gear and cover up.

Language

Language barriers can be one of the most difficult challenges when trying to choose nutritionally appropriate meals in a foreign destination. These limit athletes from making appropriate choices when choosing dishes from menus written in foreign languages as well as when asking for assistance from waiters who only speak a foreign language. It can be helpful to learn some simple words such as water, rice, pasta, fruit and, in particular, words for foods that need to be avoided or which cause allergic reactions.

24A.4 Working with athletes of different ethnicities

The ability to work effectively with athletes of different cultural backgrounds requires practitioners to be multiculturally competent. Besides being aware of factors that influence food choices – such as taste preferences, income, occupation and lifestyle, state of health, family and peer pressures, knowledge and beliefs about diet, habit and familiarity – they also need to have a strong multicultural awareness and be sensitive to the strong influence of cultures on an individual's food intakes, attitudes and behaviours.

To succeed in working with athletes of different ethnicities and cultural backgrounds, nutritionists need to acknowledge similarities and differences among cultures and be prepared to communicate and work in situations that are not typical of their own culture.

Table 24.3 Example check-list of questions to assist a sports nutritionist prepare for international travel.

What is the country of origin?
What are the major ethnic groups in this country?
What is the common spoken and written language of the country?
What is the major religion and practices of the people living in the country?
What are the food cultural practices and customs?
Are there any dress code or attire restrictions when visiting restaurants and eateries?
Are there any food taboos?
What are the main staples and common foods taken by people living in the country?
What are the typical meal timings?
What are typical methods of preparation of foods in the country of origin? For example, smoked meats, fried foods, rich sauces
What are the table manners or etiquette practices of the ethnic group?
Are utensils or hands used to consume foods?
Does the travel period coincide with any festivals?
Will the sports team be invited to any meal gatherings? What will a typical invited meal consist of?

24A.5 General skills for practitioners

The following list outlines the basic skills required for an effective approach when working with athletes of different ethnicities and cultural backgrounds (see also Table 24.3).

- It is important that respect and trust is established between the practitioners and clients. Practitioners need to be sincere when building a rapport with clients.
- Have an open view: acknowledge and accept cultural differences.
- Have knowledge of clients' food habits and health beliefs.
- Be sensitive to verbal and non-verbal communications (e.g. be observant and learn the appropriate degree of physical and eye contact in a given culture).
- Determine the primary language (oral and written) used by clients so that communication can be understood.
- Where necessary, use skilled interpreters who are sensitive to clients' cultural background and understand nutritional terminology and the concepts. When teaching interpreters the nutritional interventions and strategies, use plain language that can

be understood easily so that the nutritional messages will not be wrongly interpreted.
- Determine clients preferred communication style (direct or indirect communication). Indirect communication may mean presenting information from a third-person perspective (e.g. 'in order to decrease the salt intake, another client successfully tried to replace salt by using herbs in the cooking') or explaining the nutrition concepts or strategies through the use of illustrations and stories.
- Provide information that is most relevant to clients (i.e. what they need to know, rather than what is nice to know).
- Provide only positive messages to the clients.
- Be consistent in the messages communicated.

24A.6 Special topic: Ramadan fasting and sports performance

In recent years, there has been increased attention on Ramadan fasting and sports performance. This is due to the fact that the fasting ritual is practised by a large part of the world population and Muslim athletes adhering to this practice represent significant numbers of competitors in major sporting events. For example, the Singapore Youth Olympics 2010 and the London Olympic Games 2012 both coincide with the month of Ramadan. Hence, during these events, Muslim athletes may be observing the fast while training and/or competing. The absence of food and fluid before, during and after competition or training may impose significant implications on performance and for any training adaptations to take place. Consequently, sports scientists are looking at strategies to possibly negate any effects of Ramadan fasting on sports performance.

During Ramadan, strict Muslims, both men and women, engage in the practice of fasting during the daylight hours for 30 days. During this period, strict Muslims do not eat or drink (i.e. total abstinence from food and fluids) from dawn until dusk for 12–14 hours daily. This may be longer depending on both geographical location of the individual as well as the climatic season in which the fasting month of Ramadan falls. For example, in the peak summer months where daylight hours are extended, the duration of the day's fast may be up to 18 hours. In the coldest winter, the fasting duration may be less than 8 hours. Generally, meals are consumed at two main sittings daily: the first meal of the day around 4.30 to 5.30 am before the commencement of the day's fast (i.e. the *Sahur* meal); and the second meal at the break of the day's fast around 7 pm (i.e. the *Iftar* meal). This means Muslim athletes will have to make some changes to their sleep cycles to accommodate the shift in the pattern of food and fluid intake from daytime hours to the hours of darkness. Such fasting can result in prolonged periods without intake of nutrients or food, inflexibility with regard to timing of eating and drinking during the day and around exercise sessions, and changes to usual dietary choices due to the special foods involved with various rituals.

Previous studies have reported that in Ramadan, energy intake of Muslim athletes does not decrease despite abstinence of food and fluid during daylight hours. In fact Muslim athletes consumed either equal or more calories in total over Ramadan than they would if they had not fasted (Aziz & Png, 2008). This suggests that overall energy intake over the entire period of Ramadan is not affected, but whether the changes in food and fluid intake pattern (i.e. changes in meal timing) during Ramadan fasting affects the acute levels of muscle glycogen is not known with any certainty. Previous studies have indicated that after an overnight fast of approximately 8–10 hours, liver glycogen levels are reduced substantially (Nilsson & Hultman, 1973), whereas muscle glycogen decreased only marginally by 17–25% after 24 hours of fasting, providing that the individuals only participated in a small amount of physical activity during the fasting period (Loy *et al.*, 1986). Similarly, in a recent review by Maughan *et al.* (2010), it is reported that Ramadan fasting hours are not much different to the normal overnight fast that most people experience while sleeping. As such, it is suggested that it may have little effect on overall daily dietary intake and only small metabolic effects on lipid, CHO or protein metabolism, or hormonal levels.

With regard to the fasted individual's fluid intake, in a recent study by Aziz *et al.* (personal communication) on athletes who fasted and trained at the same time showed that although Muslim athletes presented themselves in a hypohydrated state prior to exercise due to no fluid intake for at least 10–12 hours, these athletes' body masses at the start of the training

sessions were only about 0.2–1.5% lower than values obtained in the non-fasted state. This suggests that although the fasted athletes were in an acute dehydrated state, the level of dehydration was not so severe as to be detrimental to exercise performance. However, it is unclear whether the fasted subjects would then be in a chronically hypohydrated state over the weeks towards the end of Ramadan, and whether being hypohydrated subsequently affects sporting performance warrants further investigation. Several studies have reported that exercise performance is impaired when individual are dehydrated by 2% of pre-exercise body mass, but Coyle (2004) in a review of fluid requirements during exercise suggested that dehydration only becomes a physiological concern during maximal work when fluid losses exceed 2% of body mass, with athletes generally being able to cope with body water losses of up to 2% of body mass without significant risks to performance, provided the exercise is performed in cool conditions.

Although it appears that Ramadan fasting seems to have little effect on athletes' acute dietary intake and hydration status, the accumulative effect of Ramadan fasting on athletes' overall energy and hydration status and its implications for competitive sports performance is unknown. Muslim athletes who adhere to fasting may face greater challenges when having to compete in prolonged events (i.e. longer than 45–60 min) where endogenous muscle fuel may be depleted during exercise, when performing tasks that require physical and mental coordination, when competing in multiple events within the same day, and when competing in extreme environmental conditions.

The list below provides some practical nutrition recommendations to assist Muslim athletes to optimise exercise performance and training adaptations during the Ramadan fasting month.

(1) Athletes should try to consume similar amounts of food and fluid as per the non-fasting period to meet energy requirements.
(2) Athletes could adopt a general pattern of intake that is similar to their diet when they are not fasting, with the difference being the timing of the meal sitting. For example, matching the Ramadan *Sahur* meal with the normal lunch meal, the *Iftar* meal with the dinner meal and the Ramadan night snack with the breakfast meal.

(3) The *Sahur* meal should be consumed as late as possible if allowable under the rules of fasting. This ensures that the body is then in a fasted state for the shortest period of time during the day. This strategy will help to limit the lowering of endogenous muscle glycogen stores, particularly towards the late part of the afternoon period.

(4) Athletes may want to trial low glycaemix index foods during the *Sahur* meal. Low glycaemix index food such as pasta, porridge, baked beans and multigrain breads can help prolong the release of sugars into the bloodstream and therefore may help to sustain fuel for longer.

(5) Training should preferably be carried out in the evenings after breaking fast (i.e. *Iftar* meal). In this case, the athletes can break their fast with a light meal followed with a short break of an hour to allow food to be digested and enhance blood glucose levels before performing the exercise session.

(6) The *Iftar* meal should be high in CHO and low in fat. Recommended choices include fruit loaf, toasted sandwiches, noodles or pasta (with low-fat sauces), and rice with meat and legumes/vegetables. It is inadvisable to begin exercising too soon after consuming the breaking-fast meal, as it may cause gastrointestinal problems in some susceptible athletes.

(7) Athletes should aim to consume sufficient fluid throughout the Ramadan period. The volume of fluid that the athlete requires for the entire day should account for the minimal amount needed over the day (i.e. fluid requirement for the 24-hour period plus sweat losses during exercise). For further information on fluid and electrolytes see Chapter 7. It is recommended that fluid intake should be about 0.5–0.75 l every hour after breaking fast (i.e. from *Iftar* meal onwards) in the evening until bedtime. Athletes should adopt an *ad libitum* drinking plan throughout the evening waking period, rather than within a short period of time (e.g. within 1 hour). During the *Sahur* meal, athletes are advised to ingest up to 1.0 l of fluid to top up the body's fluids and to pace this by drinking about 250 ml every 30 min.

(8) It strongly recommended that the athletes have a 'strategic' drinking plan, i.e. prepare and make the fluids readily and easily available throughout the evening.

Athletes may also need to add variety/flavour to enhance the taste of the drinks to promote voluntary consumption.

Case study: menu planning for football team training camp in Singapore during Ramadan

Scenario

The coach of a Singapore-based football team has planned to conduct a 1-week training camp in preparation for a weekend competition to be held locally. The training camp will take place in a well-known five-star hotel that the players are familiar with in past camp experiences. However, the difference this time is that the camp will be taking place during the period of Ramadan, which concerns the coach and players. The coach sought the assistance and help of a sports nutritionist to plan a suitable menu that will be appropriate for both the Muslim and non-Muslim players.

The coach emphasised that the weekend game was a crucial qualifying competition event for the team and stressed that there should not be any disruption to the planned training routine as well as scheduled recovery and rehabilitation sessions. There would be two training sessions scheduled daily, with a light morning session starting at 8 am followed by an afternoon session of tactical training starting at 4 pm. The weekly weather forecast reported that humidity would be relatively high (approximately 80%) with the temperature peaking at 30–32°C between 3 and 5 pm.

There were prior arrangements made with the hotel to provide meals at the following standardised times for the whole team: breakfast at 7 am, lunch at 12 pm and dinner at 7 pm. As the Muslim athletes had to adhere to the Ramadan fasting ritual, they are required to complete their morning meal (*Sahur*) by 5.30 am, followed by the fast of about 12 hours before they break their fast (*Iftar*) after 7 pm on the same day. There was no additional budget provided for a separate Ramadan menu except for simple snack items. The coach provided the following information on the players' demographics to the sports nutritionist to assist in the necessary meal arrangements and was also formally introduced to the head chef of the hotel, who had good expertise in international cuisine.

The demographics of the team was as follows.

- Total 27 players.
- Age range 18–32 years.
- Race distribution: 5 Chinese, 14 Malay (all Muslims), 4 Indian (1 Indian vegetarian), 1 Eurasian, 3 whites.
- White people have been living in Singapore for 5 years.
- Team training together for 2 years. Good synergy between players.

Based on the above information, the sports nutritionist was able to make the following menu planning considerations to ensure that the menu and meal timings were well accepted by the entire team.

Menu planning considerations: general

- Meal timing for the team was established as follows with consideration to the Ramadan fasting period for the Muslims athletes:
  - Breakfast: 4.30–5.30 am for Muslims (i.e. Sahur meal); 7 am for non-Muslim athletes.
  - Lunch: 12 noon for non-Muslim athletes; rest time for Muslim athletes observing fast.
  - Dinner: 7 pm for all athletes.
  Snacks and beverages were made available to athletes throughout the day in the medical/recovery room.
- The menu plan is based on a set of nutrition guidelines as provided by the sports nutritionist, which mainly addresses healthier methods of food preparation and cooking, use of low-fat items (e.g. dairy products, salad dressings), limiting use of high-fat items (e.g. coconut milk), and cooked portion sizes of the required food categories.
- Buffet menu can include the following categories of dishes:
  - soup (vegetarian)
  - salad with separate dressings
  - assorted breads and spreads
  - staples (rice to always be provided)
  - pasta
  - two protein items (one red meat and one white meat/fish/seafood)
  - one cooked vegetable item
  - two protein alternatives suitable for vegetarians, e.g. tofu (beancurd)

  - fresh fruit platter
  - traditional food items (see point 7 below)
  - Muslim sweets or local desserts/cakes
  - fruit juices and water.
- Breakfast items to include hot food items (e.g. pancakes with syrup, scrambled eggs, grilled turkey ham, baked beans), dairy items (low-fat milk, yoghurt, cheese), muesli or cereals and assorted bakery items. Some of these items can be provided as part of the night snack options for Muslim athletes to help themselves during the 7 pm to 5 am period.
- Menu should be tailored to suit athletes' general food preferences as the team includes many mature athletes who have a fixed pattern of eating (both in and out of Ramadan).
- Type of cuisine: international menu but include one or two typical Malay dishes with one gravy-based dish during dinner. Choice based on chef recommendations to maximise chef expertise.
- Inclusion of traditional food items: the *Sahur* buffet and dinner buffet will provide these additional items: dates, *Kathira* (a traditional milk-based refreshing drink), fresh fruit juice, Muslim sweets (modified healthier recipe) or other local desserts/teacakes.
- Menu for *Sahur* meal should provide appropriate and adequate dishes to match a routine lunch meal. An *Iftar* meal should match a typical dinner meal and the Ramadan night snack to match a breakfast meal.
- Both the *Sahur* and *Iftar* meals are to be high in CHO and low in fat to maximise muscle glycogen storage.
- The *Sahur* meal is to be served as late as possible as allowed under the rule of fasting to shorten the athlete's fasted state.
- Adequate choices and variety of fluid options must be provided (e.g. water, fresh juice, low-fat dairy beverages, sports drinks) to help fasting athletes meet fluid requirements.
- Seasoning such as salt can be provided alongside buffet tables for fasting athletes to increase sodium intake to aid fluid retention and replace electrolytes lost in sweat. Condiments like *sambal* (Malay traditional cooked chilli paste) can also be provided for those who favour more spice in their meals.
- A night snack corner can be set up in the medical/recovery room for athletes to collect available snacks (e.g. breads, pasta, ready-to-eat pasta sauces, dates, cereal bars, and beverages such as

sports drinks, juices, milk) which are high-CHO and low-fat foods. Also plenty of water should be made available to encourage a 'grazing' method of drinking until bedtime.

Sample of a day's Ramadan meal plan

Sahur *meal: only Muslim players (by 5.30 am)*
As well as the international breakfast items, the *Sahur* meal menu for Muslims includes:

- Malay-style chicken soup (*soto ayam*)
- oatmeal porridge
- *nasi goreng* (Malay-style fried rice, with less oil)
- hardboiled egg
- *Kathira* drink
- dates
- chiffon cake
- fresh fruits
- water.

Iftar *meal: extended to all athletes (7 pm)*

- Minestrone soup
- Assorted breads/buns
- Assorted salad with low-fat dressing
- Plain rice
- Spaghetti Bolognaise
- Grilled honey chicken
- Beef in mild black pepper sauce
- Lightly pan-fried beancurd
- Stir-fry vegetables
- *Kathira* drink
- Dates
- Glutinous rice dessert (topped with low-fat coconut sauce and brown sugar)
- Fresh fruits
- Water.

Night snack example (7 pm to 5 am): extended to all athletes

- Banana
- Muesli or cereal bars
- Wholemeal sandwiches
- Assorted low-fat muffins or sweet-filled mini buns
- Sponge cakes
- Low-fat milk
- Low-fat fruit yoghurt
- Fruit jellies
- Fruit juices.

Also see Table 24.2 regarding Muslim cultural backgrounds and dietary practices.

VEGETARIAN/VEGAN ATHLETES

Wendy Martinson

Key messages

- The reasons some athletes choose to follow a vegetarian or vegan diet may include cultural and religious beliefs, ethics, politics, economics, environmental issues and the perceived benefits to health and performance.
- Vegetarian diets tend to be higher in complex carbohydrates, fibre, fruits, vegetables, antioxidants, phytochemicals and lower in saturated fat and cholesterol than omnivorous diets.
- The potential health benefits of vegetarian diets include lower risk of heart disease, hypertension, diabetes mellitus, obesity and some types of cancer.
- It should be possible for athletes to meet their energy needs from a vegetarian diet especially as these diets tend to be high in complex carbohydrates. However, it may be more difficult on a vegan diet due to the high fibre content and bulky nature.

- It is generally accepted that athletes have higher protein requirements and these can be met on a vegetarian diet especially if egg, dairy and soy are included in the diet. Vegans need to ensure a mixture of different plant proteins during the course of the day to consume all the essential amino acids.
- The micronutrients most likely to be deficient in vegetarian diets are iron, zinc, vitamin B_{12}, riboflavin, calcium and vitamin D.
- Vegetarian athletes may benefit from creatine supplementation that increases muscle creatine levels well above what is possible with a vegetarian diet.
- There are few data available to make any definite conclusions about the performance effects of vegetarian diets on well-trained athletes.

Table 24.4 Types of vegetarian diets.

Type of vegetarian diet	Characteristics
Demi- or semi-vegetarian	Occasionally eats meat, poultry and fish
Piscatarian	Eats fish and possibly other seafood but excludes red meat and poultry
Lacto-vegetarian	Excludes all meat, fish, shellfish, eggs and ingredients derived from them, e.g. gelatin, rennet. Eats dairy products
Lacto-ovo-vegetarian	As above but eats dairy products and eggs (though possibly only of free range origin)
Ovo-vegetarian	Includes eggs but avoids dairy products, meat, poultry, fish and other seafood
Vegan	Excludes all animal flesh and products, derived ingredients and additives. Avoids animal products not only in the diet but also in every aspect of life
Fruitarian	A type of vegan diet which consists mainly of raw fruit, vegetables, nuts, seeds, sprouted pulses and grains. Usually consists only of foods which do not kill the plant of origin
Macrobiotic	Based on the Chinese philosophy of yin and yang. Aims to balance fields which contain qualities of these two opposing but complementary forces of nature. Has 10 levels, which become increasingly restrictive. Lower levels are most varied and may contain meat or fish if wild/hunted. The highest level consist of wholegrains and limited fluids

From Thomas & Bishop 2007, reproduced with kind permission from Wiley-Blackwell.

24B.1 Introduction

In the UK approximately 3–7% of the population consume a vegetarian diet, but there is little information available on the number of athletes following a vegetarian diet. The reasons some athletes choose to follow a vegetarian or vegan diet may include cultural and religious beliefs, ethics, politics, economics, environmental issues and the perceived benefits to health and performance. Some may simply dislike the taste, smell or appearance of meat and therefore exclude it from their diet. Some endurance athletes have been noted to choose this way of eating to meet increased carbohydrate (CHO) needs and keep weight under control.

Whatever the reasons, the potential effects of a vegetarian/vegan diet on an athlete's performance and overall health is of great interest, particularly since athletes generally have a higher nutrient requirement than the average population. There is therefore concern amongst some professionals working in sport that athletes following a vegetarian diet may not meet their requirements for all nutrients. There are many variations on the vegetarian diet and Table 24.4 outlines the common types, while Table 24.5 lists nutrients of special concern.

In terms of overall composition, vegetarian diets tend to be higher in complex CHO, fibre, fruits, vegetables, antioxidants and phytochemicals and lower in saturated fat and cholesterol than omnivorous diets. Studies state the benefits of vegetarian diets to include lower risk of heart disease, hypertension, diabetes mellitus, obesity and some types of cancer.

24B.2 Nutritional considerations for athletes

Energy

The energy needs of athletes depend on a variety of factors including body size and composition, gender, training programme (both volume and intensity) and type of sport. Broadly this is approximately 2000–6000 kcal/day or more and a large proportion of this energy should be composed of CHO-rich foods. Vegetarian diets tend to be high in complex CHO and quite bulky but it should be possible to meet the energy needs of athletes, although with a vegan diet it may be more difficult. The high-fibre foods typically found in a vegan diet have a reduced amount of metabolisable energy and so energy needs may be harder to achieve. In general the energy intakes of vegetarians tend to be lower than those of non-vegetarians. In particular, younger athletes going through childhood and adolescence may have difficulty meeting the energy requirements of their sport and growth demands from a vegetarian diet.

Protein

Studies have shown that vegetarian diets generally contain less protein than omnivorous diets. However, it is possible for athletes to meet their protein

Table 24.5 Micronutrients of special concern for vegetarian athletes.

Micronutrient	Function	Sources in a vegetarian diet and comments
Iron	Required for synthesis of haemoglobin and myoglobin, essential components in transport and delivery of oxygen within blood and to the muscles	Fortified breakfast cereals, bread, textured vegetable protein, dried beans, soy foods and meat alternatives, nuts, dried fruits and green leafy vegetables; vitamin C (enhances iron absorption)
Zinc	Involved in immune function, protein synthesis and blood formation	Legumes, whole grains, cereals, nuts, seeds, soy and dairy products, vitamin C and soaking beans; grains and seeds enhances zinc absorption
Vitamin B$_{12}$	Coenzyme required for normal metabolism of nerve tissue and of protein, fat and CHO	Dairy products, eggs, fortified soy milk and cereals
Vitamin D	Necessary for bone growth, promotes bone mineralisation, aids in absorption of calcium, maintains nervous tissue and normal heart action	Dairy products, eggs, fortified soy milk and cereals
Riboflavin	Coenzyme involved in production of energy, stored in muscles and used during muscular fatigue	Dairy products, soy milk, soy yoghurt, soy cheese, fortified breakfast cereals, grains and textured vegetable protein
Calcium	Necessary for blood clotting, nerve transmission, muscle stimulation, vitamin D metabolism and maintaining bone structure	Dairy products, calcium-fortified soy milk, tofu, soy yoghurt, cereals, low oxalate green vegetables such as broccoli, bok choy and kale

Adapted from Venderley & Campbell 2006, with kind permission from Wolters Kluwer Health.

requirements if they plan their food intake carefully over the course of the day. The proteins in egg, dairy and soy are all high quality and provide all essential amino acids. However, vegans exclude these foods and so may find it more difficult to meet their protein requirements. Plant proteins may be limiting in one or more essential amino acids (lysine, threonine, tryptophan or methionine) and so a variety of different plant proteins (e.g. pulses and grains or pulses and nuts/seeds) must be eaten over the course of the day to ensure the correct balance of essential amino acids is achieved.

The protein requirements of athletes are generally accepted as being higher than those of sedentary individuals, although this continues to be fairly controversial. Recommendations for protein intake exist (typically 1.2–1.7 g/kg), but athletes need to be advised on an individual basis on their required intake. The energy intake of athletes tends to be higher than average and so this in itself may mean that protein intakes are adequate. However, as plant proteins are less well digested than animal proteins, an increase in protein intake by 10% is suggested in the literature (1.3–1.8 g/kg/day).

Good sources of non-meat protein include milk and milk products, eggs, pulses (e.g. chickpeas, kidney beans, mung beans, black-eyed beans, lentils),

tofu, textured vegetable/soya protein, Quorn, nuts and nut butters, seeds and seed pastes (e.g. tahini). Grains (e.g. rice, bread, pasta, oats, quinoa and breakfast cereals) will also provide small amounts of protein as well as being a rich source of CHO.

Fat

The total fat and essential fatty acid intake of semi-vegetarians and lacto-ovo-vegetarians has been found to be similar to that of omnivorous diets. Vegan diets tend to be lower in saturated fat and higher in polyunsaturated fat than vegetarian diets. Some experts have expressed concern that vegetarian/vegan diets have a high ratio of ω-6 to ω-3 fatty acids and that this may adversely affect the types and potency of eicosanoids formed. In athletes this may translate into an undesirable effect on inflammation and immune function during and after exercise. This ratio can be improved by including ω-3 rich oils such as soya, rapeseed, linseed and walnut oil and/or monounsaturated fat such as olive oil.

Vegetarian and vegan diets are low in the long-chain ω-3 fats eicosapentaenoic acid (EPA) and docosahexaenoic acid (DHA), which have an important role in the development of brain and retinal tissue and have beneficial effects on the heart. Plant-based sources of the shorter-chain ω-3 fats can be included in the diet and these can be converted in the body to EPA and DHA, although conversion can be poor. Plant sources include linseed, hempseed, walnuts, sweet potatoes, soya beans, pumpkin seeds and green leafy vegetables. Vegan sources of DHA derived from microalgae are also available.

Iron

Iron has a major role in sports performance. It is utilised to produce haemoglobin in blood and myoglobin in muscle which carry oxygen around the body. It is also required by many enzymes system such as those involved in energy metabolism and also helps support the cells of the immune system. Physical activity leads to a greater turnover of iron and iron depletion is often reported in the literature amongst athletes, particularly endurance athletes. This can partly be explained by the increase in plasma volume that occurs through endurance training, which can then have a dilutional effect on measurements of red blood cells. In addition, it can be due to a poor dietary intake of iron and a restricted energy intake or vegetarian diet may play a role here. If a deficiency arises this may manifest itself in a reduced ability of the immune system to fight infection as well as a reduced capacity for aerobic endurance.

The iron content of vegetarian diets is similar to that of omnivorous diets but bioavailability is an issue so here is where the concerns lie. Plant foods contain non-haem iron, which is less well absorbed than the haem iron found in animal products. Haem iron represents 40% of the iron found in meat, fish and poultry and the efficiency of absorption is 15–40%. Non-haem iron has an absorption efficiency of 1–15%. Vegetarian diets contain no haem iron whereas diets with substantial amounts of red meat provide about 10–12% total iron in haem form. Semi-vegetarian diets containing chicken and fish provide less haem iron.

One study has shown that previous lacto-ovo-vegetarians who consumed red meat improved their bioavailable iron intake and haematological status over a 12-week period of resistive training. Absorption is affected by various components of the diet. Non-haem iron absorption is enhanced by vitamin C, alcohol, and possibly retinol and carotenoids. Absorption is inhibited by phytic acid in wholegrains, legumes, lentils and nuts, by polyphenols in tea, coffee, red wines and certain vegetables, and by soy protein, eggs and calcium and phosphate salts.

Although the prevalence of iron deficiency anaemia is similar among vegetarians and omnivores, many studies have found that vegetarians are more likely to have non-haem iron deficiency (depleted iron stores with serum ferritin below $12\,\mu g/l$ but normal haemoglobin concentration). Studies on vegetarian endurance athletes have also shown serum ferritin levels to be low. Lower haemoglobin levels are associated with reduced oxygen transport and impaired aerobic performance and it is well established that clinical anaemia interferes with exercise performance, and even reduced haemoglobin within the normal range can negatively affect performance. In the past the effect of low iron stores without anaemia on physical performance was thought to be minimal but now new studies using a relatively new and reliable marker of early iron depletion (soluble transferrin receptor) show that low iron stores can reduce endurance capacity and aerobic capacity.

In practice, working with athletes on a day-to-day basis, low ferritin levels without low haemoglobin can affect level of fatigue and ability to train, which is improved when ferritin levels increase through an increase in iron intake via supplementation/diet.

The iron intake of vegetarian athletes should be increased to account for the poor bioavailability of non-haem iron. New Zealand, Australia, the USA and Canada suggest that the recommended intake for vegetarian athletes should be 1.8 times higher than normal to account for this low bioavailability.

Zinc

Zinc intake is also of concern in the vegetarian diet and is required for immune function, protein synthesis and blood formation. In the omnivorous diet, 50–70% of zinc in the diet is provided by meats and dairy products and so it comes as no surprise that total zinc intake is generally lower in vegetarian athletes.

Zinc loss increases during strenuous exercise and so it may be harder for vegetarian athletes to maintain zinc status. The bioavailability of zinc is also impaired by phytate in a similar way to iron. There are some food preparation techniques that can reduce the binding of zinc by phytate, such as includes soaking and sprouting beans, grains and seeds.

Vitamin B$_{12}$

Vegan, fruitarian or macrobiotic diets do not have an active source of B$_{12}$ because plant foods, meat analogues, fermented soy products and mushrooms contain the inactive type of B$_{12}$, and so those following this dietary regimen have been found to have lower serum B$_{12}$ levels than do lacto-ovo-vegetarians or those who occasionally eat meat.

Over time an inadequate intake could lead to macrocytic anaemia, which is associated with reduced oxygen transport and hence impaired aerobic performance. Macrocytic anaemia may be masked by high folate intakes and as vegetarian diets are typically high in folic acid this may mean that signs of deficiency are not detected until after the onset of neurological symptoms. Vegan athletes should ensure they consume foods fortified with B$_{12}$ such as fortified soy and soy products, fortified vegetable or yeast extracts or fortified breakfast cereals; alternatively they should take a B$_{12}$ supplement. If small amounts of B$_{12}$ are taken frequently over the course of the day this improves absorption.

Calcium and vitamin D

Calcium intakes have been found to be low in those vegetarians, particularly females, avoiding dairy products. The bioavailability of calcium from vegetable sources including soy products is lower than from dairy sources and is due to the presence of inhibitors such as phytates and oxalates. Vitamin D improves calcium absorption, but food sources are limited and the action of sunlight on skin is the main source.

Vitamin D deficiency is on the increase in the UK and new evidence is emerging regarding the important functions of vitamin D beyond that of bone health. Even in omnivores it is difficult to obtain sufficient vitamin D through dietary sources. Ergocalciferol (vitamin D$_2$) is the non-animal form of vitamin D acceptable to vegetarians and is found in some fortified margarines, soy milk and cheese, or as a supplement. However, ergocalciferol is less effective at increasing vitamin D levels than cholecalciferol (vitamin D$_3$) and so vegetarians will need a higher intake to increase their vitamin D levels. Vegetarian athletes need to ensure a good intake of calcium-rich foods to promote optimal development of peak bone mass, particularly through the adoles-

cent years. Those athletes who train mainly indoors may be particularly at risk of vitamin D deficiency, which as well as affecting bone health can also impact on immune function and inflammatory responses.

Another consideration is that some studies show amenorrhoea to be more common among vegetarian athletes and this will affect the need for dietary calcium. Experts generally agree that 1500 mg of calcium daily is recommended for athletes with amenorrhoea and in this instance a supplement may be required to achieve this amount.

Riboflavin

Riboflavin plays a key role in energy metabolism, and for those strict vegetarians excluding dairy and soy products dietary intakes will be low. Alternative sources for vegans include yeast extract, wheatgerm, fortified breakfast cereals, almonds, pumpkin, sunflower, sesame seeds, avocado and seaweed.

Creatine

Creatine may benefit physical performance in a variety of different sports and can also facilitate gains in lean mass during resistance training programmes. Dietary intake is mainly from meat, fish and poultry and provides approximately 1 g/day and so vegetarian and vegan athletes would naturally have a reduced intake. Higher creatine levels in the muscles can increase the rate at which creatine phosphate is re-synthesised during recovery from exercise and may enhance performance during repeated bouts of maximal exercise. Many athletes supplement with creatine to increase creatine phosphate levels as it would be difficult to increase levels purely through dietary means even in non-vegetarians.

Research shows that a vegetarian or vegan diet does produce lower muscle creatine concentrations than an omnivorous diet. Vegetarians may benefit from creatine supplementation by increasing muscle creatine levels to well above what is possible with a vegetarian diet and are likely to experience an ergogenic effect. One study in untrained male vegetarians showed greater increases in bench press strength, total work output and increase in lean tissue after 8 weeks of creatine supplementation and resistance training compared with controls on placebo. This effect may be different in trained subjects but this is unknown.

24B.3 Effects on performance

Few studies have examined the effect of a vegetarian diet on physical performance. Of the studies that have been done, vegetarian diets have not been shown to be beneficial or detrimental to endurance performance. There is a dearth of data from well-controlled studies to demonstrate whether vegetarian diets have a positive or negative effect on the performance of well-trained athletes.

24B.4 Summary

With the exception of fruitarian and restricted macrobiotic diets, athletes who follow a carefully planned vegetarian diet should be able to meet their requirements for energy and essential nutrients. However, they need to be aware of the potential risks of deficiency for certain nutrients (see Table 24.5) and if possible seek the advice of a qualified sports dietitian or nutritionist to ensure their requirements are being met.

THE INJURED ATHLETE: SURGERY AND REHABILITATION

Nicola Maffulli and Filippo Spiezia

Key messages

- Mechanical or chemical injury may cause trauma and is considered a stressful event that can damage potentially all the structures of the human body. Muscles, tendons, ligaments and bones may be subject to a variety of different injuries.
- Management of injuries may require immobilisation for a variable amount of time. Even when early mobilisation is implemented, injuries continue to affect human tissues and their metabolism and therefore the homeostasis of the whole body.
- The physiological response to injury essentially aims for three goals: to decrease blood loss, to clear tissue debris and to restore

- normal function in the involved area through scar tissue formation or, in bone, production of new bone.
- Following trauma, the body's needs for nutrients differs. Trauma increases the metabolic rate, necessitating greater amounts of oxygen and nutrients such as amino acids, which are required for repair and recovery.
- Wound healing requires more energy from the diet, with carbohydrates and fats the main sources of energy normally. In the injured patient, proteins are also used to provide energy.
- After trauma, calorie requirements may be increased by up to 250–300 kcal daily.

24C.1 Introduction

Mechanical or a chemical injury may cause trauma. In this context, a trauma is a stressful event that can damage potentially all the structures of the human body. Muscles, tendons, ligaments and bones may be subject to a variety of different injuries. Management of these injuries may require immobilisation for a variable amount of time. Even when early mobilisation is implemented, injuries continue to affect human tissues and their metabolism and therefore the homeostasis of the whole body.

During the recovery period, nutrition has to be appropriately planned for the elite athlete who, for example, has undergone anterior cruciate reconstruction after a sport injury, in the same way as nutrition is planned for the older individual who has undergone a total hip replacement for hip osteoarthritis.

There are no systematic studies covering these particular issues in the literature, but several studies have cast some light on this important subject for dietitians/nutritionists, general practitioners, coaches, orthopaedic surgeons and sports medicine experts.

24C.2 Injury

Injury is a common cause of disability. To some extent, surgery can be considered a controlled iatrogenic injury with potentially the same complications. Hence, surgery deserves the same medical consideration as injury or trauma. Trauma can be blunt or penetrating, whereas burns should be considered separately. It is also possible to estimate the entirety of the trauma by taking into account the force which has caused the injury and the surface area of impact.

Penetrating trauma may have different conse-quences depending on the organ penetrated. Gunshots and stab wounds are examples of penetrating trauma. Agents that burn such as heat and chemicals may cause severe injury depending on the extent of the contact area. In electrical injuries, the surface area affected is usually very small, but these injuries may cause severe harm to the deep tissues. All types of injuries can cause metabolic imbalances. A cascade of events may lead to increased demand for oxygen transport and substrate mobilisation to attempt to regain physiological homeostasis. Trauma, depend-ing on its level, may carry short-term and long-term consequences. The aim of an appropriately planned nutrition strategy and any supplementation is to pro-mote healing and avoid the complications associated with trauma.

It has been suggested that any traumatic event may affect the body's natural metabolic balance and initi-ate a cascade of reactions aimed at the repair and res-toration of function. Human tissues respond to damage in a complex fashion. Immediately after the trauma, local reactions and systemic changes start in all systems. The physiological response to injury essentially aims for three goals: to decrease blood loss, to clear tissue debris, and to restore normal function in the involved area through scar tissue for-mation or, in bone, production of new bone.

Vasoconstriction aims to reduce blood flow to the affected area and platelets are activated to form a clot or mesh of fibrin to stop the bleeding. The platelets also release cytokines and other biologically active substances to initiate an inflammatory reaction. As soon as the bleeding is controlled by these mecha-nisms, removal of damaged tissues by this inflamma-tory response starts. When the debris is reabsorbed, production of new healthy tissue begins to replace the damaged one. Different enzyme systems and pro-inflammatory cells are activated during the inflam-matory response to injury to eliminate the damaged tissues. To allow this, in this phase of the healing response, blood flow to the affected site is increased through local vasodilation mediated by histamine, prostaglandins, and by the chemicals in the comple-ment cascade activated as an immune system response to the injury. The walls of the blood vessels in the affected area become more permeable to allow repairing substances to reach the damaged tissues. Macroscopically, this results in local swelling.

A fibrin mesh is formed with the help of fibrinogen so that the entire wound is covered. Neutrophils, monocytes, lymphocytes, eosinophils and basophils participate in the immune reaction that takes place at the site of injury. After the acute response, bleeding is stopped and there is creation of new blood vessels (angiogenesis) and formation of granulation tissue. When the debris is eliminated from the injury site, fibroblasts lay down a network of collagen that becomes granulation tissue. The collagen fibres become more interlinked, and the process of scar formation starts.

The response to the injury also involves systemic mechanisms. The sympathetic nervous system, for example, is activated through a stress reaction. The alertness of the injured subject is increased, endor-phins are released in the blood, and blood glucose levels and heart and respiratory rates are all increased. Cytokines are also released into the blood, causing several generalised effects such as fever or the increased metabolism of fats, glucose and proteins. Immune cells are also involved in the stress reactions. To support prolonged period of stress, an appropri-ate nutritional strategy is necessary.

After an acute trauma, the neuroendocrine and cytokine response start the systemic inflammatory response. This includes increased heart rate and minute ventilation to balance the higher tissue demands for oxygen. The normal anabolic state shifts rapidly to a catabolic state, with mobilisation of pro-teins, fats and carbohydrates (CHO) for energy utili-sation. Cytokines such as tumour necrosis factor (TNF), interleukin (IL)-1, IL-2 and IL-6, and hor-mones such as adrenaline, noradrenaline, glucagon and cortisol are released and are responsible for tis-sue catabolism. In addition, the level of insulin circu-lating in the blood is elevated in stressed patients, but the responsiveness of tissues to insulin is decreased, resulting in transient insulin resistance. Ischaemic injury may follow the decreased blood flow conse-quent to severe trauma.

Sepsis and haemorrhage may, for example, cause decreased blood flow and increased oxygen con-sumption. Gut ischaemia can lead to mitochondrial disruption, mucosal acidosis, progressive cell injury, and cell destruction. Mucosal acidosis, a measure of reduced intraoperative splanchnic perfusion, is asso-ciated with exaggerated local and systemic immune responses, increased intestinal permeability, an increase in septic complications and a trend toward increased multi-organ dysfunction syndrome. Ischaemia reperfusion injury (IRI) seems to be caused by reactive oxygen metabolites followed by the priming and activation of polymorphonuclear neutrophils.

Various nutrients seem to have different beneficial effects in IRI. Intraluminal glucose may increase mucosal blood flow, protect against mucosal injury and improve intestinal function after gut IRI. In addition, the amino acid alanine may amplify mucosal injury, whereas glutamine may prevent intestinal mucosal damage and enhance neutrophil function in critical illness and trauma.

24C.3 Trauma and malnutrition

Trauma causes a change in the body's needs for nutrients. Trauma increases the metabolic rate, which necessitates greater amounts of oxygen and nutrients such as amino acids, which are required for repair and recovery. The prevalence of malnutrition, or risk of malnutrition, in orthopaedic surgical patients is high. Malnutrition and risk of malnutrition in orthopaedic surgical patients contribute to the development of postoperative complications.

Research has shown that energy expenditure may rise by 10–50% in order to support the intense metabolic workload. More proteins and amino acids are needed for the formation of new tissues, for the proliferation of immune cells, and to maintain lean body mass. It has been reported that 9–44% of people with wound and surgical trauma are malnourished, a condition often unrecognised in a clinical care setting. Alternative methods of feeding, such as a nasogastric tube, are often necessary because adherence to oral nutrition supplements is poor, and dietary intake alone is insufficient to meet estimated energy requirements. Clinically significant weight loss is observed in hospitalised surgical patients. However, trauma causes many important nutrients to be channelled into the healing effort. Also, the altered levels of consciousness which may follow acute trauma may cause poor appetite, reduced digestive function and compromised blood circulation.

In the injured body, proteins, including those comprising muscle, are also used as a fuel. Therefore, patients may become hypermetabolic, with a higher need for calories and protein. Cortisol and catecholamines are released during the stress reaction consequent to trauma, a cause of the hypermetabolic state contributing to the rapid loss of lean body mass. It is therefore important that, after trauma, patients maintain an adequate supply of protein and calories to avoid loss of muscle mass.

Malnourishment following severe trauma also decreases immune system capacity, increasing the time needed for proper wound healing. Also, injured patients may be unable to consume adequate amounts of nutrients orally and other strategies of nutrition may have to be considered. Enteral nutrition (EN) or parenteral nutrition (PN) are examples. However, it should be kept in mind that there are reports of negative outcomes for PN, with systemic immunosuppression and an increased incidence of hyperglycaemia.

Strong evidence from meta-analyses comparing PN with EN after trauma shows that PN is associated with a higher risk of infection. Randomised trials comparing EN with PN showed that patients fed by EN had significantly fewer septic complications. Hence, following trauma, surgery and burns, EN should be considered first in patients with an intact gastrointestinal system. Hypercatabolism is also a typical response to trauma, so early nutrition may benefit trauma patients or those who undergo surgery, decreasing protein-energy depletion. Some studies have shown how early EN is associated with a low incidence of infectious complications. There is a definite association between nutritional status, morbidity and mortality. Subjects who received EN show a lower incidence of postoperative infections and shorter hospital stays. Conversely, preoperative PN does not reduce surgical mortality, although there have been reports of reduction in postoperative complications such as sepsis, anastomotic leaks and pneumonia.

24C.4 Nutrients for better wound healing

Wound healing requires more energy from the diet, with CHO and fats the main sources of energy normally. In the injured patient, proteins are also used to provide energy. Hence, to prevent the loss of lean body mass, there should be adequate intake of calories. After trauma, calorie requirements may be increased by up to 250–300 kcal daily.

Carbohydrate

In wounded patients, CHO is essential. Firstly, it helps fibroblast movement, which is vital in wound healing; secondly, it may also help white blood cell activity. Proteins are also essential for collagen synthesis. Glucose is the preferred fuel for the central nervous system (CNS) and blood cells. In the metabolically stressed adult, the maximum rate of glucose oxidation is 4–7 mg/kg/min, roughly equivalent to 400–700 g/day in a 70-kg person. Oxidised glucose in the hypermetabolic patient comes from amino acid substrates via gluconeogenesis and exogenous glucose administration does not inhibit this endogenous production. Hence, administration of exogenous glucose may stimulate hyperglycaemia and hyperinsulinaemia.

Also, exogenous insulin administration may increase cellular glucose uptake, resulting in lipogenesis. Hyperosmolar states have been described as complications of excess glucose administration Moreover, hyperglycaemia has been suggested as a prognostic indicator of high morbidity and mortality in trauma patients. Insulin administration via continuous infusions is useful for maintaining a euglycaemic state in trauma patients.

Protein

Trauma also increases the demand for protein. Because of the increased protein loss, a protein intake of 1.5–2.0 g/kg/day is recommended for trauma patients, with the aim of decreasing nitrogen deficit. Even though protein supplementation does not affect the high catabolic rate, the protein synthesis rate may respond to amino acid infusions.

Fat

Fatty acids are present in the cell membrane and are implicated in the synthesis of new cells. Therefore, low fat levels would delay wound healing. In the injured patient, fat metabolism can be altered because of hormonal alterations. Lipids are important substrates in the injured patient because they spare protein energy use. Between 10 and 30% of total energy requirements are recommended to come from fat in trauma patients. The omega fatty acids may exert beneficial effects in the management of such patients. For example, ω-6 fatty acids may help the production of arachidonic acid, favouring proinflammatory metabolites such as prostaglandin $(PG)E_2$, leukotriene $(LT)B_4$ and thromboxanes. The ω-3 fatty acids may help to produce PGE_3 and LTB_5.

Micronutrients

In injured patients, the need for vitamins and minerals is increased because of the high metabolic demands. However, the evidence to support supplementation is lacking. Vitamin A increases the strength of scar tissue. Vitamin A also plays a paramount role in the maintenance of an adequate inflammatory response, because it seems to counteract the catabolic effect that glucocorticosteroids exert on wound healing.

Vitamin A supplementation increases collagen cross-linking, which results in higher tensile strength of the wound. Wound healing requires higher quantities of vitamin C, which should be taken daily. Vitamin C is also important for enzyme protocollagen hydroxylase, which is involved in the production of collagen. Vitamin C helps to increase the strength of the links between the strands of collagen fibres, and helps synthesis of the intracellular matrix of bone, skin, blood vessel walls and connective tissue. Reactive oxygen species have been shown at the wound site, and vitamin C, which shows antioxidant effects, may be of help in injury management.

Zinc is required in many enzymatic reactions, such as DNA synthesis, cell division and protein synthesis, and mediates the maturation of T-lymphocytes. The requirements for this mineral are higher in trauma.

Reactive oxygen species are generated during trauma and cause tissue damage by peroxidation of plasma membranes and other detrimental effects. Low levels of circulating vitamins C and E have been also found in trauma. Administration of α-tocopherol and ascorbic acid may have beneficial effects in trauma patients. More studies are necessary to understand whether antioxidant supplementation is beneficial in patients with acute injury or trauma.

Fluid and electrolytes

The hypermetabolic state typical of the injured patient may cause dehydration. The daily water requirement for trauma patients may range from 1500 to 2000 ml/day (Leininger 2002). Electrolyte homeostasis may also be disturbed by surgery or injury, causing cardiac dysrhythmias and ileus. Fluid and electrolyte supplementation has to be provided to the injured patient to maintain adequate urine output and normal serum electrolytes. Intracellular electrolytes such as phosphorus, potassium and magnesium are also necessary for protein synthesis. For the surgeon, it is paramount to monitor the blood concentration of these electrolytes daily as they are helpful in anabolic processes.

24C.5 Fasting

Fasting before surgery is still common in many Western hospitals. Overnight fasting can induce postoperative insulin resistance, which has been shown to be related to infectious morbidity. Postoperative insulin resistance can be attenuated by preoperative intake of a clear CHO-rich beverage. Studies suggest that preoperative intake of a CHO-rich beverage can prevent surgery-induced immunosuppression and thus might reduce the risk of infectious complications. In geriatric patients, oral nutritional supplements have been recommended after orthopaedic surgery to reduce postoperative complications. Clearly, in order to manage the supplementation and nutrition strategy of injured patients, biochemical measurements play an important role. Serum prealbumin is currently used to evaluate the nutritional status of trauma patients: in an anabolic state, it correlates well with a positive nitrogen balance. However, prealbumin is synthesised in the liver, and in liver dysfunction and inflammation states the liver decreases the synthesis of proteins.

Consequently, in these situations prealbumin can no longer be considered a reliable marker of nutrition status, but more a marker of severity of liver dysfunction. Nitrogen balance measurement may also give information about clinical status in the traumatised patient. Because injury, trauma and surgery may alter body metabolism, increasing or decreasing energy expenditure, it is important to have a robust measure of nutrient requirements to avoid over- or under-feeding. The gold standard for measuring energy expenditure is indirect calorimetry and new portable devices can be used for bedside measurements of metabolic activity.

24C.6 Exercise-induced muscle damage

Strenuous physical activity and sport may cause, through eccentric contractions under high loads, disruption of the muscle ultrastructure. The trauma generated by this exercise initiates events that decrease muscle force and increase soreness. Supplementation may help to reduce exercise-induced muscle damage and/or promote recovery. Creatine monohydrate (N-aminoiminomethyl-N-methylglycine) may help improve the rate of recovery of muscle function after injury. It should be interesting to test the efficacy of creatine supplementation in patients undergoing orthopaedic surgery. Future research may show its effects in shortening the recovery time for athletes after orthopaedic surgery.

24C.7 Summary

Mechanical or chemical injury may cause trauma that can potentially damage all structures of the human body. Muscles, tendons, ligaments and bones may be subject to a variety of different injuries. The physiological response to injury essentially aims for three goals: to decrease blood loss, to clear tissue debris and to restore normal function in the involved area through scar tissue formation or, in bone, production of new bone. Vasoconstriction aims to reduce blood flow to the affected area and platelets are activated to form a clot or mesh of fibrin to stop the bleeding. The platelets also release cytokines and other biologically active substances to initiate an inflammatory reaction. As soon as the bleeding is controlled by these mechanisms, removal of damaged tissues via this inflammatory response starts.

To support prolonged period of stress, an appropriate nutritional strategy is essential. After an acute trauma, the neuroendocrine and cytokine response start the systemic inflammatory response. This includes increased heart rate and minute ventilation to balance the higher tissue demands for oxygen. The normal anabolic state shifts rapidly to a catabolic state with mobilisation of proteins, fats and carbohydrates for energy utilisation. Following trauma, the body's needs for nutrients differs. More proteins and amino acids are needed for the formation of new tissues, for the proliferation of immune cells, and to maintain lean body mass. In wounded patients, carbohydrates are absolutely essential as well as key vitamins and minerals (including vitamins A and C and zinc). Ensuring fluid/electrolyte balance is also essential.

References and further reading

Ethnic groups

American Association of Diabetes Educators. Cultural sensitivity and diabetes education: recommendations for diabetes educators. Diabetes Educ 2007; 33: 41–44.

Aziz AR, Png W. Practical tips to exercise training during the Ramadan fasting month. ISN Bulletin 2008; 1(1).

Aziz AR, Wahid MF, Png W, Jesuvadian CV. Effects of Ramadan fasting on 60 min of endurance running performance in moderately trained men. Br J Sports Med 2010; 44: 516–521.

Azrah E, Hari Raya Haji. National Library Singapore website. Available at http://infopedia.nl.sg/articles/SIP_694__2009-01-02.html. Accessed 9 May 2010.

Better Health Channel. Food culture and religion, 2009. Available at www.betterhealth.vic.gov.au/bhcv2/bhcarticles.nsf/pages/Food_culture_and_religion?open

Brown TL. Meal-planning strategies: ethnic populations. Diabetes Spectrum 2003; 16: 190–192.

Burke L. Fasting and recovery from exercise. Br J Sports Med 2010; 44: 502–508.

Burke L, Deakin V. Clinical Sports Nutrition, 3rd edn. Sydney: McGraw-Hill Australia, 2006.

Campinha-Bacote J. A model and instrument for addressing cultural competence in health care. J Nurse Educ 1999; 38: 203–207.

Cort JE. Jains in the World: Religious Values and Ideology in India. New York: Oxford University Press, 2001.

Coyle EF. Fluid and fuel intake during exercise. J Sport Sci 2004; 22: 39–55.

Curry KR. Multicultural competence in dietetics and nutrition. J Am Diet Assoc 2000; 100: 1142–1143.

Fast, A. Iraq The Culture. New York: Crabtree Publishing Company, 2004.

Genzberger C. Singapore Business: The Portable Encyclopedia for Doing Business with Singapore. Petaluma, CA: World Trade Press, 1994.

Goody CM, Drago L. Cultural Food Practices/Diabetes Care and Education Dietetic Practice Group. Chicago, IL: American Dietetic Association, 2009.

Harris-Davis E, Haughton B. Model for multicultural nutrition counselling competencies. J Am Diet Assoc 2007; 100: 1178–1185.

Hayes D, Laudan R. Food and Nutrition. New York: Marshall Cavendish Corporation, 2008.

Hutton W. Singapore Food. New York: Marshall Cavendish Corporation, 2008.

Kulkarni KD. Food, culture and diabetes in the United States. Clin Diabetes 2004; 22: 190–192.

Leiper JB, Molla AM, Molla AM. Effects on health of fluid restriction during fasting in Ramadan. Eur J Clin Nutr 2003; 57 (Suppl 2): S30–S38.

Loy SF, Conlee RK, Winder WW, Nelson AG, Arnall DA, Fisher AG. Effects of 24-hour fast on cycling endurance time at two different intensities. J Appl Physiol 1986; 61: 654–659.

Maughan RJ, Fallah J, Coyle EF. The effects of fasting on metabolism and performance. Br J Sports Med 2010; 44: 490–494.

Mujika I, Chaouachi A, Chamari K. Precompetition taper and nutritional strategies: special reference to training during Ramadan intermittent fast. Br J Sports Med 2010; 44: 495–501.

Nestle M, Wing R, Birch L et al. Behavioural and social influences on food choices. Nutr Rev 1998; 56: S50–S74.

Nilsson LH, Hultman E. Liver glycogen in man: the effect of total starvation or a CHO-poor diet followed by CHO refeeding. Scand J Clin Lab Invest 1973; 32: 325–330.

Sabaté J, Ratzin-Turner R. Vegetarian Nutrition. Boca Raton, FL: CRC Press, 2001.

Sager G. Vegetarianism and the major world religions. Society of Ethical and Religious Vegetarians website. Available at www.serv-online.org/pamphlet.pdf. Accessed 13 April 2010.

Sawka MN. Physiological consequences of hypohydration: exercise performance and thermoregulation. Med Sci Sports Exerc 1991; 24: 657–670.

Simoons FJ. Food in China: A Cultural and Historical Inquiry. Boca Raton, FL: CRC Press, 1990.

Sucher KP, Kittler PG. Food and Culture, 5th edn. Belmont, CA: Thomson/Wadsworth, 2007.

Virmani IK, Lampe K. Home Chefs of the World: Rice and Rice-Based Recipes. International Rice Research Institute, 1991.

Walsh RM, Noakes TD, Hawley JA, Dennis SC. Impaired high-intensity cycling performance time at low level of dehydration. Int J Sports Med 1994; 15: 392–398.

Waterhouse J. Effects of Ramadan on physical performance: chronobiological considerations Br J Sports Med 2010; 44: 509–515.

World and Its Peoples: Malaysia, Philippines, Singapore, and Brunei. New York: Marshall Cavendish Corporation, 2007.

Yeung, HWC. Handbook of Research on Asian Business. Cheltenham: Edward Elgar Publishing, 2007.

Vegetarian/vegan athletes

American Dietetic Association, Dietitians of Canada. Position of the American Dietetic Association and Dietitians of Canada: vegetarian diets. Can J Diet Pract Res 2003; 64: 62–81.

Barr SI, Rideout CA. Nutritional considerations for vegetarian athletes Nutrition 2004; 20: 696–703.

Borrione P, Grasso L, Quaranta F, Parisi A. FIMS Position statement 2009. Vegetarin diets and athletes. Int Sport Med J 2009; 10(1).

Burke DG, Chilbeck PD, Parise G et al. Effect of creatine and weight training on muscle creatine performance in vegetarians. Med Sci Sports Exerc 2003; 35: 1946–1955.

Cox G. Special needs: the vegetarian athlete. In: Clinical Sports Nutrition, 4th edn (Burke L, Deakin V, eds). Sydney: McGraw-Hill Australia, 2010.

Hunt JR. Bioavailability of iron, zinc and other trace minerals from vegetarian diets. Am J Clin Nutr 2003; 78 (Suppl): 633s–639s.

Jeukendrup AE, Gleeson M. Sport Nutrition: An Introduction to Energy Production and Performance, 2nd edn. Champaign, IL: Human Kinetics, 2010.

Lukaszuk JM, Robertson RJ, Arch JE et al. Effect of creatine supplementation and a lact-ovo-vegetarian diet on muscle creatine concentration. Int J Sport Nutr Exerc Metab 2002; 12: 336–337.

Nieman DC. Physical fitness and vegetarian diets: is there a relation? Am J Clin Nutr 1999; 70 (Suppl): 570S–575S.

Philips F. Vegetarian nutrition briefing paper. British Nutrition Foundation, 2005.

Position statement by the Scientific Advisory Committee on Nutrition (SACN). Update on Vitamin D. London: The Stationery Office, 2007.

Rodriguez NR, Di Marco NM, Langley S, American Dietetic Association, Dietitians of Canada, American College of Sports Medicine. American College of Sports Medicine position stand. Nutrition and athletic performance. Med Sci Sports Exerc 2009; 41: 709–731.

Schumacher YO, Schmid A, Grathwohl D, Bültermann D, Berg A. Hematological indices and iron status in athletes of various sports and performances. Med Sci Sports Exerc 2002; 34: 869–875.

Thomas B, Bishop J. Manual of Dietetic Practice, 4th edn. Oxford: Blackwell Publishing, 2007.

Venderley AM, Campbell WW. Vegetarian diets: nutritional considerations for athletes. Sports Med 2006; 36: 293–305.

Wells AM, Haub MD, Fluckey J, Williams DK, Chernoff R, Campbell WW. Comparisons of vegetarian and beef containing diets on haematological indexes and iron stores during a period of resistive training in older men. J Am Diet Assoc 2003; 103: 594–601.

Willis KS, Peterson NJ, Larson-Meyer DE. Should we be concerned about the vitamin D status of athletes? Int J Sport Nutr Exerc Metab 2008; 18: 204–224.

The injured athlete: surgery and rehabilitation

Bucci LR. Nutrition applied to injury rehabilitation and sports medicine. In: Nutrition in Exercise and Sport, 1st edn (Wolinsky I, ed.). Boca Raton, FL: CRC Press, 1994.

Cooke MB, Rybalka E, Williams AD, Cribb PJ, Hayes A. Creatine supplementation enhances muscle force recovery after eccentrically-induced muscle damage in healthy individuals. J Int Soc Sports Nutr 2009; 6: 13.

Melis GC, van Leeuwen PA, von Blomberg-van der Flier BM et al. A carbohydrate-rich beverage prior to surgery prevents surgery-induced immunodepression: a randomized, controlled, clinical trial. JPEN J Parenter Enteral Nutr 2006; 30: 21–26.

Miller MD, Daniels LA, Bannerman E, Crotty M. Adherence to nutrition supplements among patients with a fall-related lower limb fracture. Nutr Clin Pract 2005; 20: 569–578.

Ozkalkanli MY, Ozkalkanli DT, Katircioglu K, Savaci S. Comparison of tools for nutrition assessment and screening for predicting the development of complications in orthopedic surgery. Nutr Clin Pract 2009; 24: 274–280.

Websites

http://www.lef.org
http://www.nutritioncare.org

25
Training and Competition Environments

Joanne L Fallowfield, Joseph DJ Layden and Adrian J Allsopp

Key messages

- Sport undertaken outdoors will be subject to the added environmental stressors of a low barometric pressure associated with high altitude, extremes in ambient temperature and humidity, solar radiation and poor air quality.
- The decrease in oxygen partial pressure with increasing altitude means that oxygen availability to the lungs is reduced. This is associated with a decrease in maximum oxygen uptake and a corresponding increase in the relative exercise intensity of submaximal exercise.
- The dryer air at altitude also exacerbates exercise-induced dehydration, such that fluid requirements at altitude are increased.
- Acute mountain sickness (AMS) can cause loss of appetite, nausea, vomiting, headache and dehydration; following AMS, appetite can remain suppressed and higher altitudes can result in greater appetite suppression.
- A loss in body weight, in the form of lean (muscle) tissue and fat, can be incapacitating at altitude. In addition to the effects of altitude exposure on metabolism, sense of taste and food preferences can change. Food (energy) intake should be actively increased to offset the weight loss associated with a loss of appetite and hypoxia at altitude.
- The physiological challenge of exercising in the heat is the ability to maintain effective temperature regulation in the face of

compromised mechanisms of heat dissipation, where prolonged and/or intensive exercise will challenge the ability of a sports performer to maintain a thermoregulatory balance.
- The body dissipates heat through conduction, convection, radiation and evaporation (of sweat). In terms of the body's physiological adaptation to heat, the sweating response is potentially the most important mechanism of heat dissipation, although its effectiveness to reduce body core temperature is dependent upon the ambient humidity of the environment.
- Increased sweating in the heat increases body fluid losses, which are further increased by exercise, such that dehydration is a significant concern when exercising in the heat.
- Heat can have an anorexic effect such that volitional energy intake is decreased in un-acclimatised individuals on initial heat exposure.
- Under cold exposure, which is associated with a tendency for body core temperature to decrease, energy requirements increase such that dietary energy intake should also be increased.
- Both fat and carbohydrate will provide fuel for the increased energy expenditure, although the body's stores of carbohydrate are performance limiting and should be prioritised.

25.1 Introduction

Sport undertaken outdoors will be subject to the added stressors posed by the environment. With the globalisation of sporting events, these environmental stressors are more than simply the day-to-day variations in local weather. The principal environmental considerations for outdoor events are the low barometric pressure associated with high altitude, extremes in ambient temperature (heat >30°C; cold <0°C) and humidity, solar radiation and poor air quality.

Exposure to more extreme (in terms of barometric pressure and/or temperature) environments is associated with increases in physiological and metabolic stress. The actual energy cost of undertaking exercise at altitude, in the heat or in the cold, may not always differ greatly from exercise performed under temperate sea-level conditions. However, physiological perturbations leading to reduced efficiency and/or the situational aspects of exercising in more extreme environments (e.g. due to the terrain, or the weight of additional clothing) might result in a greater total

Sport and Exercise Nutrition, First Edition. Edited by Susan A Lanham-New, Samantha J Stear, Susan M Shirreffs and Adam L Collins.
© 2011 The Nutrition Society. Published 2011 by Blackwell Publishing Ltd.

amount of work being done. Increases in physiological and metabolic stress can, in turn, lead to impaired thermoregulation, altered acid–base and electrolyte balances, altered energy metabolism, more rapid depletion of muscle glycogen stores, ketosis, impaired fine motor coordination and diminished exercise capacity. At altitude, the sports performer must attend to the increased fluid and (possibly) energy demands of exercising at altitude whilst appetite might be impaired. During exercise in the heat, sensible and insensible water losses are markedly increased and thermoregulatory alterations can have important effects on eating habits and dietary requirements. Exposure to hot environments is known to impair gastrointestinal function and symptoms such as cramps, gastrointestinal reflux, vomiting, diarrhoea and nausea are not uncommon. In a cold environment appropriate nutrition is essential in the maintenance of a stable body core temperature.

This chapter outlines the physiological and nutritional challenge of the environment to exercise capability. Nutritional strategies that might be adopted to assist a sports performer in improving tolerance to the challenges of the environment such that performance is better maintained are discussed.

25.2 The physiological challenge of exercising at altitude

The effects of altitude are not universal across all sports; short-duration high-intensity sports and strength-based sports are less affected by altitude, whereas longer-duration sports where performance is dependent upon maintaining the supply of oxygen to working muscles (i.e. aerobic exercise) will be more adversely affected. This oxygen supply chain is in turn dependent upon the partial pressure gradient that drives the delivery of oxygen from the atmosphere to the mitochondria in muscle. The physiological challenge of exercising at altitude arises from the decrease in barometric pressure (and hence the decrease in the partial pressure of oxygen in the atmosphere) with increasing height above sea level: the lower the atmospheric pressure, the lower the driving force, the poorer the oxygen supply to metabolising tissues. In this regard, altitude can be stratified in relation to the degree of physiological perturbation, where low altitude would be equivalent to less than 2000 m above sea level, moderate altitude

would be equivalent to 2000–5000 m above sea level, and high altitude would be equivalent to more than 5000 m above sea level.

The decrease in oxygen partial pressure with increasing altitude in practice means that oxygen availability to the lungs per breath of the sports performer is decreased. With increasing altitude and/or increasing exercise intensity, the supply of oxygen to tissue will eventually become compromised. *Hypoxia* refers to the condition where the supply of oxygen to the tissues is inadequate to meet the requirements for energy metabolism. As a consequence, the demand for energy (and hence oxygen) must be reduced, which is associated with a reduced aerobic exercise capacity.

In addition to a reduction in oxygen supply, there are other climatic considerations associated with moderate and high altitude that may affect exercise capacity in training and competition. These include extremes in atmospheric temperatures, where ambient temperature decreases by 1°C for every 150 m (1.98°C per 1000 feet) ascent, as well as significant temperature changes between night and day; low humidity; increased penetration of solar radiation due to the thinner air; and often erratic local weather conditions.

On first arriving at altitude breathing is perceived as being more difficult. This is despite the actual energy cost of breathing being less due to the thinner air (i.e. lower density of gases). At lower altitudes, the increased ventilation frequency arises in response to changes in the partial pressure of carbon dioxide dissolved in the blood sensed by chemoreceptors. In contrast, *hypoxic drive* (i.e. changes in breathing frequency due to a decrease in oxygen availability) does not occur until the partial pressure of oxygen decreases from 21 kPa (158 mmHg) at sea level to less than 14 kPa (105 mmHg) at about 3000 m. At altitudes above 3000 m (10 000 feet) breathing frequency is increased, which will increase carbon dioxide excretion from the lungs, resulting in an increase in blood alkalinity. Those individuals who do not demonstrate an increased ventilation response on first arrival at altitude (i.e. 2000–3000 m above sea level) appear to be more susceptible to *acute mountain sickness* (AMS). This is a condition that occurs as a consequence of altitude hypoxia, and is characterised by symptoms including shortness of breath, general fatigue, headaches and nausea.

The increased breathing frequency at altitude is associated with increased water loss through evaporation of moisture from the respiratory surfaces of the airways and lungs. This is exacerbated by increased insensible water loss from the skin, as well as more effective evaporation of sweat in the dryer air at altitude. As atmospheric water content tends to decrease with increasing altitude, the air in close proximity to a sports performer's skin will more readily accept the water excreted by sweat glands, as this is evaporated to bring about a cooling effect. Thus, as relative exercise intensity increases, which in turn will be associated with an increase in ventilation, fluid losses will be increased through both enhanced ventilatory and thermoregulatory evaporation of fluid from the respiratory and skin surfaces, respectively. As such, in order to offset these increased fluid losses, an immediate strategy that a sports performer should adopt on arrival at altitude is to consciously increase fluid intake. If fluid balance is not effectively addressed, this will lead to an apparent increase in red blood cell and blood haemoglobin concentrations arising from a dehydratory loss in plasma volume. This loss in plasma volume causes an increase in blood viscosity leading to a decrease in the oxygen and carbon dioxide carrying capacity of blood, which has further implications for aerobic exercise capacity. In addition, the heart must work harder to pump the thicker more viscous blood around the body, resulting in increased cardiovascular stress.

25.3 Training and competition at altitude

Sports performers involved in events where there is a significant aerobic component may include a period of altitude training in a periodised training programme, either to achieve the physiological adaptations associated with altitude acclimatisation to benefit subsequent sea-level performances, or to prepare for competitions taking place at altitude. Acclimatisation to altitude commences as soon as a sports performer arrives, with small largely biochemical changes taking place within muscle and blood in response to a reduced inspired oxygen availability. However, it will take several weeks before any real functional adaptations are evident in sporting performances. Thus, the worst time to train or compete

is within 3–6 days of arriving at altitude where the body is still trying to adapt to the physiological challenges of this environment. In terms of the efficacy of undertaking altitude training to benefit subsequent sea-level performances, the evidence is presently equivocal: altitude training appears to offer benefits for some sports performers but not others. However, in those individuals who are positive responders, sports performers would need to remain at altitude (2000–3000 m) for a minimum of 2–6 weeks to achieve real performance benefits. There appears to be an upper limit to human tolerance of around 5000 m, beyond which acclimatisation is limited and exercise capacity progressively deteriorates.

The lower barometric pressure at altitude will reduce the oxygen partial pressure of inspired air and therefore the oxygen partial pressure in the alveolar sacs of the lungs. The process of oxygen diffusion from the alveolar sacs into blood is not changed at altitude, but the rate of diffusion will be limited by a reduced oxygen pressure gradient. This reduced pressure gradient in turn limits the ability of blood haemoglobin in the pulmonary vessels to load up with oxygen, such that the amount of oxygen transported in arterial blood is reduced. The reduced availability of oxygen in blood will limit the delivery of oxygen to mitochondria, the site of cellular oxidative metabolism. In muscle cells, this will limit aerobic adenosine triphosphate (ATP) re-synthesis, where ATP is the form of energy required by muscle cells to perform work. A decrease in the rate of supply of ATP will reduce the work output of muscle. In terms of maximum aerobic capacity, this decrease in oxygen delivery and utilisation will be evident as a reduced maximum rate of oxygen uptake at altitude. Further effects of hypoxia include a reduced ability to perform complex tasks (at altitudes <2500 m), impaired memory function (at 2500–3000 m), impaired learning of novel tasks (at altitudes >2500 m) and impaired night vision (at altitudes >1500 m).

Maximum oxygen uptake (Vo_{2max}) is defined by the Fick equation, such that:

$$Vo_{2max} = Q_{max} (Cao_2 - Cvo_2)$$

where Vo_{2max} represents maximum oxygen uptake, Q_{max} maximum cardiac output, Cao_2 oxygen content of arterial blood and Cvo_2 oxygen content of venous blood. Maximum cardiac output is defined by the volume of blood pumped by the heart with each contraction and the maximum rate of cardiac contraction (i.e. maximum heart rate). Thus during submaximal exercise the reduced availability of oxygen in arterial blood can be somewhat compensated through an increase in heart rate. However, at maximal exercise intensities the heart rate cannot exceed the maximum heart rate, which will be the same at sea level as it is at altitude. As a consequence, maximum oxygen uptake is reduced at altitude.

Maximum oxygen uptake will begin to decrease noticeably from approximately 1500 m. Initially the rate of reduction is equivalent to approximately 10% for every 1000 m above 1200 m, but will decrease at a greater rate at higher altitudes exhibiting a non-linear relationship. A sports performer's training status appears to influence this decrease in maximum oxygen uptake, with well-trained endurance athletes noticing impaired maximum oxygen uptake at altitudes as low as 900 m. Some athletes experience incomplete oxygenation of blood even at sea level, and this will become exacerbated at altitude. This condition is termed *exercise-induced hypoxaemia* and reflects a lung limitation to aerobic performance. Athletes susceptible to this condition will experience a greater than anticipated decrease in maximum oxygen uptake with altitude, as opposed to athletes limited only by cardiac output. This physiological phenomenon may partly explain the large variability in responses to altitude amongst sports performers.

A direct effect of a decrease in maximum oxygen uptake is a corresponding increase in the relative exercise intensity of submaximal exercise. Lactate is produced as a consequence of anaerobic carbohydrate (CHO) metabolism, i.e. where CHO is metabolised to yield ATP in processes not requiring oxygen. Where oxygen supply is limited, anaerobic energy production will supplement aerobic energy production, and this will be evident as an increased blood lactate concentration at altitude for an equivalent sea-level performance. This in turn would result in an earlier onset of fatigue.

As well as the effects on respiratory and cardiovascular function, and hence an indirect influence on energy metabolism, altitude hypoxia also appears to have a direct effect on muscle function. The effects of altitude on fine motor tasks is evident at altitudes above 3000 m. Impaired muscle function would be associated with a decrease in exercise economy, and a corresponding increase in the amount of oxygen required to sustain the same work output (e.g. speed sustained during running, cycling or swimming) as compared with sea-level performances.

In terms of altitude acclimatisation, the most readily observed adaptations are in the volume and composition of blood. These modifications influence the blood's ability to carry and offload oxygen in the tissue in the face of a less than optimum oxygen partial pressure gradient. At the same time there are structural modifications taking place within the capillary bed feeding tissue that improves its ability to extract oxygen from arterial blood and to make efficient use of this oxygen in oxidative energy metabolism. The physiological acclimatisation responses associated with altitude exposure are summarised in Table 25.1.

25.4 Nutrition for training and competition at altitude

From the previous discussion it is evident that there are a number of physiological and metabolic challenges to exercising at altitude – hypoxia, extremes in temperature and low humidity – which in turn will present nutritional and hydration challenges. Aside from the clinical symptoms associated with AMS, the most apparent physical changes observed at altitude are a reduced volitional energy intake and resulting changes in body composition. Indeed, there is an inverse relationship between increases in altitude and decreases in energy intake such that weight loss at altitude is very common.

Weight loss and altitude exposure

The exact mechanism or cause of weight loss is not fully understood but could be attributed to a number of factors:

- decrease in volitional food intake associated with the appetite-suppressive affects of altitude;
- mismatch between energy intake and energy expenditure which might be attributed to increased basal metabolic rate coupled with increased work rates;
- inadequate fluid intake in the face of increased fluid losses;
- changes in metabolism;
- loss of muscle mass;
- impaired absorption of nutrients from the gastrointestinal tract.

Table 25.1 Physiological adaptations to altitude exposure.

Tissue	Adaptation	Function
Blood	Increased plasma volume Increased number of red blood cells Increased red blood cell volume Increased red blood cell haemoglobin content	Improved ability of blood to carry oxygen and therefore to transport oxygen to metabolising tissue
Blood	Increase in 2,3-diphosphoglycerate (reduces affinity of haemoglobin for oxygen) concentration in red blood cells	Improves ability of blood to offload oxygen within tissue capillaries
Capillary bed	Opening of dormant capillaries Growth of new capillaries	Increased density of the capillary network supplying tissue
Muscle fibre	Reduced cross-sectional areas of muscle fibres	Increased number of capillaries per unit cross-sectional area, but will also reduce the force-generating capacity of a muscle fibre
	Increased myoglobin concentration of muscle fibres	Provides a small transient reserve of oxygen at the onset of exercise Facilitates oxygen transport from the blood capillaries into tissue
	Increased number of mitochondria per muscle fibre	Increased aerobic energy metabolism (i.e. aerobic ATP re-synthesis)

Weight loss at altitude commonly occurs during the first weeks of exposure to moderate altitude in association with dehydration, a decrease in food intake and an increase in energy expenditure. Thus a combination of altitude anorexia and negative energy balance will result in changes in body composition over time despite adequate food being made available. Indeed, there is research that makes a link between appetite and regulatory peptides, such as leptin. When anorexia occurs at altitude it is maximum during the first 3 days of exposure and may last for 12 days at moderate altitude, but may continue indefinitely if acclimatisation is incomplete. At extreme altitude (i.e. >5400 m) weight loss continues beyond any level of acclimatisation, and may also involve intestinal malabsorption of nutrients and tissue catabolism in the face of negative energy balance. Thus the mechanisms underpinning weight loss at altitude are thought to be altitude dependent: at low altitudes weight loss appears to arise, in the main, from an increase in energy expenditure; but at higher altitudes weight loss appears to be associated with intestinal malabsorption of nutrients as muscle protein catabolism also occurs. The absolute altitude that differentiates low and high altitudes with regard to these weight loss mechanisms is difficult to discern; this is likely due to differences in design of the various studies interrogating this phenomenon and

the tremendous variation in initial responses to altitude, and the acclimatisation responses, of volunteers involved in such research.

In terms of changes in body composition, during initial exposure to moderate altitude about 70% of the weight lost is in the form of fat. Individuals with higher percentages of body fat do not appear to have an advantage in this regard, as a higher body fat content seems to be associated with fat being lost at a faster rate than in leaner individuals. Furthermore, protein catabolism seems to occur before fat stores are depleted and when sufficient CHO stores remain. This balance of weight loss appears to be altitude dependent; below 5400 m weight loss is largely attributable to fat loss, while above 5400 m weight loss is, in the main, from muscle protein catabolism.

Some researchers view the weight loss associated with altitude exposure as being an inevitable consequence of chronic hypobaric hypoxia. However, others have reported that when individuals focus on the need to maintain energy balance, weight losses can be minimised. Furthermore, good physical conditioning prior to and during exposure to altitude (i.e. sports performers undertaking specific training in advance of departure to altitude as part of a progressive programme) may reduce the anorexia associated with altitude exposure. There is an established link between stress and leptin such that the two may be related. Sports performers being comfortable, and the provision of palatable (desirable) food, play an important role in maintaining adequate food intake. It is unclear whether this management of food, ensuring choice and quality of provision, would suffice to prevent weight loss during extended stays at altitude (e.g. for an altitude training camp).

Carbohydrate requirements during exercise at altitude

As discussed previously, endurance performance is impaired at altitude, partly as a consequence of an altitude-dependent decrease in maximum oxygen uptake and a resulting increase in the relative exercise intensity. This in turn will be associated with a shift in energy metabolism, where an increased proportion of the total energy demand of exercise is derived from CHO relative to the energy provision from fat and protein. It is therefore advised that endurance athletes are provided with additional CHO. This strategy is both to reduce the energy deficit through the purposeful provision of more energy in the form of CHO, but also to offset the effects of an increase in relative exercise intensity during submaximal exercise. Thus an important nutritional strategy at altitude is to ensure that the body's endogenous CHO stores are adequately maintained, which will assist in the maintenance of endurance performance.

During early altitude acclimatisation food intake is generally reduced. This is especially true if altitude exposure is sudden and leads to the AMS symptoms of anorexia, nausea and vomiting. Under these circumstances, food intake can remain very low for several days. Diets high in CHO have been observed to have direct benefits in reducing the symptoms of AMS, but this has not been a consistent observation. With acclimatisation, symptoms of AMS tend to recede and dietary intake usually increases. Nevertheless, work investigating optimal diets for maintaining exercise capability at altitude have yielded equivocal findings. Traditional views suggest that CHO metabolism is generally increased, as metabolic enzymes involved in fat metabolism are inhibited. Thus, by default CHO is the 'preferred' fuel at altitude, such that a sports performer's diet must provide adequate CHO to replace this fuel on a daily basis. Furthermore, a number of studies have reported an increase in fat utilisation and glycogen sparing during a standardised exercise bout with acclimatisation. Thus energy and nutrient requirements should be monitored, and modified if necessary, during a prolonged stay at altitude.

CHO is energetically more efficient for ATP re-synthesis at low oxygen partial pressures in comparison with fat and protein. The carbon dioxide produced during the oxidation of CHO is greater than that for a similar amount of fat or protein. However, this increased carbon dioxide dissolved in plasma can stimulate the respiratory system to better maintain blood oxygenation at altitude. Furthermore, there is considerable evidence that CHO ingestion improves physical and mental tolerance to hypoxia in humans, and diets high in CHO appear to be well tolerated. Indeed, individuals at altitude tend to self-select CHO as a preferred food source, though this is not a consistent observation; at higher altitudes, individuals tend to self-select foods with a higher fat content. Thus while there is a strong rationale for advocating a high-CHO diet at altitude, foods high in fat should not be excluded from the provision. This is especially pertinent if the energy yield per gram of fat is considered; fat is an extremely efficient storage medium, such that fat-rich foods can assist in maintaining energy balance especially if the actual volitional food intake is limited.

Fluid balance and altitude

Maintaining adequate hydration at altitude is even more important than maintaining adequate energy intake. The initial weight loss at altitude arising from dehydration reflects a significant decrease in total body water, mainly due to a decrease in plasma volume. This decrease will reflect both a decreased fluid intake in the face of adequate provision as a consequence of diminished thirst, but also the increased ventilatory losses of fluid as a consequence of the dryer (often colder) air. A cumulative dehydration through incomplete rehydration will further add to the physiological challenge of altitude hypoxia. In the worst case, inadequate hydration has been associated with an increased risk of pulmonary and cerebral oedema. Thus hydration should be a central pillar in any nutritional strategy to support sports performers training or competing at altitude, where performers are carefully monitored throughout the day and encouraged to increase their fluid intake.

Monitoring hydration status

A sports performer's hydration (fluid) status can be readily monitored to varying degrees of precision. Monitoring body weight is a ready approach to monitoring short-term fluctuations in hydration status, where fluid deficits will be reflected in rapid losses in body weight. For this strategy to be successful, it is important that a sports performer knows his or her normal body weight prior to travelling to altitude. Body weight should then be measured every morning and before and after training sessions or competitions. However, as weight loss is a potential problem at altitude, monitoring body weight as a guide to hydration status may be problematic. Thus, ideally, body weight should be monitored in conjunction with other methods of monitoring hydration status.

Other easy approaches to monitoring hydration status include monitoring urine volume and urine colour and/or odour. Infrequent urination resulting in small volumes of darkly coloured (i.e. very dark yellow, orange or brown) with a pungent odour would be associated with dehydration. For this approach to be successful, again it is important that sports performers know their normal urine production and urine appearance. However, it should be noted that sports performers taking some nutritional supplements, such as vitamin and mineral supplements, might experience atypical urine colour, such that a sports performer's supplementation regimen should also be considered in evaluating urine colour.

More technical approaches to monitoring hydration status include measurement of specific gravity or measurement of urine osmolality. Specific gravity can be assessed using chemical dipping sticks or refractometer. The interpretation of specific gravity is presented in Table 25.2. Alternatively, urine osmolality can be measured with an osmometer, or a relative measure can be obtained using a galvanometer. Whilst potentially offering a greater level of precision, these more technical approaches are more limited in their utility due to the requirement for specific measurement equipment (which will represent an additional cost) and a greater level of training and expertise on the part of the measurer.

As a sports performer moves to altitude fluid needs will increase. It is also important to remember that whilst tolerance to altitude can improve, such that

Table 25.2 Interpretation of urine markers of hydration status.

Specific gravity (g/ml)	Osmolality (mosmol/kg)	Colour	Comment
<1.020	<700	Pale yellow	Euhydrated
1.020	≥700	Dark yellow/brown	Under-hydrated

the physiological effects are less stressful, the body cannot improve its tolerance of dehydration. As a consequence, monitoring fluid status and replacing lost fluid should be an important part of any nutritional strategy to support training and competition at altitude.

25.5 Training and competition at altitude: summary

From the above discussion, the key points to be attended to in a nutritional strategy to support sports performers training and competing at altitude are as follows.

- Loss of fluid from the body is more rapid at altitude.
- Monitoring fluid balance and actively replacing lost fluid should commence before sports performers move to altitude.
- Altitude exposure is associated with a loss in appetite.
- AMS can cause loss of appetite, nausea, vomiting, headache and dehydration. Following AMS, appetite can remain suppressed and higher altitudes can result in greater appetite suppression.
- Sense of taste is reduced and food preferences can change at altitude, which can decrease tolerance to monotonous foods.
- Actively increase food (energy) intake to offset weight loss associated with a loss of appetite and hypoxia at altitude.
- The loss of body weight in the form of lean (muscle) tissue and fat can be incapacitating. Allow time for gentle training on arrival at altitude and prior to competition.
- Energy requirements for altitude increase such that dietary energy intake should be increased by at least 10%.
- CHO is the preferred energy source at altitude. Maintaining the body's CHO stores will prevent excessive protein catabolism to meet the body's energy requirements.

Table 25.3 Physiological mechanisms of heat dissipation.

Mechanism	Action
Conduction	The transfer of heat from one material (e.g. body core) of a relatively higher temperature to another (e.g. skin) of a relatively lower temperature through direct contact
Convection	The transfer of heat from one location (e.g. skin) to another (e.g. environment) through the motion of a gas or liquid. This would be achieved through the movement of air over the surface of a sports performer's skin, where the rate of heat transfer is proportional to the rate of air movement
Radiation	The transfer of heat by the emission of infrared rays
Evaporation (of moisture)	The transfer of heat through the evaporation of moisture (sweat) from the skin (i.e. latent heat of vaporisation). Increase in core temperature relative to the set point of the hypothalamus initiates the sweating response; heat (energy) is drawn from the surrounding area of skin to evaporate the sweat

25.6 The physiological challenge of exercising in the heat

The physiological challenge of exercising in the heat is the ability to maintain effective temperature regulation in the face of compromised mechanisms of heat dissipation. *Thermoregulation* refers to the combined physiological processes regulating body temperature within a relatively narrow range. Under normal resting conditions in a temperate environment, body temperature will rarely fluctuate by more than 1.0°C from an average body core temperature of 37°C. The ability of a sports performer to effectively thermoregulate will be influenced by:

- physical characteristics such as body weight, body height (i.e. body size) and body composition;
- heat acclimatisation status;
- aerobic (endurance) training status;
- fluid (hydration) status;
- type of clothing worn.

Prolonged and/or intensive exercise will challenge the ability of a sports performer to maintain thermoregulatory balance. If the rate of heat production is not matched by the body's ability to dissipate heat, core temperature will rise. The ability to thermoregulate will also be influenced by illness and/or infection, such that even mild infections can significantly increase a sports performer's susceptibility to suffering some form of heat illness.

The body's thermostat is the hypothalamic region of the brain. Like the thermostat in a domestic house, the hypothalamus will initiate heat production and heat dissipation mechanisms to maintain a stable *set point* temperature. Neurones in the preoptic area of the anterior hypothalamus monitor the temperature

of blood passing through the brain (i.e. central thermoreceptors). These receptors respond to changes in the temperature of blood; a decrease in blood temperature will initiate mechanisms to conserve or produce heat, and an increase in blood temperature will result in the initiation of heat loss mechanisms. Peripheral thermoreceptors in the skin monitor skin and local environmental temperature, and similarly relay their temperature messages to the hypothalamus to assist in the central processing of physiological temperature information such that the body's response is appropriately modified. The mechanisms of heat dissipation from the body are described in Table 25.3.

During exercise, a sports performer's body will produce heat as a by-product of energy metabolism. As such, body core temperature will start to increase. This change in core temperature is detected by the hypothalamic central thermoreceptors, which will send signals to the smooth muscle that acts as cuffs in blood vessels to regulate blood flow to the skin. The smooth muscle relaxes such that the aperture of blood vessels dilates and blood flow to the skin is increased. Thus the dissipation of heat from the (high temperature) core to the (lower temperature) skin brings about a cooling effect.

From a thermoregulatory perspective, the onset of sweating (i.e. when sweat is secreted from sweat glands onto the skin's surface) is related to changes in body temperature, though it should be remembered that a sweating response is also associated with a general sympathetic stress response. Under ambient conditions there is a delay in the onset of sweating following the start of exercise as heat-producing metabolic and mechanical processes associated with exercise are initiated, and as such there is an increase in body core temperature sufficient to initiate a thermoregulatory response. If exercising in the heat, depending on the ambient temperature, it is likely that the sports performer will already be sweating. Thus the sweating response of individuals (in terms of onset and the extent of sweating) will depend on such factors as the ambient temperature, the training status of the sports performer and his or her heat acclimatisation status.

The effectiveness of the sweating response to reduce body core temperature depends on the ambient humidity of the environment. For sweating to work efficiently, the water vapour pressure (i.e. the water content of atmospheric air) gradient between the skin and surrounding air must be high. In a hot dry environment (e.g. desert regions) where ambient humidity is low, the sweating response will work at its most effective to rapidly lose heat from the body. However, this heat loss will also be associated with a high rate of fluid loss, such that the sports performer will be at risk of dehydrating if hydration status is not monitored and fluid intake is not consciously increased. Conversely, in a hot wet environment (e.g. tropical regions) the effectiveness of the sweating response is reduced. This is because the water vapour pressure gradient between the skin and the surrounding air is very small or non-existent. Sweat will therefore drip from the skin rather than being evaporated.

25.7 Training and competition in the heat

Whilst training or competing in the heat, the cardiovascular system must manage two competing challenges: the challenge to maintain a supply of oxygen and nutrients to working muscles (and the removal of carbon dioxide and metabolic waste products) to sustain exercise performance, and the challenge of increasing peripheral blood flow to increase heat dissipation. If either challenge is not met, at best exercise capacity will be compromised, although in the worst case the sports performer is at risk of experiencing metabolic tissue damage or thermal injury.

Sports performers who are intending to participate in competitions located in hot environments would benefit from a period of heat acclimatisation in order to better maintain exercise capacity. The body can undergo a certain amount of physiological adaptation to the combined environmental stressor posed by heat and humidity. The time course of heat acclimatisation is much more rapid than the adaptive responses to altitude, with the majority of adaptation taking place within the initial 12–14 days of exposure. There is good evidence to suggest that the acute acclimatisation response (i.e. changes in core temperature, heart rate response and endocrine adaptations) occurs between 2 and 5 days of exposure, whereas the chronic acclimatisation response (i.e. changes in the onset of sweating and the sweating rate) requires longer, being about 75% complete within 9–12 days. The degree of acclimatisation, and the pattern of acclimatisation, is variable between individuals; indeed some sports performers may never significantly adapt to a hot environment. Thus sports performers competing in the heat should arrive *at least* 7 days prior to competition to both habituate and acclimatise to conditions prior to competition. Some of the adaptive responses to the heat may persist for a number of weeks on returning to more temperate environments; however, there is a significant loss of general heat tolerance within 3–4 days of removal from the heat stimulus. The process of de-acclimatisation is relatively rapid, taking place at a rate of 15–30% per week.

Passive exposure to heat is associated with only small adaptive responses. Aerobic exercise *per se* undertaken under temperate environmental conditions is associated with adaptive responses that will improve a sports performer's heat tolerance. However, optimal acclimatisation is achieved by a combination of exercise (moderate intensity for 60–100 min/day) and heat of 32–35°C (90–95°F). The relative humidity of the environment will also influence the acclimatisation response. Ambient vapour pressure may limit sweat evaporation through *hydromeiosis*; under conditions of high humidity the skin's outer layer of dead squamous cells of the stratum corneum can swell, closing or reducing the lumen of sweat glands and hence reducing the sweating rate. However, sweat evaporation can be limited in humid conditions in the absence of hydromeiosis (i.e. sweat rate stays high but the sweat either drips from or runs off the body). In this instance, the effectiveness of the sweating response to bring about a cooling of the body is reduced, such that large volumes of sweat may be lost as the body tries, and possibly fails, to control core body temperature. In terms of acclimatisation, a dryer environment (i.e. lower relative humidity) would

Table 25.4 Physiological adaptations to heat exposure.

Tissue	Adaptation	Function
Brain	Lowering of hypothalamic set point	Earlier initiation of heat dissipation mechanisms
Heart	Increased stroke volume	Increased volume of blood pumped by the hear per beat, such that resting and submaximal exercising heart rate is reduced
Circulation	Increased venous return	Better maintenance of central blood pressure
Blood	Increased plasma volume in response to increased plasma protein concentrations	Contributes to better blood pressure stability at rest and during exercise
	Increased total blood volume	
Sweat gland	Earlier onset of sweating	An earlier, greater and more efficient sweating response will better facilitate heat dissipation
	Increased density of sweat glands per unit area of skin	
	Increased sweat volume per unit time	
	Decreased salt (sodium) concentration of sweat	

provide a more efficient stimulus to the sweat glands to adapt. An acclimatisation programme should be progressive in terms of exercise intensity, exercise duration and temperature exposure. The specific details of the starting load and the programme's progression will depend on the initial training and heat-acclimatisation status of the sports performer, but should be increased towards optimal levels as quickly as is appropriate for each individual. Duration and frequency of training is of greater importance in facilitating adaptive responses than the intensity of training. Acclimatisation sessions should start at an easy pace, where the aim is to raise body core temperature by about 1°C and to maintain this elevated temperature over a sustained period of time (60–90 min). To achieve the desired physiological adaptations, the purpose of the exercise intensity and exercise duration is to initiate and to maintain the sweating response. The progression will gradually increase both the intensity of sessions and the duration of training throughout the 1–2 weeks of acclimatisation. Table 25.4 details the physiological adaptations associated with heat acclimatisation.

25.8 Nutrition for training and competition in the heat

Energy expenditure, energy metabolism and energy intake

The relationship between ambient temperature and energy requirements was initially addressed during military studies undertaken in the 1940s. These early investigations observed that acute exposure to hot environments was associated with a suppressed appetite, where this effect might be further compounded by gastrointestinal distress associated with exercising in the heat. Appetite suppression was most evident in un-acclimatised volunteers upon initial heat exposure. Volitional food (energy) intake in physically fit military personnel was inversely related to ambient temperature; as ambient temperature increased, volitional energy intake decreased. In 1950 the Committee of Caloric Requirements of the Food and Agricultural Organisation (FAO) of the United Nations reported an approximate linear relationship between energy expenditure and mean external (ambient) temperature. These early studies commented that the large difference in volitional energy intake could not be simply explained by differences in basal metabolic rate, body mass, or specifics related to the type of activity being undertaken, as these factors were standardised across the different groups. Indeed, these early studies have been confirmed by more recent investigations which have shown in hot wet environments that hunger decreases independently of energy expenditure. The FAO tentatively recommended that daily energy requirements should be adjusted by 5% for every 10°C departure from a reference mean temperature of 10°C, with a 5% increase in energy intake for lower temperatures and 5% increase in energy intakes for higher temperatures. The nutritional requirements for sports performers in the cold are discussed later in this chapter.

Training and competition in the heat is associated with an increased rate of energy expenditure in comparison to undertaking the same exercise challenge in more temperate environments. However, it should be noted that this is not a consistent finding amongst all researchers, where some studies have reported no change in energy expenditure with ambient temperature and a few have reported a reduction in energy expenditure. This variation may be due to differences in training and acclimatisation status of study volunteers, the specific details of the exercise challenge (i.e. in terms of intensity and duration), and possible differences in clothing and equipment. Where an increased rate of energy expenditure has been observed, this was greater for hot wet (humid) environments compared with hot dry environments. This is partly due to a necessarily higher sweating response in a hot wet environment to dissipate the heat as a consequence of the reduced efficiency of the sweating response, and partly due to alterations in the circulatory system associated with maintaining an appropriate heat exchange. The possible reasons for this increased energy requirement in hot environments are detailed in Table 25.5.

In terms of the balance of aerobic and anaerobic energy metabolism, there appears to be an increased contribution of anaerobic metabolism to the total energy expenditure for a standard exercise challenge in the heat compared with a more temperate environment. This shift in energy metabolism is likely a consequence of reduced muscle blood flow, and hence oxygen delivery, following a thermoregulatory reprioritisation of systemic blood flow to the skin. This balance between aerobic and anaerobic metabolism will be further compromised by dehydration, such that failure to replace fluid losses is associated with increased blood lactate concentration, which in turn will reflect an increased dependency on endogenous CHO reserves. It is likely that these increases in anaerobic metabolism would become greater if exercise performance was maintained over a prolonged period.

Thus a sports performer's energy intake must be increased in order to offset the increased energy expenditure in the heat. If energy intake is not systematically increased in exercising individuals, then a sports performer will soon be in energy deficit. In the short term this will be associated with compromised exercise capacity. However, over the longer term sports performers will experience weight loss. It is recommended that individuals engaged in moderate-intensity physical activity should increase energy

Table 25.5 Possible physiological processes involved in increased energy expenditure in hot environments.

Inefficient physical activity and/or psychomotor stress
Q10 effect on metabolism associated with elevated body core temperature[a]
Increased sweat gland activity
Tachycardia (i.e. elevated rest and submaximal heart rate)
Increased pulmonary ventilation
Increased anaerobic metabolism
Increased oxygen debt[b]
Increased lactate production
Increased muscle glycogen utilisation
Increased blood glucose utilisation
Decreased skeletal muscle blood flow

[a] The Q10 effect is the adjustment in metabolic rate in relation to temperature change; for higher temperatures (within physiological norms) the rate of metabolism is increased.
[b] The amount of oxygen required to repay the oxygen deficit accrued during intensive exercise or exercise where the oxygen supply is inadequate to meet tissue needs. This additional amount of oxygen is required for the removal of lactic acid and other metabolic products that accumulated when the supply of oxygen was insufficient.
Adapted from Buskirk ER. Energetics and climate with emphasis on heat: a historical perspective. In: Nutritional Needs in Hot Environments. Reprinted with permission from National Academies Press, Copyright 1993, National Academy of Sciences.

intake by about 0.7% per degree Celsius rise in ambient temperature above 30°C. For example, if the mean daily energy intake of a sports performer was 3000 kcal, this would increase by 21 kcal for every 1°C rise in ambient temperature above 30°C. However, daily energy requirements under extremely hot environments (>40°C) may reach 56 kcal/kg (i.e. 3920 kcal for a 70-kg sports performer), due to the increased energy requirements of thermoregulating and maintaining exercise performance.

Fluid balance in the heat

Previously this chapter has detailed simple and more technical approaches to monitoring fluid status in sports performers. As was the case at altitude, exercising in the heat is associated with increased rates of fluid loss compared with exercising under temperate conditions. This is of particular concern on early arrival as the body is coping, and then adapting, to the added stress imposed by the heat. Over this period, fluid losses, and associated electrolyte losses, are at their greatest, and as such maintaining adequate hydration (and possibly under conditions of extreme rates of fluid loss, electrolyte intake) is essential for maintaining health and exercise capacity.

The major routes of fluid loss during exercise are from the respiratory surfaces and in the form of sweat. The higher the exercise intensity, the higher the ventilatory rate and the greater the respiratory fluid losses; concomitantly, the greater the exercise intensity, the greater the metabolic heat production and the greater the requirement to dissipate heat as efficiently as possible, hence an increase in the sweating response.

Dehydration will impair sporting performance, and the longer the duration of an event, the potentially greater the performance decrement arising from dehydration. Any level of dehydration is potentially performance limiting in a trained sports performer, but the exercise science literature often quotes a level of dehydration equivalent to 2% of body mass (i.e. equivalent to 1.4 kg in an 70-kg sports performance, or approximately 1.4l of fluid) as being associated with a significant reduction in exercise capacity. Under temperature conditions, submaximal exercise of moderate intensity is associated with an average sweating rate of the order of 1.0l/hour, and this can easily increase twofold with increasing ambient temperature but rarely beyond 2.0–2.5l/hour.

Maintaining fluid balance and factors influencing effective rehydration of the sports performer has been addressed in Chapter 7.

Gastrointestinal function in the heat: implications for fluid balance

Gastric emptying and intestinal motility decrease as ambient temperature and body core temperature increase. Although the mechanism is not clear, it is thought that thermal strain associated with hypohydration and heat stress results in reduced splanchnic blood flow and elevated plasma β-endorphin concentrations. Sports performers under heat stress often report gastrointestinal symptoms including stomach cramps, belching, reflux, bloody stools, vomiting, diarrhoea and nausea. Severe heat exposure simulates haemorrhage and intestinal ischaemia as a consequence of blood pooling in the cutaneous capitance vessels. Central blood volume and sphlanchnic blood flow decline and mean arterial blood pressure falls as the heart rate cannot fully compensate for a declining stroke volume to maintain cardiac output. The effects of heat stress on gastrointestinal function and sports performance can range from mild discomfort to serious impairment. It is thought that severe hyperthermia is associated with mucosal lesions in the small intestine as a consequence of tissue hypoxia, which will increase capillary permeability and result in endotoxaemia.

Whilst gastric emptying is impaired during exercise heat stress, it is unclear whether intestinal absorption is also compromised. Early studies suggested that there was an inverse relationship between exercise intensity and rates of gastric emptying and intestinal absorption. However, with regard to intestinal absorption this is not a consistent finding; some of the more recent studies have reported that neither exercise intensity (30–70% Vo_{2max}) nor exercise duration (60–90 min) had a negative effect on intestinal fluid absorption. The majority of studies investigating gastric emptying, intestinal absorption and gastrointestinal damage have involved exercise models of relatively short durations (<90 min). The effects of exercise lasting longer than 90 min, in association with heat stress, on the gastrointestinal tract are unknown. There is also contradiction with regard to whether mode of exercise influences gastric emptying and/or intestinal absorption. Some studies have observed a slowing of gastric emptying and/or intestinal absorption in running compared with cycling exercise, whereas others have observed no effect. The differences in such studies may simply reflect differences in individual tolerance to exercising with fluid or food in the gastrointestinal tract. Indeed, this appears to be a trainable attribute, where tolerance can be progressively improved in most individuals over time.

Thus in terms of the implications for fluid balance, smaller boluses over time of lower-osmolality (lower CHO concentration) beverages would be more preferable than larger single boluses. It is advisable for sports performers to experiment with different beverages during training so that an insight into their personal preferences in terms of palatability and drinking strategy is gained. Care should be taken in terms of the flavouring (not too strong), temperature and consistency (not too sticky or viscous), to ensure that, should gastric emptying and/or intestinal absorption be compromised in the heat, the beverage formulation will not further confound rehydration and maintenance of fluid provision.

Effects of heat acclimatisation/acclimation on energy intake

Following acclimatisation the dietary requirements are similar in hot dry and temperate areas. Volitional dietary intake may remain suppressed in hot wet environments due to the sustained high sweat loss and anorexia. Exercise metabolic rate during a standard submaximal exercise bout is decreased following heat acclimatisation (compared with performance during initial exposure), and this is associated with a decreased rate of oxygen uptake. However, the mechanisms of this reduced metabolic rate remain unclear.

25.9 Training and competition in the heat: summary

From the above discussion, the key points to be attended to in a nutritional strategy to support sports performers training and competing in the heat are as follows.

- Increased sweating increases body fluid losses, which are further increased by exercise.
- Monitoring fluid balance and actively replacing lost fluid should commence before sports performers travel to the heat.
- Heat can have an anorexic effect such that volitional energy intake is decreased in un-acclimatised individuals on initial exposure to the heat.
- Sense of taste may also change in the heat, decreasing tolerance to monotonous foods.
- During initial exposure to the heat, actively increase food (energy) intake to offset weight loss associated with loss of appetite.
- If the sports performer's hydration strategy includes sports/energy beverages, these will provide additional energy to support any potential energy deficits.
- Following acclimatisation the energy requirements for exercising in the heat are no different to exercising under temperate conditions.
- However, the greater stress on the body in the heat may be associated with increased use of CHO to fuel exercise.
- A sports diet to support training and competition in the heat should specifically attend to replacing the body's CHO reserves of muscle and liver glycogen stores.

25.10 The physiological challenge of exercising in the cold

Sports performers would rarely find themselves subject to a cold environment without the appropriate protection. However, in considering the nutritional challenges of training and competition environments, it is important to address the effects of cold on the body, the potential performance impairments, and the nutritional strategies that might be adopted to maintain body core temperature and hence performance.

The human body is less able to adapt to the challenges of cold environments than it is of hot environments. In the main, humans depend upon behavioural changes (e.g. wearing more clothes and moving to shelter) for protection against cold exposure. The rate of body core temperature reduction when exposed to a cold stress is proportional to both the duration of exposure and the temperature gradient between the body and its immediate environment. If body temperature falls below 35°C, physical and mental performance rapidly deteriorate; this condition is referred to as *hypothermia*. If body core temperature continues to fall to less than 32°C, the mechanisms of heat production become inadequate; this level of cold exposure will very quickly become life-threatening. Nevertheless, even modest decreases in ambient temperature are associated with changes in physiological function and performance.

Physiological mechanisms for either conserving heat or generating more heat are less effective than mechanisms for heat dissipation. Mechanisms to preserve body core temperature are initiated when the temperature of blood passing through the hypothalamus falls below the set point. Immediate responses include shivering thermogenesis, non-shivering thermogenesis (i.e. heat production through increased cellular metabolism) and peripheral vasoconstriction (i.e. a decrease in blood flow to the skin). When individuals are not sufficiently insulated during cold exposure at rest or during light-intensity exercise, shivering thermogenesis will contribute to an increase in total energy expenditure and hence heat production. The peak intensity of shivering is of the order of five times resting metabolic rate, which corresponds to 42–50% Vo_{2max}. Carbohydrates and lipids provide the main sources of fuel for shivering, with only a minor

Table 25.6 Effects of cold exposure on sports performance.

Tissue	Response	Physiological effect	Performance effect
Skin capillaries	Vasoconstriction	Reduced oxygen supply to active muscle, increased dependency on anaerobic metabolism	Earlier onset of fatigue
Heart	Reduced contractility	Decreased maximal heart rate and hence Vo_{2max}	Increased relative exercise intensity
Muscle	Reduced contractility	Decreased economy	Decrease in endurance
	Reduced velocity of contraction	Decreased muscle speed and muscle efficiency	Decrease in maximal speed
	Reduced power of contraction	Decreased muscle force and muscle efficiency	Decrease in maximal strength
Nervous system	Slowing of action potential propagation	Reduced fine motor control	Decreased technical (skill) ability

contribution from protein. The contribution of each substrate (CHO or fat) during shivering is not predictable and is most likely influenced by differences in the nutritional status of the sports performer, shivering intensity, and the severity and type of cold exposure. Individuals exposed to cool air tend to preferentially use CHO, whereas cooling arising from cold-water immersion is associated with increased use of fat. Increasing exercise intensity, such that the rate of energy metabolism (and hence heat production) to sustain exercise is associated with an increase in body core temperature, will inhibit shivering, as both processes originate from muscular contractions.

Cold-induced increases in metabolic heat production, arising from sympathetic stimulation of energy metabolism, will also contribute to the defence of body core temperature. Sympathetic stimulation of the smooth muscles in arteries (i.e. vasoconstriction) decreases peripheral blood flow, which will effectively improve insulation at the skin layer. In addition, vascular heat exchanges ensure that warm blood leaving the core will exchange its heat with cooler blood returning from the skin.

In terms of energy metabolism during cold exposure, it is not simply an increase in total energy turnover; a number of studies have also reported associated shifts in metabolic substrate utilisation. Indeed, shifts in metabolic substrate oxidation are evident even with moderate cold stress that is associated with a decrease in skin temperature but not a decrease in body core temperature. During rest and during moderate-intensity exercise under such conditions, the rate of oxygen uptake increased such that the respiratory exchange ratio (i.e. the ratio of the rate of carbon dioxide production to the rate of

oxygen uptake), which provides an index of substrate utilisation, was reduced (indicative of increased fat oxidation). However, some researchers have observed increases in CHO oxidation during exercise in the cold. Thus, the balance of substrate utilisation may be dependent on the severity of the cold exposure (which will influence peripheral vasoconstriction and oxygen supply to muscle) and the intensity of the exercise being undertaken (and hence an inhibition or attenuation of vasomotor tone encouraging vasodilation and maintenance of peripheral blood flow).

Physical factors influencing a sports performer's ability to cope with cold exposure include body composition (i.e. ratio of body fat mass to lean muscle mass), body size (i.e. ratio of skin surface area to body volume) and possibly training status. These factors define the insulation of the body and its capacity to dissipate heat relative to heat storage.

25.11 Training and competition in the cold

The physiological responses to cold exposure will affect the functioning of the respiratory system, the cardiovascular system, energy metabolism and muscle function (see Table 25.6). During submaximal exercise, the rate of oxygen uptake for an equivalent exercise challenge will increase in the cold relative to a temperate environment. This reduced economy reflects a temperature-dependent reduction in skeletal muscle contractility, but also a decrease in contractility of cardiac muscle that will be associated with a decrease in maximal heart rate. Thus, during maximal intensity exercise (as discussed previously according to the Fick equation), maximum oxygen uptake will be reduced, though this is not a consistent observation. Initial cold exposure will be associated with vasoconstriction of skin capillaries in an attempt to conserve body core temperature. If body core temperature is not adequately conserved, a decrease in blood temperature is associated with a reduction in the amount of oxygen unloaded from blood as is passes through muscle capillaries. However, with increasing heat production during submaximal and more intensive exercise, shivering is suppressed and muscle demand for blood flow overrides cold-induced vasoconstriction.

As well as a decrease in muscle contractility with cold exposure, the velocity and power of muscle contraction are also reduced and the pattern of muscle fibre recruitment is changed. The combined effect of these temperature-dependent modifications in muscle function is a reduction in muscle efficiency. This decrease in efficiency will further increase the oxygen requirement for maintaining exercise performance, at a time when oxygen supply to muscle is less than optimal. In addition, the effect of cold on both neural and muscular processes is such that fine motor control will be impaired, and there will be a decrease in the quality of skilled performance. Thus performers involved in more technical sports may experience greater performance decrements.

Independent of exercise effects, cold exposure leading to a decrease in body core temperature will lead to an increased metabolic rate to increase heat production. Thus a sports performer undertaking an exercise challenge in a cold environment will have an increased rate of energy turnover for the same exercise challenge relative to a temperate environment, partly by virtue of the energy cost of exercise and the added energy cost of the ambient temperature-dependent increase in metabolic rate. Thus, the total energy cost of submaximal work is greater in the cold than at neutral temperatures, and this increase in energy expenditure is not totally attributable to cold exposure *per se*. Indeed, the exact causes of a higher energy expenditure during exercise in cold environments is not fully understood. In addition, any reduction in muscle blood flow associated with cold-induced vasoconstriction, which will reduce oxygen and nutrient supply to working muscles as well as removal of carbon dioxide and waste metabolites, will increase anaerobic energy production. A consequence of such an increase in anaerobic metabolism would be increased lactate formation and associated hydrogen

ions. This sequence of events, which will be exercise intensity dependent, will be associated with a more rapid utilisation of the body's endogenous CHO reserves, as well as buffering capacity to manage the hydrogen ions, potentially resulting in an earlier onset of fatigue.

Nevertheless, cooling during exercise has also been shown to result in improvements in exercise performance. In general, these improvements have been attributed to a reduced thermoregulatory and cardiovascular strain during exercise (as evident by a lower body core temperature and lower skin temperature at similar work rates) and an enhanced capacity for heat storage. In addition, improvements in performance during exercise in environments of a lower ambient temperature could be attributed to shifts in energy metabolism (i.e. increased fat oxidation and decreased CHO oxidation). However, such a rationale is likely linked to the severity and type of cold exposure, and would be exercise-intensity and exercise-duration dependent; lower-intensity longer-duration events, where heat storage and substrate utilisation would become limiting, are more likely to benefit in cold environments than higher-intensity shorter-duration events.

A further consideration of training and competing in the cold is that of dehydration. Dehydration can reduce appetite and lead to lethargy (fatigue and weakness), where lethargy is not good in the cold as physical activity will assist in heat generation. As a consequence of the increased clothing sports performers will wear, performers will continue to experience high fluid losses through sweating. However, the drive to drink and maintain hydration is not as strong in the cold as it is whilst exercising in the heat. In addition, in extreme cold, the air will be relatively dry, which would increase respiratory fluid losses. In addition to its impact on systemic function, dehydration may exacerbate the risk of cold injury. Thus, as at altitude and in the heat, sports performers should be educated to understand the importance of maintaining fluid balance, how to monitor their hydration status in the cold, and how to ensure that their fluid intake is adequate.

Acclimatisation to the cold is very limited. A sports performer exposed to cold on a regular basis might experience a reduction in the body core temperature associated with the onset of shivering, whilst the extent of shivering might also be reduced. However, these are relatively small adjustments that would not significantly offset performance decrements associated with cold exposure.

25.12 Nutrition for training and competition in the cold

Adequate energy intake is essential for maintaining body core temperature and maintaining sporting performance in the cold. From the above discussion cold exposure is typically associated with an increase in energy expenditure to maintain the same level of exercise performance as in more temperate environments. The daily energy requirements for a sports performer may be of the order of 5% higher in a cold (<14°C) environment compared with a warmer environment. This increase requirement is normally associated with a compensatory increase in energy consumption by individuals in the cold, where decreased ambient temperatures have generally been seen to stimulate appetite. Thus any nutritional strategy to support training and competition in the cold should provide additional energy, and the greater part of this energy, if possible, should be provided in the form of CHO.

Nevertheless, it is accepted that the volume of food that can be consumed within a dietary day will limit some sports performers, and as such some of this additional energy could be provided in the form of more energy-dense foods that will have a higher fat content. Nevertheless, unsaturated fats should be preferred over saturated fats from a health perspective, and care should be taken that the overall balance of the diet is maintained. There is no requirement for sports performers to increase their fat intake prior to transiting to cold training or competition environments in order to offset any potential energy deficits. Such a strategy is likely to be associated with a decrease in performance and may result in gastrointestinal distress. Indeed, it takes several weeks to adapt to a high-fat diet and the benefits presently remain unclear. Similarly, there is no evidence that cold exposure increases the body's requirements for vitamins and minerals.

In terms of the pattern of energy intake, it appears that individuals receiving smaller but more frequent meals throughout the day were more *thermogenic* than individuals receiving the same total energy provision but as three main meals across the day. This thermogenic effect was associated with a greater use of fat as opposed to CHO. The mechanism to favour increased lipid metabolism over CHO metabolism with more frequent meals appears to be due to a flattened insulin response, such that insulin's inhibition of lipolysis was reduced. The implications for exercise performance are that, through modifying energy intake across the training or competition day, a more favourable balance of substrate utilisation could be maintained.

In terms of maintaining sporting performance, the whole day needs to be considered in terms of training and/or competing, refuelling, active and passive rest, and also the quantity and quality of sleep. Being away from home, a break in the normal training routines, and away from the social support of family and friends will be disruptive in itself. It is therefore important to re-establish some kind of routine when relocated to a training/competition camp, and this is even more important if that location is multiple time zones away from a sport performer's home country and/or has a challenging environment.

There is a complex relationship between sleep, nutrition and well-being. Given that factors associated with hypothermia include energy depletion, weight loss and sleep deprivation, the importance of adequate and appropriate nutrition in the cold is very evident. Sleep deprivation on its own is unlikely to impair temperature regulation, but when combined with poor nutrition and cold exposure the risks of hypothermia are significantly increased. The neural mechanisms regulating sleep appear to interact with thermoregulation. During rapid eye movement (REM) sleep, neither the cold-sensing nor hot-sensing thermoreceptors of the hypothalamus are activated. As a consequence, the body does not thermoregulate during REM sleep. During non-rapid eye movement (NREM) sleep, some thermal information is received, and shivering can occur if an individual is exposed to a cold stress. During REM sleep the reduction in metabolic activity reduces nutritional (energy) requirements. However, the decrease in metabolism is associated with a decrease in body core temperature. Thus, the balance of REM and NREM sleep will influence night-time thermoregulation. On waking, any fall in body core temperature occurring during sleep is generally reduced by thermogenesis. However, if sleep is disturbed then further decreases in body core temperature can occur. Prior exercise, energy intake and the menstrual cycle can all affect body core temperature during sleep. A travelling sports performer is likely to experience disrupted sleep and loss of appetite, in association with disturbed thermoregulation, if multiple time zones are crossed. Providing meals at set times, and re-establishing normal routines, can assist in re-synchronising the sleep and temperature-regulating clock.

The key to cold weather nutrition is to provide hot palatable food, providing a warm sensation, satisfying the appetite and maintaining morale, at regular intervals throughout the day. Eating regular meals and hearty snacks help maintain higher skin temperatures and prevent excess shivering. In addition, eating a small meal before bed helps maintain body core temperature and prevents sleeplessness. From a training and/or competition camp perspective, eating meals together also helps improve group morale.

In terms of maintaining hydration status, it is important that sports performers are aware that cold suppresses thirst. As such, drinking should be scheduled at regular intervals and the volume should be based on individually assessed rates of fluid losses. Fluid losses will be dependent on the intensity of exercise being undertaken, the duration of exercise, ambient temperature, and the clothing worn. Daily and pre- and post-exercise body mass assessment should be used to provide an estimation of training and/or competition fluid losses, from which an individualised drinking strategy should be developed.

25.13 Training and competition in the cold: summary

From the above discussion, the key points to be attended to in a nutritional strategy to support sports performers training and competing in the cold are as follows.

- Under cold exposure, which is associated with a tendency for body core temperature to decrease, energy requirements increase such that dietary energy intake should also be increased.
- Both fat and CHO will provide fuel for the increased energy expenditure, although the body's stores of CHO are performance limiting and should be prioritised.
- Monitor fluid balance in the cold and actively replace lost fluid.
- Quickly re-establishing routines is important from a nutritional perspective, but also from training and/or competition, sleep and well-being perspectives.

25.14 Other environmental challenges

As well as altitude, heat and cold, there are other environmental challenges that interact with these principal stressors to add to the environmental burden placed on a sports performer. In the modern world perhaps the most pervasive and threatening challenge is that of poor air quality. Air pollution has implications for sporting performance, but also for longer-term health. The potentially harmful effects of air pollution are dependent on:

- type of pollutant;
- pollutant particulate size;
- how readily the pollutant can dissolve in water;
- effects on pulmonary function;
- concentration relative to dose–response characteristics.

Pollutants will most readily impact on the lungs (influencing mechanical function and gaseous exchange) and the cardiovascular system (influencing oxygen transport). Ozone, sulphur dioxide and nitrogen dioxide impair lung function and irritate the lung lining, such that ventilatory efficiency is reduced. Carbon monoxide competes with oxygen in binding to haemoglobin, such that blood oxygen delivery is impaired. More common pollutants, such as pollen or suspended dirt particles, will affect sports performers with underlying respiratory conditions.

The extent to which air carries particulate matter will depend on local environmental conditions such as air temperature, relative humidity and air movement. Thus global regions of higher ambient temperature, high humidity and limited air movement, and where there is less regulated industrial and domestic pollution, will present the greatest environmental challenge to a sports performer. Photochemical reactions of airborne pollutants, which are more readily carried in warmer air, with ultraviolet radiation from the sun result in increased levels of ozone. Ozone is a toxic gas, and the summer smogs surrounding industrial cities are evidence of these dangerous chemical reactions. Ozone is associated with oxidative damage to the respiratory tract that will impact on respiratory efficiency.

There are similar dangers arising from interactions between airborne pollutants and cold air. These reactions will present problems for sports performers with relatively sensitive airways who are susceptible to exercise-induced asthma. The physiological reaction will result in constriction of the airways that would limit ventilation.

Further reading

Armstrong LE. Performing in Extreme Environments. Champaign, IL: Human Kinetics, 2000.

Burke LM. Nutritional needs for exercise in the heat. Comp Biochem Physiol A Mol Integr Physiol 2001; 128: 735–748.

Cheung S. Advanced Environmental Exercise Physiology. Champaign, IL: Human Kinetics, 2009.

Committee on Military Nutrition Research, Food and Nutrition Board. Fluid Replacement and Heat Stress. Washington, DC: Committee on Military Nutrition Research, Institute of Medicine, 1994.

Doubt TJ. Physiology of exercise in the cold. Sports Med 1991; 11: 367–381.

Galloway SD. Dehydration, rehydration, and exercise in the heat: rehydration strategies for athletic competition. Can J Appl Physiol 1991; 24: 188–200.

Hamad N, Travis SP. Weight loss at high altitude: pathophysiology and practical implications. Eur J Gastroentrol Hepatol 2006; 18: 5–10.

Jacobs I, Martineau L, Vallerand AL. Thermoregulatory thermogenesis in humans during cold stress. Exerc Sports Sci Rev 1994; 22: 221–250.

Marriott BM (ed.). Nutritional Needs in Hot Environments: Applications for Military Personnel in Field Operations. Washington, DC: Committee on Military Nutrition Research, Institute of Medicine, 1993.

Marriott BM, Carlson SJ (eds). Nutritional Needs in Cold and High-Altitude Environments: Applications for Military Personnel in Field Operations. Washington, DC: Committee on Military Nutrition Research, Institute of Medicine, 1996.

Shephard RJ. Metabolic adaptations to exercise in the cold. Sports Med 1993; 16: 266–289.

Westerterp KR. Energy and water balance at high altitude. News Physiol Sci 2001; 16: 134–137.

Young AJ. Energy substrate utilisation during exercise in extreme environments. Exerc Sports Sci Rev 1990; 18: 65–117.

Index

Page numbers in *italics* denote figures and tables.

Sport and Exercise Nutrition, First Edition. Edited by Susan A Lanham-New, Samantha J Stear, Susan M Shirreffs and Adam L Collins.
© 2011 The Nutrition Society. Published 2011 by Blackwell Publishing Ltd.

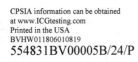

CPSIA information can be obtained
at www.ICGtesting.com
Printed in the USA
BVHW011806010819
554831BV00005B/24/P